Case Management

A Practical Guide for Education and Practice

THIRD EDITION

Case Management

A Practical Guide for Education and Practice

THIRD EDITION

Suzanne K. Powell, RN, BSN, MBA, CCM, CPHQ
Editor-in-Chief
Professional Case Management:
The Leader in Evidence-Based Practice
Lippincott Williams & Wilkins
Philadelphia, Pennsylvania

Hussein A. Tahan, DNSc, RN
Executive Director of International Health Services
NewYork-Presbyterian Hospital
New York, New York

Wolters Kluwer | Lippincott Williams & Wilkins
Health
Philadelphia • Baltimore • New York • London
Buenos Aires • Hong Kong • Sydney • Tokyo

Executive Acquisitions Editor: Elizabeth A. Nieginski
Product Managers: Helen Kogut and Rosanne Hallowell
Production Manager: Beth Martz
Marketing Manager: Kimberly Schonberger
Design Coordinator: Holly Reid McLaughlin
Interior Design: Lisa Delgado
Cover Design: Larry Didona
Manufacturing Coordinator: Karin Duffield
Production Services: Cadmus Communications

Third Edition

9 8 7 6 5 4 3 2 1

Printed in the United States of America

Library of Congress Cataloging-in-Publication Data

Powell, Suzanne K.
  Case management : a practical guide for education and practice / Suzanne K. Powell, Hussein A. Tahan. — 3rd ed.
       p. ; cm.
  Includes bibliographical references and index.
  ISBN 978-0-7817-9038-3
  1. Hospitals—Case management services. 2. Primary nursing. I. Tahan, Hussein A. II. Title.
  [DNLM: 1. Case Management. W 84.7 P886c 2010]
  RA975.5.C36.P69 2010
  362.17′3068—dc22   2009014375

Care has been taken to confirm the accuracy of the information presented and to describe generally accepted practices. However, the authors, editors, and publisher are not responsible for errors or omissions or for any consequences from application of the information in this book and make no warranty, expressed or implied, with respect to the currency, completeness, or accuracy of the contents of the publication. Application of this information in a particular situation remains the professional responsibility of the practitioner; the clinical treatments described and recommended may not be considered absolute and universal recommendations.

The authors, editors, and publisher have exerted every effort to ensure that drug selection and dosage set forth in this text are in accordance with the current recommendations and practice at the time of publication. However, in view of ongoing research, changes in government regulations, and the constant flow of information relating to drug therapy and drug reactions, the reader is urged to check the package insert for each drug for any change in indications and dosage and for added warnings and precautions. This is particularly important when the recommended agent is a new or infrequently employed drug.

Some drugs and medical devices presented in this publication have Food and Drug Administration (FDA) clearance for limited use in restricted research settings. It is the responsibility of the health care provider to ascertain the FDA status of each drug or device planned for use in his or her clinical practice.

LWW.COM

This book is dedicated to my mother, Leah,
and
to the memory of my father, Harry Kotlicky

—*Suzanne*

This book is dedicated to my mother, Fatimeh, and father, Ahmad,
and
to those who make a difference in people's lives every day

—*Hussein*

We also dedicate this book to the patients—
may your quality of life be optimized because of case management;
to our wonderful friends and colleagues
who always encourage us to achieve our dreams
and remind us to have fun along the way;
and to the current and future case managers
who give their lives every day to those in need—
may God bless you!

FOREWORD

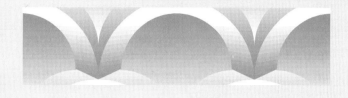

The case manager in the U.S. healthcare system has evolved into an essential and invaluable member of the healthcare team. The case manager's role is multifaceted and unique; however, it is executed with the patient as the central focus of care activities, rather than the agency where services are provided. The roles and functions of an outstanding case manager include, but are not limited to:

- Education, primarily about healthy lifestyle behavior and self-care.
- Quality and safety.
- Throughput and safe transitions of care.
- Financial management and appropriate allocation of resources.
- Relationship building with those receiving care and those involved in its provision.
- Patient and family satisfaction.

Case managers have their hands in every aspect of patient care. They may ensure the patient receives the needed medications or durable medical equipment; has an effective transitional plan in place, including safe transition to the next level of care or home; or is able to assume responsibility for self-care. They also may assist the healthcare agency where they work (e.g., hospital, skilled nursing facility, managed care organization) in meeting regulatory, accreditation, quality, and safety requirements. Involvement of the case manager in coordination, facilitation, and management of patient care activities provides other healthcare professionals, especially physicians, with the support necessary to proactively deal with the numerous and competing clinical or administrative needs, to effectively care for patients, and to successfully develop the multidisciplinary team that is essential for the provision of patient-centered care and achievement of safe and cost-effective outcomes.

The case manager is hands-on for patient needs; is holistic in his or her approach to managing the situation and environment; is empathetic to the patient, family, and other healthcare providers; and is strategic in achieving performance standards and desired outcomes. At the University of California, Irvine Medical Center, I developed a unique council called the *Inpatient Leadership Council* (ILC). This council was formed to meet the goals of patient satisfaction, quality, and throughput within the institution in a manner that achieves our five legacy goals:

1. Patient Satisfaction.
2. Quality of Care and Patient Safety.
3. Financial Strength.
4. Healthcare Employer of Choice.
5. Specialty Referral Growth.

The purpose of the ILC was to *build teams, set vision, problem-solve,* and serve as a *think tank.* It became immediately clear that if the ILC, which represented about eight patient care units in our hospital, wanted to be successful, it would need effective leadership—not just from physicians and nurses, but also case management. As a result, I established an approach to care provision that focused on a special state of partnership between physicians, nurses, and case managers. This was successful in that it achieved 12 milestones in its first year, moving our institution forward in accomplishing our five legacy goals. Some of these milestones included:

- Workshops dedicated to leadership training and teamwork among the 21 members of the ILC.
- Achievement of Press Ganey inpatient satisfaction scores of >82% for at least two quarters by implementation of this collaborative team involving physicians, discharge coordinators, and nursing leadership.
- Reducing the time to get discharge medications from the pharmacy to the patient's bedside, in order to facilitate discharge turnaround from several hours to minutes.
- Implementing communication vehicles to ensure that the financial status of the patient reaches case management on the day of admission or the day after. In the past, this took several days thus delaying discharge planning coordination.
- Implementation of dedicated official rounds among the leadership, at least twice a month and sometimes weekly, on the six units of the hospital.

- Initiation of staff retention rounds on some floors.
- Implementation of call-backs to patients discharged from the hospital.

The initiative helped the UC Irvine Case Management Department at the University of California become nominated for the prestigious Joint Commission and American Case Management Association (ACMA) national Franklin Award. Even though we were the runner-up, the experience of receiving a nomination for such a prestigious award showed the institution the importance of case management in our daily patient care practices.

The successful case manager is one who provides comprehensive oversight over the patient care process and serves as a patient/family advocate. The case manager's role is so complex that it requires special training and mentoring. *Case Management: A Practical Guide for Education and Practice* offers the necessary tools and knowledge for case managers to achieve success in their role. This textbook is written in a particular style that makes it conducive to developing, improving, or maintaining the knowledge, skills, and competencies essential for the effective performance of case managers. It is not only a resource guide, but also a ready reference case managers may use as an "on-hand" consultant. The new format of this textbook, including continuing education posttests at the end of the book and study questions at the end of each chapter, as well as the problem-based learning case studies found in Chapter 12, offers numerous opportunities for ongoing learning and exchange of information among case managers in an effort to promote case management practice which achieves desired outcomes. Clinicians, administrators, or academicians can easily use this textbook in a formal or informal education setting, as well as while mentoring, guiding, leading, and educating new and existing case managers.

Alpesh Amin, MD, MBA
Professor and Chair, Department of Medicine
Executive Director, Hospitalist Program
University of California, Irvine

PREFACE

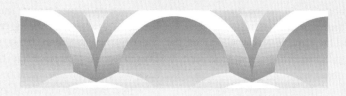

The late Dr. John Miller was an old-fashioned physician in the truest sense. With a medical practice typical of those of the 1960s and 1970s, he was devoted to his patients and always looked out for their best interests. He was accustomed to making patient decisions and dispensing curatives in a single-handed fashion. Conversely, he was not used to being second-guessed or "policed" by insurance companies. When the face of healthcare began to change in the early 1980s, it was difficult for Dr. Miller to come aboard. When "managed care"—with its ominous implied restrictions—no longer loomed as a threat, but became reality, he fought back. In classic Gandhi-like tradition, Dr. Miller carried out his own brand of "civil disobedience," leaving his patients in the hospital longer than what was becoming acceptable by utilization management standards. He also penned his disapproval of the "new ways" to several large newspapers and got himself bounced out of favor with a few managed care insurance plans. As a self-professed "medical dinosaur," he did a lot of charity work, made frequent house calls, and taught me a lot about patient advocacy.

The older physicians, who remembered "how it used to be," felt frustrated because of a severing of the patient-physician relationship; many of those physicians have since retired. It seemed that case managers were evolving as the link between the beleaguered healthcare system and the crucial need for patient advocacy. The first edition of this text was initiated in the early 1990s. At that time, case management was poorly defined; in fact, many health professionals could not yet distinguish between the concepts of "case management" and "managed care." It was becoming crystal clear that case managers were a critical asset to what was termed the *healthcare crisis*, but their impact was diluted by poor training, quick burnout (and subsequent turnover of case managers), and lack of definition and guidelines.

By the late 1990s, case management had grown at an astounding rate. Not only were there journals, books, seminars, and college courses about case management, but there were now professional associations, standards, guidelines, accreditation opportunities, and credentials with increasing credibility. Clearly, the second edition of this text no longer needed some of the "baby steps," but it did require a tremendous amount of new information to guide case management into the adolescent and adult evolutionary stages. In fact, the case management knowledge became so profuse that books on advanced case management practice published by various agencies are a testament to the enormous development that case management had gone through in a few short years.

In addition to the core elements of the first edition, the second edition included information on evaluation and steps to create or change your current case management model; trends in international case management and case management academia; the *Case Management Code of Professional Conduct*; and an entire chapter on credentials, organizations, and standards. The second edition also included information necessary for the case manager to function with all the new managed care, legal, and insurance changes, including the Balanced Budget Act of 1996; updated versions of utilization management modalities that incorporate "through the continuum" concepts; case management approaches to expedited and standard appeals, reconsiderations, and grievances; and critical ethical issues that have surfaced since the early 1990s. The intent was that the second edition would function as a teaching tool and useful reference on pertinent issues for case managers from all health professions.

Many of healthcare's problems have shifted, but they still represent an inequitable and raging economic tidal wave. The price tag for healthcare in 1993 was a staggering $903 billion—$233 billion *more* than in 1990; $2.4 *trillion* in 2007; and projected to reach *over* $4.3 trillion by 2017[*]. The need is still great, and case management remains an exciting challenge, as case managers are in a unique position to continue to be recognized for their contributions to healthcare.

You may wonder why we have published a third edition of this book. Well, we decided on it for several reasons, among which are the current and increasing popularity of case management as a strategy for ensuring that individuals receive quality, safe, and cost-effective healthcare services; the continued confusion

[*]National Coalition on Healthcare. (2009). (accessed 4/21/2009). *Facts on health care costs*. [Online]. Available: http://www.nchc.org/facts/cost.shtml.

about case management models and roles; and a limited number of available training and education programs for case managers. This time, however, we had education and practice in mind and a special return to the basics of case management practice.

We noticed that most of the available case management literature falls in the "advanced" knowledge category; the number of academic and training programs in case management has been declining; and more health professionals are expressing interest in becoming case managers but uncomfortable with their knowledge of case management practice. Therefore, we decided to contribute a case management book that addresses these concerns—one that is an invaluable resource for those who desire to become case managers as well as those who are interested in enhancing their case management knowledge, skills, and competencies. In addition, our intent is to offer case management experts involved in training, educating, or mentoring others a book equipped with up-to-date information about case management. A major characteristic of this third edition is the approach we took to enhance the development of case management knowledge and advance the field. The list of objectives at the beginning of each chapter frames the learning opportunities. The list of key terms assists case managers to become familiar with the case management language spoken in the various practice settings and highlights the essential aspects of learning the chapter addresses. The study questions at the end of each chapter enhance learning through reflection and application. These study questions encourage readers to reflect on the content they reviewed in the chapter and ask them to apply the gained knowledge into practice. Finally, the posttest for each chapter available at the end of the book furthers the learning opportunity and at the same time rewards the reader with continuing education (CE) credits. One must complete the posttest and submit the answers to Lippincott Williams & Wilkins to receive credits that can, for example, be used toward recertification.

The last chapter of the book focuses on *problem-based learning* (PBL) to allow health professionals to practice case management by proxy. Different from the traditional approach to learning, this chapter is designed for teamwork: a group of individuals can gather in a formal or informal setting and work through a PBL case. Through interaction, discussion, questioning, curiosity, and sharing of knowledge and past experiences, group members can begin to mentor each other, or a case management expert can facilitate group learning with an ultimate goal of spreading the knowledge through active exchange of experiences, information, skills, and competencies.

It is our hope that the third edition of this book, coupled with a solid training program, will help develop case managers both who are new to the profession and who have demonstrated peak job performance. Another benefit that can be realized by healthcare institutions and providers is developing a new case management model (or improving the conditions of an existing one) that can ensure quality and safe patient care practices and improve the satisfaction of those who receive health services—the patients and their families. Such also will ensure the satisfaction of those who provide these services—the case managers who will be recognized as shining lights, pulling the fragmented pieces of healthcare together.

Suzanne K. Powell
Hussein A. Tahan

CONTENTS

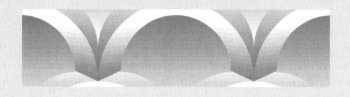

PART 1 ▸ INTRODUCTION TO
CASE MANAGEMENT 1

1 Overview of Case Management 2
2 Essential Case Management Job
Responsibilities and Skills 35
3 Reimbursement Concepts 69

PART 2 ▸ CASE MANAGEMENT
PROCESSES AND ACTIVITIES 99

4 Utilization Management 100
5 Transitional Planning: Understanding
Levels and Transitions of Care 161
6 The Case Management Process 205

PART 3 ▸ KEY CONCEPTS IN CASE
MANAGEMENT 241

7 Quality Management and Outcomes 242
8 Legal Issues in Case Management 267
9 Ethical Issues in Case Management 303

PART 4 ▸ PRACTICAL APPLICATIONS 325

10 Case Management Credentials,
Organizations, and Standards 326
11 Job Stress and Success Factors in Case
Management Practice 349
12 Practicing Case Management by Proxy 368

Index 383

Continuing Education Enrollment Forms
and Posttests 397

PART 1

Introduction to Case Management

"Foolish is the doctor who despises the
knowledge acquired by the Ancients."

HIPPOCRATES, C. 460–C. 377 B.C.

CHAPTER 1

Overview of Case Management

"Give a man a fish and you feed him for a day; teach him how to fish and you feed him for a lifetime."

LEARNING OBJECTIVES

Upon completion of this chapter, the reader will be able to:

1. Define case management.
2. State the difference between case management and managed care.
3. List four milestones in the history and evolution of case management systems.
4. Name five models of case management.
5. Describe the role of the nurse versus the social worker in case management.
6. Recognize five strategies in ensuring the effectiveness of case management models.
7. Determine the value of telehealth and information systems in the practice of case management.

ESSENTIAL TERMS

Acute Care Case Management • Beyond-the-Walls Case Management • Care Management • Case Management • Case Management Model • Case Manager • Entrepreneurial Case Management • Home Health Case Management • Hospice Case Management • Insurance Case Management • International Case Management • Managed Care • Nurse Case Manager • Social Worker Case Manager • Vocational Case Management • Within-the-Walls Case Management • Workers' Compensation Case Management

▶ THE REALITY OF THE HEALTHCARE ENVIRONMENT

"What is case management?" "What is a case manager?" "What is managed care?" We are asked these questions weekly by staff nurses, attending physicians, residents, interns, patients, families, other healthcare professionals, and nursing students, who are especially eager to learn about their future career options. Often, what is being asked is, "What does a case manager do?"

This question is not easily answered, given the plethora of job descriptions, licensures, certifications, and models of case management available. Lack of standardization and the void of widely agreed-on definitions has made answering such a question more complex and challenging. However, this book attempts to describe what a case manager does, keeping in perspective the diversity of case management practice and the roles assumed by case managers. For about three decades, the terms *case management, nursing case management*, and *managed care* are still being used interchangeably, even though case management experts agree that they are not exactly synonymous. Add to these terms all the other expressions for this endeavor (such as care management, care coordinator, case coordination, service coordination, transitional planning, and continuity coordination), and much confusion results. In general:

▶ *Managed care* is *systems*-oriented and focuses on health insurance plans and the management of member benefits.
▶ *Case management* is *people*-oriented and negotiates the managed care systems in a way that, ideally, benefits everyone, particularly the patient.

Managed care was a natural response to a healthcare system of waste and expanding, expensive technology. In the 1950s and 1960s, healthcare was paid for on a fee-for-service basis; essentially, this meant that a bill was rendered and paid without limitation of any kind. In the 1970s and 1980s, Medicare reimbursement changed to the Diagnosis-Related Groups (DRGs)/Prospective Payment System, which set the following standard: each diagnosis carried with it a set prearranged reimbursement, whether a patient stayed in the hospital 2 days and cost the hospital $1,000 or stayed 2 weeks and cost the hospital $15,000. This system changed the face of healthcare forever. With new limitations being placed on reimbursement for care, everyone started scrambling to improve the management of that care. Even now—three decades later—the ripple effects are still being felt by everyone: the payor, the provider, and the recipient of care.

Managed care systems sprang up in insurance companies and hospitals and in virtually all agencies affected by healthcare dollars. Health maintenance organizations (HMOs), preferred provider organizations (PPOs), and traditional healthcare plans managed the care through various forms of restrictions such as prior authorization for services, use of networks or panels of providers, preadmission authorization, utilization management and review, capitation, DRG reimbursement, per diem payments, and gatekeepers (see Chapter 3 for a discussion of these issues).

Managed care is a mutating and dynamic force—economically driven—that is constantly trying out new delivery systems. The goal of managed care is to encourage consumers, providers, and payors to all become accountable for the wise use of limited and ever-expensive healthcare resources. The definitions of managed care—perhaps because they are changing at such a velocity—often focus on strategies used in managed care and the restrictions placed on healthcare dollars. This is exemplified in the following two definitions:

1. Managed healthcare, according to Kongstvedt (2003) is a regrettably nebulous term. At the very least, it is a system of healthcare delivery that attempts to manage the cost of healthcare, the quantity and quality of that healthcare, and access to that care. Common denominators include a panel of contracted providers (network of participating providers) that is less than the entire universe of available providers; some type of limitations on benefits to subscribers (enrollees or consumers of care) who use noncontracted providers (unless authorized to do so); and some type of authorization system (certification for services prior to being provided). Managed healthcare is

actually a spectrum of systems, ranging from so-called managed indemnity, through PPOs, point of service (POS), open-panel HMOs, and closed-panel HMOs.

2. "Managed care is defined as a set of techniques used by or on behalf of purchasers of healthcare benefits to manage healthcare costs by influencing patient care decision-making through case-by-case assessments of the appropriateness of care prior to its provision. The implementation of managed care strategies follows a series of other cost control measures including insurance benefit limitations and exclusions, prepaid health plans, prospective payment systems, and fee schedules" (Williams & Torrens, 1993, p. 226).

Another perspective of managed care that provides a global view has elements of disease/case management. Managed care refers primarily to the management of the funding of services. It is an arrangement that gives the healthcare agency responsibility for ensuring that a given population receives a defined set of services in a coordinated and continuous fashion. Ultimately, the services should improve the health of the population by appropriately managing the existing disease entity (for example, heart failure or diabetes), preventing or delaying the progression of disease and the need for acute care and therefore, reducing the cost and improving the quality of care.

Managed care conjures up different images to different people. Some see it as an overbureaucratization, which will lead to rationing of services, limitations on access to care, poor quality of care, and loss of choice and autonomy. Others see managed care as a necessary evil that will provide healthcare coverage to a larger segment of the U.S. population. The simple days when the physician decided on patient care, ordered it, billed for it, and was paid are over. The new reality of requirements, restraints, restrictions, authorizations, gatekeeping, and rationales have catapulted the healthcare environment into ever-increasing complexity. Issues never before thought of must now be addressed. Such issues include the following:

▶ What services will Patient A's insurance company allow? When and by whom?
▶ What will Patient B's pharmacy benefit cover and which pharmacy must he or she use?
▶ What patient is reimbursed under a DRG versus a risk contract or a per diem rate?
▶ What extended care facility or home health agency can be used?

▶ What physician is contracted with the health plan?

▶ Is the Medicare coverage of the traditional type or a risk contract type?

▶ How can the case manager provide a safe discharge plan if the insurance company wants the patient discharged quickly and while the patient is supposedly still ill?

▶ How can the case manager secure necessary durable medical equipment if it is not covered in the health plan?

▶ CASE MANAGEMENT

Nursing was quick to recognize the constraints healthcare was under, and nurses viewed the dilemma as an opportunity to expand their practice and patient advocacy roles. They became the response to managed care. The nature of managed care dictates that healthcare services are limited; it is economics-driven. Case management balances this concept by ensuring caring, access, and quality. For this reason, nurses are proving themselves to be the most effective equalizers to managed care.

Historically, the definitions of case management found in the literature often confused rather than clarified the issue for several reasons. Some of these reasons still exist today and contribute to case management role confusion and in some instances, role overload.

▶ There are numerous models of case management; in fact, there are as many models and definitions as there are healthcare organizations in the United States. Each model looks at case management from its own perspective and therefore defines its own goals, processes, and type/context of case management rather than supplying a definition that applies universally. Often this definition describes what works for that particular facility or setting.

▶ The definition often merely restates the case management process—what a case manager does—rather than contributing a definition.

▶ Many still simply confuse case management with managed care or utilization review.

▶ Some definitions make it difficult to differentiate between individual case management functions. Like managed care, the case management role is evolving and dynamic. Once a purer role, the case manager is now often a hybrid of the clinical care provider, utilization reviewer, and quality improvement specialist-case manager.

▶ Some definitions are influenced by the specialty or profession of the person who assumes the role of case manager. For example, nursing primarily reflects management of clinical care in its case management practice; social work focuses on psychosocial counseling and brokerage of community resources; utilization management emphasizes resource consumption and allocation; and vocational rehabilitation stresses return to work.

To prevent confusion, some professional case management organizations continue to advocate for national and standardized definitions of case management. The Case Management Society of America (CMSA), the Commission for Case Management Certification (CCMC), the American Nurses Association (ANA), and the National Association of Social Workers (NASW) are four organizations that have done much work over the years to bring clarity to case management. CMSA, a multidisciplinary organization, defines case management as:

a collaborative process of assessment, planning, facilitation, and advocacy for options and services to meet an individual's health needs through communication and available resources to promote quality cost-effective outcomes (CMSA, 2002).

The Commission for Case Management Certification, established in 1992 to administer the first certification exam in case management, the Certified Case Manager (CCM) credential, defines case management as:

a collaborative practice that assesses, plans, implements, coordinates, monitors, and evaluates the options and services required to meet the client's health and human services needs. It is characterized by advocacy, communications and resource management and promotes quality and cost-effective interventions and outcomes (CCMC, 2005a).

The American Nurses Association defines case management as

a healthcare delivery process whose goals are to provide quality healthcare, decrease fragmentation, enhance the client's quality of life, and contain costs (ANA, 1994).

The National Association of Social Workers defines case management (using the term *social work case management*) as:

a method of providing services whereby a professional social worker assesses the needs of the client and the client's family, when appropriate, and arranges, coordinates, monitors, evaluates, and advocates for a package of multiple services to meet specific client's complex needs (NASW, 2007).

Other important definitions are included here because (1) they contain essential elements of case management or (2) their simplicity (as in example number one) is refreshing.

1. "Case management is the process of getting the right service to the right client" (Yee, 1990, p. 31).
2. "The purpose of care coordination is to work directly with clients and families over time to assist them in arranging and managing the complex set of resources that the client requires to maintain health and independent functioning. Care coordination seeks to achieve the maximum cost-effective use of scarce resources by helping clients get the health, social, and support services most appropriate for their needs at a given time. It guides the client and family through the maze of services, matches service need with funding authorization and coordinates with clinician and provider organizations" (Williams & Torrens, 1993, p. 202).
3. Case Management—A method of managing the provision of healthcare to members with catastrophic or high-cost medical conditions. The goal is to coordinate the care so as to both improve continuity and quality of care as well as lower costs (Kongstvedt, 2003).
4. "Case management is a coordination of a specific group of services on behalf of a specific group of people. Case management can also be defined by listing its component processes. By widespread agreement, these processes include screening or case finding; comprehensive multidimensional assessment; care planning; implementation of the plan; monitoring; and reassessment..." (Kane, 1988, p. 161).

By combining aspects of these definitions, the reader can focus on a bigger picture of what case management is all about. Case managers are the pivotal, prime movers of the managed and health care environment. Their presence adds humanity to an otherwise overwhelming system. More important than the definition of case management or what case managers accomplish is the heart of their role: the holistic, advocacy, and humane care of both patients and their families.

Case management and *care management* are two terms that tend to be used interchangeably; however, they are not exactly the same. Case management is a way of managing unique and high-risk health conditions, often associated with costly acute care and hospital stay. Patients who require case management services are of diminished/compromised self-capacity

and with complex medical conditions. Care management, on the other hand, is a system of care for patients with particular conditions where services are delivered across the continuum of care; it ensures seamless transition to the right provider at the right time. In case management, healthcare services are delivered primarily applying the medical model; in care management, services are delivered applying the psychosocial model. In either model, care is facilitated by a case manager (Bodie-Gross & Tahan, 2008).

▶ CONSUMER DEFINITION OF CASE MANAGEMENT

Several years ago, the Case Management Leadership Coalition (CMLC) developed a consumer-friendly definition of case management. This was a product of comprehensive research of the varied definitions published in the case management literature as well as the views of experts in case management, including a few public advocates. The main purpose of this research effort was to develop a definition of case management the consumer of healthcare services (including case management services) would understand. This development was an important milestone in the evolution of case management. Case managers are encouraged to share this definition with their patients and their families when attempting to explain what case management is and what case managers do. The CMLC (2007) definition is as follows:

> *Case management assists people to navigate through the healthcare and community systems to find solutions that work.*

▶ HISTORICAL PERSPECTIVE

Case management concepts and approaches to healthcare delivery and resources are not new. However, as a healthcare delivery system, case management is a fairly recent phenomenon. It has been in use for almost a century (Display 1-1). In the early 1900s, case management was applied by public health nurses and social workers in the form of coordination of healthcare services and resources for patients and families while in the community-based setting. In the 1920s, professionals in the fields of psychiatry and social work applied case management concepts in the management of the care of the behavioral health patients, especially in the ambulatory/clinic and community-based settings.

Case management practice and models as we know them today proliferated in the mid-1980s after implementation of the prospective payment system

SELECT MILESTONES IN THE EVOLUTION OF CASE MANAGEMENT

Early 1900s (turn of the 20th century)—Coordination of healthcare services in the public health sector by public health nurses and community social workers.

1920s—Coordination of services for chronically ill behavioral health patients by psychiatric specialists and social workers in the outpatient care setting.

1930s—Community-based case management approaches applied by public health visiting nurses in the community care setting.

Early 1940s—Case management approaches used as cost-saving measures in workers' compensation.

Post-World War II—Coordination of services by insurance companies for soldiers with complex injuries or health conditions and requiring multispecialty services.

1970s—Workers' compensation insurers develop and implement case management programs focusing on "return-to-work."

1970s—Coordination of services (health and human/medical and social services) by social workers and human service specialists in the community care setting funded through Medicare and Medicaid demonstration projects.

1978—Older Americans Act authorizes the use of case management services for elder patients through Area Agencies on Aging.

1980s—Case management of the catastrophically ill or injured with main focus on cost containment.

Mid-1980s—Case management programs in acute care settings mainly as a nursing initiative.

1990s—Hospital-based case management programs became multidisciplinary in nature and similar programs proliferated into other care settings.

Late 1990s to Early 2000s—Case management is practiced in every setting across the healthcare continuum and in almost every healthcare organization. Role of the case manager is performed by various healthcare professionals including nurses, social workers, physical therapists, vocational rehabilitation counselors, pharmacists, and physicians.

2009—Number of case managers exceeds 100,000 and at least one-third hold a certification in case management.

(i.e., the DRG system) in the acute care setting. They witnessed increased popularity in the 1990s as a result of the rise in managed care organizations and the use of capitation as the desired reimbursement method for healthcare services. Today, case management models are applied in almost every healthcare organization or setting regardless of type (acute, subacute, rehabilitation, ambulatory, community-based, long-term care, home health, palliative and hospice care, and so on). Case management practices flourished as a result of the implementation of prospective payment systems beyond the acute care setting (e.g., acute and subacute rehabilitation facilities, long-term care, and nursing homes, etc.) as well as due to their proven value in healthcare quality and safety.

▶ WHO SHOULD BE CASE MANAGERS?

Every discipline today seems to have case managers. Depending on the agency, the educational preparation varies from a high school diploma (GED acceptable) to master's level and beyond. The level of academic completion continues to be a hotly debated topic in some circles. The professional license is the other issue defining who should be a case manager. In today's health-

care market, the main and most common contenders for the role of case manager are nurses and social workers; however, that is broadening to include many other professional disciplines. Traditionally, social workers held the position of discharge planners in most hospitals until the mid- to late-1980s. With the advent of the prospective payment system and managed care (i.e., with the goal of getting the patient through the cost-intensive acute care setting as efficiently as possible), the trend in that level of care is the use of nurses as case managers. Nevertheless, the "nurse versus social worker as case manager" debate still remains a touchy subject. Turf wars have ensued over it, articles have been written about it, and jobs have been lost over it.

Who is more appropriate for the role of case manager? Critical to answering this question is assessing the type of population needing case management. This will help to determine the professional background that will most suitably meet the patients' needs. For example, foster children as the target population reflect a predominantly social model, thus needing the expertise of a social worker case manager. Respiratory therapists have been hired as case managers for patients with chronic pulmonary diseases such as cystic fibrosis, chronic obstructive lung disease, or asthma. The cognitively fragile population may also benefit from the use of social workers or from psychiatrically experienced registered nurses (RNs). Rehabilitation facilities may use RNs, social workers, or physical/occupational therapists individually or as teams. Gerontology practitioners may be best suited for the fragile elderly. In the workers' compensation arena where the main focus is return to work of the injured employee, vocational rehabilitation or disability managers are best fitted for the case manager role.

Getting more specific, in a disease management program for diabetes, dietitians have been effectively utilized. Certified Diabetes Educators (CDE) have successfully managed that population for years. In an asthma program, respiratory training is invaluable; in behavioral health programs, social worker case managers have been successful.

Acute hospital care, at first glance, appears to be a purely medical model; thus, at that level of care, the obvious choice would appear to be professional registered nurses. Consider some of the responsibilities of a hospital-based case manager:

- ▶ Astute assessment skills are necessary to aid in recognizing ominous changes in medical status, whereby timely interventions can divert an impending medical crisis; often these changes in patient status may also necessitate a change in the service plan.
- ▶ Direct bedside care may be performed.
- ▶ Thorough systems assessment, documentation, and placement into utilization management language are needed for insurance authorization and reimbursement purposes.
- ▶ Descriptions of wounds and surgical interventions often must be reported to the insurance company for negotiating hospital stay authorization.
- ▶ Coordination of durable medical equipment and other resources for home use will often necessitate a medical perspective. For example, tracheostomies may require a range of supportive equipment from suction catheters and suction machines to home oxygen or aerosol masks. Colostomies require colostomy bags and skin care products. Diabetes monitoring needs blood glucose monitoring devices and related supplies.
- ▶ Knowledge of medications and of the safe and appropriate time to change from an intravenous route to an oral route is important.
- ▶ The meaning of various laboratory and test results must be understood when looking at the total medical picture.

- ▶ Teaching may include any aspect of medical care, from teaching the patient (and or family/caregiver) the side effects and correct administration of specific medications to suctioning a tracheostomy or packing and redressing a wound in a sterile manner.
- ▶ Understanding of patient flow and throughput is a necessary skill for today's case managers. Flow and throughput focuses on assessment and evaluation of patients' conditions and treatment plans in an effort to ensure that care is received in the most appropriate setting, that is, the patient is provided care at the necessary level. For example, patients may transition from the emergency department to the intensive care unit (ICU) or from the telemetry unit to a regular floor as their conditions warrant.
- ▶ Knowledge of insurance plans and health benefits is essential and allows case managers to be effective at utilization management, assuring that acute care is the most appropriate level of care for the patient based on his or her health condition and required care.
- ▶ Identification of actual or potential delays in care or treatment allows them to be addressed with the goal of resolving the issues and preventing deterioration in the patient's condition; therefore improving outcomes of care and enhancing patient's satisfaction.

For these types of responsibilities, nurses, as specialists in holistic bioassessment and functional health planning, are ideally suited as case managers.

In reality, the acute care setting is often not a purely medical model. Trauma units routinely overflow with various patients, from those who have been in motor vehicle accidents, to those who have sustained gunshot wounds, to those who have been victims of gang violence. ICUs house patients who have attempted suicide or drug overdoses. Personnel on medical floors treat cellulitis and abscesses from intravenous drug abuse; those on obstetric floors routinely witness "babies having babies"—14-year-olds who are already multigravida moms. Staff on all units treat catastrophic conditions and diseases that can bring the strongest families to their knees. All inpatient care units need the assistance of social workers as well—for social assessments, psychosocial counseling, and social discharge planning. However, the intensity of involvement of the social worker in care is dependent on the individual patient/family need. Often, the social worker case manager tends to focus on the patient's social, financial, and complex discharge planning needs.

A person's professional training elicits its own unique perspective; a nurse case manager and a social worker each have a different point of view about what a patient's needs might be on discharge. Both contribute important data for a patient's successful rehabilitation, illustrating that perhaps the best solution is a nurse case manager–social worker team approach. This is ideal in many settings, not only in acute care but in subacute levels such as hospice or spinal cord rehabilitation centers.

▶ WHAT MAKES THE NURSE CASE MANAGER–SOCIAL WORKER TEAM WORK?

Superimposing nurse case managers on already existing social worker-discharge planners can create turf wars until both professionals realize their importance and necessity. The nurse case manager–social worker team members may initially appear to have some overlapping roles as well as their more obvious, distinctly separate responsibilities. However, these overlapping gray areas do not necessarily mean duplication. Good communication within the team and mutual trust regarding follow-through can eliminate the risk of wasted effort from repetition. Some nurse case manager–social worker teams have had difficult times because of attitudes about roles "carved in stone" or an individual need to "do it all." These attitudes make one of the basic tenets of teamwork—pitching in for one another—very difficult. Ensuring that the most qualified professional gets involved in the care of a patient is important. One way of achieving this objective is by having the nurse case manager provide case management services if the patient's prevailing needs are clinical or educational in nature and a social worker case manager do so if the prevailing needs are financial or social.

The case management–social worker team has now had several years to test its efficacy. It has proven to be essential in many settings. Important suggestions given by facilities with five or more years of this team (dyad) model are as follows:

1. Strategically place case managers and social workers under one department; this will minimize territorial issues.
2. Teach and facilitate the team concept. Success is reflective of the team effectiveness rather than the individual contribution alone.
3. Stress the three "Cs"—communicate, communicate, communicate. Communication is the key to success.
4. Document, in writing, the basic components of each job description. However, there are many gray areas that overlap because of covering for one another or because of the sequence of events in an individual's case. "How to" and resource manuals specific to the local cultures, community resources, and facilities should be kept updated. This includes updating addresses, telephone numbers, contacts, and any new resources. This also will allow for more independence of the team members.
5. Outline the selection criteria for nurse versus social worker case manager. For example, a nurse case manager may be needed for teaching the patient and family about complex wound care while a social worker case manager gets involved in counseling a family regarding their coping pattern in response to their premature newborn. Even when such criteria are spelled out, there will always be situations where both the nurse and social worker case managers are involved, as in the case of conducting a patient and family conference or participation in interdisciplinary patient care management rounds.
6. Implement in-service programs. This is a good strategy to keep the team current. For example, social workers require training on the basics of utilization review; case managers require more in-depth practice in grief counseling; both case managers and social workers need to know the latest changes in regulatory and legal issues.

Perhaps the element most responsible for making nurse case manager–social worker teams work best is the elusive factor known as chemistry.

When all the components of a good nurse case manager–social worker team are in place, the patient wins, the family wins, the facility wins, the healthcare team is pleased, job satisfaction peaks, and managed care becomes quality, cost-efficient care.

▶ CASE MANAGEMENT CODE OF PROFESSIONAL CONDUCT

Case managers are expected to act based on case management-related ethics principles and standards as well as those of their original profession or specialty. For example, in addition to the case management code of ethics, nurse case managers would also adhere to the nursing code of ethics, and social work case managers would comply with the social work code of ethics.

Those who abide by the professional code of ethics are able to protect the best interest of their patients, are accountable and responsible, are effective advocates, and recognize ethical dilemmas and address them.

In 1996, the Commission for Case Manager Certification (CCMC, 2005b) adopted a Code of Professional Conduct for Case Managers. Compliance with this code is mandatory for all applicants of the CCM certification examination. The code can be obtained from CCMC's Web site (www.cmcertification.org). This code was written to protect the public and represents another step needed for credibility and accountability of case management. The Code of Professional Conduct for Case Managers has been revised multiple times since 1996, most recently in 2005. The code consists of seven sections:

1. Preamble.
2. Scope of Practice for Case Managers.
3. Principles (fundamental assumptions to guide professional conduct).
4. Rules of Conduct (prescribe the level of conduct required of every CCM).
5. Guidelines for Professional Conduct (offer information with regard to various aspects of an individual's professional conduct).
6. Guidelines and Procedures for Processing Complaints.
7. Complaint Form.

The code is ethically oriented, and according to CCMC enforcement (CCMC, 2005b), offers the following advantages:

▶ It constitutes a response to the professional obligation to provide only quality services to clients (note: the definition of "client" in the code refers to the individual to whom a CCM certificant provides services).
▶ It safeguards clients by identifying unethical practitioners and disciplining them through censure or, when warranted, the revocation of their professional credential.
▶ It serves as a form of self-regulation that helps protect practitioners from ill-considered or overly restrictive regulations that might be imposed by other entities.
▶ It protects the public interest by providing guidance to both the public at large and case managers as to what constitutes ethical conduct, how to adhere to ethical practice, and what to do in case ethical standards and principles were overlooked.

The code is quite extensive and worth reviewing. With all the complexities of case management, including ethical and legal dilemmas, it serves as another reminder of staying focused on the patient/family while maintaining professional responsibilities. There is another necessity for understanding this code. As lawsuits increase, there is always a remote chance that a case manager may end up in court; standards, codes, and protocols can always be held up as a "sword or a shield." Whether the code, or *Standards of Practice for Case Management*, are protective may depend on a case manager's knowledge of these texts and adherence to them.

▶ OPPORTUNITIES IN NURSING CASE MANAGEMENT

As the managed care environment tightens, more positions for case managers are becoming available in both the public and private domains. The massive changes in reimbursement strategies in the late 1990s by the Health Care Financing Administration (HCFA, known today as the Centers for Medicare & Medicaid Services [CMS]) has served to increase the opportunities for case managers not only in the acute care settings but at the postacute level as well. Because managed care strategies are constantly changing, it is reasonable to speculate that some of the current case management job responsibilities may become more diverse, some may no longer be considered necessary, and new ones may be emphasized. At any rate, the basic functions of case management—ensuring quality of and access to care in a cost-efficient manner—will not become less relevant.

Case management began as either a community-based model with a focus on the community or a hospital-based model with a focus on one acute episode of care. Now the trend is managing the patient through the continuum of care, which includes acute and postacute levels of care, including the patient's home. In this integrated system, there is more continuity for the patient when a single case manager oversees all levels of care. Disease management, or managing a patient population that is defined by a specific medical condition, is a good example of case management that follows a patient throughout the continuum of care and services. The multidisciplinary team for a single patient includes all the key players in the patient's individual case, although some of the players may change depending on the patient's needs. The team may also include case managers from various portions of the care plan such as insurance companies, third-party payors, skilled nursing facilities (SNFs), hospices, physician groups, hospitals, home healthcare agencies, the patient's employer (if the case has to do with workers' compensation), and the family or caregiver.

Some medical soothsayers predict that in the near future hospital care will consist mainly of ICU treatments, and the trend does appear to be going in that direction. The largest portion of every healthcare dollar is spent in acute hospitals, which provides the financial incentive to move care out of the costly hospital setting and into the community. Therefore, new models of case management continue to be generated. The vision of keeping patients out of the hospital may become reality through still unexplored case management strategies.

Case management across all levels of care has several advantages:

▶ Its primary focus is on wellness and optimizing quality of life, autonomy, independence, and optimal patient/family functioning.
▶ Detour of potential problems can be accomplished through preventive practices.
▶ There may be foreseeably fewer readmissions to the acute level of care (inpatient or emergency department episodes of care).
▶ There may be less acuity when a patient is readmitted through early identification of medical changes, thus resulting in less costly hospitalizations and reduced lengths of stay.
▶ Unnecessary admissions may be prevented. This may include low acuity admissions or those known as "social admissions," primarily for disposition problems.
▶ A contact person for patients to help them access and navigate the complex healthcare system is provided.
▶ Careful medical monitoring may decrease complications.
▶ There may be fewer visits to emergency departments and fewer 911 calls.

When a case manager (in any setting) follows patients in this way, many emergency department visits are appropriately avoided. A study performed in 1992 by the U.S. Department of Health and Human Services revealed that of the 90 million emergency department visits that year, only 45% were deemed urgent or emergent (Anonymous, 1994). Almost as many people went to emergency departments for coughs and sore throats as for chest pain and level I traumas. These trends continue to be evident today. Rather than sending a patient to an emergency department, a case manager—on assessment—may send the patient to his or her primary care physician (PCP) or an ambulatory care site, or may call in an extra home health nurse

visit, a respiratory professional, a social worker, or a psychiatric nurse to visit the patient. Perhaps the far-sighted payor source is contracted with one of the new, futuristic, entrepreneurial physician groups who specialize in the age-old activity of house calls. Surely, even a physician-assisted house call is less expensive than a 911 ambulance charge plus the emergency department treatment charges.

▶ MATCHING PERSONAL GOALS AND BELIEFS WITH THE APPROPRIATE CASE MANAGEMENT MODEL

There are many types of case management models in the contemporary healthcare environment. Those interested in case management as an employment opportunity are advised to evaluate the job description and responsibilities carefully to see whether the model of case management offered is compatible with personal beliefs and professional goals. Some might prefer the episodic version of case management, whereas others would find long-term relationships with patients very satisfying. If home-based case management services are included in your job description, would you be at ease going into others' homes and assessing their medical and psychosocial needs? Are you comfortable and effective with issues such as self-neglect, noncompliance, or abuse (child or elder)? Are you clinically astute enough to safely triage a patient at home and make appropriate care decisions? If you have a nursing specialty that you find gratifying, perhaps a disease management position in that area would be a perfect fit, especially if you also like to follow "your" patients throughout the continuum of care.

Another issue for your discernment is whether you feel that direct care is part of the nursing case management role. In varying degrees, some nursing case management delivery systems, although rare today, combine the nursing case management role with bedside nursing care. In this combined role, the case management–bedside nurse may assess acute care and discharge planning needs for the patient. A plan of care would be developed by the nurse; included in it would be the clinical interventions necessary based on the patient's condition as well as the postacute care/services required on the patient's discharge back to the home setting or transfer to a less-acute-care facility. The plan of care would then be sent to the multidisciplinary team for additional recommendations, then sent back to the nurse for evaluation. The team assists the nurse in the implementation and evaluation of the plan.

Variations on this type of case management-staff nurse model exist, but universal acceptance of this style of case management is lacking. Case management experts tend to feel strongly that case managers should not perform direct bedside nursing care. Combining these roles may present a main cause of frustration, burn-out, and the eventual demise of the case management model.

When assessing job openings in case management, note that many employment opportunities are available for various aspects of the total case management role; these are not the whole picture but can provide valuable experience in the management aspects of healthcare. Some of these areas are preadmission case management, utilization management, quality improvement, risk management, telephone triage, and transitional planning. When interviewing or during a preinterview telephone call, it is wise to ask about the expected job responsibilities because some job advertisements may be misleading. For example, an advertisement for utilization reviewers may actually be more akin to a case management position or vice versa.

Experience in the above roles is important, because considerable skills and an extensive knowledge base are useful to perform case management functions well. In the evolving role of what a case manager *is* and *does,* more of these functions are being included in the hybrid interpretation of a case manager. Many case managers who come into the profession with utilization management or quality improvement backgrounds have made the transition with more ease than even the most clinically competent staff nurses. All experiences are valuable and will add to your knowledge, skills, and competencies. They also are essential for career advancement and professional development.

▶ MODELS OF CASE MANAGEMENT

It is not the intent of this section to describe various case management models in detail or to present a comprehensive list of all the models that exist today. Current models are well detailed in some of the invaluable case management journals that are available. Innovative case management models are being attempted in every phase of managed care, every setting of healthcare delivery, and current publications describe them and articulate their successes and barriers to success.

Thinking broadly, case management models have been described in either of two approaches: within-the-walls and beyond-the-walls case management. Within-the-walls case management models are those that are implemented in the acute care/hospital setting and focus primarily on managing the care of patients during an

acute episode of illness. Beyond-the-walls case management models are those that are implemented in settings other than acute care such as outpatient, community, payor-based, and long-term care. The role of the case manager in these models varies depending on the settings in which it is implemented. For example, the case manager in within-the-walls models plays an active role in transitional/discharge planning; in the outpatient and community settings he or she may focus more on management of chronic illness and prevention of disease progression; in the long-term settings, the focus may be more on supportive or rehabilitative care; while in the payor-based setting, case management may emphasize management of member benefits and triaging patients to the appropriate level of care when needed.

It is recommended that those who develop a new case management department review the current literature for ideas and lessons learned to avoid committing similar mistakes or wasting their efforts. More importantly, it is essential that each organization evaluate its individual needs and the population it serves before instituting a specific case management model. This is key to case management success. The right case management model will maximize reimbursement, lower the total costs of providing care, and satisfy an organization's internal and external customers (i.e., patients, patients' families, and payors). A case management model that does not complement the internal structure and satisfy identified critical needs is likely to fail.

The proliferation of case management models is not without problems. The integration of case managers continues to be an emerging challenge. Historically, acute care case managers performed their responsibilities in an episodic manner, focusing on the safe discharge of a patient to the natural next level of care. Case managers external to the acute care setting performed their job responsibilities according to their job descriptions. There was essentially no communication between the two except for, perhaps, a brief time during the actual "handing over" of the patient. Like managed care, case management became very fragmented.

Problems with this fragmented case management model ensued, and "through the continuum" case management models developed, especially when an organization had integrated systems. There are still multiple coordination challenges about who does what, where, and when. When all case managers are under one organizational umbrella, however, it makes it easier to coordinate the communication; in such a setting, the patient benefits with more continuity of case management coverage. In those organizations without the integrated systems of acute care, home healthcare, SNF care, ambulatory and rehabilitation care, and so on, case management still remains fragmented. Now that there are so many external and internal case managers, an emerging challenge is to find an efficient method of everyone working together.

One suggestion for complex and integrated systems is that one case manager must assume accountability and responsibility for being the central point of contact. If an integrated system includes HMO case managers, acute care case managers, home health case managers, rehabilitation case managers, and SNF case managers, the model still remains fragmented, unless, for example, the HMO case manager is accountable for the coordination of the big picture of care; the other case managers (or "attending case manager") will manage the crises and details while that patient resides in their respective level of care.

In this instance, the HMO case manager is chosen as the primary case manager. Other case managers can also take on the role of the coordinating case manager; a payor-based case manager or a case manager for a group of several self-funded plans may be the primary case manager. This case manager is responsible for ensuring that the care meets acceptable standards, that the care is within the benefits guidelines of the health plan, and that the care is provided through a PPO when possible. This case manager essentially becomes the consultant for the case, coordinating all levels of care and overseeing the resource utilization. Nevertheless, this case manager cannot provide all the aspects of care needed at all levels of care; the time-intensive responsibility of coordinating the day-to-day care, education, and social services will go to the case manager of whatever setting the patient resides in.

It is imperative that at the beginning of a case, all case managers agree on the coordination efforts. Whether the pivotal case manager will be called the primary case manager, the case management consultant, or the case management coordinator, is something that will work itself out in case management history. The important thing is that the assignment is made. If this case management challenge is not attended to, case management will eventually get a reputation as being a cause, rather than the cure, of healthcare fragmentation, poor quality, and unsafe experiences or medical errors. In general, the consultant case manager will assist the other case managers with important issues with which only one who has followed the patient through the chronic illness may be familiar. In addition to issues such as allowable benefits and PPO providers, this case manager will supply others with patient-specific information on important psychosocial and financial aspects of the case or areas in which the patient needs more education and instruction about the illness, injury, or disability.

The assignment is a bit more complex than just choosing the "least busy" case manager. The choice has legal and regulatory ramifications. For example, CMS regulations state that a hospital's personnel are responsible for the safe discharge of its patients; therefore, it is the responsibility of the hospital social work–case management team to provide this service. *The Conditions of Participation for Medicare Hospitals—CMS Discharge Planning Regulations* (CMS, 2009a, No. 482.43) state that the hospital must arrange for the initial implementation of the patient's discharge plan. In this instance, the HMO or payor-based case manager will communicate with other case managers by providing the names of PPO facilities or speaking with the patient/family. However, this may be further complicated if there is an HMO-risk Medicare plan (as an example); the hospital/HMO contract may require the HMO case manager to perform the discharge planning duties. Does the regulatory or contractual agreement take precedence? This is a decision for hospital administration to make. In general:

1. First, assess contractual and regulatory agreements. If administration or legal counsel needs to be involved, get their expertise and advice.
2. Second, if there are no legal restrictions, then communication is the key. Always keep focused on the bottom line: the patient.

The following reflect some of the general classifications of case management models that are available in our contemporary healthcare environment. Broadly stated, case management models can be differentiated by setting, disease type, and domain (the provider domain and the payor domain). Providers include hospitals, nursing homes, subacute and rehabilitation facilities, physician offices, home health agencies, hospices, or mental health settings. Payors include any insurance setting (workers' compensation, HMOs, PPOs, Medicare, Medicaid, employer groups, etc.). Regardless of where case management is practiced along the healthcare continuum, the complexity, intensity, and major characteristics of the model depend on the following factors: the care setting/level of care, patient population, reimbursement methods, and the care provider (Display 1-2).

In addition to being common case management models, the following also represent potential areas of case management employment.

▶ Acute Care Case Management

Acute care case management is usually time limited, episodic nursing case management at the hospital level. This model integrates clinical care management,

display 1-2

FACTORS THAT IMPACT MODELS OF CASE MANAGEMENT

1. The CONTEXT of the care setting where case management is practiced; for example, ambulatory, community-based, acute care, subacute/rehabilitation, long-term care, and nursing homes.

2. The PATIENT POPULATION served and its needs; for example, critical/acute episode of illness, specific disease such as asthma or heart failure, long-term supportive care, or chronic illness.

3. The REIMBURSEMENT METHOD applied; for example, managed care, capitation, discounted rate, prospective payment system.

4. The CARE PROVIDER needed for care provision; for example, generalist, specialist, individual, multidisciplinary team, internal or external to the healthcare agency.

Adapted from Tahan, H. (2008). Case management practice settings and throughput. In S. Powell & H. Tahan (Eds.), *CMSA core curriculum for case management* (2nd ed., pp. 39-73). Philadelphia: Wolters Kluwer/Lippincott Williams & Wilkins.

utilization management, and transitional planning functions. Acute care case management may be managed in five different ways. First, it may be unit-based, in which case managers manage patients while on a particular unit such as ICU, orthopedic, medicine, or telemetry. In a second scenario, acute care case management may mean that case managers follow patients from admission to discharge. These case managers often do prehospital teaching if the admission is nonemergent and planned. The same case manager will follow up with a patient in whatever level of care/unit is required, thus ensuring continuity of care. Third, acute care case management may be disease-based, following up with patients according to their primary illness. Each setting requires unique components, skills, and knowledge for effective care. Fourth, case management may be practiced based on an individual physician or group of physicians within a specialty. In this case, the case manager follows patients who are cared for by such physician(s) regardless of diagnosis or unit with the hospital where care is provided. Finally, acute care case management may be represented through primary nursing case management.

Case managers may also practice hands-on care of the patient. They identify acute care needs and discharge needs as well as help develop the treatment plan with the multidisciplinary team. This is not an either/or phenomenon; successful hospitals have found that a combination of case manager roles best meets the needs of the organization and patients.

Case managers in acute care settings usually are registered professional nurses. Most often and at a minimum, they are prepared at the bachelor's degree level. Recently, it is becoming more common to have case managers with graduate-level education. The combination of nurse and social worker case managers is another more recent occurrence in the acute care setting; in fact, such a combination is not popular in other health care settings.

Adjunctive to acute care, many facilities are recognizing the importance of providing throughput areas such as the emergency department, admitting office, and perioperative services, with designated case managers. This case manager can steer a patient into a more appropriate setting before being admitted into acute care; the process of case management should begin at the earliest possible time.

EMERGENCY DEPARTMENT CASE MANAGEMENT

Since the emergency department is a common entry point to the hospital setting, it is important for case managers to provide gatekeeping oversight there. In the emergency department case management model, the case manager interfaces with physicians, nurses, social workers, admitting office staff, payor-based case managers, and others to ensure cost-effective and medically necessary care. Emergency department case managers deal with various groups of patients including those who are to be treated and released, admitted to the hospital, discharged but require services such as home care, and observed for a period of time before a final decision is made whether to admit or release. They also are involved in the care of patients who present mainly with social rather than medical problems, such as homelessness and domestic violence or abuse.

ADMITTING OFFICE CASE MANAGEMENT

Today's mature case management models of the acute care settings recognize the importance of gatekeeping at the point of admission to the hospital. Case managers in the admitting office evaluate the patient's condition (primary and secondary reasons for admission to the hospital) and the preliminary expected plan of care (e.g., type of diagnostic and therapeutic procedures) for appropriateness for care provision in the acute setting.

The main focus of the case manager's assessment here is the patient's severity of illness and intensity of services requirement. If the patient's condition does not meet the standard or criteria for admission to the acute care setting, the patient is diverted to an alternate level of care that is appropriate to the patient's condition. The case manager in this case contacts the patient's physician, explains the situation, including the findings of the assessment, and negotiates agreement on the alternate care setting. The use of the admitting office case manager has proven effective in reducing reimbursement denials or the conversion of an acute hospital stay to an observation status instead.

PERIOPERATIVE SERVICES CASE MANAGEMENT

The perioperative services case manager cares for surgical patients during the preadmission testing phase, the day of surgery as the patient goes through the surgical phase, and/or in the recovery area postsurgery and during recovery from anesthesia. The case manager ensures that the patient has been authorized for surgery by the health insurance plan, underwent appropriate preadmission testing and the findings deemed the patient ready for surgery, received medical clearance for surgery, signed necessary consents, and had no questions that remained unanswered.

▶ Large Case Management

In another type of service-based case management, known as large case management, the case selection includes patients who are at risk for extremely high healthcare costs (e.g., patients with AIDS; premature infants in neonatal intensive care units; and patients with possible kidney/liver/heart/bone marrow transplant, high spinal cord injury, or end-stage renal disease receiving hemodialysis). Almost any setting can support a large case management model: insurance companies, hospitals, disease management carve-outs, home health, rehabilitation facilities, etc.

Large case management focuses not only on patients with chronic illness but on those with disabilities and catastrophic illnesses as well who require intensive short- or long-term management of services. The focus of the case manager in these populations is rehabilitation (physical and vocational), occupational therapy, return to work, prevention of deterioration in the patient's condition, and management of health care resources.

▶ Disease Management

The success of disease-based case management in the acute setting and large case management probably had much to do with the current evolution of disease management. Unlike case management for a particular condition or disease in the acute care setting and for only one episode of illness, disease managers follow their population through all levels of care. Some disease managers are required to follow their patients for a limited time, as in high-risk pregnancy. Other disease managers may follow their patients for longer periods, such as heart failure disease managers. Disease management programs are often developed in sites such as physician practices or insurance companies.

Disease-state case management is a relief! For those case managers who have been expected to know all things about all disease states, being an expert in one disease (including pathophysiology and potential comorbidities) is a comfort. Physicians are not expected to be expert in every specialty; that is the intent of referrals to specialty care providers. Yet, historically, case managers and nurses have been required to "do it all." In one study about nurses on a medical floor, it was found that these nurses cared for patients whose health conditions fell in 109 DRGs in a 6-month period. Medical case managers do the same. Add the integrated medical-surgical units some work on, and the number of DRGs escalates. The information needed to perform excellent medical case management is overwhelming. The diabetes or heart failure case manager is emerging as the true "physician assistant."

In disease management case management models, case managers apply evidence-based guidelines or protocols. These protocols are nationally recognized standards of care that describe the necessary care and treatments (diagnostic and therapeutic interventions) for patients with a specific chronic health condition such as heart failure or end-stage renal disease and based on the severity of illness. These protocols also include the expected outcomes of care that are easily measured and tracked over time. Case managers assess patients and classify them, based on specific criteria, into low-, moderate-, or high-risk groups. They then manage the care of the patients, applying treatments and interventions indicated by their risk group. Treatments include medications, lifestyle changes, and health education. Such models of care have proven effective in preventing the need for emergency department visits or acute care hospital stays.

▶ Insurance (Third-Party Payor) Case Management

Case managers must balance quality of care and patient advocacy with the responsibility for carefully shepherding that health plan's dollars. If there is a conflict between the expectations of the insurance company and the facility to which the member is currently admitted for care, the case manager must depend on communication and negotiation skills in resolving such conflict. The case manager is the company's liaison. Third-party payor case managers often have the power to authorize services and levels of care. Their main focus is managing members' benefits effectively and ensuring that members receive healthcare services in the most appropriate level of care/setting justified by the presenting health condition. Case managers may perform their job responsibilities in two ways: telephonically and on site.

TELEPHONICALLY

Some case managers for large insurance companies have patients all over the United States and must rely on telephone review. Because their assessment and planning are only as good as the information they can extract from the facility/member, they must be skilled in asking tough, pertinent questions. If they do not get the right answers, coverage for a hospital admission (or specified days) may be denied.

ON SITE

On-site case management is often preferable to telephonics. The member's medical record can be reviewed, members of the involved healthcare team can be interviewed, if necessary, and the patient (health plan member) can be seen and assessed. Proximity to the patient is an advantage. It allows the case manager to develop a therapeutic relationship, see a patient's condition first-hand, and make personal observations when assessing the patient's interactions with family members for discharge assessment purposes. Sometimes a picture is worth a thousand words.

Regardless of whether insurance-based case managers perform their job responsibilities telephonically or on site, the focus of the role is the same. Case managers in this model assess the patient's condition, determine the type and level of setting in which the patient should receive care, and ensure that the discharge plan (postepisode care) matches the patient's and family's needs. Additionally, they manage the patient's health benefits as stipulated in the health plan and promote compliance with the standards and procedures of the insurance company and as agreed on in the plan.

▶ Palliative Care and Hospice Case Management

Case managers in the palliative care and hospice case management model coordinate the care and comfort of the dying patients and their families. Often, the nurse becomes the primary manager of the case; the physician becomes a consultant. A special focus in this model is the care of patients suffering from a terminal illness and who have a limited life expectancy, that is, care at the end-of-life. Case managers here deal with the complex consequences of illness as the patient's death nears, as well as postdeath during the family's bereavement stage.

Hospice care takes place either in an institutional setting (e.g., hospital, skilled nursing facility, or freestanding hospice facilities) or in the patient's home. In either setting, the focus of the case management model is the same: respectful, comfortable, and dignified death.

▶ Home Health Case Management

In home health case management, case managers service the needs of the chronically ill in the home setting. Coordination of several therapeutic modalities may be necessary in an individual case. These may include wound care, infusion therapy services, physical therapy, speech therapy, occupational therapy, coordination of durable medical equipment, tube feeding, medication monitoring, assessments, tube/tracheostomy care—almost anything done in hospitals. If the patient is stable, home care can also include such intensive services as ventilator assistance. These case managers monitor for early warning signs, contact the patient's primary physician for treatment, and can thereby prevent or lessen the severity of exacerbation of the illness and reduce the frequency of readmissions to the hospital. The therapeutic home health case manager's relationship usually begins and ends with insurance authorization. However, acting as a patient advocate, the case manager can help to extend authorization from the insurance company if tangible reasons can be cited and the case manager is adept at negotiation.

▶ Physician Groups

As large physician practice groups become more common, case management positions in this area are being seen more frequently. Clinical nurse specialists or highly experienced nurses are often placed in a case management role in physician specialist offices (e.g., cardiology, respiratory, neurology, gastroenterology, oncology, orthopedics).

▶ Skilled Nursing Facility Case Management

When patients' self-care needs exceed their self-care capabilities after an episode of acute illness, SNF placement may be necessary. Case managers act as liaisons between the acute care and subacute care levels. They also assist during the convalescent period by determining appropriate needs and services and obtaining required payor funds for the SNF care. Many other responsibilities that resemble those of an acute care case manager may be required during the patient's SNF admission. This level of care has opened up case management opportunities in large numbers because of the federal reimbursement changes that have taken place recently (e.g., implementation of the prospective payment systems) and that continue to occur. Gerontologists, nurses, physical or occupational therapists, and social workers are good choices for this case management position.

▶ Public Health/Community-Based Case Management

This model helps families and patients access appropriate services needed for independent functioning. A wide range of target populations may receive services, depending on the focus of the agency. Community health nursing, such as that on Indian reservations or with high-risk/low-income maternal/child health, has long been taking care of families' health on a case-by-case basis. Other areas or populations needing case managers include mental health, geriatrics, catastrophic diseases such as AIDS, homeless families, or substance abuse patients. Some populations can be well served with a social service professional; others require medical knowledge, especially in the HIV and geriatric populations. Like home health nursing, community-based case management also works to prevent exacerbations of illnesses by early assessment of changes in patients' conditions and early interventions.

▶ Rehabilitation Specialists

Many rehabilitation units (both freestanding and those in acute or subacute care facilities) have discovered the efficacy of the case manager–social worker team concept. Patients enter rehabilitation units for many reasons, such as cerebral vascular accidents, motor vehicle accidents, traumas, gunshot wounds, head injuries, and spinal cord injuries. Most patients are not even allowed on rehabilitation units unless they are functioning at a low enough level to require intensive rehabilitation services. Inherent in the criteria for acceptance onto this unit is a precipitating illness or event that requires a full-scale biopsychosocial assessment, planning, and intervention. The goal is to bring that person back to a functional level that matches his or her baseline level as much as possible. Depending on the precipitating event, this type of case management may require the utmost in creativity, pulling in both private and community resources.

▶ Vocational Case Management

Vocational case management may be a component of rehabilitation case management, a part of workers' compensation case management, or a separate form of employment. Vocational case managers assist patients in returning to meaningful employment, given their new limitations as a result of injury in the work setting. A thorough knowledge of disability and workers' compensation laws and excellent assessment skills (both of functional and cognitive ability and employability) are necessary.

▶ Workers' Compensation

Case management is the key strategy in management of a workers' compensation cases. The goals are to proactively prevent injuries, when possible, and to manage injuries when they occur. Workers' compensation case management stresses early recognition and referral of the injured patient and provides a comprehensive evaluation, assessment, and care plan. The primary focus of workers' compensation case management is return to work. Another aspect of case management is prevention of work-related injuries or illnesses. As in all types of case management, workers' compensation lends itself to abuses; therefore, the case manager must be aware of the red flags of malingering while maintaining a strong patient advocate role.

▶ Case Management Firms

Case managers working in private case management agencies need a national network of resources. Patients are often willing to travel to receive the best care for their particular illness. Case managers may need to identify the most up-to-date treatment for a specific disease and locate the facility where that treatment is offered. Patients may be admitted to hospitals anywhere in the United States or even worldwide. This type of case management holds the same limitations as telephonics review (i.e., reliance on asking the right questions and receiving accurate information from a nurse on the other end of the line, who may have little time to spare for telephone consultation).

Private case management focuses on managing the care and resources of patients with chronic illnesses, disabilities, or injuries that have resulted in long-term and complex physical, cognitive, or psychosocial problems. Patients with such conditions tend to consume expensive healthcare resources and require care that is intensive and time-consuming. Their conditions are long-term; most often, they are not resolved, and sometimes last until the patient's death.

▶ Entrepreneurial Case Management

Several brave nurses have been willing to risk starting their own case manager businesses. Also known as case management consultants, these independent case managers may be contracted by patients, family members, physicians, or insurance companies. Entrepreneurial case managers need good business skills and the ability to work autonomously. There are some perils involved in this type of case management; if a patient sustains a poor outcome from a referred physician or treatment, the company may be sued for liability. On the positive side, independent case managers often have increased freedom to fulfill the patient's desires and needs, especially if the patient has funds to supplement private insurance. Without financial constraints and insurance policy restrictions, patient choices can be implemented to the benefit and satisfaction of the patient, family, and physician.

As in other forms of case management, independent case managers coordinate all aspects of care, in the home and in any level of care needed. Specialties such as geriatrics or rehabilitation may dominate a professional group practice, depending on the skill and experience of the case managers. Patients may reside in various parts of the country, and travel may be part of the job description.

Before considering entrepreneurial case management, assess whether you have both the background skills required for the job and the personality makeup. Successful case managers benefit from some of the entrepreneurial characteristics listed in Display 1-3 (Tassel, 1994, p. 143).

In 1990, some entrepreneurial nurses employed by St. Mary's Hospital in Tucson, Arizona, seized an opportunity to contract case managers and community nursing services to a medical HMO, forming a nursing HMO group. Their vision included a better way to manage patients, enter the managed care arena, strengthen business opportunities for case managers, and advance the nursing profession (Michaels, 1992). With the fast-changing healthcare climate, opportunities for entrepreneurship abound. An unselfish vision in the proper hands can benefit the patient, the nursing profession, and all those touched by the dilemmas inherent in the managed care arena.

▶ Hospitalists

Although not a case management model per se, this current hospital structure has been showing initial success in many locations. Most often, there is at least one case manager on the hospitalist team; a social worker is included in the more evolved models and where the patient population managed by hospitalists is of increased acuity and complexity. Hospitalists are physicians who take over care for the primary care provider (PCP) when the PCP's patients are admitted to the hospital. Many physicians like this arrangement because they can then focus on their office patients without running from their office to a hospital on the west side of town, then to another on the east side of town. It also allows physicians to get some rest, as there are physicians in-house at the hospital during the day and night to handle medication changes or emergencies. There are some problems, as with all new innovations. Not all patients feel secure without their "own" physician, and not all physicians are willing to "give up" their patients during hospitalizations. Much variation exists among those trying out this model. Case managers act in a capacity similar to any hospital-based case manager.

▶ EVALUATION OF A CASE MANAGEMENT MODEL

Evaluation of the case management needs of your organization and the patient population is germane to both the development of new case management departments and to situations where the current case

---

display 1-3

▶ ENTREPRENEURIAL CHARACTERISTICS

- *Opportunist*—Sees opportunities but also the risk involved in pursuing them.
- *Risk taker*—Accepts risk and attempts to manage it effectively and proactively.
- *Visionary*—Sees a better way of doing things and takes advantage of the situation.
- *Actor*—Is action-oriented with little patience for frequent committee meetings.
- *Strategist*—Focuses on the best solutions, especially those that ensure meeting the goals.

- *Innovator*—Is unafraid to try a new way of doing something.
- *Learner*—Is open-minded and asks questions to develop new strategies and advances own knowledge.
- *Confident*—Assesses opportunities comfortably, confidently, and produces favorable changes and results.
- *Flexibility*—Adapts to fast-paced changes and able to rearrange priorities.

Tassel, M.V. (1994, August). Case managers use entrepreneurial skills. *Hospital Case Management*, 143.

management department is not meeting its goals. This strategic planning activity will direct the organization toward the target and possibly save time, money, resources, and staff burn-out from unnecessary failure.

One large inner-city hospital identified case management services as a means of responding to changes in reimbursement strategies. They appeared to do all the right things; they reviewed the literature, visited other hospitals and studied what worked for those sites, and appointed a multidisciplinary team to implement the chosen model. What they did not do was evaluate their needs and match a model that worked with a similar population of patients. They were in a big city and most of their patients had a low income with little family or financial support. The model hospital that they chose to emulate was a small, community hospital with affluent patients and sufficient family and financial support. When choosing a case management model or evaluating one that is less than satisfactory, consider the following areas in your organization:

▶ The geographic location. An organization/facility in a large city with adequate acute, postacute, and community services support has very different needs than the challenges faced by a rural organization/facility with limited or distant resources.

▶ The demographics of the patient population served. In the example above, one hospital had very different patient needs than the other it attempted to emulate. The inner-city hospital likely had more Medicaid and Medicare patients; the community hospital likely had more private insurance patients. Transitional and discharge planning also might have posed different challenges. The inner-city hospital had a greater number of emergency department visits because a lower percentage of its admissions were managed care patients who had PCPs. Denied reimbursement levels were crippling, high-risk patients were not being expediently identified, and disease management programs were not available.

This scenario will change with the growing numbers of managed care Medicare and Medicaid plans, but it clearly illustrates the importance of evaluating your patients' demographics.

▶ Collect and analyze data.
1. Discern the patient mix.
2. Assess the payor mix commonly seen in your organization/facility and the percentage each type accounts for: Medicare, Medicaid, private pay, workers' compensation, private insurance.
3. Evaluate the major types of reimbursement: managed Medicare versus fee-for-service, DRG reimbursement, capitation, per diem, etc.
4. Discern which diseases or medical conditions (e.g., traumas, organ transplantation) compose a large portion of the patient population. List the high-volume, high-cost, high-risk diagnoses encountered.
5. Assess recidivism. Which patients with which diseases frequently get readmitted to the hospital, go to the emergency department, call/visit the physician? What is the acuity and chronicity of the population?

▶ Assess gaps in staff education and training. A well-trained case management staff will contain all the ingredients for success. To case manage in an environment that yields quality of care, the case manager must be clinically astute. To affect patient, provider, and payor satisfaction, the case manager must be adept in communication and negotiation skills and be knowledgeable in all areas covered in this text. To develop the best strategies for maximum reimbursement with minimal denials, case managers must clearly understand the ramifications of insurance benefit designs and reimbursement systems (see Chapter 3: Reimbursement Concepts).

▶ Set organizational goals. It is important that the organization is clear about what it wants to achieve with case management services. Set short-term, intermediate, and long-range goals as part of a strategic planning activity.

▶ Consider the standards of regulatory agencies. Regulatory and accreditation agencies play a major role in the decisions a healthcare provider or administrator makes. Case management can fulfill many requirements for several of these agencies, while also improving quality and satisfaction as well as balancing costs and revenue.

▶ Operationalize case management at the patient level; that is, ensure that the model is patient- and family-centered and would apply to the care of every patient regardless of location in the organization: clinic, ICU, regular floor, observation in the emergency department, home setting, and so on. To achieve this, all staff must be familiar with the model and educated on how to implement it while they are involved in the care delivery to their patients. One important aspect of the model is that it must be relevant to all patient populations served to facilitate consistency and conformity in care provision.

▶ Redesign implementation processes. Because the implementation of the case management model impacts the way care is delivered and its related context and processes, redesigning these processes is essential. Otherwise, it may appear that the model is implemented in a vacuum, presenting the staff with great challenges in implementation. For example, staff, including physicians, must be aware of the role of the case manager and its contribution to patient care management. Examples of the processes that would require redesign are care provision/management such as transitional/discharge planning, financial processes such as resource allocation and utilization review and management, and quality/outcomes measurement such as compliance with core measures and reporting of significant events to the risk management department.

▶ Determine the system of measurement of the effectiveness of the case management model. It is important to identify the metrics to be used for evaluation of the model prior to implementation. It is also advisable to determine the process of data collection, analysis, and reporting. The metrics should be determined based on the goals and expectations of the model. This avoids unnecessary and costly efforts, especially if the metrics identified can serve multiple purposes. For example, core measures, if chosen, are also required by CMS.

▶ SUGGESTED STEPS FOR CHOOSING OR CHANGING YOUR CASE MANAGEMENT MODEL

1. Develop your organizational compass by listing important goals. Perhaps your organization decided on the following goals:
   ▶ To balance the cost of care with the reimbursement.
   ▶ To be a world-class hospital/managed care organization/home health agency (other) through achieving clinical and administrative benchmarks in selected areas.
   ▶ To develop an integrated system for a seamless flow of patients across the continuum of care.

2. Prioritize the goals that are most important to the organization. Balancing the cost of care with available reimbursement is essential for survival, so your organization may choose this as its number one goal. Clinical excellence is also important, so the organization may choose this goal as number two. A seamless, integrated system may be on the "wish list" for the future.

3. Evaluate your present strengths and weaknesses as they affect your ability to accomplish those goals. There are many avenues to increase cost-efficiency, decrease waste, and continuously improve quality of services and care. What are your current systems that are good or salvageable? Use the evaluation data you gathered above to address this step. For your first goal, you may determine that you already have a preadmissions nurse or a solid utilization management department. However, your length of stay is long because of weakness on the transitional/discharge planning end. Unreimbursed care and denials are a serious problem. Do you have readmissions in a few targeted conditions? Will you benefit from a disease management structure in these specialties? Do you have staff expertise that can fill needed roles? Do you have the technology to support the changes planned or will this be a major expense that must be budgeted?

   Decide which goals can be accomplished with minimal changes versus those that may be in your future. Do not try to do everything at once; for example, before community integration is attempted, hospital-based or internal case management should be well defined and operational. The internal case management system should be developed with a vision of ultimately extending its scope into the community and caring for the patient throughout the continuum of care.

   Consider the example of the large inner-city hospital that tried to use a small community hospital model; it did not fail in its case management attempt, but rather learned some very important lessons. It continued with a new, customized case management pilot program that included training case managers in transitional/discharge planning; educating physicians, nurses, and other staff members in the case management process; and implementing aspects of disease management for targeted patient populations such as individuals with asthma.

4. Evaluate future trends that will affect patient care and reimbursement. Are you expecting more Medicare and Medicaid managed care patients? Are the demographics of your community changing? Are you well-positioned to get enough business in the healthcare future?

5. Plan how you will monitor for success. In the large inner-city hospital, monitoring was done in several ways:

   ▶ Lag days were identified and monitored.

   ▶ Areas tracked to ascertain if there was improvement included denied payments, recidivism rate for identified patient populations, and length of stay for targeted DRGs.

   ▶ Satisfaction with the case management process was measured for physicians, nurses, and other care providers.

6. Adapt aspects of current case management models to your needs and requirements. Customize what you see and read to best meet the needs of your organization and patients. Apply various designs of case management and disease management if that will move you toward your goals of quality and cost-efficiency. When possible, improve the model. Anything that is done can be done better. If your organization has requirements that have not been addressed by others, be creative! Go where no healthcare organization has gone before, and your facility may write the next "best practice" article on case management models.

▶ INFORMATION TECHNOLOGY AND CASE MANAGEMENT

Historically, case managers kept track of their daily activities using a "paper and pencil" approach; a manual and laborious process. Their work was viewed as "top secret;" they documented their involvement in patient care in a file that was kept out of the patient's medical record; no one had access to the file except for the case management program administrators. The primary focus then was utilization review and reimbursement for care rendered. Currently however, contributions of case managers in patient care are no longer secret; in fact, they are transparent to all who are directly or indirectly involved in patient care and the role has expanded beyond utilization management. Additionally, the documentation of case managers' activities is kept permanently in the patient's medical record and accessed daily by other members of the healthcare team.

The use of the "paper and pencil" approach to case management documentation presents some problems, especially for organizations that have implemented electronic medical records. Accreditation and regulatory agencies require a seamless multidisciplinary approach to patient care planning and management, with evidence of compliance present in the patient's medical record. If case management documentation is kept unautomated, the result is a fragmented medical record that jeopardizes adherence to accreditation and regulatory standards. Health information technology companies began to address this issue over a decade ago; however, the software applications developed only recently are becoming useful to case managers, with accurate depiction of what case management practice is about.

Recently, the use of information technology in case management practice has been on the rise. This is especially true because of the various case management software applications currently present in the market. Initially, case management information technology development focused on the utilization review and management aspect of the role of the case manager; today, however, applications have grown to allow effective approaches to clinical care management; quality and patient safety; variance management; patient flow management; cost analyses; and data collection, aggregation, and reporting. Such improvement in case management information technology is an evidence of the maturation of case management programs and their value in healthcare delivery and management.

In the absence of case management information technology, case managers engaged in numerous manual and labor-intensive activities that were considered "busy work" or "clerical work" and resulted in increased job-related stress and dissatisfaction. Examples of these activities are duplicate documentation; photocopying parts of the medical record to keep in own files or share with others; using a "to do list" or placing stickers (Post-It notes) everywhere as reminders to complete certain activities, or for others, asking them to follow up on things or answer certain questions; filing of forms; and using a list/tool for tracking delays in care (i.e., variances). McGonigle and Mastrian (2008) claim that case management information technology presents case managers with solutions to these problems. It allows them to be more efficient and efficacious in their role. For example, information technology facilitates data collection (e.g., variances, outcomes measures), report generation, and dissemination. It also functions as an effective tool for bringing people, data, and procedures together for the betterment of patient care, especially in the area of managing information to support case management functions and decision making at the individual, team, and organization levels.

The benefits of case management information technology are numerous; examples are as follows (McGonigle & Mastrian, 2008):

1. Work flow: Support of case management process; reduction of duplicate documentation; elimination of double data entry; improvement of data entry, retrieval, access, storage, and dissemination; generation of reminders of due tasks; and generation of alerts, especially those that are patient-safety oriented.

2. Patient care: Keeping patients safe, monitoring progress, use of best practices and evidence-based care, use of nationally recognized standards and guidelines, standardization of care patterns, reduction or elimination of medical errors, and compliance with core measures.

3. Organizational: Improving the efficiency of care activities, better job satisfaction, increased accountability, improved relationships among care providers, and return on investment measures for case management.

▶ TELEHEALTH AND CASE MANAGEMENT

The use of telehealth is not new; however, its application in case management is fairly recent. When telehealth approaches are used in case management practice, it is referred to as *tele-case management*. Tele-case management is simply the provision and management of healthcare services from a distance. It has become more common because of disease management programs that require the use of telecommunication technologies for improving patients' adherence to medical regimens, health education, and psychosocial/emotional support.

The use of tele-case management also means the sharing of information with others for the better management of patient care and employing the assistance of telecommunication technologies such as the telephone, fax machines, and electronic communication via the Internet. Sharing of information in this fashion was the first aspect of tele-case management used by case managers, especially after an increase in the use of managed care health insurance plans. Examples of tele-case management activities include authorizations of services, telephone triage, concurrent reviews of patient care and progress, and handling of reimbursement of denials and appeals.

▶ A DAY IN THE LIFE OF A NURSE CASE MANAGER

This section, beginning with the next paragraph, is written based on the experiences of a hospital case manager in the early-1990s. We tell the story of this case manager using the first person pronoun just to keep it real and personal. This case manager describes her story as follows:

For several years, I have case managed clients (patients) belonging to self-insured plans in a five-state area. Although sometimes this is on site, it is mostly telephonic—and very different from case management within facilities. The pace is not as intensive; however, the knowledge base of each client's benefit package must be exact. Each model of case management has its challenges and its joys.

Several years ago, I attended a case management seminar given by one of the pioneer case management teams in the southwestern United States. When the speakers asked for audience questions, I asked each speaker to describe a typical workday. Their stories were interesting and educational, but what surprised me was how varied their individual experiences were. Only one case manager's day resembled my own! After some reflection, I realized that even my own tasks differ dramatically from day to day. As I listened, I realized that there are many forms of case management, with different managers putting emphasis on different facets of the case management system. To some, discharge planning is a priority. Others act as utilization review nurses. One nurse case manager appeared to be involved with basic staff nursing (direct patient care) but had strong ties to the multidisciplinary team. No singular set of role definitions could describe this group. Soon I realized the reason: case management was in its adolescence, complete with identity crisis and a growing, awkward form. Case managers attempt to do everything for everyone—an impossible task—while insurance regulations, state laws, and professional standards are ever changing.

I believe our identity as case managers will arise out of our own field. Certification examinations are already a reality, and standards on case management practice as well as legal and ethical guidelines will be written to guide us through life as case managers.

I am a hospital case manager. My patient population is a medical mix, with some surgical patients. My patients are all ages and may have multisystem failure, pulmonary disease, HIV, suicide gestures, gastrointestinal bleeding, cancer, pancreatitis—in other words, almost any medical problem. When other units are full, orthopedic, neurologic, obstetric, cardiac, surgical, or even older pediatric patients may appear in my ward and need case managing.

▶ An Ideal Day in the Life of a Nurse Case Manager

An ideal day in the life for me would be to use the morning to review patient charts, especially new admissions, input utilization review data, check on any quality of care issues, set up transfers and equipment needs, and elicit plans from physicians during their morning rounds and then pass these on to insurance company liaisons (perhaps third-party payor case managers) and others who are part of the plans. After these preliminaries are handled and as needs arise, I would visit patient rooms, talk to patients, and catch family members for brief consultations. Then I would, if I was lucky, enjoy an ideal 30-minute lunch without shop talk.

The afternoon would be the time to tie up loose ends, finish utilization review from the morning, complete transfers to other facilities, and do patient rounds. Patient rounds are room-to-room visits designed for introduction, initial assessment of possible discharge needs or further plans for discharge, patient education on various topics, emotional support for impending invasive procedures or surgeries, assessment of patient satisfaction, and handling the many different issues that pop up unexpectedly.

This is my ideal day, not my typical day.

▶ An Actual Day in the Life of a Nurse Case Manager

I have picked a day to share that is without long meetings, because such a day would not provide the educational intent of this section, which is to draw a clear picture of the nurse case manager serving on the front lines. However, long meetings are often a vexing reality; therefore, setting daily priorities is essential.

6:30 AM—I pick up my laptop computer and patient census. I delete discharged patients from the computer and make sure all new admissions are programmed in. I quickly look at new admissions for ages and admitting diagnoses and log in obvious and necessary social service referrals. Then, I attend to the notes taped to my door!

7:00 AM—Shift report. I set my first priority list for the day, which frequently changes. Today's list looks like this:

▶ Speak to physicians about a do-not-resuscitate (DNR) order for Mrs. Adams—impending code.
▶ Visit Mr. Innes—multicomplaints to staff.
▶ Transfer Mr. Block to SNF. Dr. T to follow.

▶ Transfer Mrs. Cohn to SNF. Find a physician to follow.
▶ Call mental health agency—is it possible to do an involuntary transfer of Ms. Diamond today? Make sure psychiatric sitters are available.
▶ Possibly transfer Mrs. Elliot to SNF tomorrow. Finish plans.
▶ Review arterial blood gas values for Mr. Frank. Does he need home oxygen?
▶ Put in for social referrals for Mrs. Garrett and Mr. Harris.
▶ Talk with physical therapist about Mr. Harris— is it safe for him to go home?
▶ Probably discharge Mr. Johns today or tomorrow. Arrange for home intravenous antibiotics; get authorization from insurance company.

7:45 AM—I leave hurriedly to attend a short daily case manager meeting. I ask the charge nurse to please make a notation to ask Mrs. Adams' physicians (if they come by) about the DNR order (if they do not show up by the time I get back, I will call them.)

8:10 AM—Back on the unit. The physicians called Mrs. Adams' daughter. She wants "everything done." I expect the worst in this case (i.e., that she will code shortly) but hope that my gut feelings are wrong.

I am moving along on my priority list:

▶ I look at Mr. Block's chart. His temperature spiked last night. Physicians wish to hold patient transfer and culture blood and urine. This may take 24 to 48 hours. The following calls need to be made about change of plans:
   1. Patient/family.
   2. Social worker.
   3. SNF—will they hold the bed? (yes, thanks!).
   4. Transportation—cancel stretcher van.
   5. Insurance company—need hospitalization coverage for additional hospital days.
▶ I document all of the above in the computer or the patient's chart.

The psychiatric nurse phones me. The mental health agency has completed the paperwork for an involuntary admission to a mental health facility for Ms. Diamond. The sheriff should be arriving to pick her up around 9:30 AM (not much time!). Ms. Diamond is unaware of the plan. Her physicians feel it is not in her best interest to tell her beforehand because she has a history of suicide attempts and adamantly refuses help. The psychiatric nurse will be there but recommends a call to security, because this procedure sometimes gets "ugly." I alert security and the attending and resident physicians of the plans. All are relieved that after 4 days in this hospital Ms. Diamond will finally be in a proper setting for her problems.

The unit secretary gives me Mr. Frank's arterial blood gas results, which show a PO_2 of 49. I call the physician for a verbal order for home oxygen, then the durable medical equipment company for delivery of two portable oxygen tanks to the hospital for Mr. Frank's ride home (he lives 50 miles away). I coordinate the home oxygen setup with the company and the patient's family.

Better check to see whether Mrs. Cohn is stable for transfer. Yes. I have not yet found a physician to follow her up at the nursing home. Priority: find one!

Now facing me are four large men in civilian clothes. They are here to "escort" Ms. Diamond to the mental health facility. They have come early. Why four? They explain that two are in training. Ms. Diamond is a fragile, petite woman; I do not want her to be frightened. I ask "the boys" to be patient, then call the psychiatric nurse, who arrives to speak with Ms. Diamond about the plan. I call security. Ms. Diamond is visibly upset, crying. She is making loud accusations, heard throughout the ward, toward the staff and her significant other. I comfort the significant other, realizing that he has tried to do what is best. Meanwhile, the psychiatric nurse works magic in calming the patient. Finally, Ms. Diamond, escorted by the four deputies, leaves peaceably, quietly crying. We are all left with a little sadness. Ms. Diamond is a pretty, intelligent, young woman in a lot of emotional pain. I document each detail into the computer.

Back to Mrs. Cohn. Which physician goes to the SNF? I look in my files and pick one with whom I often have success.

Emergency! Before I have a chance to make the call, I hear a Code Blue. It is for Mrs. Adams! I run to her room. Compressions have already started. I cut open the code cart while the code team rushes in. I begin recording. We get a fleeting heartbeat 5 and 8 minutes, then lose it. Every advanced cardiac life support medication is used. The chaplain, already alerted, has called Mrs. Adams' daughter, who is on her way to the hospital. I ask the chaplain to try to stop the daughter before she arrives at the room. At 20 minutes, the heartbeat is erratic, but Mrs. Adams is intubated. A bed in the ICU is available. (Thank goodness the daughter did not walk in on this.) Mrs. Adams is transferred to ICU. I look up to see the physician speaking to Mrs. Adams' daughter. In tears, she accompanies him to the ICU. I document the transfer into the computer.

Back to the nurses' station. I hear someone say, "Is this a full moon?"

Another answers, "It looked full last night."

A resident physician turns his head skyward and howls like a wolf. Laughter breaks some of the tension.

10:30 AM—Back to finding a physician for Mrs. Cohn. I page the physician I have chosen. He calls back and agrees to follow up Mrs. Cohn at the nursing home. Relief! (Sometimes finding a physician to follow up at an SNF is an all-day task.) I call the resident to write transfer orders and dictate the discharge summary. I call the family; they are pleased with the transfer news. The SNF is close to home, making visiting easy. Mrs. Cohn also is happy to be "graduating" from the hospital. The social worker sets up transportation; I inform the SNF of the physician's name and phone number, Mrs. Cohn's health status today, and her time of departure. The charge nurse and staff nurses are told of the transfer and time. I document.

I am starting to feel pressured because I have not yet done any utilization review or looked at my new patient charts.

Mr. Johns' physician tells me that he can leave the hospital today if I can set up twice-daily intravenous ceftriaxone at home. The physician has already spoken with his patient about leaving today, and Mr. Johns will not take "tomorrow" for an answer! Okay. I can do that! I check the facesheet for the name of the insurance company and call them. The insurance representative likes the idea of sending him home; it saves 5 hospital days. I am also given the okay to use our hospital's home health agency. I call the home health agency, and the agency's coordinator does the rest. I enter Mr. Johns' room and tell him to be patient and that we will get him out as soon as possible. Does he have transportation home? No problem. I document.

I look at my list again—social service referrals. These will take only a few minutes so I get them done.

Finally, I have time to do some "admission" reviews on my new patients. I add a few thoughts to my priority list: one patient may not be able to return to independent living; another is being worked up for probable new diagnosis of cancer, with possible referrals to chaplain services and oncology life enrichment; another patient is a 19-year-old new admission, entering for diabetic ketoacidosis. I make a note to call the diabetic nurse educator to start teaching. I document everything.

The charge nurse lets me know Mr. Frank's oxygen has not arrived. I make another call; it is in the truck, on its way.

From overhead, I hear: "Any trauma surgeon to medical ICU." I call to see whether this is about Mrs. Adams. Yes. She coded again in the ICU. She has one chest tube inserted and needs another. The daughter still wants every effort made. It looks grim.

12:00 PM—Telephone call for me. Lunch, already! Ready in 15 minutes. I want to squeeze in some admission reviews, then a quick lunch. The luncheon rule is no shop talk allowed. It seeps through at times, anyway. I sit down and take a deep breath. At what time this morning did I stop breathing?

12:30 PM—Back to the front lines. I had better see to Mr. Innes' multicomplaints while I am refreshed. Mr. Innes has chronic obstructive pulmonary disease, and the staff knows him from previous, recent hospital admissions. Usually a pleasant patient, this time he is different. He also has a new diagnosis—severe anemia. I review Mr. Innes' chart for updates: at admission, his hemoglobin and hematocrit levels were very low. He received 3 units of blood, and his condition is fairly stable now. After several procedures and tests, no source of bleeding can be identified. Mr. Innes recognizes me when I enter. I tell him that I hear that he is unhappy with some aspects of his care and suggest that perhaps I can help. Mr. Innes has many concerns, ranging from the wrong diet on his meal trays to too much noise from the nearby nurses' station. Other, more important, clues to his discontent emerge subtly as we continue our talk. He is concerned about how his debilitated wife is getting along, with his being so often in the hospital. Finally, after so many tests, "Why won't they tell me what's wrong?"

We take each issue one at a time. A call to the dietary department (actually, three calls) fixes the dietary problem. I suggest a room change (if available) to a quieter part of the unit. He is pleased with this idea. Together, we call his wife, and they agree to have home nurse and social worker visits. With the approval of their family physician, I set this in motion. The next major hurdle is Mr. Innes' health concerns. I ask him if he feels that no one is telling him the truth. He answers, "Yes," and expresses fear that bad news is on the way. I know that his tests are negative. I explain that it may feel like he is not being told the truth, but the tests truly do not show a bleeding source anywhere. I also explain that his laboratory test values are stable; he is doing well. He agrees to allow me to discuss his concern with his physician, which I do. The physician then spends time with him, showing him the written test results and making plans for further work ups if his hematocrit and hemoglobin levels drop again. The complaints stop; Mr. Innes seems more relaxed and remains that way for the remainder of his stay.

1:00–2:00 PM—Weekly multidisciplinary patient rounds. Each patient on the unit is discussed. The focus is on the entire range of needs for each patient and how well we (as a team) are meeting these needs.

I call back down to the ICU. Mrs. Adams has a grim prognosis, with three chest tubes now in place. There are no family members present at this time.

I recheck Mr. Frank's oxygen. It has arrived, and he has departed.

I recheck Mrs. Cohn's transfer. The transport team is in the room now.

I recheck Mr. Johns. Home health intravenous antibiotics are set up, and he is a happy guy.

I review Mrs. Elliot's chart; she is scheduled for possible transfer to SNF tomorrow. Her chart looks good. I call the SNF; her bed is available. Social services can call for transportation tomorrow. A taxi is appropriate, relevant to discussions with the physician, patient, and family. I document and proceed to the next priority.

I check Mr. Harris' chart; is it safe for him to go home? I look at the physical therapist's notes—excellent progress today. Perhaps one more day of physical therapy. I did not think Mr. Harris would do this well. He is spunky, though!

A family member finds me and needs to talk. We go into the family room. Dad is deteriorating more each month. He has Parkinson's disease, and the family is feeling overwhelmed with the care. This family feels guilty about putting Dad in a nursing home. What other options do they have? We explore insurance benefits, financial ability to get home health aide care, increase in respite care time, and family/neighbor/church support. I ask the social worker to speak to this family about possible community resources. We plan to have a family meeting the next day with the social worker to explore options further. This gives me time to find out more about insurance benefit possibilities. I add this patient to my priority list.

I review more charts until it is time for my 3:00 PM monthly case managers' meeting.

▶ Discussion

The nature of the written word necessitates telling a story in a linear fashion. However, I can attest to the fact that many of these events actually occur simultaneously during a busy day in the life. What this account does not depict are the many other interactions and interruptions: support for staff members; answering telephone calls and pages; discussing patient plans with dozens of physicians, nurses, social service personnel, physical therapists, home health professionals, and more. Each day, there are reports to and negotiations with insurance companies regarding length of stay and patient needs. Education of patients in areas pertaining to their own individual needs is a key component. Also, many individual problems and concerns arise that are unique to an individual patient's diagnosis and life support.

The pace is often breakneck. Boredom is not in a case manager's dictionary. I frequently look at the clock and wonder what happened to the day. This type of case management is not for everyone and could leave some on the ragged edge. I once overheard a job description in which the employee appeared to be able to do one activity at a time. Discussing it with the charge nurse on the unit, I said that it was a unique concept, doing one thing at a time. She smiled at me and said, "Don't get any ideas. You love this pace." She was right.

Although this account was written back in the 1990s, it continues to be relevant and depict a day in the life. With shortening length of stay hospitals, pressure to comply with the utilization management practices of insurance companies (especially managed care), and increasing demands from accreditation and regulatory agencies, the pace of case management has turned from fast to faster and now fastest. Multidisciplinary patient care rounds have become a daily rather than weekly occurrence; complex discharge planning is evident in every patient currently seen in the hospital setting; and the need to carefully review and manage compliance with publicly reported quality data such as acute myocardial infarction, heart failure, and pneumonia core measures has only increased the complexity of the role of the case manager and filled the day in the life with competing priorities and activities that cannot be managed in a linear fashion, but require resolution in the most efficient and effective manner despite the time and resource constraints case managers may face while caring for their patients.

▶ TRENDS IN CASE MANAGEMENT

There are exciting trends in case management. First, it has become a managed care strategy in its own right. It is even an integral aspect of any healthcare delivery environment today. The CCM credential has added credibility; the work of the CMSA has moved case management into international waters; accreditation of case management programs/models has also added consistency and accountability; and the outcomes movement with the Center for Case Management Accountability (CCMA) will sustain case management through the consumer and employer demands for documented "results." The executive summary of CMSA (1998) addresses the changing nature of case management.

> The environment in which case management is practiced, and thus, case management itself, is in transition. The healthcare climate has changed

dramatically in the 1990s, necessitating a change in the way case management is viewed and practiced. The case manager's role is transitioning from negotiator of cost to negotiator of care. Its role in the education and empowerment of the patient as well as its proactive and preventative nature have increased.

Case management opportunities are expanding. The case management trend is from individual case management to managing a disease-specific population. Disease management and chronic care programs are carving the way for disease-specific case management experts. An advanced level nursing degree may fill this need in the future.

Major changes in both human demographics and healthcare funding and reimbursement will open up opportunities inclusive of all areas of healthcare. The coordination skill of case management is needed everywhere: hospitals, SNFs, insurance companies, physician hospital organizations (PHOs), HMOs, home health agencies, rehabilitation hospitals, etc. The older portion of the population is expected to increase sevenfold from 1980 to 2050. The pattern of illness and disease has made a dramatic shift from predominately infectious disease in the early 1900s to diseases that require case/disease management (chronic diseases). These chronic conditions, coupled with managed Medicare and Medicaid, make a perfect marriage for the skills of a trained case manager.

Other trends that will be detailed are the changes in healthcare definitions and the trend of international case management.

▶ Confusing Terms and Definitions

In 1996, a class action lawsuit was filed in a district court, claiming that the HCFA (now known as CMS), arbitrarily and capriciously interpreted Medicare's "confined to home" requirement to deny severely disabled Medicare beneficiaries needing home health services (Bureau of National Affairs, 1998). This is not surprising, given the ambiguous definitions that abound in many areas of healthcare. This is certainly one trend that will change; healthcare terminology must become more distinct and accurate to avoid lawsuits. In many ways, insurance-related definitions that are still open to interpretation drive the authorization of healthcare services. Nebulous terminology can no longer be acceptable when more adverse outcomes are entering the courtrooms. The case manager, as a patient advocate, must be alert to vague interpretations of benefits. Recent attempts at improving this situation have been made, and specific criteria are now being attached to some of the more vague definitions. Time, and possibly litigation, will define this trend (for more on terminology, see Chapter 7).

MEDICAL NECESSITY

Sometimes care is denied based on it being "not medically necessary." This is a time bomb case managers have dealt with since the birth of managed care. Often the basis for medical necessity is based on political or economic factors, rather than on clinical reasons. Because the definition of medical necessity has caused more than a few problems, it has evolved a bit further than some other managed care definitions. This trend will continue with other vague wording. The detail to which it will evolve to is a matter of practicality; in this example, it would not be practical to specify the following criteria for every service or equipment that is covered in the benefit design. That would truly be "cookbook medicine" and would not allow for new developments in disease treatment without a major overhaul in the benefit design.

Several definitions of medical necessity can be found in the literature and benefit books. The most comprehensive of them, and considered a classic, included the following criteria (Anonymous, 1998):

▶ The services or equipment were consistent with the individual's diagnosis or medical condition.
▶ The services or equipment were prescribed or rendered by a physician or other qualified healthcare professional.
▶ The services or equipment were generally accepted as effective (that is, consistent with nationally accepted and recognized standards of practice).
▶ The services or equipment were not primarily based on the recipient's convenience.
▶ The more economical choice (rent versus buy) is chosen when there is more than one alternative available.

From a case management standpoint, it must be realized that there is an economic benefit to the insurance company if the claim for medical necessity is not appealed. If a patient/family strongly feels that a service or piece of equipment should be covered, explain the appeals process according to the state laws and insurance policy and procedures (see section on appeals in Chapter 6). This frees the case manager from a potential legal mess; it shows good faith. It also frees the case manager from an ethical tangle; if the case manager is also an employee of the insurance company making the rules, at least there is another step that can be provided while acting on behalf of the patient.

REASONABLE AND NECESSARY

This one piggybacks off the medical necessity concept. The intention may have been to add a little more definition to the term *medical necessity* (and it did), but very little useful information was added! According to one expert, if a treatment meets the following conditions, it will rarely provoke an argument about being reasonable and necessary, except in cases in which it returns the patient to a lesser quality of life (Banja, 1997).

▶ A general agreement exists on the meaning of the treatment's or service's success.
▶ The treatment or service in question not only results in an outcome meeting that definition, but does so most or all of the time.
▶ The treatment or service is affordable or inexpensive.

The efficacy of treatments and services is being scientifically determined and defined through the many disease management and outcomes management projects occurring throughout the United States and the world. As empirical results are agreed on, vague definitions will be replaced by best practice criteria.

This concept opens up an ethical Pandora's Box. According to John Banja, PhD, "no treatment is reasonable if delivering it imposes intolerable burdens on others. Thus it would not be reasonable for a hospital to routinely deliver treatments whose costs could not be recovered because doing so would propel the hospital to bankruptcy" (Banja, 1997, p. 35). At what point is the cost or the burden unreasonable? I had one patient who needed a heart transplant. No one could refute the necessity or the reasonableness; she did not have enough left ventricular ejection fraction to sustain life. She also had a stipulation in her insurance policy that excluded heart transplants.

Reasonable and necessary treatment has changed numerous times throughout the centuries. What were considered best practices in the 1800s would be considered "witchcraft" today or malpractice; what is considered unscientific and unconventional today may be the key to true health in a few short decades. Reasonable care today means that health care services are provided based on the patient's medical condition, acuity, and severity of the illness, and that the course of treatment conforms to what is nationally recognized and agreed on as the standard of care.

INTERMITTENT SERVICES

Intermittent services is another term that gets confused. It is mainly used in the home health setting and means that care is provided on a part-time basis, for portions of the time such as a few hours in a day and for a few days of the week.

SKILLED VERSUS NONSKILLED CARE

There continues to be confusion among healthcare professionals as to what constitutes skilled or non-skilled care and services. Some agencies commit the mistake of confusing aspects of care that require the involvement of a licensed professional/care provider and those that do not. Skilled healthcare services are those that require delivery by a licensed professional such as a registered nurse, a social worker, or a physical, occupational, or speech therapist (e.g., wound care, vital signs assessment and monitoring, physical rehabilitation). Nonskilled healthcare services are those that can be provided by an unlicensed healthcare paraprofessional such as a home health aide or a homemaker (e.g., bathing, feeding, preparing meals).

ACTIVITIES OF DAILY LIVING

Traditionally, activities of daily living (ADLs) have focused on the basics of functional life: eating, dressing, bathing, toileting, and other life essentials of self-care. ADLs are often defined according to range-of-motion, muscle strength, or mental clarity. Case managers have broadened this definition to include other important aspects of a patient's life. Is the ability to participate in chosen spiritual activities less important than the ability to bathe oneself? However, few benefit designs allow support for this one critical example, and there are many more like it.

HOMEBOUND

Under Medicare guidelines (CMS, 2009b), homebound generally means that the patient's condition is such that:

▶ It confines him or her to the home setting all (or almost all) of the time;
▶ It restricts his or her ability to leave home without the aid of supportive devices such as canes, crutches, wheelchairs, or walkers, the use of special transportation, or the assistance of another person. Leaving the home is very infrequent and for a limited period of time; or
▶ Leaving the home is medically contraindicated.

Homebound is one term that can be badly misused. Essentially, the spirit of the guidelines states that it would be a hardship for the homebound person to leave the home to get medical care.

One patient had multiple sclerosis. At the time she was admitted to case management, she was essentially bed bound; with much difficulty, she could transfer to the wheelchair. The primary insurance company repeatedly stated that she was not homebound because she was able to get to her physician appointments every other month. However, this was done only at great hardship and some risk. The definition of homebound as interpreted by this company was that it was "impossible to leave the home; as long as there were a way to transport the patient, the patient was not homebound." This company's definition of homebound would not hold up and with the aid of some education and negotiation, the patient was authorized for home care.

ADEQUATE PATIENT EDUCATION

Adequate patient education is defined as the provision of appropriate teaching or transmission of pertinent information to meet the patient's needs, including any necessary postoperative instructions, lifestyle changes (healthy behaviors), and activity or nutritional counseling. These activities must always be reflected in the patient's medical record. This is a key role in case management. It is critical for good and desirable outcomes in disease management or chronic care programs. Many accreditation agencies require case management programs to provide adequate patient education. Criteria that are specific to the education desired must be added to make accreditation more meaningful and compliance with the standards more manageable.

CARE OR LACK OF CARE

This is defined as inappropriate or untimely assessment, intervention, or management of care. Again, this is too vague to hold up. "Inappropriate" and "untimely" may mean different things to different people.

IN A TIMELY MANNER

The ability to receive care or appeal decisions in a timely manner is a basic patient right. Specific, set time frames for obtaining services are the ideal but not always the reality. In the absence of predetermined intervals, the case manager should look for unreasonable delays in obtaining care or precertification for care. This problem is becoming more common, and even the best case managers have probably been personally frustrated at some point while caring for patients. However, when the situation is endangering a patient's health, action must be taken. More providers are receiving accreditations from such organizations as The Joint Commission (TJC), the American Accreditation Health-Care Commission/Utilization Review Accreditation Commission (URAC), and the National Committee for Quality Assurance (NCQA). Within the standards of many accreditations are strict time frames that must be adhered to; accreditation status depends on it.

Access to care is also a standard that is scrutinized during some accreditations and directly related to providing care in a timely manner; providers are accountable for reasonableness in providing access to care in a timely manner. All this also directly relates to customer satisfaction. There are customer satisfaction reports published for all to see; the media can be a powerful tool to assure that patients receive attention in a timely manner, or consumers will merely pick another provider.

▶ International Perspective on Case Management

There was a time in the mid-1990s when some experts thought that case management had a life span of about 5 more years; they were more than a little bit wrong. In the United States, it has become the link between managed care, other type payors, and patient care. It is not only here to stay, but expanding internationally, as evidenced by the Case Management Society International (CMSI) (see CMS International in Chapter 10), as well as the numerous publications in case management that are of an international nature.

We believe that the United States has some of the best care—and the most complicated care—in the world. Many countries have more socialized medical healthcare structured systems than the United States. Three important characteristics of the socialized medicine approach are that the systems (1) usually provide universal coverage for basic healthcare needs, (2) are relatively simple to administer, and (3) are therefore inexpensive. Great Britain has a national health service; France has a national insurance system; The Netherlands has a system based on private practice physicians, community- and church-affiliated hospitals, and nonprofit and for-profit insurers; and Australia has publicly funded universal coverage for basic medical services with approximately 30% of the population also carrying private insurance for access to private hospital services and other services not covered by public funding. However, as the private, for-profit insurers penetrate the healthcare industries of the various countries, more complex healthcare rules can be expected. In Australia, an increasing percentage of public services are being provided by for-profit healthcare corporations. In almost every country, all services (both public and private) are coming under increasing pressure to provide high-quality and cost-effective care, leading to increasing complexity and cost-consciousness; therefore, case management systems and models are needed. In fact, most of these countries either have already implemented case management demonstration projects or are in the process of examining the value of such programs.

Healthcare complexity was the major catalyst for case management's growth in the United States; the complex insurance benefit packages and reimbursement rules that overtook our healthcare industry led to the use of nurses and other licensed professionals as case managers. Unlike the "good old days," physicians do not have the time to juggle all the necessary aspects of a patient's case; they sincerely appreciate the efforts of case managers sorting out the benefit designs and discharge planning possibilities.

Many countries are looking to the United States for lessons (both positive and negative) that are applicable in their own rapidly changing environments. Universal coverage is common in other countries. Often these countries do not actively promote health or disease prevention, but rather specifically exclude services unless they are "curative." However, significant health promotion programs were provided, yet were not always tied to health insurance. Although the rank order may be slightly different, most countries have the same major disease epidemiology, including cardiovascular disease, cerebrovascular disease, cancer, depression/mental health, and infectious diseases. This has led to a growing interest internationally in evidence-based disease management programs that integrate all aspects of health. As a consequence of the economic imperatives in the United States, considerable work has been done here in research and evaluation. Consequently, as interest in this area grows and as successes in disease and chronic care management programs become more public, the international exchange of evidenced-based information has become an ongoing occurrence.

The Dutch healthcare system has been chosen as one example demonstrating similarities and differences among other countries' healthcare systems and is discussed in detail below. The Dutch started with a social structure like many other countries, attempted many models, learned some of the same lessons, and responded to some of the same challenges as the United States, England, Australia, and others. Case management in Australia and Canada is also highlighted below.

The Dutch are a healthy population, as a whole, and are capable of delivering the most modern forms of healthcare. Historically, the issue of "rights" was rarely discussed; rather, The Netherlands had a system of "obligations." Essentially, there is an obligation that physicians, hospitals, and other providers care for all patients; there is also an obligation that all patients pay for the care rendered (through various public and private systems). Persons with high incomes are obligated to purchase health insurance, with some employer contributions; persons with low incomes are also obligated to purchase insurance, and their employers contribute to the fund. The bottom line in The Netherlands is that all members of the society receive care, all providers receive compensation for their efforts, and all people with limited means can afford insurance.

In The Netherlands, general practitioners fulfill a gatekeeper role like the PCP in managed care. Patients are free to choose their general practitioner but must have a referral before seeing any specialist. The patient can then choose any physician within the licensure of the referral specialty; hospitals are another free choice in this model.

Healthcare has been facing changes and challenges in The Netherlands. There are essentially three systems of insurance in The Netherlands: sickness funds, private insurance, and the Exceptional Medical Expenses Act. This has created administrative complexities when coordinating services for the elderly, the chronically ill, and other groups such as the mentally ill. Upper-income elderly persons are subject to very high insurance premiums. Some programs are funded by the local government out of direct tax revenue and are not part of any of the three insurance systems, causing the fragmentation we know so well in America. On the other hand, "mergers" among sickness funds and private insurance systems are occurring. These alliances are resulting in selective contracts with specialists and hospitals. The capitated agreements with the health insurers are being shared with the specialists and hospitals (risk-sharing), and specialists and hospitals have formed umbrella organizations not unlike America's PHOs. Patients pay higher out-of-pocket expenses if generic medications are not used.

At this time and in the traditional healthcare system, formal referrals to home care services are not needed; the patients initiate contact themselves. An initial visit for assessment purposes commences. Then a care plan is developed that includes care/treatment goals and a listing of services and frequency of the visits planned. The assessment visits are often done by a team primarily composed of nursing and social work professionals. Even this does not go on without resistance and turf battles.

Demographically, Dutch healthcare and home care face challenges similar to those in other countries: the population is aging, the number of single family households is rising, and more women are working outside the home, leading to less available family support. The challenges cross all country boundaries: structural and financial changes, risks of potentially misaligned incentives, increasing costs of healthcare, and fragmentation. As a result of the changes, many countries are more focused on patient rights.

In 1994, a concept called *transmural care* was introduced in The Netherlands. This is similar to the *shared care* of England, and the *integrated care delivery* of the United States. The concept of an integrated delivery system was especially challenging to The Netherlands, a country that has traditional divisions between hospital and primary and specialist care delivery systems. In addition, the population, like in the United States, was becoming increasingly demanding about what they expected from a healthcare system. Technology was allowing minimally invasive surgeries and safer equipment in the home setting, and the resulting trend toward shorter lengths of stay in the hospital was another inevitable change. The Dutch leaders recognized that something had to be done, and transmural care was chosen as a means to realize more efficient, higher-quality healthcare.

In 1995, the National Advisory Council on Health-Care defined transmural care as care geared to the needs of the patient, provided on the basis of cooperation and coordination between general and specialized caregivers, with shared responsibility and specifications for delegated responsibilities (Van der Linden, 2002). Transmural care can range from merely improving patient transfers from hospital to home, to a complete redesign of a specific patient group. There are essentially seven categories of transmural projects; each project is reminiscent of case management, either through coordination of care efforts or working toward an efficient length of stay in hospitals. Most probably, the lessons learned from these projects would be something all countries can relate to as well as benefit from.

1. Home health: The evolution of home care technology has advanced the use of home healthcare in lieu of hospital stays. This is similar to home health models everywhere, with the exception that in The Netherlands (and possibly in other countries), general practitioners also receive special training to handle the bedside technology for patients. Specially trained nurses provide the around-the-clock care, with these physicians on-call as back-up.

2. Before-and-after care in the primary care setting: These transmural projects focused on performing prehospital diagnostic workups to shorten lengths of stay and increasing the use of home care postoperatively. It was found that this approach increased patient privacy and often led to a more rapid recovery.

3. Consultation of medical specialists in the primary care setting:. These projects moved specialists

outside the walls of hospitals and into diagnostic centers. These centers demonstrated a 35% reduction in laboratory tests.

4. Specialized transmural nurses: These projects developed specialized training programs for nursing that are very similar to case management/disease management as it is evolving everywhere. These nurses are responsible for care that had traditionally been in the general practitioner's domain. For example, in diabetic outpatient clinics, the transmural nurses would provide diabetic education to patients. Other types of clinics may see cancer or asthma patients. Cancer patients would receive various intravenous therapies from nurses; and asthma patients would receive respiratory treatments by specialty nurses.

5. Rehabilitation units/wards: In many countries, posthospital care requires lengthy waiting lists or complex admission procedures. In an attempt to streamline transfers for patients requiring posthospital care, a growing number of hospitals have either opened their own rehabilitation wards or facilitated special contracts with nursing homes.

6. Discharge planning: Specialized "liaison" or "transfer" nurses were promoted to facilitate expedited discharges. These nurses are actively involved in identifying high-risk or potentially difficult discharges.

7. Pharmacological transmural care: Pharmacy boundaries widened in these transmural projects, ranging from provision of medications posthospitalization to a model similar to specialty pharmacy companies that provide mail-in medications for either patient administration or home nurse administration.

The transmural care projects opened up a Pandora's box that is probably familiar to most people working in the healthcare sector of any country. Some of the challenges include:

▶ Cooperation issues:. Transmural care involved a new way of healthcare professionals working together. Traditionally, general practitioners and specialists have operated independently of each other, without much direct communication. New skills were required to work effectively in multidisciplinary teams.

▶ Training programs: Like case management, transmural care has been added to and currently is being offered in training programs.

▶ Development of transmural care protocols: Like clinical pathways in specific settings and through-the-continuum, The Netherlands realized that transmural care requires new protocols and practice standards.

▶ Length of stay challenges: When utilization review became a constant companion of the managed care industry in the United States, the lengths of stays shortened; the patients in acute care came in sicker and were discharged sicker; families were burdened with these responsibilities; and the sicker patients led to increased workload for hospital staff, often leading to higher employee turnover. The story and the lessons are the same all over. Some Dutch experts looked on transmural care as a self-defeating system. How many case managers have not felt that way about managed care, from time to time?

▶ Financial incentives: The staff is working harder, discharging patients quicker. The families are more burdened. The general practitioners are losing autonomy. The challenges and after-effects of transmural care continued on an ever-increasing scale. Nevertheless, the reimbursement system did not support any incentives for all this trouble. Empty beds and/or increased production did not produce revenues. Until 1995, medical specialists were paid on a fee-for-service basis; therefore, they were inclined to see patients longer rather than sending them back to the general practitioner.

Initially, healthcare experts in the Netherlands seemed skeptical that anyone other than physicians needed to be case managers. There has been some conflict between the general practitioners and specialists about patient control and case management. The general practitioners are paid a capitated wage. They feel it is their role to be the managers of their patients and are supporting the idea of treating fewer patients and getting reimbursed at a higher capitated rate. This would give them the time to do case management/disease management, without a lower overall salary. Some Dutch experts were skeptical of the experience with trained transmural nurses. Nevertheless, the interest in disease management, case management, occupation and workplace wellness, quality improvement, and quality assurance in the health system is growing. On an optimistic note, the Dutch—as a society—value collaboration; this is an excellent foundation for their goals.

The Dutch experience is similar to the evolving healthcare industry globally. However, attitudes about case management differ. The welcome that case management receives varies widely within any healthcare system, usually depending on the observer's role within the system and what people think case management is. For example, in Australia there is a reasonable degree of interest and acceptance of case management, but there is a great deal of resistance to managed care. The interest, acceptance, and recognition of case management's potential value has been positive in Australia, and one consequence of this has been the development of a postgraduate course in case management at the University of Melbourne (one of Australia's most prestigious universities). The course is taught over the Internet and has attracted students from as far away as New Zealand and Hong Kong. CMSAustralia was the first group to branch out from the CMSA. New Zealand, Israel, Spain, Canada, Puerto Rico, South Africa, Argentina, and the Pacific Rim send representatives to U.S. case management annual conferences. Some have spoken at these conferences, and Australia now has its own annual major case management conference.

The primary focus of case management may be different in various countries. The catalyst for case management as a strategy occurred in the United States because of managed care challenges, but the initial bottom line was cost containment, with quality and safety being a close second. Perhaps this rank order has changed, at least in some organizations, but the reality is that healthcare is expensive and must be contained within a budget. Because of differing reimbursement structures in other countries, cost-containment strategies were not always the primary reason for case management. In Australia, which spends approximately half as much on healthcare per capita compared with the United States, the emphasis has been more on quality. This is not to say that cost issues are being ignored, but as a result of a different financial structure and overall lower expenditure, the incentives are quite different from those in the United States. Some private hospitals are looking to case management not so much to save money, but rather to increase the satisfaction of patients, which will in turn help attract people to the private system. Public hospitals in Australia have been looking to case management as a way of performing better in an environment that has (in most areas) shifted to a case-mix funding base. In Australia the largest area for growth in case management is in the community-based aged care sector, where for at least the past 20 years, significant efforts and public resources have been put into helping people stay at home longer. This has included a significant commitment to case management as the way of coordinating and organizing these services.

In countries such as England, New Zealand, and Australia, community case management occurred first, with hospital case management following; they are distinctly different case management roles. Perhaps community case management evolved first because these countries have had community nursing for decades. For example, in New Zealand, community case management merely added service accessing and coordination functions to the job descriptions of the nurse specialists already practicing in the community setting (Litchfield, 1998).

Even with different reimbursement structures, varying perspectives of nursing, and diverse demographic and geographic needs, case management definitions evolving in other countries do not fall far from those currently promulgated in the United States, such as the CMSA's official case management definition. In New Zealand, case management as practiced by the Professional Nurse Case Manager (PNCM) is described as "a scheme for professional nursing practice in which the client is pivotal, a caring partnership between the client and the case manager is essential, and where attending to client's health as expression of the whole life process is the norm. The organization and management of case management provide for continuity and integration of healthcare services crossing primary, secondary, and tertiary settings, attending to the diversity of people's need where it arises or is anticipated" (Litchfield, 1998, p. 31). Although this is a more nursing-based definition, it emphasizes the patient as being of pivotal importance and management of the needs of the patient throughout the continuum of care as essential.

▶ Case Management in Canada

The following, starting with the next paragraph, was written by Genelle Leifso, RN, BSN, CPN(C), Senior Nurse Advisor for the Workers' Compensation Board (WCB) of British Columbia (BC). Like the Dutch healthcare experience, this overview provides both similar and different perspectives on case management. It is exciting to see case management globally evolving in such a caring and balanced way.

The Canadian healthcare system operates under the federally enacted Canada Health Act (1984). This legislation enshrined the principals of a universal, accessible, portable, comprehensive, and nonprofit/publicly funded healthcare system that is now as synonymous with Canada as apple pie is with America. Universal means that all Canadians are covered, and accessible means that no particular area or region will be deprived of routine service. Canadians moving from one province to another are provided for because their coverage is portable, and the care is comprehensive because everything except that which is deemed cosmetic is covered. The entire system is publicly funded, and any province instituting user fees is penalized.

Taxes are collected federally, and proportional transfer payments are made to the provinces that are charged with disbursements and implementation of healthcare services. This level of healthcare has required increasing amounts of the Canadian gross domestic product (GDP). In 1975 it required 7.1%; in 1980 it went to 9.1%; in 2006 it was 10.4%; in 2008, it was 10.8%, and it is expected to continue to rise. Provincial governments currently spend one-third of their budgets supporting healthcare. In Canada each province has a Workers' Compensation Act; the provincial WCB develops its own policy and guidelines that interpret the Act. Thus coverage can differ from province to province. Each Board is fully funded by that province's employers.

Increasing interest in efficient, cost-effective healthcare delivery has led to the development of centers of excellence. The intent is to avoid expensive service duplication when possible. In BC, the government has focused on "closer to home" service delivery in the past several years. This has resulted in the increased need for community-based services and home care—services that we are still struggling to provide adequately.

Resource allocation at the WCB of BC is determined by the nature or seriousness of the injury and the pre-injury salary of the injured worker. The case manager at the WCB of BC operates within established guidelines that determine how many treatments will be covered (e.g., chiropractic, physiotherapy). Likewise, vocational rehabilitation consultants provide input geared to reestablishing pre-injury salaries. Case managers do not prescribe treatment; therefore, the worker's attending physician (who is considered to be the PCP), is consulted, and approval is sought for proposed treatment plans. At the WCB of BC the development of a case management model has been driven by the need to improve the quality of service to injured workers in the province in a more cost-effective fashion.

Case managers deal with several cultural issues that affect their ability to provide service. BC has a large immigrant population, with many of the new arrivals coming from the Far East. For many, fluency in English takes some time to develop. If a member of this population is injured, ongoing interpretation needs to be provided to ensure service delivery and to aid in identifying all the barriers to successful problem resolution. We must also be sensitive to those cultural perspectives related to injury and rehabilitation. Certain cultures have particular ways of viewing disfigurement or disability. For example, a South Asian man with a partially amputated hand has immense culturally driven body image problems, which often separate him from the social supports (i.e., temple activities), that contribute to ongoing stability in the life of a newer immigrant. In addition, different cultural groups have preferred treatment modalities. At the WCB of BC, injured workers from an Asian background often have requests for acupuncture approved as a culturally sensitive therapy even if, in those circumstances, current medical literature would not support its use.

Case management is practiced under many other monikers in Canada. In hospital settings, nurse clinicians, clinical nurse specialists, or clinical resource nurses are involved in ongoing case management of their specific patient/client groups. In some facilities, utilization review is being done in collaboration with physicians. Currently, it is a politically sensitive area with nurses involved in the day-to-day work, and physicians doing the "enforcing" with their peers. Nurses and, in some settings, social workers are also involved in discharge planning—another form of case management. Similarly, in a community health environment, nurses may share the case management role with social workers.

In the WCB of BC setting, there is multidisciplinary provision of case management services. Although the medical advisors, nurse advisors, and psychologists may develop the actual clinical care plan that will be the "critical pathway" for the worker's return-to-work plan, the adjudicator (at the WCB this person is called the case manager), vocational rehabilitation consultant, therapists (e.g., occupational, physiotherapy) who are part of the treatment/rehabilitation network, and the individual's PCP are all considered members of the case management team.

Recruitment of new case managers entails targeting professionals with bachelor's degrees in health or social science fields. There was no such requirement for adjudicators who have been grandfathered into this new and demanding role. It is difficult to say how many case managers are in Canada. Titling of practitioners as case managers differs from that in the United States. Therefore, some hospital staff members who would be called clinical nurse specialists in Canada would be called case managers in the United States. Within the WCB of BC, the claims adjudicators all became case managers in 1997. Current recruitment is trying to attract individuals with a health science background (e.g., nursing, occupational therapy, kinesiology). In Ontario, the WCB has recruited and hired a large number of nurses who are trained as case managers.

Canadians are afraid of the managed care concept. Managed care is equated with cookie-cutter medicine, which is something quite different from the evidence-based, clinical guideline-driven care that case management advocates. There is resistance among current medical and claim staff members who lack understanding of these different concepts and fail to see the need for, or benefit from, the change into case management models. Further, case management outcomes measurement is not being done; however, nurse advisors are continuing to explore ways to track the success of their interventions.

Case management is a solution to the Canadian healthcare system and its challenges when it can:

▶ Offer earlier intervention;
▶ Avoid service duplication;
▶ Provide a primary point of contact for injured workers and their healthcare providers; and
▶ Offer efficiencies to the employer community and an earlier return-to-work for their injured workers.

Case management in Canada is a huge quantum leap, given the attitude toward managed care. However, it is a leap whose time has come.

STUDY QUESTIONS

1. How do case management and managed care differ? In what ways are they similar?
2. Explore various target populations. Who should case manage these populations?
3. Who would be on your ideal case management team? Why?
4. What would motivate you to pursue a position in case management? What type of case management appeals to you? Why?
5. How do national/domestic and international case management practices compare and contrast?
6. What are some of the contributing factors to case management becoming an international phenomenon?
7. What are some of the applications of tele-case management? How valuable are they to case management and patient care?
8. What are some of the benefits of case management information technology systems? What should one look for when considering implementing such systems?

▶ ACKNOWLEDGMENTS

We thank Bradford Kirkman-Liff, DrPH, Professor of Health Administration and Policy at Arizona State University, for the opportunity to be part of The Netherlands visit and for much of the specific Dutch healthcare information in this chapter; Genelle Leifso, RN, BSN, CPN(C), Senior Nurse Advisor, Workers' Compensation Board of British Columbia, for the excellent Canadian overview; Joanna Harper from New Zealand; and my friends from Australia, Anita Grindlay and Michael Summers, for their support.

▶ REFERENCES

American Nurses Association. (1994). *Nursing case management.* Kansas City, MO: Author.

Anonymous. (1994). Emergency departments visits mostly non-urgent. *Arizona Hospital Association Weekly Newsletter, 8*(33), 1.

Anonymous. (1998, Spring). Not medically necessary. *Rehab Review, 37,* 4.

Banja, J. (1997). Reasonable and necessary care. *The Case Manager, 8*(6), 34–36.

Bodie-Gross, E. & Tahan, H. (2008). Roles and functions of case managers. In S. Powell & H. Tahan (Eds.), *CMSA Core curriculum for case management* (2nd ed., pp. 159–176). Philadelphia: Wolters Kluwer/Lippincott Williams & Wilkins.

Bureau of National Affairs. (1998). Homebound Medicare beneficiaries file lawsuit against HCFA for denial of benefits. *BNA's Medicare Report, 9*(20), 513.

Case Management Leadership Coalition. (accessed 12/27/2007). Consumer Friendly Definition and FAQ. [Online]. Available: www.cmleaders.org/activities/definition.html.

Case Management Society of America (CMSA). (1998). *Center for case management accountability (CCMA).* [Online]. Available: www.cmsa.org.

Case Management Society of America. (2002). *Standards of practice for case management* (2nd ed.). Little Rock, AR: Author.

Centers for Medicare and Medicaid Services. (2009a). (accessed 4/13/2009). Conditions of participation for hospitals, chapter IV: Discharge planning. [Online]. Available: www.cms.hhs.gov/CFCsAndCoPs/06_Hospitals.asp#TopofPage.

Centers for Medicare and Medicaid Services. (2009b). (accessed 4/13/2009). Conditions of participation, home health services. [Online]. Available: www.cms.hhs.gov/HomeHealthPPS/01_overview.asp.

Commission for Case Manager Certification. (2005a). *CCM certification guide.* Rolling Meadows, IL: Author.

Commission for Case Manager Certification. (2005b). *Code of professional conduct for case managers.* Rolling Meadows, IL: Author.

Kane, R.A. (1988). Case management: ethical pitfalls on the road to high quality managed care. *Quality Review Bulletin, 14*(5), 161–166.

Kongstvedt, P.R. (2003). *Essentials of managed health care* (4th ed.). Gaithersburg, MD: Aspen Publishers.

Litchfield, M. (1998). Case management and nurses. *Nursing Praxis in New Zealand, 13*(2), 26–35.

McGonigle, D., & Mastrian, K. (2008). Information systems and case management. In S. Powell & H. Tahan (eds.), *CMSA core curriculum for case management* (2nd ed., pp. 292–323). Philadelphia: Wolters Kluwer/Lippincott Williams & Wilkins.

Michaels, C. (1992). Carondelet St. Mary's nursing enterprise. *Nursing Clinics of North America, 27*(1), 77–85.

National Association of Social Workers (NASW). (accessed 12/27/2007). NASW *standards for social work case management.* [Online]. Available: www.socialworkers.org/practice/standards/sa_case_mgmt.asp.

Tahan, H. (2008). Case management practice settings and throughput. In S. Powell & H. Tahan (Eds.), *CMSA core curriculum for case management* (2nd ed., pp. 39–73). Philadelphia: Wolters Kluwer/Lippincott Williams & Wilkins.

Tassel, M.V. (1994, August). Case managers use entrepreneurial skills. *Hospital Case Management,* 143.

Van der Linden, B.A., & Rosendal, H. (2002). The birth of transmural care in the 1990s. In E. van Rooij, L. Droyan Kodner, T. Rijsemus, and G. Schrijvers (Eds.), *Health and health care in the Netherlands. A critical self-assessment of Dutch experts in medical and health sciences* (pp. 191–197). Maarssen, The Netherlands: Elsevier Gezondheidszorg.

Wikipedia. (2009). (accessed 4/13/2009). Health care in Canada. [Online]. Available: http://en.wikipedia.org/wiki/Health_care_in_canada.

Williams, S.J., & Torrens, P.R. (1993). *Introduction to health services.* New York: Delmar.

Yee, D.L. (1990, July). Developing a quality assurance program in case management service settings. *Caring Magazine, 9*(7), 30–35.

CHAPTER 2

Essential Case Management Job Responsibilities and Skills

"A life isn't significant except for its impact on others' lives."

JACKIE ROBINSON

LEARNING OBJECTIVES

Upon completion of this chapter, the reader will be able to:

1. Explain five optimal and five undesired outcomes of case management.
2. Describe the roles and responsibilities of case managers.
3. Differentiate between a case manager's leadership roles and personality traits.
4. Describe three approaches to training and education of case managers.
5. List the various necessary topics to be covered in a case management education program.

ESSENTIAL TERMS

Advocacy • Advocate • Collaboration • Confidentiality • Coordinator of Care • Cost–Benefit Analysis • Discharge Planner • Fiscal Responsibility • Inadequate Outcome • Integrator • Negotiator • Optimal Outcome • Privacy • Responsibilities • Skills • Traits • Transitional Planner • Utilization Manager

▶ GOALS OF CASE MANAGEMENT

It is necessary to be clear about the purpose of case management and its related outcomes to understand the context of the case manager's job responsibilities and required skills and knowledge. The first section of this chapter describes the outcomes of case management programs and services; the second section discusses the job responsibilities and skills. The lists of outcomes, responsibilities, and skills covered here are by no means comprehensive, nor does every case management program focus on all of the items included in this chapter. Healthcare organizations vary in their case management focus, purpose, and goals, and in their design of the case manager's role.

▶ Optimal Versus Inadequate Outcomes

The three main target goals (or tenets) of case management are quality care, access to healthcare services, and cost efficiency. Many smaller goals contribute to these ultimate aims and, when achieved, culminate in "good case management." When these goals are not met, the consequences are poor quality of care or poor and costly utilization of healthcare resources.

Unmet case management goals may occur for many reasons. The following are some examples:

- No formal case management program in the facility or agency.
- Unclear roles and responsibilities of case managers and other professionals impacted by the introduction of case management.
- Poorly trained case managers.
- Inadequate case management staffing and the assumption that case management is a Monday to Friday and 9:00 AM to 5:00 PM job.
- Inadequate social service staffing to support the psychosocial aspect of the care needed.
- Case loads that are too heavy to permit all details to be attended to adequately.
- Patient/family resistance.

▶ Staff resistance—especially physicians.
▶ Patients who are incorrigibly noncompliant with care regimen and medications.
▶ Unrelenting patient/family dissatisfaction.
▶ Lack of cooperation from the payor source.
▶ Lack of payor source.
▶ Lack of understanding among members of the healthcare team regarding case management principles.
▶ Substandard care in the facility/agency.

The tables included in this chapter display outcomes of the case management process. On the left of each table are optimal outcomes—characteristics resulting from competent case management practice. The right side of each table lists consequences that occur when those objectives are lacking or inadequately met. As the issues and game rules of the healthcare environment change, the goals must also transform to match new priorities. It is certain, however, that quality, effectiveness, and efficiency will never go out of style.

▶ QUALITY OF CARE ISSUES

OUTCOMES FROM OPTIMAL CASE MANAGEMENT	OUTCOMES FROM INADEQUATE CASE MANAGEMENT
▶ Increased patient/family satisfaction	▶ Patient/family dissatisfied with care; possible increase in lawsuits
▶ Optimal clinical outcomes through monitoring of and adhering to quality standards of care	▶ Increased quality of care issues; possible risk management scenarios, complaints, and grievances
▶ Comprehensive and accurate assessment of clients' deficits, needs, health status, resources, formal and informal support systems, and outcomes	▶ Increased complications/ineffective care, medical errors, and unsafe situations
▶ Matching assessed needs to valuable services/resources	▶ Duplication, fragmentation or gaps in services, and unmet client's needs
▶ Continuity of care emphasized, thus reducing or eliminating fragmentation, duplication, or gaps in treatment plan and/or services	▶ Fragmented, inefficient, and costly care
▶ Careful monitoring of safety issues	▶ Missed risk factors that lead to risk management issues (e.g., falls, avoidable deterioration in health condition)
▶ Reduced adverse patient outcomes	▶ Increased adverse outcomes and errors
▶ Proactive: prevention of adverse occurrences when possible or initiation of interventions quickly if prevention is not possible, thereby minimizing poor outcomes	▶ Adverse occurrences maximized before anyone recognizes them
▶ Maximum recovery; minimum complications	▶ Minimal recovery; maximum complications

▶ COLLABORATION AMONG HEALTHCARE TEAM MEMBERS/PROFESSIONALS

OUTCOMES FROM OPTIMAL CASE MANAGEMENT	OUTCOMES FROM INADEQUATE CASE MANAGEMENT
▶ Physician satisfaction with the case management process and the quality of patient care	▶ Alienation and frustration of physicians; undesired outcomes
▶ Healthcare team member satisfaction with the case management process and the quality of care	▶ Lack of team work; uncooperative clinicians; undesired outcomes
▶ Roles are clearly defined	▶ Role conflict; frustrated professionals
▶ Effective collaboration and coordination strengthened among all members of the healthcare team	▶ Treatment delays; fragmented care; frustrated and obstructed efforts to improve health status of the patient
▶ Communication enhanced among the multidisciplinary team	▶ Each discipline singing in a different key resulting in discordant care for the patient; miscommunications and misunderstandings among the team alienates team members

▶ FISCAL RESPONSIBILITIES

OUTCOMES FROM OPTIMAL CASE MANAGEMENT	OUTCOMES FROM INADEQUATE CASE MANAGEMENT
▶ Provider-payor satisfaction	▶ Uncooperative providers
▶ Balancing fiscal responsibility for the client, the facility/agency, and the reimbursement source	▶ Conflicts of interest; mixed or inequitable loyalties; poor or unethical allocation of resources
▶ Appropriate and efficient use of benefits and resources; care provided at the appropriate level and setting	▶ Suboptimal use of healthcare resources; unnecessary waste; over- or underutilization of resources
▶ Cost-efficient care through timely use of appropriate level of care for the client's needs	▶ Expensive and inappropriate level of care; may not be reimbursed by payor source; may leave facility or client fiscally responsible for excess payment
▶ Appropriately reduced length of hospital stays	▶ Increased length of hospital stays
▶ Reduced number of intensive care days	▶ Increased number of intensive care days
▶ Reduced visits to emergency department	▶ Increased number of emergency department or unscheduled clinic visits
▶ Unnecessary admissions prevented; acuity on admission reduced; number of admissions reduced	▶ Preventable admissions; higher acuity on admission; frequent readmissions
▶ Careful identification and matching of clients' needs with resources available (both public and private resources)	▶ Suboptimal use of healthcare system and public or private resources
▶ Maximizing reimbursed services at all levels of care by meeting established criteria, performing precise utilization reviews, accurate and thorough documentation, and timely discharges	▶ Agencies/facilities at increased financial risk because of lost revenue for the facility from uncompensated patient care; increased charges to clients; clients unable to pay or left financially destitute
▶ Successful negotiation of cases for appropriate continuation of lengths of stays or extension of services	▶ Same as above
▶ Accurate interpretation of benefits for the client and the facility	▶ Same as above

▶ PATIENT AND FAMILY ADVOCACY

OUTCOMES FROM OPTIMAL CASE MANAGEMENT	OUTCOMES FROM INADEQUATE CASE MANAGEMENT
▶ Personal attention in a large, complex, and impersonal healthcare system	▶ The client (patient and family) is alone, frustrated, and afraid
▶ Case manager as advocate for client/family	▶ No one to advocate for client/family
▶ Patient's quality of life, autonomy, and, if possible, independence optimized through thoughtful, appropriate placement at discharge	▶ Patients warehoused in inappropriate environments; poor quality of life
▶ Fostering educated, independent choices in all aspects of care and services	▶ Uninformed decisions
▶ Education on disease processes, allotted services, rehabilitation techniques, self-care; education matched to individual needs	▶ Poor education resulting in noncompliance with treatment plan, "out-of-control" feelings, decreased self-care capabilities, and inability to avoid or allay the disease process
▶ Patient and family empowerment through participation in informed decision making	▶ Paternalism; decreased freedom of choice; decreased autonomy of client
▶ Optimal function of patient-family unit	▶ Frightened, exhausted, stressed-out families
▶ Optimizing self-care capabilities by assisting patient to become fully functional as quickly as possible; if return to independence is not possible, assisting family unit and client in obtaining supportive care	▶ Minimal time for patient to become independent and optimally healthy; family may become exhausted or dysfunctional and utilize excessive healthcare services

(continued)

▶ PATIENT AND FAMILY ADVOCACY (*Continued*)

OUTCOMES FROM OPTIMAL CASE MANAGEMENT	OUTCOMES FROM INADEQUATE CASE MANAGEMENT
▶ Ensuring patient/family understand the direction of the plan of care and knowledge of the disease process through education, clinical pathways, and so on	▶ Confusion, anxiety, and out-of-control feelings of patient and family
▶ Careful monitoring of and advocating for a clinically appropriate treatment plan	▶ Duplication of services, gaps in treatment plan, wasteful services, inappropriate levels of care, excess costs being billed to client
▶ Assisting client/family in accessing the complex healthcare system, thus utilizing available and necessary resources	▶ Underutilization of resources, leaving some needs unmet; services ordered not covered by the health plan, creating wasted effort and possibly extensions of hospital stays because of delays in accessing needed services for a safe discharge
▶ Finding solutions to noncovered services; accessing charitable agencies and services	▶ Families' funds exhausted through noncoverage of services, necessitating private payment

▶ OUTPATIENT/COMMUNITY-BASED CARE MANAGEMENT

OUTCOMES FROM OPTIMAL CASE MANAGEMENT	OUTCOMES FROM INADEQUATE CASE MANAGEMENT
▶ Thorough identification of discharge needs including medical, educational, durable medical equipment, and social support	▶ Frustrated and exhausted families who are suboptimally caring for patient
▶ Facilitation of timely, coordinated, safe, and appropriate discharges	▶ Unsafe, incomplete dispositions; lack of postdischarge resources/services
▶ Linking the client with appropriate level of care and services: acute, subacute, supervisory, homebound, or community-based services	▶ Service gaps; higher readmission rate and emergency department visits
▶ Comprehensive and consistent posthospital or post–extended-care facility follow-up	▶ Complications during convalescent phase of care with setbacks and possibly readmissions for acute hospital care
▶ Optimal outpatient management that reduces or avoids acute hospital readmissions through early identification of health status changes or changes in self-care capabilities	▶ Poor outpatient management leading to increased complications and increased utilization of acute facilities
▶ Chosen level of care for client matches client's need and financial capability	▶ Client's/family's financial resources are exhausted through nonreimbursed placement of client in an expensive care facility

▶ PROFESSIONAL PRACTICE

OUTCOMES FROM OPTIMAL CASE MANAGEMENT	OUTCOMES FROM INADEQUATE CASE MANAGEMENT
▶ Promotion of professionalism by creatively and proactively finding solutions to the problems facing the healthcare system	▶ Case management in a subordinate and supportive role, rather than in a collaborative partnership with other healthcare professionals
▶ Enhanced research opportunities about efficient, effective care for the chronically and acutely ill	▶ Diminished credibility due to lack of serious research

OUTCOMES FROM OPTIMAL CASE MANAGEMENT	OUTCOMES FROM INADEQUATE CASE MANAGEMENT
▶ Increased job satisfaction	▶ Job stress and burn-out
▶ Established scientific base for case management practice; evidence-based practice	▶ Unclear science behind effective case management practice
▶ Dissemination of best practices; case managers feel the need to disseminate knowledge and share their experiences with others	▶ Best practices kept within individual organizations; lack of desire to share knowledge with others
▶ Increased membership in case management-related professional organizations; strong and well-respected professional societies	▶ Weak case management professional organizations

▶ ESSENTIAL JOB RESPONSIBILITIES AND SKILLS

Not long ago, the task of case management belonged to the family physician. Choices were simple; insurance companies usually paid for the services that the doctors deemed necessary. Enter the age of convoluted insurance plans (or no insurance plans at all), multiple specialists for a single patient, absent primary owner of care (lack of a case manager), multidisciplinary teams that include dozens of members of varied backgrounds, the rush to get patients through the system and into less cost-intensive settings, increasing chronicity and acuity of health problems, ethical dilemmas, increased patient and family expectations, and the list goes on.

Much of the management of acute care patients has been transferred to the nursing arena. Nurses assume a key role in ensuring that patient's needs are met and that other healthcare professionals contribute to the care and treatment plan as indicated by the patient's health condition and the choice(s) of treatment. However, staff nurses, already overloaded with daily nursing tasks, barely have time to read a patient's chart, let alone fill in the gaps between the patient's needs and his or her reality, assess the availability of resources and support systems, and figure out insurance benefits. As Figure 2.1 shows, the case management role is a pivotal one. This chapter discusses essential characteristics that affect how well the case manager performs the role. This section explores what a case manager does. Although the list is extensive, it should be noted that the role of the case manager continues to evolve and, therefore, the list may still be incomplete or may vary from one organization to another. Because case management responsibilities are extensive, on some days case managers may feel that they are "dancing as fast as they can!"

The roles and responsibilities of case managers continue to change and evolve similar to the way our healthcare system is constantly changing. Case management roles also vary according to the patient population being served, the setting in which the case manager is employed, and the case management perspective (i.e., program structure, goals, and processes). The job priorities of each case management position must also be weighed. A hospital case manager may have a perspective (e.g., clinical care management) different from one who is employed by an insurance company (e.g., member benefits management); a case manager for a private insurance company may encounter different issues than one who works for Medicaid or long-term care. An entrepreneurial case manager may have a different point of view and priority set compared to one who works for a privately owned or state-run company; a case manager who is responsible for patients across a continuum of healthcare settings may have a different perspective from one who is responsible for episodic (i.e., one episode of illness and one care setting) case management.

Roles and responsibilities also differ because of the case mix of patients for whom the case manager is responsible. Geriatric patients have different needs than high-risk obstetric, AIDS, cancer, or cystic fibrosis patients; virtually each clinical category has its own needs. At times, the case manager may find the various roles complementary and necessary; at other times, conflicting. As a patient advocate, the case manager wants the best of everything for the patient and family; as the procurer of healthcare resources, the case manager may not be able to obtain all that the patient wants or needs. Perhaps a service is not covered or the patient has already used up that particular benefit; perhaps the insurance company does not feel the patient

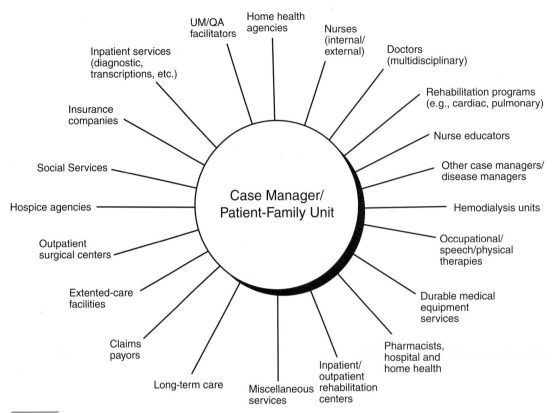

Figure 2.1 Case manager/patient–family unit.

is entirely homebound and denies home nursing services, claiming the services are unnecessary and unjustified (see Chapter 9). Fortunately, however, other resources can come to the rescue. Knowledge of alternative and community resources—and the case manager's own creativity—can often ease such ethical dilemmas and offer some options.

After considering all the roles, responsibilities, and challenges listed in the first two chapters of this book, it is no wonder that student case managers have difficulty seeing "the big picture" of what case management is all about. As sometimes happens, *within the question lies the answer*. The question is, "What is the big picture of case management?" The answer is, "Case management is the big picture of the patient's entire universe!" Nurses and other professionals such as social workers have traditionally been task oriented; the physician wrote the orders, and the nurses had to finish all the tasks on all their patients within the allotted time. If the tasks were accomplished in the time specified, using the correct method and applying the correct amount to the correct patient, the nurse could go home and sleep restfully that night. Case management is not task oriented in the same

way. The case manager must look at the big picture—an expanded version of the whole universe of the patient. This includes the patient's past capabilities (physical, cognitive, emotional, financial, and psychosocial), the patient's current condition, and an anticipation of the patient's future needs and abilities. It includes not only the patient, but all those closely affected by the patient's current and future world—the family, caregiver, or significant other. Lastly, a case manager must also take into consideration everything that could affect the patient: the strength or lack of psychosocial support, financial support, insurance benefits, cognitive abilities, physical condition, and every important aspect of the patient's universe.

The case manager then takes this one step further. When case managers act in the capacity of disease managers, they are not only looking at the whole universe of an individual patient, they are also looking at the universe of an entire disease-specific population of patients. Care of all patients with congestive heart failure, for example, must be coordinated; within that, each patient/family unit has its own unique needs. Although there is a primary focus on population care management, individualizing the care provided to each patient is necessary.

The following characteristics, roles, and case management skill requirements are important strengths to develop and will greatly aid all case management daily activities, no matter what the setting. Not everyone is organized or is a "detail person" or a "top-notch" negotiator, and not every case manager needs all these characteristics. Many excellent case managers are weak in some areas and compensate adequately with other talents. Nevertheless, if any shortcoming is causing problems, the case manager should look for ways to grow; all the characteristics can be enhanced or developed if desired. Not all the roles and responsibilities that follow may apply to one's clinical area of expertise, practice, or type of case management; yet, many are essential in every form of case management. Some of these roles are so complex that one or more chapters were required here, e.g., utilization management, risk management, legal and ethical issues, transitional and discharge planning, and insurance issues. Critical elements of some of the roles are discussed in this chapter, e.g., cost-benefit analysis, negotiation skills, and assertiveness. Discussions of many of these roles will overlap throughout the book, as case management is not a set of distinct job actions; rather, it is a tapestry of many aspects of life woven together.

▶ ROLES, RESPONSIBILITIES, AND CHARACTERISTICS OF CASE MANAGERS

The roles, functions, and responsibilities of case managers are defined by professional organizations such as the Case Management Society of America (CMSA), the American Nurses' Association (ANA) and the National Association of Social Workers (NASW). They are defined based on scientific evidence, experiences and opinions of case management experts, and the lessons learned from organizations that have implemented case management programs. Roles and responsibilities of case managers are also found in the employing agency's or facility's job descriptions.

There is no standard or nationally recognized case management job description. The literature published on this topic, similar to this book, tends to list all possible roles and responsibilities; however, an organization's specific job description lists those responsibilities it finds relevant to its program of case management. Regardless, if one reviews the available literature, one will find that it contains the core aspects of case management practice and the common roles of case managers.

These include five broad categories (domains) that describe the primary responsibilities of case managers: (1) clinical care management, (2) management and leadership, (3) financial and resource management, (4) information management, and (5) professional responsibilities (Tahan, 2005). Display 2-1 lists examples of specific roles and responsibilities in each of these broad categories.

The Commission for Case Manager Certification (CCMC), the oldest and largest multidisciplinary certifying agency for case managers, offers certification in case management practice and conducts research on the practice of case management with special focus on the case manager's role. It also publishes its findings; the most recent research was completed in 2004 and published in 2006 (Tahan, Huber, & Downey, 2006; Tahan, Downey, & Huber, 2006). CCMC reported in these publications six essential domains of practice for the case manager: (1) case finding and intake, (2) provision of case management services, (3) outcomes evaluation and case closure, (4) utilization management, (5) psychosocial economic issues, and (6) vocational concepts and strategies. Examples of case managers' roles in each of these domains are listed in Display 2-2.

The roles, responsibilities, and job/personal characteristics shared in Display 2-1 and 2-2 and those described in the remainder of this chapter should be used as a guide for understanding or designing the role of a case manager. They should be studied carefully and considered based on what is required or essential for a specific care setting of case management practice.

▶ Patient Advocate

Think for a moment about a time when you felt especially vulnerable, when few elements of your life were within your control. Perhaps you were told you had an inoperable tumor, or the dreaded test came back positive, or a loved one was seriously ill. Times such as these leave people feeling overwhelmed, uncertain, and afraid. Those who can ask pertinent questions are already on their way to healing, but many are too overcome with the enormity of their situations to even articulate their needs; they become paralyzed.

The role of patient advocate is one of the most important of the case manager's charges; it is also one of the greatest challenges. Advocacy is integral to every action case managers take and every decision they make, regardless of the care settings or the patients in their care. It is most necessary when dealing with patients and families who are unable to speak for or represent themselves. Historically, nurses and social workers have always acted as patient advocates to some extent. Today's healthcare climate presents some

ROLES AND RESPONSIBILITIES OF CASE MANAGERS

display 2-1

1. **Clinical Care Management**
   a. Patient selection and identification.
   b. Assessment and problem identification (actual and potential).
   c. Plan of care/case management plan development including the transitional plan.
   d. Implementation and reassessment of the plan.
   e. Patient and family education.
   f. Assessment of the patient's and family's social support network, coping skills.
   g. Assessment of the patient's health insurance status.

2. **Management and Leadership**
   a. Coordination, facilitation, and expedition of care activities.
   b. Scheduling of and following-up on tests, procedures, and treatments.
   c. Brokering of community resources.
   d. Negotiation of care options.
   e. Evaluation of quality of care.
   f. Facilitation of communication among healthcare team members.
   g. Teaching and mentoring of others.
   h. Advocating for patients and families.
   i. Participation on committees.

3. **Financial and Resource Management**
   a. Addressing under- and overutilization of resources and services.
   b. Management of length of stay.
   c. Utilization review and management.
   d. Management of variances/delays in care.
   e. Management of denials.
   f. Appeal of denials.
   g. Engagement in cost reduction activities/projects.

4. **Information Management**
   a. Data collection, analysis, management, and reporting.
   b. Communicating and disseminating information (healthcare team, organization-wide, external).
   c. Documentation.
   d. Sharing of information about patients' care and progress with representatives of managed care organizations (utilization review).

5. **Professional Responsibilities**
   a. Conduct of research and utilization of findings.
   b. Promotion of evidence-based practice.
   c. Participation in professional organizations.
   d. Public speaking.
   e. Publishing.

challenges to that role. "Advocacy for the patient was given highest priority unless it conflicted with advocacy for the physician or advocacy for the employing institution" (Leddy & Pepper, 1989, p, 378). Today, advocacy for the payor source (which may also be the employer) often muddies the issue. It is the case manager's primary responsibility—an obligation, if you will—to remember that the patient is the most relevant unit, not the payor, not the utilization review modality, not the service offered or not offered, not the other providers of care, and not the institution. Advocacy is being patient/family-centered and focused in one's approach to care.

How does a case manager act as a patient advocate? In a sense, this whole book readies the case manager for that role. By understanding the principles of case management and managed care, the case manager can best position the patient to maximize his or her chances for optimal services and outcomes.

One tenet of advocacy is to assist patients to achieve autonomy and self-determination, to assist them to become empowered and independent. This is done by helping patients or families with an incapacitated family member to articulate their views and choices and to make informed decisions. The case manager is obligated to act in the patient's best interest, but the patient will determine what the definition of "best interest" will be, according to personal wishes, beliefs, and values (Prins, 1992).

Autonomy in decision making and self-determination also requires informational support. The quality and relevancy of the information are important, and the quantity of data must be delicately balanced. Giving information that the patient did not seek and is not ready to hear, and that is too detailed—causing information overload—violates the basic principles of patient advocacy. Giving too little information may be considered paternalistic and prevents self-determination and informed consent.

One of the biggest challenges the case manager often has to face is the ethical dilemma of the conflicting roles of patient advocate versus gatekeeper (see Chapter 9). It is difficult to balance the demands of these two strict taskmasters—one necessitates optimal patient care and services and the other demands cost-containment and stringent allocation of resources. Wise allocation of resources fulfills the requirement for the role of gatekeeper but may violate the concepts of advocacy; on the other hand, if case managers can successfully perform the role of patient advocate, they can

SIX DOMAINS OF CASE MANAGER'S ROLES AND FUNCTIONS

1. **Case Finding and Intake**
   a. Identifying patient who would benefit from case management services.
   b. Obtaining informed consent for services to be provided.
   c. Communicating patient's needs to others.
   d. Identifying patients who would benefit from alternate levels of care such as subacute or skilled nursing facilities.

2. **Provision of Case Management Services**
   a. Facilitating and coordinating services and care activities.
   b. Assuming responsibility for communication with care providers, patient and family, and others external to the organization.
   c. Monitoring care activities and patient's progress toward expected outcomes.
   d. Reviewing and modifying as needed the delivery of healthcare services.
   e. Collaborating with stakeholders in establishing an appropriate case management plan.
   f. Serving as a patient and family advocate.
   g. Assuring adherence to ethical, legal, regulatory, and accreditation standards.

3. **Outcomes Evaluation and Case Closure**
   a. Collecting, analyzing, and reporting of outcomes data.
   b. Evaluating the quality of case management services and the effectiveness of the case management plan.
   c. Ensuring access to timely and necessary services.
   d. Applying evidence-based practice guidelines in the development of a case management plan.
   e. Closing the case manager–patient relationship.
   f. Communicating termination of services to stakeholders.
   g. Educating the patient about wellness behaviors and illness prevention.

4. **Utilization Management**
   a. Evaluating appropriateness of the level of care.
   b. Communicating with payors and other providers of care.
   c. Allocating resources based on patient's needs and as indicated by the health condition.
   d. Managing reimbursement denials and appeals.
   e. Reviewing patient's condition for appropriateness of hospitalization.
   f. Identifying cases that are at high risk for complications and instituting actions to prevent complications.

5. **Psychosocial and Economic Issues**
   a. Reviewing patient's social and financial resources and identifying problems if they exist.
   b. Assessing patient's social support network.
   c. Considering patient's cultural characteristics in planning and delivering care.
   d. Addressing behaviors that affect patient's health status.
   e. Evaluating the availability and ability of a designated caregiver to assist patient when outside the hospital setting.
   f. Determining patient's eligibility for insurance coverage (e.g., Medicaid) or charity services and funding.

6. **Vocational Concepts and Strategies**
   a. Identifying the need for changes in patient's home environment.
   b. Eliminating access barriers.
   c. Determining the need for specialized services such as physical rehabilitation to achieve optimal level of wellness and functioning.
   d. Arranging for vocational assessment and services.
   e. Coordinating patient's job analysis to implement job modifications and accommodations.
   f. Recommending job modifications to patient's employer.
   g. Managing return-to-work activities.

often "become the levelers" for inequities in the system (Dubler, 1992, p. 85). The best way to deal with such dilemmas is by asking yourself, "What is in the best interest of the patient and family?" Answer such questions by always ensuring that the patient's and family's autonomy and freedom of decision making are maintained; their needs/wishes/interests are met, and their rights are protected. This confirms your role as an effective patient advocate.

The essence of advocacy is caring for another human being. If we lived "in a perfect world with equal access to healthcare resources and patients who are powerful players in the healthcare system, advocacy would not be necessary" (Hein & Nicholson, 1994, p. 166). The reality is that inequities in our healthcare environment exist, and most of the population does not have the knowledge or the savvy to access this convoluted system. Through the case manager's caring, attention, and support, perhaps one more patient will be prevented from "slipping through the cracks," will receive the help needed for one more try at independent living, or will have a last wish acknowledged and granted. Supporting a patient's own choices with available means and services is the gift of advocacy. Examples of how a case manager engages in patient advocacy activities are presented in Display 2-3.

EXAMPLES OF CASE MANAGER'S ADVOCACY ACTIVITIES

1. Doing the right thing at the right time and in the right amount.
2. Maintaining patient's and family's privacy and confidentiality, and protecting their rights.
3. Educating patient and family about healthcare services, benefits, medical condition, and medical regimen.
4. Seeking patient's and family's informed consent to treatment.
5. Seeking patient's and family's involvement in care planning and selection of treatment options.
6. Making referrals to necessary services on behalf of the patient.
7. Informing members of the healthcare team of patient's and family's wishes, interests, and needs.
8. Assuring authorizations by insurance company for services to be rendered to avoid denials and appeals.
9. Ensuring provision of evidence-based care.
10. Coordinating a case conference to resolve conflict and solve problems.
11. Facilitating access to needed services.
12. Identifying variances (delays) of care and addressing them as indicated; preventing the occurrence of variances.
13. Assuring that care provision is fair, just, and equitable.
14. Coordinating services across the continuum of care and settings.
15. Providing patient and family with emotional support and psychosocial counseling, especially during situations of anxiety, apprehension, and confusion.
16. Answering patient's and family's questions and guiding them through the healthcare maze.

▶ Protector of Privacy and Confidentiality

In today's age of technology, including telephonics, computers, electronic communications, and the Internet, maintaining privacy and confidentiality is no easy task. It seems as if everyone has access to the medical record, including many types of medical caregivers, quality improvement specialists, insurance companies, auditors, billers, case managers, governmental representatives, and others. "Indeed, much of modern medicine, with the computerized passing of data, is designed to preclude privacy, not to protect it. Healthcare providers regularly set aside the patient's needs for secrecy in pursuit of the kind of communication that permits all to strive together toward a shared goal of care" (Dubler, 1992, p. 84). The reader is referred to Chapter 8 for recommendations on the preservation of privacy and confidentiality. However, these are not sure measures. "The lawyer/client relationship is more protected, more fully confidential, than the physician/patient relationship. Unlike a hospital chart, records of the attorney/client dialogue cannot be subpoenaed. They are guarded and protected" (Dubler, 1992, p. 84). New problems are arising because of computer charting; fail-safe ways must be provided to keep patients' medical records from computer hackers, employers, and others without a right or a need to know.

The case manager has an obligation—as a patient advocate—to protect the patients' privacy as much as possible. By doing so, the case manager is protecting that person's dignity and is practicing within the standard and scope of care and adhering to the case management professional code of conduct. Case managers in their daily practice ensure that those involved in the patient's care and who have access to the medical record are the appropriate healthcare professionals based on the patient's health condition and treatment plan, and that the patient has agreed to their involvement. The case manager also adheres to the Health Insurance Portability and Accountability Act (HIPAA) of 1996 when engaged in a release of information activity.

▶ Case Screening Expert

It would be overwhelming, unrealistic, and unnecessary to case manage all patients in any facility or diagnostic group. It is often the case manager who identifies those patients who would most benefit from case management services. A more thorough discussion on case screening can be found in "Stage I: Case Selection" in Chapter 6. Case managers use predetermined criteria when screening patients during the initial encounter to determine whether their condition and needs necessitate case management services.

▶ Coordinator of Care

Coordinaton of care is the umbrella role under which all other roles fall; it is "where the rubber meets the road" in case management. If done well, case management provides a seamless and smooth-running system in which everyone benefits: patient, family, provider, and payor. If done poorly, case management is a rough ride, with team members colliding into one another and desired outcomes remaining unmet. Coordinating many care providers (with their different perspectives, orders, suggestions, and roles), facilitating collaboration among these professionals, and then matching it all to the patient's and payor's permissions constitutes no small task. The "what," "when," and "how" of the coordination of services make up an individual sequence that depends on the nature of each patient's illness, psychosocial support network, insurance coverage, and many other factors.

Procuring resources and services is sometimes called brokering of services; it is part of the overall coordination of care role. The first place to look for resources that will meet the patient's needs is the patient's own support system. If skilled services are required, most insurance companies cover them. However, there are limits either in the number of homecare visits allowed or in a dollar cap. Community resources may be needed to fill in gaps that the family and insurance company cannot cover. However, many people do not have the support of family, friends, or church; some do not have health insurance, because universal coverage is not a reality in the United States. Sometimes the only option is charity care. Many hospitals and social service departments have some funds in reserve for these tough cases. Usually, persistence and creativity eventually yield enough services for a safe discharge or transition. Here, the case manager acts as a general problem solver. To have an experienced, knowledgeable social worker on board is probably the closest thing to case management heaven. The social problems of many patients are overwhelming, and many would benefit from a good social worker's expertise. However, social service support is sometimes unavailable; therefore, the case worker's knowledge of community resources, including ways to access them, is a necessity.

▶ Assessing, Reassessing, and Reassessing

The needs of patients can change daily, sometimes even hourly. Constant reassessing of a patient's physical status, psychosocial support system, mentation, and spiritual needs is important. The patient's financial resources must also be monitored. Attention to the patient's and family's goals will keep the care and treatment plan on track; therefore, the case manager must be alert for changing goals, needs, and interests. Good case managers keep a flexible attitude about each patient's situation, allowing creativity to flow when tough and sudden changes occur.

With the multitudinous levels and facets of assessment that are necessary, missed details at this critical juncture can delay or imbalance the whole care plan and outcomes. Assessing and reassessing are essential skills. (Details are addressed in "Stage II: Assessment/Problem Identification" in Chapter 6).

▶ Discharge Planner and Facilitator in Level of Care Changes

Many case managers have entered the world of case management through either the role of discharge planner or utilization reviewer. Regardless, these tasks require an assessment of the total medical, psychosocial, and financial elements of each patient's situation. Although some cases may be similar, no two are exactly alike. Discharge planning should be started at admission or, if possible, during preadmission screening (see "Stage III: Development and Coordination of the Case Plan" in Chapter 6).

Two examples of discharge planning that involve transitional changes in levels of care are discharges from a hospital to a skilled nursing facility or to home, and from a subacute facility to home. Sometimes, the level of care may go to a more acute phase. If a home patient is found to be quickly deteriorating, will a skilled nursing facility prevent further decline and avoid an acute hospitalization? Case managers must also be alert for a patient's readiness to change levels of care, such as transfers from the intensive care unit to a step-down unit or a standard patient floor. The case manager must often alert and gently prompt the physicians that the patient may be ready for this change. As case managers coordinate the transition of patients from one level of care to another, they rely on their knowledge and skills in utilization review to appropriately manage these transitions.

Changes in the level of care can go in either direction. If a home health case manager finds the patient's condition deteriorating and the home situation is no longer safe, a call to the physician may elicit some home modalities to attempt, an order for a move to a skilled nursing facility, or a hospital admission. Home care case managers often facilitate the change from home healthcare to hospice care when appropriate and when the patient and family are ready.

▶ Follow-Up and Follow-Through

Fewer case managers perform strictly episodic case management every year, because the trend is toward case management through a continuum of care. Episodic case management involves following the patient through a single episode of acute illness. More and more case managers follow up their patients wherever they reside, whether acutely ill in a hospital or chronically stable at home. Others perform intermittent postdischarge hospital follow-up on a need-to basis. How often a case manager needs to follow up after discharge depends on the acuteness or chronicity of the patient's condition and assessment of the following:

- ▶ Is the care optimum? Is the patient receiving quality care? Is the patient receiving the services that were brokered prior to discharge?
- ▶ Does the patient's condition still match the level of care he or she is receiving?
- ▶ Is the patient/family still satisfied with the arrangement and care, or is modification needed?
- ▶ Are the treatment goals being met, or are new goals needed? Are the desired outcomes achieved?
- ▶ Are the appropriate care providers involved in the delivery of care and services? (More information about postdischarge is discussed in "Stage VI: Continuous Monitoring, Reassessing, and Reevaluating" in Chapter 6.)

Following patients through the continuum of care has become common practice. However, there will always be acute care case managers and case managers whose jobs are to follow the patient wherever he or she may be. The type and extent of follow-up will depend on the job description and the organization's case management program design.

A related skill for a case manager is good follow-through. Gaining either patient or physician trust is not always easy, but perhaps the most important activity as an inroad to trust is follow-through once a plan has been finalized. If something impedes the plan, a telephone call to the patient or physician to discuss the problem and to offer a potential solution or new course of action keeps the trust level high.

▶ Utilization Manager

Historically, utilization review referred to the process of monitoring intensity of service and severity of illness (ISSI) (see "InterQual" in Chapter 4: Utilization Management), medical necessity, and appropriateness of the level of care the patient was receiving. Case managers do not simply monitor or review the utilization of services; they manage them. Thus, the more appropriate terminology to be used is *utilization management*. Using utilization tools, such as ISSI, reveals the patient's changing condition and the necessary level of care and setting. For acute care case management, this provides a cue to the case manager to speed up a discharge plan if the patient is doing exceptionally well or change a discharge plan if the patient is deteriorating or remains debilitated. Tools correspond to different healthcare environments. Many organizations are experimenting with tools that follow a patient through a continuum of care; these tools have shown some success, although they present several challenges, as seen in the case management literature.

Utilization management is the language that an insurance company can understand; authorization for extensions of hospital days is often based on utilization modalities (see Chapter 4). Utilization management functions in another capacity, too: reviewing for appropriate utilization of services and resources can reveal overutilization of tests and services. Overutilization may arise from many causes of this, including the following:

- ▶ The facility is a teaching hospital in which medical students, interns, and residents are trying to find the balance between good and complete care.
- ▶ Patients insist on expensive, high-tech procedures.
- ▶ Physicians are cautious if a litigious event arises (e.g., a patient falls).
- ▶ Physicians practicing defensive medicine overcautiously order multiple tests to prevent lawsuits.
- ▶ A test has a duplicate order and no one caught it.
- ▶ The monitoring frequency (e.g., of hemoglobin/hematocrit or prothrombin/partial thromboplastin time) could be changed due to patient's stability, but no one has done so.
- ▶ A medication given intravenously can be changed safely to an oral route.

There are situations where resources are underutilized, including the following:

- ▶ Delays in performing a necessary test or procedure.
- ▶ Denial of certain services by insurance companies even when clinicians feel those services are warranted.
- ▶ Lack of monitoring of a patient's response to treatment resulting in lack of performing indicated tests (e.g., assessing hemoglobin/hematocrit levels after administering blood and blood product transfusions; assessing prothrombin/partial thromboplastin time when patients are on anticoagulation therapy).
- ▶ Not placing a patient on skin care precaution although he or she is at risk for skin breakdown.
- ▶ Transferring a patient to subacute rehabilitation when he or she could benefit from acute rehabilitation services.

The utilization management role can be touchy. Conflicts may arise if the physician feels the case manager is telling him or her what to do or is "policing" the patient and patient care. Utilization tools such as clinical pathways are sometimes helpful. When a care plan goes off the path, that clinical pathway—and the patient—can be the focus of the discussion, which directs the conversation away from any personal physician practice and maintains the focus on the patient.

▶ Knowledge of Insurance Structures: The Insurance Benefit Analyst

Many types of case management require intensive analyzing of benefit allowances. This is especially true for entrepreneurial case managers, and for those working with union groups, self-funded plans, or payor-based organizations. This skill is least important for acute care case management; essentially, as long as a patient requires acute care, most plans cover the expense up to the maximum of the plan's dollar allowance. However, other case managers, and certainly those who follow a patient through all levels of care and home, must be aware of benefit limitations.

Case managers often describe this role as a *game keeper*. Each insurance company has its own rules, covered services, interpretation of utilization management modalities, and type of reimbursement. To obtain the full hospital stay authorization, to maximize the chance of a successful discharge plan, to minimize last-minute surprises, and to be legally correct in any type of case management, *know the game rules for your patient's insurance plan.*

Consider home health benefits. Some plans allow 60 visits per year; others allow $10,000 per year; still others may allow a set dollar amount per visit or any combination of the above. For this case management responsibility, a call to the claims payor or a careful study of the most recent benefit book is the safest route. Each plan design is unique, and patient care must be customized to adhere to the set of rules and regulations of the plan to which the patient belongs. Case managers must know every detail of the benefit book. It is essential that case managers understand strategies behind insurance structures (see Chapters 3 and 4).

Another important consideration for case management is that in the realm of insurance benefits, case managers are often looked to for new trends in reimbursement. Sometimes, case managers are not aware of why they are asked for their "opinions." One payor requested that the case manager research preventive screening for high-risk colon cancer patients. During the conversation, it became clear that this company's benefit design allowed for preventive screening for high-risk beneficiaries for prostate cancer and breast cancer; it disallowed the same consideration for beneficiaries with a high risk for colon cancer. This situation was remedied after detailed information on this topic was provided and the necessary organizational protocol was initiated. Over the years, we know of case managers who fought for a particular service to save a patient's life. Although that life was not always spared, benefits changed and future patients were offered the benefits. Did these pleas, telephone calls, and meetings really help future patients? Something changed the minds of those who make the rules—perhaps credible case managers and court judgments were the necessary combination.

▶ Cost-Benefit Analyst

Beyond analyzing insurance benefits, many case managers will be asked to do a cost analysis of a case. Occasionally, family members need comparative financial information or insurance companies (inclined to refuse payment for a requested plan if they feel that a less cost-intensive solution is available) may request prices. Many case managers are required to make a formal documentation of savings per case for accounting purposes. Disease management case managers may be required to contribute to the savings information for an entire population of disease-specific patients.

Many case managers shun this responsibility. There may be several reasons for this dislike.

▶ They do not go into a "warm and fuzzy" helping profession to do accounting work. Case managers improve the quality and safety of a patient's life.

▶ Case managers already know that they improve quality and decrease costs per case; justifying their existence is someone else's responsibility or considered unnecessary.

▶ It is difficult to understand accounting and budgeting concepts.

▶ It is often tedious and time-consuming to address and report financial details.

All of these "reasons" aside, case managers are as real an expense to the payors and facilities who hire them as are physician services, hospital costs, and medications. Everything has its price and must prove its worth in the business world. "Warm and fuzzy" case managers are no exception. In fact, this skill is so important that the case management crystal ball reveals that basic accounting, or a course in analyzing costs in healthcare, will eventually be a case management curriculum event. It is understandable that case managers are not always comfortable doing this task;

the main licenses that comprise case managers certainly do not stress accounting principles. It is also very time-consuming to justify how dollars were saved in a case for reporting purposes, and time is a commodity that few case managers have in excess.

Case managers must periodically write reports on each case they manage. At times, when costs were clearly saved (often in huge amounts) this budgetary portion of the report is felt to be fun, almost exhilarating; at other times, when payors want dollars saved more than they want improvement in quality of life, this part of the report usually is a challenge and felt to be stressful.

HARD SAVINGS

Costs that are clearly saved or avoided in a case are the *hard savings* or *avoided costs*. A new client once asked the case manager to attempt negotiation on a large hospital bill that was several months old and in another state. The client and case manager agreed that it was a long shot. Knowing that some companies extend contracted rates to specific facilities in other states, they did some homework. As luck would have it, this was a match! The new client saved more than $78,000 on the hospital bill, and case management time was less than 2 hours. This is a hard savings—the result of strong case management.

Some examples of hard savings are the following:

▶ Change in level of care facilitated by the case manager to one that is most appropriate based on the patient's condition and treatment plan.
▶ Change in length of stay facilitated by the case manager.
▶ Change to a contracted preferred provider organization (PPO) healthcare professional facilitated by the case manager.
▶ Negotiation of price of services, supplies, equipment, or per-diem rates facilitated by the case manager.
▶ Negotiation of frequency of services facilitated by the case manager.
▶ Negotiation of duration of services facilitated by the case manager.
▶ Prevention of unnecessary bed days, supplies, equipment, services, or charges, facilitated by the case manager.
▶ Discovery of unauthorized charges that are unwarranted.

SOFT SAVINGS

Soft savings are also called *potential savings* or *potential costs/charges*. If no case manager is assigned to a patient, the potential costs incurred might be much higher than with case management. Soft savings are not as concrete as hard savings. They are, however, very real savings; they represent costs that are avoided most likely because of case management intervention and follow-up by the case manager. The reason they are not considered hard savings is that no one can be absolutely certain what the outcome of the case would have been if a case manager had not been on board. These are the savings that take time and patience to document. High-risk pregnancy case management is a good example. If a 16-year-old pregnant teenager, known substance user, and diabetic is not case managed, the baby could end up in the neonatal intensive care unit (NICU) for 2 months at a minimum and cost $100,000 or more. However, with support and intervention, there is also a chance that the baby could be fairly healthy and may require a short hospitalization. Miscarriage is another possibility that would incur no NICU charges.

Case managers are not always comfortable playing the "what if" scenario. It is more challenging and time-consuming to document these types of cases. With hard savings, it is a simple equation: *the total hospital bill, minus the contracted rate that should have been billed, equals the hard savings*. With soft savings, each case manager must research potential charges to document potential avoided costs. The potential charges are often specific to a location, type of facility, and contracted rates the payor would have allowed had the services been provided. Then the case manager must guesstimate factors such as the length of time in the NICU (how premature was this baby?). Each case is unique, and so are the potential savings. Therefore, each cost-benefit report for soft savings will require a customized set of numbers. It helps to keep a file of these numbers and use them for references in future cases. As more outcomes data on case/disease management become available, case managers will be clearer about what is actually a case management impact.

Some examples of soft savings are the following:

▶ Avoidance of potential hospital readmissions.
▶ Avoidance of potential emergency department visits.
▶ Avoidance of potential medical complications.
▶ Avoidance of potential legal exposure.
▶ Avoidance of potential costs (equipment, supplies, etc.).
▶ Avoidance of potential acute care days.
▶ Avoidance of potential home health visits.
▶ Avoidance of unscheduled clinic visits.
▶ Prevention of medical errors.

Other soft savings relate to quality and satisfaction. It is difficult to put a dollar amount on these, and they are sometimes priceless to the patient and family. Examples may include the following:

▶ Improved quality of care and outcomes.
▶ Improved patient/family satisfaction with case management services.
▶ Improved patient compliance with care regimen.
▶ Improved patient's quality of life.
▶ Improved patient's social support network.

The detailed research is the tough part; the math is quite simple.

1. How much did the care cost? $20,000.
2. How much would the care have cost without case management services? $30,000.
3. Subtract number two from number one. The difference is the costs saved. $30,000 – $20,000 = $10,000 saved.
4. Lastly, consider all miscellaneous costs and subtract them from the costs saved. What other costs did the payor incur for the case management fee, physician fees, other expenses? $1,500.

Total costs saved: $10,000 – $1,500 = $8,500 savings *because case management was involved.*

There is a lack of research about cost efficiencies and savings as a result of case management. When the limited published literature is reviewed, one may observe that such research is not generalizable and that it is limited to the setting where it was conducted. Additionally, such research lacks standardized approaches, which prevent its explicability in other settings. Despite these concerns, case management experts have been able to document the value of the programs to their organizations and have been able to sustain these services. Healthcare organizations that employ case managers save money and improve their bottom line as a result of the unnecessary hospital days, ambulatory visits, or healthcare resources case managers prevent every day. This translates into millions of dollars annually for each organization. These numbers are important for case management survival. Case managers work hard for cost savings; documentation of the results of these efforts will continue to ensure the future of case management by speaking in terms that business people can understand. For those who resist this accounting skill, remember that sometimes case managers have saved much more than a 30:1 ratio, and the savings were in terms more dear than dollars.

▶ Negotiation Skills

In the current healthcare environment of scarce resource availability and declining benefits, the art of negotiation is extremely important. Negotiation is essentially a communication exchange for the purpose of reaching an agreement. It is a daily activity of case managers and used with all parties: patients/families, payors, care providers (internal or external to a healthcare organization), vendors of durable medical equipment, transportation agents, and so on. Cost containment, often through negotiation skills, was one of case management's well-known attributes. However, with the proliferation of contracted rates, negotiation opportunities are diminishing and are shifting from a primary focus on cost to a focus on quality and safety. It is important to continue to look for these opportunities and have the skills to make each negotiation opportunity count. Few people are natural-born negotiators, and to become an expert and effective negotiator requires practice. The effort is well worth it, because advocating for a patient's needs frequently requires this skill. Things will rarely happen for a patient unless the case manager makes them happen, and that usually takes negotiation. Negotiation serves the following important purposes:

▶ It facilitates reaching an agreement. Case managers use negotiation to solve problems and conflicts as they arise in the course of caring for a patient and family.
▶ It has the capacity to control costs—one of the primary reasons case managers negotiate.
▶ It has the capacity to gain medically necessary benefits for the patient that the patient would otherwise not receive. This is the other primary reason case managers negotiate: access to services.
▶ It can avoid chaos (Jones, Skelton, & Hochuli, 1998). Many case managers attempt to obtain services or equipment for a patient, knowing full well that the patient needed what was being requested to maintain stability. Many case managers live through frustration and chaos when the patient's condition deteriorates, at least partly because the negotiation for the requested service or equipment is denied or treatment is delayed.
▶ It can be a learning experience. Case managers may learn why the request is denied (sometimes there *is* a valid reason). They may also reveal weaknesses in the "No!" argument, which could lead to further strengths in the case manager's negotiation stance.
▶ It can improve the quality of care. Case managers frequently assess patient's needs and monitor care and services. When a potential delay in treatment, test, or procedure is identified, such as a delay in completing a

magnetic resonance imaging (MRI), the case manager negotiates expedition of such test. This ultimately provides clinicians with the ability to better diagnose a health problem and to institute appropriate action.

❱ It can improve communication. As case managers negotiate, they interact with members of the healthcare team (formally or informally). During such interactions, case managers keep the team well informed of the status of the patient's plan of care, decisions of insurance companies (payors) about authorizations for care to be provided, and changes in the patient's condition (progress or deterioration). Additionally, the interactions ensure that all team members are on the same page with the plan of care, the goals of treatment, and outcomes to be achieved.

Some case managers are hesitant to take on the big guys. There are five stages of negotiation that will take some of the fear out of this task.

1. Do your homework. Be optimally prepared to present the facts clearly. Before negotiation begins, it is wise to do some research and understand the other side. For example, know what services are covered, know the approximate readmit rates if a patient does not receive a particular service, and be prepared to ask for a supervisor—by name, if possible—if you feel strongly about a particular service need. Standards of care and practice, written protocols, written criteria, and community care guidelines should be established before the first telephone call or contact. Also, assess yourself for any hidden agendas that may push the negotiation into conflict.

2. Start your engines. Negotiation starts by stating the problem(s) and the goal and stating what is needed to solve the problem. For example, explain the reasons why the services are imperative and the benefits of the services to all concerned (i.e., less costly readmissions to the acute care setting). State the request in a positive and thorough way. Allow the courtesy to the other party; negotiation is a two-way street and facts need to be shared. Areas in which there is agreement can be put aside; then, begin to search for mutual compromise (Rehberg & Sullivan, 1997).

3. Use the three "Cs"—communicate, communicate, and communicate. Always have clear, factual, and pertinent data to share and avoid losing sight of the goal of negotiation while communicating. Cultivate an interactive,

collaborative relationship rather than an antagonistic one. Wait for the right moment to make your pitch and avoid talking too much. Use active listening and acknowledge the other side's concerns; ask how some of the problems may be overcome. Unless there is some indication that a message has been received, true communication has not taken place. Common mistakes can create a defensive environment not conducive to negotiation. Some behaviors that may be problematic include poor listening skills, poor use of questions, improper disclosure of ideas, mismanagement of issues, becoming emotional, inappropriate stress reactions, too-quick rejection of alternatives, misuse of a negotiating team member, failure to disclose true feelings, improper timing, and being aggressive rather than assertive (Hein & Nicholson, 1994) (see "Assertiveness Skills" later in this chapter). Sometimes, if the flames are getting too hot, it is time to take a break and resume at a later date.

4. Be realistic. Attempting to negotiate for a service, medical equipment, or a price that absolutely will not be covered or met wastes everyone's time and energy. Approach negotiation as a process, not an event or one-time task. Focus on interests rather than positions. Appreciate small wins; they are as important as the large ones. Always have alternate solutions or options for use when necessary.

5. Put it in writing. Once an agreement has been reached, write it down and have all parties sign it. This can avoid future problems when, months down the road, the claims payor calls you with a question about this situation or the other party "forgot" what was agreed.

Another reason that case managers are sometimes reluctant to start negotiations is that they have run up against some rather unreasonable characters. There are two types of negotiators: the aggressives and the cooperatives. Aggressive negotiators use psychological maneuvers such as intimidation and threats to make their "opponent" feel disparaged. Cooperative negotiators try to establish trust. Knowledge of the differences can arm a case manager in powerful ways. If, to your dismay, your negotiation tactics resemble the more aggressive or manipulative model, study the weaknesses and evaluate yourself.

THE AGGRESSIVE NEGOTIATOR (JONES ET AL., 1998)

❱ This negotiator moves psychologically against his or her "opponent." Note the key word *psychologically.* If the case manager feels that something is amiss, that he or she is being toyed with, the case should be brought back to facts.

◗ Common tactics include intimidation, accusation, threats, sarcasm, playing games, and ridicule.
◗ There is an overt or covert claim that the aggressive negotiator is superior and never loses a negotiation.
◗ The aggressive negotiator makes extreme demands and few concessions.
◗ There are frequent threats to terminate negotiations.
◗ False issues are brought up time and again. Once more, the case manager needs to bring the case back to the facts.

STRENGTHS OF THE AGGRESSIVE MODEL Any perceived strengths are diminished by a lack of trust in future negations.

WEAKNESSES OF THE AGGRESSIVE MODEL Some weaknesses include:

◗ It is more difficult to be a successful aggressive negotiator.
◗ Tension and mistrust that develop may increase the likelihood of misunderstandings.
◗ Deadlock over one trivial issue may escalate other issues.
◗ The "opponent" may develop "righteous indignation" and pursue the case with more vengeance.
◗ The reputation as an aggressive negotiator hurts future negotiations.
◗ Aggressive tactics increase the number of failed negotiations.
◗ The trial rate for aggressive negotiators is more than double.

THE COOPERATIVE NEGOTIATOR
(JONES ET AL., 1998)

◗ The cooperative negotiator moves psychologically toward his or her "opponent."
◗ The cooperative negotiator establishes a common ground. For case managers, the common ground is the patient.
◗ The cooperative negotiator is trustworthy, fair, objective, open-minded, and reasonable. This is very important. Respect and trustworthiness are critical for negotiations and for self-respect as a case management professional.
◗ The cooperative negotiator works to establish credibility and unilateral concessions. The attitude is one of win-win.

◗ The cooperative negotiator seeks to obtain the best joint outcome for everyone. This requires respect, empathy, and active listening as described in other sections of this text.
◗ Future negotiations are made easier.

STRENGTHS OF THE COOPERATIVE METHOD Some strengths include:

◗ The cooperative method promotes mutual understanding.
◗ Agreement is generally produced in less time than with the aggressive approach.
◗ There is a larger percentage of agreement in cases than with aggressive approaches.
◗ The cooperative method often produces a better outcome than aggressive strategies.
◗ The percentage of "successful" negotiations is much higher.

WEAKNESSES OF THE COOPERATIVE METHOD Some weaknesses are:

◗ Aggressives view cooperatives as weak, so they push harder.
◗ Cooperative negotiators risk being manipulated or exploited because of the assumption that, "If I am fair and trustworthy and make decisions with all parties in mind, then the other side will feel an irresistible moral obligation to reciprocate."

If negotiations start sounding like something from a professional wrestling match, use the following techniques to overcome the deadlock. Try resummarizing ideas, discussing the remaining alternatives, asking hypothetical questions, evaluating the differing points of view, and analyzing past and future needs of all concerned. Some people, when they feel angry and backed against the wall, say nothing; unexpressed emotions can result in misunderstandings and detours. Always remember that *the most important focus is the patient and family and what they require for safety and health purposes.* When negotiating, case managers can increase the likelihood of achieving desired outcomes by avoiding the behaviors listed in Display 2-4.

◗ Clinical Expertise-Disease Management Expert

Keeping up-to-date on new treatments and technologies in your area of case management is a necessary edge, and it is important to update clinical knowledge regularly through seminars and texts. It is impossible to completely case manage in a medical environment

---

BEHAVIORS TO AVOID DURING A NEGOTIATION

display 2-4

1. Making the other side feel guilty, distrusted, or disrespected. Using sarcasm, cynicism, or putdown statements.
2. Becoming emotional or losing temper.
3. Threatening the other side.
4. Rushing the process or becoming impatient with progress or the lack thereof.
5. Playing games or tricks.
6. Distorting the facts.

7. Jumping at the first offer.
8. Refraining from asking questions for fear of appearing stupid.
9. Losing sight of the bottom line, the long-term goal.
10. Cultivating an aggressive, antagonistic relationship.
11. Talking too much.
12. Giving up prematurely.
13. Appearing unprepared.

---

without clinical expertise. Many extra days have been authorized by insurance companies because important clinical data were provided by the case manager. Accurate assessment of discharge needs depends on knowledge of the disease process and treatment regimens. Practice standards also change as safer and improved methods are discovered. A clinically sharp case manager offers an important advantage, and it is necessary to apply the most up-to-date knowledge, evidence, and standards to the care of your patients.

As the managed care industry expands the role of disease management, clinical expertise and critical thinking is the expectation. The disease-specific case manager must have intimate knowledge of the population he or she is serving. In essence, a disease management case manager is a case management specialist in a particular clinical area or disease entity. The case manager is familiar with the pathophysiology of the disease, its progression, diagnostic and therapeutic tests and procedures, treatment options, and desired outcomes. All of this knowledge mainly benefits the patient and family.

▶ Knowledge of Complementary and Alternative Medicine

What started out as a grass roots movement in the early 1970s is now big business, and case management must be aware of the ramifications of their patients' use of complementary and alternative medicine (CAM). Some modalities such as acupuncture have been used for thousands of years in other cultures. Herbal medicine has been proven to assist in many chronic conditions. Magnetic therapy is being studied by credible organizations. Like Western medicine, CAM is powerful and must be respected. Many of the complementary modalities are an excellent adjunct to Western medicine. Sometimes, the two traditions do not coexist harmoniously. This is such a complex situation that the famous *Physician's Desk Reference* (PDR) has come out

with an herbal version. It is well documented that many patients use complementary medicine without telling their healthcare provider. The reason is often fear of ridicule; physicians have traditionally balked at non-Western approaches to healthcare.

The use and acceptance of CAM is one of the most far-reaching changes in healthcare. Insurance plans are already covering certain modalities, and the changes have just begun. The National Institutes of Health (NIH) has allocated millions of dollars for the Office of Alternative Medicine's budget. The White House Commission on Complementary and Alternative Medicine Policy has also done the same (Dean, 2001). These credible forums promote scientifically rigorous research into various modalities. The results may change the face of healthcare.

Case managers as patient advocates promote what is in the best interest of their patients. Doing so means that the case manager respects the patients' wishes, values, and beliefs, including their attitudes about CAM. If a patient is using any CAM modality, it must be communicated to the healthcare team, incorporated in the plan of care, and considered for its impact on care progression and options.

▶ Critical Thinker and Problem Solver

In nursing, this skill is often referred to as critical thinking; in business, the same type of skill is referred to as problem solving. In both, it is being a creative thinker or "thinking outside the box." It is the ability to

▶ Put together the known components of the problem
▶ Anticipate the potential issues and concerns
▶ Research possible solutions
▶ Find a way to improve the condition.

Critical-thinking case managers, especially nurses, have the capacity to walk into a patient's room, look at the patient, perhaps ask a question or two or do a quick assessment, and then make an emergency move that could save a patient's life. This relates to clinical expertise; it is also problem solving. Such nurse case managers are able to put together all the known components, add medical knowledge and intuition, identify a problem, and initiate a solution. Business problem solving does not usually require that speed of action, but thinking on one's feet may be needed in many situations case managers face. Components of a case management problem may be more complex; the sheer number of considerations that must be taken into account may be dizzying. Case managers must have this ability to function in the complex world of healthcare. (Chapter 11 contains more information on conflict resolution and problem solving.)

▶ Competent Professional

Being a competent professional translates into doing things well and taking responsibility for the outcomes. In her book, *From Novice to Expert,* Patricia Benner discusses competency using the Dreyfus Model of Skill Acquisition (Benner, 1984). This model theorizes that a student must pass through five levels of proficiency when acquiring and developing a skill. Stages I and II, Novice and Advanced Beginner, describe those who have little, limited, or no experiences from which to draw when performing their new responsibilities. This stage may describe a staff nurse who enters the role of case management with little understanding of insurance principles, utilization review modalities, quality issues, or discharge planning.

The other three stages—Competent, Proficient, and Expert—describe a progression of advanced skills and perceptions. This holistic understanding goes beyond a merely analytical response to a situation to an intuitive grasp of the events taking place. According to Benner, an intuitive grasp is not wild guessing; it is a direct comprehension of a situation that is only available when a broad base of knowledge, experience, and a deep understanding has been encountered. Therefore, advanced competency is often more visible in its absence and thus may go unnoticed and unrewarded. Experienced case managers learn to organize, plan, and coordinate multiple patient needs and requests and to reshuffle their priorities in the midst of constant patient changes (Benner, 1984, p. 149).

KNOWLEDGE AND USE OF LEGAL AND QUALITY ISSUES AND STANDARDS OF PRACTICE

Quality outcomes are a main goal of case management. Astute case managers routinely avert potential disasters by recognizing potential problems and resolving them before they get too far out of line. Related to this is the responsibility to monitor quality of care issues. Monitoring for quality of care issues is required in all aspects of patient care. One of the main tenets of case management is quality care, and identifying deviations from standards of care or practice is an important obligation. Case managers, being on the front lines, often pick up potential or actual variances (e.g., delays, errors, or omissions) from standards of care; this is another potential way in which case managers can avert a full-blown crisis (see Chapters 7 and 8).

ACCOUNTABILITY

Competency and accountability go hand-in-hand. The simplest definition of accountability is "being responsible." Case managers are responsible for myriad outcomes (results) from the case management interventions they perform daily. Through the sponsorship of CMSA, an outcomes initiative was created in 1996: The Center for Case Management Accountability (CCMA). With the assistance of prominent and respected scientists in the field of quality and outcomes research, CCMA is establishing evidence-based measures consistent with the *Standards of Practice for Case Management* and providing a mechanism for the measurement, evaluation, and reporting of case management outcomes. CCMA's goals (CMSA, 1998) are to:

▶ Demonstrate the impact of case management on healthcare.
▶ Develop a consistent framework for measuring and reporting case management outcomes.
▶ Add to the body of knowledge on case management practice and outcomes.
▶ Identify methods to increase case managers' capacity to participate in quality improvement and outcomes measurement.

This is a formidable task that will require the cooperation of case managers everywhere.

Dennis O'Leary, former president of The Joint Commission (TJC) discusses the "cascade of accountability." This cascade can begin with an individual who, through a union contract or some other leverage, holds his or her employer accountable for offering a range of high-quality healthcare coverage options. The employer, in turn, holds the health plan accountable; the health plan holds the provider organization accountable for delivering services that result in good outcomes. The provider organization will hold physicians, case managers, and other clinicians accountable to the individual patient.

▶ Physician Support

Case management has evolved to the point that some experts have called case managers the true physician's assistant. In clinical settings and offices, the case manager assesses problems, follows up with the patient/family, sets up equipment or home health services, teaches, and at the same time may also infuse chemotherapy. Hospital case managers accompany physicians on rounds, informing them of the patient's status and progress. This informational role may repeat throughout the day when any change in a patient's condition or critical value (laboratory test results, vital signs, radiology test results) occurs. A case manager may suggest a consultant if he or she feels it may help in the case. For example, a case manager may hear a disturbing report or comment from a patient (e.g., suicidal ideation) and suggest a psychiatric consultation, thereby averting a full-blown crisis. Each setting has a different perspective, but all case managers provide support to the contemporary physician's complex role.

▶ Facilitator of Multidisciplinary Patient Care Rounds

Various types of multidisciplinary rounds may take place; these include daily rounds with physician groups and other healthcare professionals, weekly rounds discussing all cases on the case manager's caseload, and patient care conferences that focus on one particular patient with extensive needs or special problems. The case manager is often responsible for facilitation and coordination of these rounds. A few tips for well-coordinated rounds are included in Display 2-5.

▶ Team Player

This is a multidisciplinary world; all players are important. Currently, in the healthcare environment, several types of teams are required for the practice of case management, accreditation, and quality initiatives. A team is a group of people who have come together for a specific purpose; ideally, teams are empowered to assess problems, institute actions, initiate changes, and evaluate the impact of those changes. Case managers are well acquainted with multidisciplinary teams. Continuous quality improvement (CQI) and cross-functional teams have a different focus and are often run quite differently than patient care teams. For example, patient care teams may be planned for daily, weekly, or biweekly meetings. The agenda and purpose is focused around patient care. Sometimes, patient care conferences are impromptu, almost emergent, in their timing. Often, the team members depend on which patients need attention and what the underlying problems may be; this necessitates a constant changing of important team players.

A CQI team, on the other hand, most often has a set schedule, a specific goal or goals, an assigned group of team members (with occasional experts called in on ad hoc basis) that will change only infrequently, and the initial luxury of a meeting or two to get to know the team members and establish meeting guidelines. The cross-functional team members can include almost anyone (physicians, case managers, biostatisticians, computer programmers, data analysts, administrators, financial personnel, etc.), depending on the reason for the initiation of the team. The team members are chosen for their ability to contribute to solving the problem.

---

display 2-5

TIPS FOR PATIENT CARE ROUNDS

1. Know the case histories of the patients being discussed in as much detail as possible. Be able to give a good overview of the patients' present status and state the problems that need discussion clearly and completely.

2. Focus on the plan of care, including the transitional and discharge plan. Communicate outcomes of interactions with payor-based case managers.

3. Involve everyone on the patient's healthcare team. Each member knows the patient from a different perspective, and the sum total of all the perspectives allows a more complete picture. As the patient advocate, do not forget the patient's and family's perspective and communicate what is in their best interest.

4. Try not to allow interruptions during conferences with the healthcare team. If possible, hold calls and pagers until completion of rounds.

5. Anticipate problems that might arise with all the solutions discussed and have a second possible course ready in case the first one falls through.

6. Bring each case to closure with a plan with which everyone can work if possible. Be in the habit of making rounds an effective use of time.

7. Set time limits to help make rounds an efficient use of time.

8. Conclude the rounds after making sure that items that require follow-up have been delegated among the team members and that each item had a designated responsible party. Make sure that expectations are made clear.

▸ CQI and Outcomes Management

Case management accreditation requires initiation of CQI efforts and continuous monitoring of the improvement. This has been the case in all other accreditations from the American Accreditation HealthCare Commission/Utilization Review Accreditation Commission (URAC) to the National Committee for Quality Assurance (NCQA) (see Chapter 10 for more on accreditation). Initiation and participation in quality improvement projects has become a necessary activity in which case managers are involved and an important skill and job responsibility of case managers.

The same is true for outcomes management. Outcomes are results. Case management outcomes are the results of case management interventions. Outcomes management is a scientific system of assessing, evaluating, and managing the results; the results demonstrate the effectiveness of the actions. The evolution of accreditation processes has changed the face of healthcare, and almost every accreditation or regulatory body now requires outcomes in some form. Case managers are intimately involved in many of these mandated requirements and are increasingly requested to participate in these projects. This is a complex job responsibility.

▸ Strong Interpersonal Communication Skills

The case manager, as the hub of the wheel (Figure 2.1), must channel information to and from all other parties. Almost every case management task requires some form of communication. This is a mandatory, not to be compromised, case management skill. The ability to communicate and work well with people is a characteristic that many employers place among their top three priorities when hiring case managers; therefore, many case management firms assess applicants for these skills. Each patient may have several agencies on board and many individuals involved in the care plan. The case manager must not only work with all of these agency members, but also coordinate them and the services they represent. This is not always easy when there are conflicting ideas and priorities about what is right and best for the patient.

Communication can be verbal, nonverbal, or written. There are four primary purposes of communication: (1) to inquire, (2) to inform, (3) to persuade, and (4) to entertain (Leddy & Pepper, 1989). Three of the four are essential in the case management process. Inquiring can be done through written communication or verbally, either in person or by telephone. Written communications must be succinct and unambiguous; verbal communication often involves tact and diplomacy.

Informational communication is a large part of case management transactions. Insurance companies must be informed and updated about their members' health conditions, treatment plans, and progress; thoroughness and creative persuasion are often important here. Physicians and other team members need frequent information about how patients are faring according to the other modalities (coordinating information). Patients need information about their disease process and treatments. An important case management communication skill is the ability not only to understand complex and technical information, but to be able to translate this information into layman's terms so that it is understandable to a patient. This is not always easy, because other factors may block the exchange of information. The patient may have suboptimal receptive and retention abilities due to shock, illness, high anxiety level, fear, depression, developmental age, language or cultural barriers, already being on "information overload," or the harboring of an "I don't care" attitude.

According to some experts, nonverbal communication relays more of the message than the verbal component. Posture, tone of voice, facial expressions, and nervous mannerisms provide clues that enhance or confuse the message. This information may assist the case manager in "reading" the real message. Nonverbal gestures may also help or hinder the case manager in his or her role. Ask coworkers to critique your style, or use a tape recorder or video to assess this powerful element of communication.

Perhaps the most important communication act is that of listening. A wise person once directed, "listen twice as much as you speak. That is why you have two ears and one mouth." The ability to listen sends a message that the case manager places the needs of the patient before his or her own needs or those of the organization.

▸ Assertiveness Skills

Assertiveness skills are an important part of the case manager's communication repertoire. Not infrequently, case managers are placed in tense situations; any case manager who has *never* been told off by a physician is either an expert at assertiveness or is topping the scale of wishy-washy passivity. Historically, those in the helping professions have always tried to please everyone. "We hate to offend anyone. We pride ourselves on being fair, flexible and open minded. Someone quipped that we try to be so open-minded our brains fall out" (Chenevert, 1988, p. 69). Flexibility is necessary in some situations; backbone is necessary in others. Passive behavior (e.g., giving up your seat when a doctor enters the room) is no longer applauded or condoned.

Substituting self-doubt with self-assurance is the first step in assertiveness and takes patience and practice; after changing your outlook, you can change your behavior (Hein & Nicholson, 1994). First, an understanding of the differences among passive behavior, aggressive behavior, and assertive behavior is helpful.

▶ In passive behavior, you may violate your own rights by ignoring them (i.e., self-denying) and allowing others to infringe on you (Bradley & Edinberg, 1986); doing as you are told can lead to feelings of anxiety, helplessness, and depression.

▶ In aggressive behavior, others may be violated, dominated, humiliated, intimidated, or put down (Bradley & Edinberg, 1986); one usually is taking advantage of another or enhancing oneself at the expense of the other (i.e., self-enhancing). Aggressive behavior may lead to feelings of guilt, bitterness, and loneliness.

▶ In assertive behavior, one is direct, honest, and lacking in excuses. One usually pushes hard without attacking and is expressive and able to influence the results and effect desirable outcomes. To be assertive, you must trust your feelings, like yourself, respect your own hunches and feelings, and be willing to accept the consequences of your assertive behavior.

Assertiveness is a tool, not a weapon (Chenevert, 1988). It is a desired communication style for the case manager. However, other less-favorable styles could be used if the specific situation requires such an approach. Fundamental to assertiveness practice is the substitution of "I" messages for "you" messages (Hein &Nicholson, 1994). "You" messages often put the recipients on the defensive. Simple questions such as "Why did you...," "When do you plan to...," "What did you intend by..." immediately cause people to put on their armor. "I" messages such as "I feel...," "I understand that...," "I want...," "I expect...," "I choose...," "I plan...," or "I am..." provide a clear, honest, and direct expression of one's feelings, thoughts, opinions, and beliefs. Other verbal techniques include choosing words carefully, speaking clearly, using a full, well-modulated voice, and projecting the message boldly, confidently, positively, frankly, and concisely. Nonverbal techniques include good posture, head held up, good eye contact, and hands quiet and relaxed (Chenevert, 1988).

Assertiveness allows you to act instead of react in a given situation. It is the perfect tool to get not only your own needs met, but those of your patients; it is the perfect tool for the patient advocate to use. A rule of thumb is "focus on the patient and you will be amazed at how the petty, peripheral things will float away, and your work will seem less complicated and cluttered" (Chenevert, 1988, p. 156).

▶ Management and Leadership Skills

As the title implies, case management requires a wide array of management skills: delegation, conflict resolution, crisis intervention, collaboration, consultation, coordination, identification, and documentation. However, case managers are no longer just managers of care, they are leaders—and there is a difference. *Managers manage systems; leaders lead people.* Case managers do both; they manage cases (patients' care) and lead or guide people (the healthcare team). Leadership is one step up on the ladder of professional growth. As case management continues to grow in responsibility, leadership qualities will necessarily be presumed.

The jury is still out about whether leaders are born or made. However, experts have noticed specific attributes that successful leaders share, regardless of the type of organization they lead. Effective leaders exhibit the following characteristics:

▶ Make others feel important. They emphasize the strengths and utilize the talents of others in the organization. Then they share in the success and give credit where it is due (Anonymous, 1997).

▶ Promote a vision. People need a vision of where they are going. Leaders provide that vision (Anonymous, 1997).

▶ Follow the golden rule. Anyone who has been demeaned or treated with disregard knows what effect that treatment has on the work (Anonymous, 1997).

▶ Admit mistakes. Everyone makes them. According to Will Rogers, "We're all ignorant. Only on different subjects."

▶ Praise others in public. Criticize others only in private.

▶ Stay close to the action. In case management, it is the administrator who goes to the "front lines" occasionally to get back to "reality." This also means that the leader is visible and accessible.

▶ Say, "I don't know" when confronted with a case management problem, then assist with a solution.

▶ Get the whole story before making a decision.

▶ Focus on what is right, not who is right.

▶ Develop a plan and execute effectively.

▶ Think and act in a goal-oriented manner.

▶ Conflict Resolution Expert and Referee

Fear and anger are emotions commonly expressed by patients and families. Attentive listening is often all that is needed to defuse the anger. Some simply need validation or a bit of control over their seemingly uncontrollable situation. Honest and thorough answers are often what are required. The skills used for crisis intervention and conflict resolution may be similar. However, crisis intervention often revolves around pure grief, whereas conflict resolution requires detective work to get to the core problem, which is often hidden behind various acting-out behaviors. Also, the case manager should be prepared to play referee when conflict enters the multidisciplinary team; patients and families are not the only dispensers of acting-out behaviors. The case manager needs to stay objective and bring the focus back to the patient (see Chapter 11 for further information on conflict resolution and problem solving).

▶ Coach

Lest this list starts to sound like an athletic arena, case managers coach and support their patients on a daily basis. Consider complex and chronic conditions such as diabetes. Several times a day, small invasive procedures (i.e., finger sticks for monitoring of blood glucose level) must be performed. Aspects of life such as diet and exercise that many people take for granted must be scientifically balanced against insulin and other factors that affect diabetes. Nonadherence to medical regimens is often the result of this daily battle. The case manager realizes that approximately 95% of a diabetic's care is self-care; for true empowerment, the patient is the center of the universe, with the case manager as a supportive coach and a catalyst for change in the individual's lifestyle habits.

Case managers also coach members of the healthcare team. They share with them the latest information about a patient's condition and plan of care. They teach them about the procedures and reimbursement methods of insurance companies, transitional and discharge planning rules and regulations, hospital-related administrative procedures and standards, and so on. In some situations, they also mentor newly employed or novice case managers.

▶ Organizational Skills

With all the details that must be attended to, organizational skills are a must. Also, time is prime; time constraints are frequent, and often everything must be accomplished precisely and quickly. Since the evolution of the CQI movement, seminars on organiza-tional and leadership growth abound. Many case managers are already organized people; if you are not, or if your organizational skills need improvement, seek out these seminars (also see Chapter 11 for more on this topic).

▶ Commitment and Desire to Be a Case Manager

Each professional will have his or her own personal reasons for wanting to become a case manager. Perhaps it is to help level some inequities observed as managed care regulations, and healthcare regulations in general, have become tighter; perhaps it is the unique nature of the case manager–patient relationship that is appealing. A clear view of your commitment may get you through challenging cases and stressful days.

▶ Ability to Prioritize

This is simply doing the most important task first. In general, good case managers excel at prioritizing. Each hour and each day has its own priorities. Meetings have been missed because of a Code Blue, and interfacility transfers have been delayed to meet the safety needs of a suicidal patient. Ability to shift gears instantaneously is also as important, knowing that case management priorities are moving targets. Priorities shift with changing patients' conditions, needs, and interests. Distinguishing between urgency and importance is vital. Urgent tasks must be attended to immediately, no matter what. Important tasks come next. The ability to decide what is important and what is more or less routine is often a matter of common sense. Having a "feel" for the pacing and sequencing of a case is important; sometimes intuition plays a role and pushes a case farther "up the list," which averts an urgent scenario later. For example, getting a code status or calling a family meeting may ward off a crisis situation. Delegation of tasks often helps to get several tough jobs done.

▶ Documenter of Plans and Report Writer

As in any of the healthcare professions, case managers are accountable for their actions. Documentation is important for obvious legal reasons. Thorough documentation is necessary when, for example, the case manager is not present and a situation arises in which contacts must be made immediately; therefore, all important contact telephone numbers and plans should be visible on the patient's chart for quick reference. The documentation theme is important and recurs often throughout this text.

Many case managers are also responsible for writing case management patient reports. Depending on the contract, this may be required biweekly, monthly, or whenever a patient's condition changes dramatically. The length of the reports and what should be included is a matter of organizational procedure. Essentially, the report should include an overview of the patient, case management concerns, case management activities, and a hard-versus-soft savings analysis. Thorough day-to-day documentation provides the material with which to write these reports, as no case manager will likely remember the details in every case.

❯ Ability to Read Poor Penmanship (or Tracking Down the Perpetrator!)

One day a case manager was squinting herself nearly blind trying to read an important note on a patient's chart, when Dr. Finehand walked in. He gave the chart a bemused look and threw up his hands; even he could not read his own script. Fortunately, he remembered what he had written. If all else fails, offer the physician a laptop! This issue is decreasing these days due to the increased popularity of electronic medical records. Despite this, there are still numerous organizations that have not computerized physician documentation.

❯ Respect and Trust by Peers

Peer respect and trust do not come with the job title, but are earned! Acquiring and demonstrating the skills described in this chapter and the knowledge shared in this book will promote respect and trust. As a rule of thumb, you must treat others the way you prefer to be treated yourself. You must take your job seriously and demonstrate that through your daily interactions with patients, their families, and other professionals—regardless of whether those interactions are internal or external to your organization.

❯ Self-Esteem, Confidence, and Risk-Taking

Case management is not a job for the meek. In fact, it involves quite a bit of risk-taking. At times, being a patient advocate requires going toe-to-toe with everyone from physicians to insurance companies. Self-confidence often comes from a good knowledge base and a history of solid, successful case plans. Novice case managers should be gentle with themselves and realize that it takes time to learn how to fit together all the pieces of the healthcare jigsaw puzzle.

❯ Diplomacy

Diplomacy is a skill and an art. When several of the team players are singing in different keys, the case manager must possess the tact and finesse to bring the group through negotiation and help them to decide which key is best for the patient.

❯ Attention to Detail

If you are not a detail person, bone up. Each case has so many variables, multiplied by the number of patients you have, that your total is perhaps thousands of details. Again, missed details can destabilize the whole case, compromise the outcome, and leave patients, families, and other healthcare professionals dissatisfied.

❯ Flexibility, Resourcefulness, and Creativity

Case managers must adapt to different units, facilities, doctors, patients' cultures, other case managers, changing medical conditions, and changing transitional plans. Sometimes a care plan must turn on a dime; this requires flexibility and creativity so that no hospital day or resource is wasted. Rigidity can lead to poor case management, bad outcomes, and stress or burn-out.

When the case manager may be called on to provide everything from a translator for an obscure European dialect to a macrobiotic diet, flexibility may turn into creativity. Creativity is often the first step in solving unusual problems. Tenacity and persistence are the other keys. Creativity is the ability to think "outside the box." Case managers are challenged with unique situations every day and previous experiences may not directly apply to resolving these situations. Therefore, to think and act creatively is a necessary skill case managers must all possess.

Creativity is so important in case management that administrators who do the hiring may want to use a case management version of the Edison test of creativity. Before hiring engineers, Thomas Edison would hand the applicant a light bulb and ask how much water it held. Edison had at least two methods to attain the answers. An engineer could use gauges, measure all the angles, and calculate the surface area; this took an average of 20 minutes. Or an engineer could fill the light bulb with water, pour the contents in a measuring cup, and obtain the answer in less than 1 minute. Edison politely thanked the first group for their time; the second group was hired.

❯ Self-Directedness

Case management is not a position for someone who needs constant direction and supervision. Case managers must make many independent and autonomous decisions each day and must prioritize their caseload according to their own judgment. For those who love autonomy, case management is a real fit.

❯ Caring Attitude and Behavior

Caring involves being concerned about another's welfare; it is the root of the role of patient advocacy and the heart of nursing, social work, and other helping professions. Caring between the case manager and patient requires reciprocal communication, trust, respect, understanding, and commitment (Hein & Nicholson, 1994). Almost every task a case manager performs is done out of involvement with, and caring for, the quality of care and patient safety. Specific caring actions include being present in a reassuring manner; providing information; assisting with pain; spending time with the patient; promoting autonomy (Hein & Nicholson, 1994); listening; nurturing hope and faith; cultivating sensitivity to promote comfort, recovery, and wellness in others; extending altruistic behaviors such as empathy and kindness; accepting others; using creative problem-solving processes for the patient's best outcome; providing a supportive or protective environment; assisting with gratification of basic human needs; and allowing each person to express himself or herself spiritually as he or she chooses (Wadas, 1993). Negotiations to achieve the optimal resources for a patient and the scrutiny of the case for quality of care and safety issues are expressions of caring.

Establishing a caring connection may be the first line of case management business, because "People don't care how much you know until they know how much you care" (Anonymous, 1997). One basic tenet of case management, and a very caring part of the job description, is facilitating patient autonomy, empowerment, and involvement in their care. To assist others in building self-reliance in their own lives is one of the greatest gifts a case manager can give.

❯ Sense of Humor

Used with taste and in discriminating proportions, laughter and humor add an important dimension to a case manager's work and increase job satisfaction (see "Humor" in Chapter 11).

❯ Information Guide

There are times when patients and families do not know what they need, what is available to them, or even what they want, because the situation they have found themselves in is simply too overwhelming. Eliciting preferences and priorities from patients or their families is a great relief to them; it also steers the case manager in the right direction. In turn, the case manager keeps the family/patient unit updated and informed on how plans are progressing. Changes and detours can be discussed when the need arises.

❯ Crisis Intervention/Grief Counselor

Most hospice case managers and social workers are well trained and prepared for this role, but some nurses may need to seek training. Not everyone is comfortable with this assignment; yet in the healthcare field, it is inevitable that case managers will be involved when loved ones deteriorate or when death occurs. Some situations may be more difficult for a particular case manager to feel comfortable with than others. We personally find it easier to comfort children of an aged parent than parents who have lost their child—no matter what the age. On some level, parents feel that for a child to die first is not the natural order of things. Yet pediatric patients, young trauma victims, and young AIDS patients are "disrespectful" of that order. Inherent in the populations that require case management are those who are dying. Case managers should attend seminars or peruse the literature on grief counseling to become more proficient in this area.

❯ Integrator

Murphy's law of medicine says that the more medical specialists on a case, the less they speak to one another. The case manager is often the integrator and collaborator of the fragmentation of care caused by this. The complexity and increased acuity and need for intense resources of patients who are selected by the case manager for case management services make it necessary that multiple healthcare professionals (sometimes including several physicians) be involved in the care. Add to this scenario the payor-based professionals (e.g., case manager) and other external agents such as those from medical transportation companies, skilled nursing facilities, home care agencies, and so on, with whom case managers interact daily regarding coordinating care for these patients. Keeping the lines of communication open across these professionals and agencies is a monumental task that, if not coordinated properly, may result in poor patient outcomes and unsafe experiences. The role of case manager as integrator is a necessary responsibility in these situations. Not having a designated person to assume this role is a "recipe for failure" with its poor results experienced primarily by the patient and family.

❯ Staff Development and Informational Resource

The case manager is a resource person for all levels of the staff. In teaching hospitals, this extends to medical students, interns, and residents, as well as attending physicians, who will look to you to help them develop the best transitional plans for their patients. Nurses, too, appreciate the case management perspective in such foreign areas as insurance idiosyncrasies and utilization review. Time spent in developing staff and helping doctors and nurses understand the concepts of managed care will be repaid in cooperation, timely changes in levels of care, reduction of time spent trying to make excuses to the payors as to why that patient is still there, and improved patient care and patient satisfaction.

▶ Case Presenter

A case manager may be asked to present a particularly challenging case to the nurses, interns, and residents during teaching rounds for educational purposes. It is a wonderful opportunity to explain the concepts of utilization review, go over the case's budget (and losses if necessary), and explain potential ways improvements in the case plan might have been initiated. Case presentations can be used equally effectively among seasoned case managers to elicit new insights and further hone case management knowledge, skills, and competencies.

▶ Educator

The opportunities for case managers to teach are unlimited. Topics for education of patients, families, or significant others are wide-ranging and varied, including medication administration and side effects, disease processes and treatment, insurance coverage and noncoverage, tube/catheter care, lifestyle changes/behavior modification, and any other needs that have been individually assessed. Staff nurses often help with medical topics, but patients also ask insurance questions, such as what pharmacies they are allowed to use, how much is their deductible and copay, how can they change Medicaid plans, or if they can change doctors. The case manager is the expert in these areas.

Careful assessment of teaching needs and education of knowledge deficits is cost-effective and leads to greater patient satisfaction and adherence to medical regimen. Readmissions due to lack of adherence are reduced when the patient understands the disease process and the importance of the treatment needed. If a patient has a newly diagnosed condition, it is critical to thoroughly educate the patient; insufficient understanding can lead to a deteriorated medical condition, more emergency department visits, complications, and hospital readmission.

Case managers often see patients who, after a long discussion with their physician, are more confused than ever. The ability to clearly explain difficult concepts in

simple, easy-to-understand, lay terminology is an asset to the case manager–patient relationship. It helps to build trust, and the patient does not feel embarrassed or condescended to. A ready-made file of handouts and information is a time-saver; bilingual handouts are also needed in many populations.

The teaching process may require repetition. It is unrealistic to teach a new tracheostomy patient all the care needed on the day of discharge (see the case studies presented in Chapter 12). Other factors can hinder learning: too much information in too short a time, fear, anger, shock, depression, medications, or any number of things patients in hospitals routinely go through. When preadmission or preoperative teaching can be carried out, this is an excellent choice. Some insurance plans may attempt to deny readmission payments if they feel the hospitalization was caused by poor discharge preparation (i.e., education).

Education about what case managers do and what case management is can sometimes be the most challenging of topics. Patients are not the only ones who require education about case management; even payors who retain case management firms are at a loss to articulate what they want from case management in specific cases. Just as it is up to case managers to describe to patients the case manager's capabilities and limitations, they must also do the same for companies who hire them.

▶ Liaison Between Payor and Patient

The first step here is often the identification of the primary and secondary payment sources. In this position, the ability to speak the insurance company's language is very useful when requesting extended hospital days (see Chapters 3 and 4). A good case manager-utilization reviewer can save financial stress for both the patient and the facility. Sloppy reviews can lead to reimbursement denials, appeals, and grievance trials, which would be unnecessary if the insurance company had all the facts in the first place. Attention to detail and a thorough knowledge of utilization modalities are important for the role of liaison.

▶ Concurrent Coding, DRG Assignments, ICD-9-CM Coding Issues

Case managers occasionally have, as one job responsibility, concurrent coding using International Classification of Diseases (ICD-9-CM) or other coding structures, or diagnosis-related group (DRG) assignments. Although this usually is done elsewhere (most of the time in the coding division of the medical records department), knowledge of concurrent coding is advantageous. Coding is done in a timely manner, allowing hospital reimbursement to take advantage of quick pay discounts. Because the case manager knows the medical details of a case, few potential charges will be missed. Coding also encourages physicians to document thoroughly the disease process, using appropriate and necessary terminology, which decreases the risk of insurance companies or Medicare and Medicaid denying hospital reimbursement. Case managers engaged in concurrent coding are able to ask physicians specific questions and recommend certain documentation be present in the patient's chart. This is done in an effort to improve documentation and to ensure it is appropriately reflective of the patient's condition, the diagnosis, and the treatment plan and its related outcomes. This function is essential for improving reimbursement for the care provided. The case manager engaged in documentation improvement activities must be knowledgeable of fraud and abuse issues so that the improvement made in documentation and reimbursement is compliant with Medicare and Medicaid rules and regulations as well as local and state laws.

▶ Selecting and Monitoring Clinical Pathways

Many institutions have been using clinical pathways for several decades now. Patients with a "pure" diagnosis (e.g., pneumonia, total hip replacement, asthma, acute myocardial infarction) have a clear and definite pathway to choose from. This is not always the case. Multimedical mix patients or those who develop severe complications may require more careful choices; sometimes the case manager may choose to change pathways if a new complication overpowers the original diagnosis. Clinical pathways have many advantages and are discussed in more detail in Chapter 4.

▶ Technology User

The use of information technology has become an essential tool for the case manager. Knowledge of case management information technology systems is a necessity today. The case manager uses telecommunication devices daily and almost all the time. Examples of such devices are the telephone, fax machines, computers, Internet, electronic mail, PDAs, and videoconferencing. These devices assist the case manager to communicate in a timely fashion with insurance representatives (external and payor-based case managers), other healthcare providers, and agents involved in patient care directly or indirectly.

Case managers also use electronic medical records for documentation of patients' assessments, plans of care, case management activities, and findings from the monitoring of patients' progress. In addition, they use information technology to keep tabs on decisions made about patients' care and use of resources, to develop and disseminate reports on care outcomes, as well as to communicate with patients and their families postdischarge from a hospital or termination of an episode of care.

Understanding the use of information technology by the case manager is a necessary skill and a prerequisite job requirement. Case managers are encouraged to become familiar with available information systems and their applicability for parts or all of the case manager's role responsibilities (e.g., how information systems are used to track patient flow, work flow, variance management, utilization review and management, and quality improvement).

▶ Devil's Advocate

It takes a healthy dose of objectivity and "chutzpah" to play this part, but often, like engaging in brainstorming, acting as a devil's advocate breaks apart any stagnant thinking and helps to provide a fresh new review. It also facilitates open mindedness, creativity, and brainstorming for solutions to complex problems. Acting as a devil's advocate allows case managers to critically think about an issue, consider the unobvious, and be prepared with a "plan B" if an intervention does not lead to desired outcomes. Additionally, such an attitude enhances the quality of care, improves outcomes, prevents medical errors and unsafe experiences, but most importantly, keeps the plan of care and decisions made patient and family centered.

▶ Have Fun

It's an attitude! Some fun is essential for survival, especially after a long and challenging day of case management.

▶ Basic Versus Advanced Case Management Skills

The skills discussed above cannot easily be separated into basic and advanced case management. Certainly, many of the aspects of case management discussed above are mandatory even for a beginner. So what constitutes advanced case management skills? Does the individual with a nursing degree or a social work degree overshadow a respiratory therapist, physical therapist, or occupational therapist? The core licensure is determined by the best match to the patient population; it is not something to be placed in a hierarchy. Some case management experts attempt to define the difference between advanced and basic skills by level of academic degree, rather than by experience and skill. However, those with doctorate degrees who have never done more than cursory case management (although well presented at case management seminars) may have difficulty handling an actual patient caseload. The Certified Case Manager (CCM) credential is held by associate degree (and all other degrees) registered nurses, physicians, social workers, and almost every healthcare licensee in between. Therefore, the CCM is not what places the advanced practice badge on the lapel.

Although it may be difficult to articulate what constitutes an advanced case management practice, advanced case managers have certain attributes and skills in common. Advanced case managers:

▶ Have published their works in magazines, peer-reviewed and nonreviewed journals, trade publications, or books. They are committed to advancing the case management industry with valid, pertinent, and useful information and evidence-based knowledge (Llewellyn & Moreo, 1998).

▶ Have a creative sense that allows thinking outside the box. This talent is a combination of experience, knowledge of outcomes, and intuition.

▶ Typically have had case management experience in several healthcare settings (perhaps with health maintenance organizations (HMOs), hospitals, workers' compensation, and self-funded plans); they have case managed patients through a continuum of care, not just an episode of illness.

▶ Understand the basic principles of management, leadership, outcomes (including how to put together a simple case management outcomes management project), and CQI.

▶ Keep up with the upcoming trends in healthcare and plan strategies for future needs; this may range from the whirlwind increase in the use of CAM to regulatory and fiscal changes happening at the regional or national level.

▶ Possess a good working knowledge of technical support systems (Llewellyn & Moreo, 1998).

▶ Are the ones peers typically call on when assistance with difficult cases is needed (Llewellyn & Moreo, 1998).

▶ Often hold management positions in their organizations (Llewellyn & Moreo, 1998).

▶ Have thorough autonomy, as well as a thorough understanding and use of the core case management components (assessment, problem identification, planning, implementation, coordination,

monitoring, evaluation, and advocacy) (Llewellyn & Moreo, 1998).

▶ Possess a core national certification (Llewellyn & Moreo, 1998).

▶ Hold a bachelor's or master's degree in healthcare fields that are related to case management (e.g., RN, MSW, MHSA, etc.) (Llewellyn & Moreo, 1998).

▶ Engage in the conduct of case management-related research, dissemination of findings, and the utilization of research outcomes in their own practices and for the benefit of patient care.

▶ Mentor other novice case managers or those interested in becoming case managers. They also act as consultants to others interested in improving their case management programs.

After completing this list, it occurred to us why case management has grown so fast that many are uncomfortable with its vast expansion. It had to—for survival. No one else had taken up the flag and run with it, and the patients needed help. Just when people are most vulnerable, they are thrown into a complex and convoluted system with a reputation for rationing care that requires a tremendous amount of information to blaze through. We heard a joke at one of CMSA's annual conferences that brings this point home.

There was a group of NASA scientists trying desperately to work out a problematic area in the space program. After weeks of struggling, one of the rocket scientists threw up her hands and said, "Come on. It's not like this is *case management!*"

▶ SKILLS AND PERSONALITY TRAITS OF CASE MANAGERS

The characteristics of the case manager's roles and responsibilities as described previously are in essence the skills and **traits** required for success and effectiveness of the role. The skills (Display 2-6) and traits (Display 2-7) make the case manager capable of carrying out the role responsibilities and the case management activities. It is not a prerequisite that candidates for the case manager role possess all these skills and traits. It is, however, important that candidates demonstrate potential for developing these skills and acquiring these traits. Moreover, it is necessary to differentiate between those traits that are innate and those that can be developed over time and with appropriate mentoring. When evaluating whether a case manager job is made for you, it is worthwhile to first examine yourself through reflection and assess whether you possess these traits and whether you

display 2-6

▼ **EXAMPLES OF CASE MANAGER'S SKILLS**

1. Expertise in clinical care provision
2. Patient and family teaching
3. Coordination and facilitation of care activities
4. Assessment, monitoring, and evaluation of care
5. Advocacy
6. Crisis intervention and counseling
7. Problem solving and conflict resolution
8. Critical thinking
9. Project management
10. Delegation
11. Negotiation
12. Priority setting
13. Time management
14. Utilization management
15. Cost-benefit analysis
16. Quality improvement
17. Outcomes management
18. Gatekeeping
19. Customer relations
20. Communication
21. Documentation
22. Writing reports and publications
23. Active listening
24. Team work and collaboration
25. Networking
26. Public speaking
27. Use of information technology
28. Use of telecommunication devices in patient care

will be able to develop those that are lacking. Having a sense of the case manager's role demands before assuming such responsibility allows you to determine whether this role is made for you, if you will be able to succeed in it, and whether you will feel satisfied with it.

▶ CASE MANAGEMENT ACADEMIA

In the 1980s and early 1990s the only way to learn case management was "trial by fire." For better or worse, many case managers developed and performed the case management role with little (or poor) training. The trend now is for case managers to develop or improve case management knowledge, skills and

competencies in many ways. First, a few journals, magazines, and books moved the educational level up a bit. On-the-job training helped provide case managers with knowledge of organization-specific responsibilities and mentoring by those who were experts in the role or had done it for several years. Next, journals, magazines, books, and seminars proliferated; major accreditation bodies added case management, and in 1998, the NCLEX examination that licenses RNs included questions about case management. Today, case management is included as a top as a topic on other professional licensing examination (e.g., social work and vocational rehabilitation counseling). College courses and university-based programs (degree- and non-degree granting) now take place all

▼ **EXAMPLES OF CASE MANAGER'S PERSONALITY TRAITS**

1. Caring attitude
2. Sensitivity, especially to cultural issues
3. Resourcefulness
4. Commitment
5. Creativity
6. Autonomy
7. Emotional intelligence
8. Self-directedness
9. Assertiveness
10. Motivation and initiative
11. Practicality
12. Willingness to learn
13. Comfort in admitting mistakes or areas of deficits
14. Openness and flexibility
15. Ability to ask questions or seek assistance
16. Pleasant
17. Sense of humor
18. Risk taking
19. Tolerance
20. Confidence
21. Respect
22. Attention to details

over the globe. Some are even available online as distant learning programs.

▶ Levels of Case Manager Education

Essentially, there are four levels of education for case managers.

1. On-the-job training. This can be done within a specific practice setting. It is useful for training new case managers, even those with experience, because it can be tailored to the needs of the organization.
2. Continuing education programs. These include local, regional, national, or international conferences specializing in or specifically designated for case management. Examples include the annual CMSA conference and contemporary forum. Continuing education offerings vary in length from one day to week-long programs. At the conclusion of these programs, an educational certificate of attendance is granted.
3. School-based, nondegree granting programs. These consist either of a single case management course or a few courses about case management within another program. They include the basic strategies and issues necessary to function in a case management role.
4. Graduate level. This is a full case-management program for professionals with another licensure such as registered nurses or social workers. A total package of theory, leadership, and practical skills is taught. Some programs are offered as postgraduate or postbaccalaureate certificate programs; others are full degrees (i.e., master's degree) at the graduate education level.

▶ Importance of Case Manager Training

Everyone is in agreement that solid training for case managers is imperative. Without training, many potentially talented case managers have quickly become discouraged. At what level should a nurse (as an example of a professional case manager) have case management training—with an associate, a baccalaureate, or a master's degree? Certainly, a good debate can be made for disease-specific case managers having an advanced practice degree in nursing. However, the truth is that case management skills are needed well before the graduate level. Staff nurses in hospitals, home health agencies, and skilled nursing facilities (SNFs) require the skills of a case manager, whether they are an RN with an associate or a doctoral degree. The same applies for social workers as case managers.

▶ Core Competence for Case Management Training

Areas of core competence for case management training have been occupying several speech slots at national case management seminars. They also have been discussed and debated in the case management literature. Display 2-8 shows some of the current thinking on what is important for inclusion in case management training, whether that training is on-the-job, a single course, or a university degree. The details in each core competence will change as new models are designed and as disease management and outcomes management discover the best practices of case management.

The following breaks down the core competence areas into more detail.

CASE MANAGEMENT: INTRODUCTION, HISTORY, AND CHARACTERISTICS

▶ Professional organizations such as CMSA and URAC
▶ First attempts at case management guidelines, CCM and other accreditations
▶ Definitions, history, and trends in case management such as the historical Individual Case Management Association (ICMA)
▶ In advanced courses, use theories and conceptual frameworks that guide practice

CASE MANAGEMENT PROCESS

▶ Steps of the case management process
▶ If a single case management course, use case management by proxy as an adjunctive exercise
▶ If advanced and on-the-job training courses, clinical practicum with an actual caseload of patients

CASE MANAGEMENT ROLES/FUNCTIONS

▶ Evolution of the case manager's role in the United States and globally
▶ Case manager's skills and personality traits
▶ Assessment of various job descriptions

CASE MANAGEMENT MODELS

▶ Descriptions of an organization including its case management program, like the one the student works in
▶ The whole case management picture in advanced training courses

UTILIZATION MANAGEMENT

For this very large and important aspect of case management, examine

display 2-8

CORE AREAS OF CASE MANAGEMENT COMPETENCE

Core Areas of Competence	On-the-Job Training	Continuing Education/ Graduate Course	Graduate Level—Full Case Management Program
Case management: introduction, history, and characteristics	✓	✓	✓
Case management process	✓	✓	✓
Case management roles/functions	✓	✓	✓
Case manager skills and personality traits	☆	✓	✓
Case management models		☆	✓
Utilization management	✓	✓	✓
Reimbursement methods, managed care and other insurance lines	✓	✓	✓
Legal issues	✓	✓	✓
Ethical issues		✓	✓
Disease management: strategies and process	✓	✓	✓
Assessment of high-risk populations	✓	✓	✓
Transitional and discharge planning/levels of care	✓	✓	✓
Social services/community resources	✓	✓	✓
Life care planning	*		✓
Quality management and risk management	✓	✓	✓
Outcome measurement/variance management/ guidelines	*	☆	✓
Stress: case manager's and patient's/family's	☆	☆	✓
Case management by proxy	*	✓	
Case management internship	*		✓
Cost-benefit analysis	*	☆	✓
Negotiation skills	☆	☆	✓
Communication/collaboration/leadership skills	☆	☆	✓
Information systems and telehealth	*	☆	✓
Case management research		☆	✓
Theoretical framework		☆	✓
Health policy, legislation, case management trends			✓

✓, Recommended; ☆, at least some discussion recommended; *, depends on the needs of the organization.

▶ Different utilization management modalities, such as clinical pathways, InterQual and Milliman guidelines, and length of stay. Look at the pros and cons of each.
▶ Denials, reconsiderations, expedited/standard appeals, precertification, concurrent review, retrospective review, etc.
▶ Utilization: management–related accreditations.

REIMBURSEMENT METHODS INCLUDING MANAGED CARE AND OTHER INSURANCE LINES

▶ Reimbursement methods and their differences (This is the foundation within which a case manager must function. The student cannot case manage without a good working knowledge of reimbursement methods and the managed care world; insurance provides the game rules and the starting parameters of each case.)

▶ Indemnity, managed indemnity, HMOs, PPOs, DRGs, capitation, coinsurance, Medicare and Medicaid (managed versus fee-for-service, new Medicare product lines), and all other types of contracts and risk-sharing methods of managed care

▶ Who the insurance players are (e.g., utilization managers, claims payors, reinsurance carriers)

▶ Use of strategies of different insurance types (Practice and role play can be valuable; focus on the student's ability to use effective strategies and tactics.)

LEGAL ISSUES

▶ Documentation, medical records, privacy, confidentiality, fraud and abuse, special mental health/HIV issues, medical directives, medical power of attorney, Americans with Disabilities Act issues, regulatory issues, surrogates and guardians, do-not-resuscitate (DNR) orders, autopsy, informed consent, Patient Bill of Rights, Patient Self-Determination Act, utilization management grievance and appeals laws, and anything from birth injuries to liability from negligent physician care or case management recommendations

ETHICAL ISSUES

▶ Confidentiality, especially with increased use of computers

▶ Withholding versus withdrawal of life support, nutrition, fluids

▶ Physician-assisted suicide and right to die

▶ Rationing of healthcare

▶ Advocacy

▶ Conflicting roles (e.g., the case manager as gatekeeper versus patient advocate)

▶ Ethical theories and tools; helping students evaluate their own ethical compasses

▶ Use of the CMSA's *Ethics Statement on Case Management Practice* and the CCMC's *Code of Professional Conduct for Case Managers* as the basic foundations from which to apply ethical principles to the practice of case management

DISEASE MANAGEMENT: STRATEGIES AND PROCESS

▶ The disease management process

▶ The chronic care model

▶ Clinical indicators for various disease processes

▶ Wellness and empowerment through education—a key component in disease management

▶ Clinical expertise (can be extensive in more advanced courses)

ASSESSMENT OF HIGH-RISK POPULATIONS

Assessment of high-risk or vulnerable populations is another big area! Students must be taught the following:

▶ How to perform thorough, accurate assessments of all details of medical, psychosocial, financial, and insurance benefits

▶ How to avoid being task-oriented

▶ How to look at the whole "universe of the patient"

▶ How to identify a high-risk population

TRANSITIONAL AND DISCHARGE PLANNING/LEVELS OF CARE

▶ Assessing needs: different needs for acute care versus through-the-continuum care

▶ Understanding levels of care: what is paid for or not paid for; matching level to patient needs

▶ Understanding the relationships between transitional planning and utilization management

SOCIAL SERVICES/COMMUNITY RESOURCES

▶ Referrals to community resources

▶ Complete psychosocial assessment of the patient/family

▶ Conducting a community analysis for a specific population to determine if the community resources can meet needs of the community (advanced practice)

▶ Social systems theories, cultural diversity

LIFE CARE PLANNING

▶ Ability to project the physical, financial, and medical needs of the patient in years to come

QUALITY MANAGEMENT AND RISK MANAGEMENT

▶ Indicators to look for when doing quality reviews

▶ Documentation

▶ CQI/total quality management (TQM) theories (advanced): Deming, Crosby, Juran

▶ Accreditations and quality credentials (e.g., NCQA, TJC)

OUTCOME MEASUREMENT/VARIANCES/GUIDELINES

▶ How to measure and assess outcomes; processes of evaluation; tools for process and performance improvement (pareto charts, statistical process control charts, flowcharts, etc.)

- Accreditations such as *Health Plan Employee Data Information Set (HEDIS)*, in which health plans are compared using the same set of indicators (comparing apples to apples)
- Use of guidelines such as the CMSA's *Standards of Practice for Case Management*
- Use and application of software programs to track and trend data

STRESS: CASE MANAGER'S AND PATIENT'S/FAMILY'S

- Coping strategies, problem-solving methods
- Theories: loss and grieving, change theories
- Self-care concept, empowerment
- Roles, role conflict, and role overload: strategies on how to prevent them from happening

CASE MANAGEMENT BY PROXY

- This is role-playing using sample case studies. It can be used:
  - in a single case management class
  - before giving actual cases to a novice case management student
  - in evaluating and brainstorming an unusually tough case
  - in assessing knowledge, skills, and competencies as well as improving them.

CASE MANAGEMENT INTERNSHIP

- Application of knowledge into practice; clinical experiences, especially in advanced courses (Offer a variety of practice settings that may help students identify a preferred case management niche area/practice setting.)

COST-BENEFIT ANALYSIS

- Fiscal management studies: how to figure true case management savings
- What constitutes hard-versus-soft savings
- Report writing
- Budget basics

NEGOTIATION SKILLS

- Assertiveness
- Conflict resolution and problem solving
- Accurate assessment of what is available to the patient

COMMUNICATION/COLLABORATION/ LEADERSHIP SKILLS

- Multidisciplinary team management, team building, delegation, conflict resolution, problem solving

- Leadership versus management; qualities of a leader are needed for performing case management

INFORMATION SYSTEMS

- Computer literacy: familiarity with software systems, literature searches, word processing, project planning, data entry, graphics, and flowcharts
- Necessity for outcomes management projects
- Computers and confidentiality
- Telehealth

CASE MANAGEMENT RESEARCH

- Advanced critical thinking using the research process
- Evidence-based practice
- Research utilization and dissemination

THEORETICAL FRAMEWORKS

- Nursing theories, quality management theories, change theories, systems theories, behavioral theory

HEALTH POLICY, LEGISLATION, CASE MANAGEMENT TRENDS

- United States healthcare delivery system and its rapid changes, crisis in Medicare and Medicaid budgets, changing healthcare policy, universal coverage issues, global impact of case management
- Future of case management

Teaching case management involves an immense amount of understanding. Few who have only taught, without having been on the front lines, can understand the total commitment necessary for this enormous job. Some further suggestions include:

- Keep lessons fun and useful.
- Plan assignments that can be tailored by the students to areas of practice (specialty or setting) in which they are interested; help the students find their niche.
- Facilitate creativity in every class; students will need it in the real case management world.

Case management by proxy is suggested for many levels of education, and in various practice settings. We cannot say why any better than with this anonymous verse:

Tell me....I'll forget
Show me....I'll remember
Involve me....I'll understand.

STUDY QUESTIONS

1. Cite an example in which case management was done poorly. Explore reasons and illustrate ways in which improvements could be made next time.

2. Do the characteristics necessary for a case manager differ from those needed for a direct care nurse? If so, how?

3. How do the job responsibilities of case management differ from traditional direct care nursing?

4. Cite an example in which you demonstrated the role of patient advocate. What might have resulted if you were not there to advocate for the patient?

5. Evaluate your own strengths and weaknesses in terms of essential characteristics of a case manager. How would you turn weaknesses into strengths?

6. What personality traits contribute to success as a case manager? Why? How does each trait add value to the case manager's role effectiveness?

7. What leadership skills are necessary for successful case management? How does each skill contribute to the case manager's role effectiveness?

▶ REFERENCES

Anonymous. (1997). *The manager's intelligence report.* Chicago, IL: Lawrence Ragan Communications.

Benner, P. (1984). *From novice to expert. Excellence and power in clinical nursing practice.* Menlo Park, CA: Addison-Wesley.

Bradley, J.C., and Edinberg, M.A. (1986). *Communication in the nursing context.* Norwalk, CT: Appleton-Century-Crofts.

Case Management Society of America (CMSA). (1998). *Center for case management accountability (CCMA).* [Online]. Available: www.cmsa.org.

Chenevert, M. (1988). STAT—*Special techniques in assertiveness training for women in the health professions* (3rd ed.). St. Louis: CV Mosby.

Dean, K.L. (2001). White House Commission on Complementary and Alternative Medicine Policy town hall meeting: Practitioners and patients speak up. *Alternative and Complementary Therapies,* 7(2), 108–111.

Dubler, N.N. (1992). Individual advocacy as a governing principle. *Journal of Case Management,* 1(3), 82–86.

Hein, E.C., & Nicholson, M.J. (1994). *Contemporary leadership behavior.* Philadelphia: Lippincott Williams & Wilkins.

Jones, Sketlon, & Hochuli. (1998). Seminar in Phoeniz, AZ.

Leddy, S., & Pepper, M. (1989). *Conceptual bases of professional nursing.* Philadelphia: Lippincott Williams & Wilkins.

Llewellyn, A., & Moreo, K. (1998). Transitioning from basic to advanced case management. *Nursing Case Management,* 3(2), 63–66.

Prins, M.M. (1992). Patient advocacy: The role of nursing leadership. *Nursing Management,* 23(7), 78–80.

Rehberg, C., & Sullivan, G. (1997). The art of negotiation: A delicate balance. *Nursing Case Management,* 2(4), 177–179.

Tahan, H. (2005). The role of the nurse case manager. In E. Cohen & T. Cesta (Eds.), *Nursing case management* (4th ed., pp. 277–295). St Louis, MO: Elsevier.

Tahan, H., Downey, W. & Huber, D. (2006). Case manager's roles and functions, Part II. *Lippincott's Case Management,* 11(2), 71–87.

Tahan, H., Huber, D., & Downey, W. (2006). Case manager's roles and functions, Part I. *Lippincott's Case Management,* 11(1), 4–22.

Wadas, T. (1993). Case management and caring behavior. *Nursing Management,* 25(9), 40–46.

CHAPTER 3

Reimbursement Concepts

LEARNING OBJECTIVES

Upon completion of this chapter, the reader will be able to:

1. Describe the various methods of reimbursement for healthcare services.
2. Define prospective payment system.
3. Define managed care organizations.
4. Differentiate between governmental and private (commercial) insurance.
5. Differentiate between Medicare and Medicaid benefit programs.
6. Determine the role of case managers in managed care contracting.
7. List five reimbursement-related responsibilities of case managers.

ESSENTIAL TERMS

Aid to Families with Dependent Children (AFDC) • CAP • Capitation • Carve-Out • Catastrophic Claims • Catastrophic Coverage • Catastrophic Reinsurance • Categorically Eligible • Centers for Medicare & Medicaid Services (CMS) • Coinsurance • Competitive Medical Plans (CMPs) • Consolidated Omnibus Reconciliation Act (COBRA) • Coordination of Benefits (COB) • Copayment • Coverage Gap • *Current Procedural Terminology, 4th edition (CPT-4)* • Days per Thousand • Deductible • Deferred Liability • Diagnosis-Related Groups (DRGs) • Direct Contract Model • Eligibility Worker • Employer Mandate • Fee-for-Service • Gatekeeper • Grievance • Group Model • Health Maintenance Organization (HMO) • Indemnity Plans • Independent Practice Association (IPA) • *International Classification of Diseases, 10th revision (ICD-10)* • Lifetime Reserve Days • Long-Term Care (LTC) • Managed Care Contract (MCC) • Managed Care Organization (MCO) • Managed Indemnity Plans (MIP) • Management Information System (MIS) • Medicaid • Medical Assistance Only (MAO) • Medically Needy/Medically Indigent (MN/MI) • Medicare • Medicare Benefits Periods • Medicare Advantage Plan (MAP or MA) • Medicare Part A—Hospital Insurance • Medicare Part B—Medical Insurance • Medicare Part C—Medicare Advantage Plans • Medicare Part D—Medicare Prescription Drug Coverage • Medicare Risk Contracts • Medicare SELECT • Medigap Plans • Network Model • Open Enrollment Period • Office of Prepaid Health Care Operations and Oversight (OPCOO) • Other Weird Arrangement (OWA) • Outliers • Pay-for-Performance (P4P) • Physician Hospital Organization (PHO) • Point-of-Service (POS) • Preferred Provider Arrangements (PPA) • Preferred Provider Organization (PPO) • Premiums • Primary Care Physician (PCP) • Prospective Payment System (PPS) • Quality Improvement Organization (QIO) • Reinsurance • Sixth Omnibus Budget Reconciliation Act (SOBRA) • Specialist Care Provider (SCP) • Social Security Disability (SSD) • Social Security Income (SSI) • Spend Down • Staff Model • Stop Loss • Third Party • Third-Party Liability (TPL) • Tricare • Viatical Settlements • Workers' Compensation

Insurance provides the financial motor that runs the medical/healthcare system. Although it may be the most confusing part of case management practice, it is perhaps the most important aspect of the role the case manager needs to understand. Each insurance company has its own rules, standards, and by-laws. Some companies carve these rules in stone, whereas others modify them slightly on a patient-by-patient basis, especially if they foresee a favorable chance of lessening the prospect of a future expensive hospital admission. If at times you feel like the master of ceremonies in the insurance game, you will be in good company. However, without a solid knowledge of benefits and covered services, a case manager's best intentions, plans, time, and energy will be wasted if he or she hears the words "insurance refused to pay" for this plan (patient's plan of care). It is better to know up front what the limitations are and to try to negotiate from there, than to have to throw away the entire plan.

Working closely with a knowledgeable social worker provides valuable information and may also prevent a true disaster for some patients. More than one HIV-positive patient has been lured into accepting Medicare's Social Security Disability (SSD) category instead of the Social Security Income (SSI) category; the latter pays out less money. In these instances, when the financial statement was checked by Medicaid, it was found that those who were paid the SSD rate no longer qualified for medical insurance under Medicaid. Their monthly income was slightly higher than what qualifies a person for Medicaid coverage. Therefore, these ill members had no money to buy expensive medications, and if they needed hospitalization, it would have to be through hospital charity until they could spend down (see "Spend down" later in this chapter) into a Medicaid plan.

This type of scenario can be more than just confusing and financially troublesome. For some, it means life or death. Consider the case of a single mother in her late twenties from Arizona. The woman worked full-time as a clerk and went to school part-time to improve her future prospects for a better-paying job. When she was diagnosed with leukemia in 1992, she eventually qualified for AHCCCS (Arizona's form of Medicaid). She was receiving Aid to Families with Dependent Children (AFDC), which allowed her the right to the state's Medicaid coverage and a chance at a bone marrow transplantation. However, when she became too ill to work and was persuaded to apply for SSD at $456.80 per month, the SSD payments put her and her son $86 over the limit for AFDC. She was taken off the AFDC rolls, and with it the AHCCCS rolls. Her chance for a bone marrow transplantation was gone, and she died of leukemia a short time later. Because of this type of outcome, there has been some reform in the rules; however, as a patient advocate the case manager must balance the requirements of the patient with the "rules of the game."

The information in this chapter does not cover all that a case manager must know about insurance and reimbursement methods, because each health insurance plan has its own standards for coverage or interpretation of coverage and procedures. In addition, the rules change yearly or sometimes more frequently. When describing different types of plans such as a health maintenance organization (HMO) or a preferred provider organization (PPO), it must be understood that even their basic structures are constantly changing. As the insurance company's vision of healthcare becomes clearer, the definitions of these plans become more blurred; this is in an effort to become more efficient.

From mathematics to physics, every classification of knowledge has its own terminology. Case managers learned to be fluent in "medicalese" in nursing school. Now we must also be fluent in "insurance-ese"; therefore, some of this chapter is in glossary form. As patient advocates, case managers must understand the convoluted system that insurance is and be wary so that our plans do not saddle patients and their families with unexpected bills or, worse, place them in Catch-22 scenarios like the bone marrow transplantation case and others mentioned above.

As seen in Chapter 1's section on "International Perspective on Case Management," each country has its own types of health laws and regulations, standards, insurance benefits, policies, and reimbursement methods. The United States has tried many reimbursement strategies, and each leads to a different incentive for plans of care. Other countries certainly have used strategies that the United States has borrowed and learned from; other countries have also learned from the United States (in terms both of what works and what may best be left alone).

▶ TYPES OF HEALTHCARE INSURANCE

The healthcare system in the United States includes two main broad types of insurance companies: commercial and governmental. Commercial insurance is also known as private insurance and includes programs such as the following:

1. Liability insurance: Benefits are paid for bodily injury, property damage, or both.
2. No-fault auto insurance: Benefits are paid for bodily injury, property damage, or both, incurred while driving a car. The policies and regulations of this type of insurance vary by state.
3. No-fault workers' compensation: Benefits are paid for bodily injury and replacement of lost wages due to an injury that occurred while in the workplace. This type of insurance is

regulated by state; in some states, it is regulated by the federal government.

4. Accident and health insurance: Benefits include payments for healthcare costs and may include short- or long-term disability.
5. Indemnity insurance: Benefits are in the form of payments rather than healthcare services, provide security against possible loss or damages, and are paid based on predetermined amounts in the event of covered loss.
6. Stop loss insurance: Benefits are used to cover cases that are costly; that is, that may require a large dollar outlay (see "Protective Strategies for Insurance Companies" later in this chapter).
7. Managed care insurance plans: Provide a generalized structure for the management of use, access, cost, quality, and effectiveness of healthcare services, and link patients to providers of healthcare. Reimbursement is based on the arrangement agreed on between the insurance plan, the patient, and the provider of care, and defined in the health plan.
8. Union health: Offers coverage for healthcare services for the employee of one or a group of organizations where the employees belong to a collective bargaining unit.

Government insurance plans are public programs and include Medicare, Medicaid, and Military.

1. Medicare: Financed by Social Security; benefits those age 65 or older, those under age 65 with certain disabilities, and those of any age with end-stage renal disease who are entitled to Social Security benefits. The Centers for Medicare & Medicaid Services (CMS) provides administrative oversight for this program.
2. Medicaid: Financed by state and federal governments through tax structures; benefits those who are considered indigent, with income at or below poverty levels, the uninsured, or those with inadequate medical insurance.
3. Military: Benefits active duty and retired members of the military, their families, and survivors. It is in the form of either TRICARE or Veterans Administration.
4. Federal employee: Benefits current and retired federal employees and covered family members.
5. Indian's health: Benefits Indians; usually offered in the form of Indian Health Services, Tribal Health Program, or Urban Indian Health Program.

▶ REIMBURSEMENT AND PROTECTIVE STRATEGIES

▶ Cost-Sharing Strategies for Insurance Companies

The following four terms relate to cost-sharing strategies used by most insurance companies. The beneficiary is usually responsible for copayments, coinsurance, and deductibles.

PREMIUMS

Premiums are the monthly fees that most insurance companies charge the member for insurance coverage. This fee is paid regardless of whether a beneficiary or plan member accesses healthcare services.

COPAYMENT

Copayment is a set amount of money specified by each health plan that the member must pay at the time healthcare services are rendered (Kongstvedt, 2003). This out-of-pocket payment may range from $1 (for Medicaid recipients) to $15 or more. Pharmacy copayments also are common. They tend to be paid per prescription (e.g., $5 per prescription filled). Some patients are unable to pay even small copayments, so many physicians and emergency departments waive them.

COINSURANCE

Coinsurance is another type of out-of-pocket expense for the health plan member. This type of cost-sharing limits the amount of coverage by a health plan to a certain percentage, commonly 80% (Kongstvedt, 2003). The member is responsible for the remaining 20%, but normally there is a ceiling dollar amount (usually $5,000). Private/indemnity plans often use coinsurance strategies.

DEDUCTIBLE

A third type of out-of-pocket expense for a health plan member is the medical deductible; typically, this must be paid every year before the health insurance becomes active. In the 1990s, deductible amounts were frequently $100 to $300. With the rising cost of healthcare, high deductibles of $1,000 to $1,500 are now offered to keep monthly premiums lower. Deductibles are common in private plans and PPOs; HMOs rarely use deductibles.

▶ Protective Strategies for Insurance Companies

CAP

Not to be confused with capitation, a CAP is the maximum dollar amount allowed in an insurance policy. Some policies are capped at $25,000, whereas others are capped at $1 million or more for a lifetime. Yearly caps are occasionally (although rarely) specified. Some insurance sources have no maximum cap, such as most Medicaid plans.

REINSURANCE (AKA "STOP LOSS")

Reinsurance, or stop loss, is purchased by an insurance company to protect itself against extremely expensive cases. Just as an individual may purchase an insurance plan with a $500 deductible for protection from high medical bills, health plans also purchase reinsurance with deductibles. A stop loss is a form of reinsurance that protects a health plan when a medical case exceeds (for example) $100,000 (Kongstvedt, 2003); any charges over $100,000 are paid at 80% from the reinsurance company. The remaining expenses (the 20%) are the responsibility of the health plan. Stop loss amounts differ, just as an individual may purchase higher or lower deductibles on their insurance plan. These high dollar claims are known as catastrophic claims. Because certain diagnoses or injuries carry proven statistics of being expensive cases, *catastrophe reinsurance* may be tied to diagnoses such as AIDS and human organ transplants.

DEFERRED LIABILITY

Deferred liability offers Medicaid plan protection in specific circumstances. Suppose a patient is admitted through the emergency department without medical insurance and spends down to a level at which he or she is eligible for membership in a Medicaid plan. Under deferred liability, a portion of the medical expenses is deferred by payments from federally funded coffers. This helps the plan to maintain some financial control, especially if the new member is very ill. In many states, sick newborns (e.g., premature babies) are an automatic deferred liability category.

THIRD-PARTY LIABILITY

Third-party liability (TPL) can best be understood by an example. Suppose an automobile accident victim is admitted to the hospital. Mr. Victim was sitting at a red light when Mr. Careless hit him from behind. Mr. Victim had lacerations and facial swelling caused by his head hitting the steering wheel. He had to be monitored for a possible cardiac contusion. Mr. Victim and Mr. Careless both had medical and automobile insurance plans. Most likely, Mr. Careless' auto insurance would be the liable third party for Mr. Victim's hospital bill.

Insurance companies keep a close eye on certain red flags (warning signs or symptoms that warrant caution or careful attention) that may signal TPL.

Some target diagnoses may include motor vehicle accidents, multiple trauma, near-drowning, and unnatural events such as explosions, burns, assaults, fractures, and lacerations. Insurance sources that may be liable include automobile, homeowners', workers' compensation, malpractice, and product liability insurance.

CARVE-OUT

A carve-out plan "carves out" or replaces a portion of the insurance coverage provided to beneficiaries (health plan members). Carve-outs are usually explicitly excluded from a provider managed care contract and tend to include expensive procedures or catastrophic conditions such as organ or bone marrow transplantation or AIDS care coverage. Carve-out services are those covered through arrangements with other providers. Healthcare providers are not responsible for services carved out of their managed care contracts. The companies who provide the services usually have case managers managing expenses and members' benefits. However, it is wise to continue to oversee the case. Many little rules for coverage in carve-out portions of a plan need attention. For example, in one plan autologous bone marrow transplants are covered. The policy starts 30 days before the actual transplant. This means that the bone marrow must be both harvested and transplanted within a 30-day time frame. On the other end, some policies will pay for all services including medications for 12 months after the procedure. If an organ transplantation requires life-long antirejection medications, the primary case manager must coordinate care after the carve-out policy expires.

LIMITS

Limits in a health insurance plan describe the types of services covered (including a list of providers an enrollee may use for healthcare services), delineate the enrollee choice for services (e.g., within or out-of-network), and explain the costs and premiums.

▶ Types of Reimbursement

PROSPECTIVE PAYMENT SYSTEM (PPS)

In 1983, Social Security amendments initiated the Medicare Prospective Payment System. Under this system, hospitals are no longer reimbursed on a fee-for-services basis; that is, for inpatient services, on the basis of what services were performed, how long the patient stayed in the hospital, or the costs of care. Rather, hospitals are reimbursed for certain types of insurance, most notably Medicare, according to diagnosis-related groups (DRGs) (see discussion in the following section). DRGs set predetermined rates of reimbursement; the hospital is permitted to keep excess dollars if the patient does not incur the limit of cost. Conversely, the hospital is required to absorb losses for patients who are more resource-intensive than given in the DRG allotment (Williams & Torrens, 1993). The DRG system also prospectively allocates the average number of days a patient will stay in the acute care setting; this allocation is stipulated by diagnosis or procedure. Another aspect of the DRG system is a predetermined expected acuity (called relative weight) that also is by diagnosis or procedure, which together with the length of stay, impact the amount of reimbursement a hospital receives for care rendered.

PPS has now moved into almost all care settings including the subacute care arena, long-term care, skilled care facilities, home care, rehabilitation, and others. This change has brought about the most far-reaching transformation in healthcare since the 1983 initiation of PPS. These settings and case management strategies are discussed in detail in Chapter 5.

PPS in the ambulatory care setting is called ambulatory payment classification (APC). It originated in 2000 and includes a fee schedule for bundled outpatient services. It is encounter-based and similar in philosophy to the DRG system. However, unlike the DRG system, a single outpatient encounter may result in the payment of one or more APCs depending on the services provided.

PPS in the rehabilitation care setting is called case mix groups (CMGs). It includes a patient assessment instrument (PAI) that is completed for every rehabilitation patient. Based on that score, the patient is placed in a CMG. The CMG then establishes the reimbursement rate for care rendered. Similar to the DRG system, CMG rates are predetermined and an organization is reimbursed that amount regardless of the cost incurred caring for the patient. The CMG classification is determined based on clinical and medical characteristics as well as on expected resource consumption; those patients who have similar problems and require similar resources are grouped together into a CMG.

PPS in the skilled nursing facility (SNF) is called resource utilization groups (RUGs). Minimum datasets for large numbers of SNF patients were reviewed to determine the RUG system. The final product was a system of 7 major hierarchies and 44 RUGs. Data reviewed to establish the RUG system included medical and clinical conditions, resources, and services required for care. The hierarchy and RUG were then allocated a specific reimbursement rate that the SNF receives as reimbursement for care rendered.

PPS in the home care setting is called home health resource groups (HHRGs). Reimbursement for home care services, unlike all other PPS systems, is determined based on a nursing assessment that is completed at the time a patient is admitted (during first visit) into home care. Reimbursement is determined based on a score the patient receives after the nurse completes the Outcomes and Assessment Information Set (OASIS). This instrument consists of clinical, financial, administrative, and service utilization data, as well as specific outcome indicators. The resulting score places a patient in one of 80 HHRGs. Each HHRG has a predetermined dollar amount associated with it and the home care agency is reimbursed that amount regardless of the actual number of visits rendered to a patient. Reimbursement occurs based on an episode of care or every 60 days.

DIAGNOSIS-RELATED GROUPS

A group of Yale researchers developed DRGs in the 1970s based on hospital-based historical data on thousands of patients. They were originally designed as a patient classification system, not as a reimbursement method (InterQual, Inc., 1993). A total of 494 diagnoses are listed and divided into 25 major diagnostic categories. Several variables account for the choice of DRG for a patient, including the primary diagnosis, comorbidities (preexisting conditions), treatment procedures (including diagnostic or surgical), age, sex, complications, secondary diagnosis, secondary procedure, length of stay (LOS), and discharge status. Each DRG is scored according to its potential consumption and intensity of resources. Each DRG category has a specific expected acuity rating (or relative rate) and an expected LOS that is presented as a range.

A dollar amount is placed on each DRG, and hospitals are most often reimbursed a flat rate for all patients who fall within each DRG category. If a particular case has been extremely cost-intensive or had a very long LOS (one that exceeds the upper range) when compared with other cases in the chosen DRG, extra reimbursement is possible for these outlier cases. Extra reimbursement is determined based on the number of extra days a patient spends in the hospital, as long as these days are justified by the patient's health condition and the care/services required. For example, a simple appendectomy would not be considered an outlier case until the patient stayed for 15 days. Then the case may cost the hospital more than two times the DRG rate of payment, or $44,000, whichever is greater (Williams & Torrens, 1993). As a comparison, Milliman Care Guidelines (see Chapter 4) has a goal LOS for a simple appendectomy of 1 day; with abscess or peritonitis, the goal LOS is 4 days. The number of allocated days usually changes annually based on historical data; sometimes it increases, other times it decreases.

Perhaps more than any other factor, DRGs provided the impetus for hospitals to utilize case managers. With the exception of the above outlier cases, the hospital will receive the same basic DRG reimbursement whether the case is managed well or poorly and regardless of the costs incurred.

Compare the two following cases:

1. Patient A with Medicare coverage came into the emergency department with abdominal pain. An ultrasound performed in the emergency department showed gallstones. An open cholecystectomy was performed on the evening of the patient's first hospital day. She was tolerating clear liquids on the evening of postoperative day 1 (POD 1). On POD 2, she tolerated full liquids and was ambulating short distances. Her diet was advanced as tolerated. On POD 3, she tolerated a soft diet, her bowels were functioning, and she was taking oral pain medications. She was discharged in the evening of POD 3, her fourth day in the hospital.

2. Patient B with Medicare coverage came into a different emergency department with abdominal pain. Again, an ultrasound performed in the emergency department showed gallstones. The next afternoon, an open cholecystectomy was performed. This patient received nothing by mouth for 2 days postoperatively. On POD 3, the doctor wrote orders for a clear liquid diet. On POD 4, the patient was allowed to advance his diet as tolerated. He tolerated a full liquid diet at lunch and a soft diet for dinner. His bowels were functioning, he was ambulating in the hallway, and he was taking oral pain medications. The following day, POD 5, the physician discharged the patient—on hospital day 7.

These two disparities are not uncommon. Both hospitals received the same DRG reimbursement. Studies have shown that case management has made a difference in cases such as these. Hospitals can no longer afford not to manage their resources wisely, and case managers are proving to be one of the best resources for this. They follow up on care progression and manage the LOS based on the patient's condition and required services.

LENGTH OF STAY

Some insurance companies allow the hospital a standard number of days for a patient's condition. A laparoscopic cholecystectomy may be given a 1-day LOS. An uncomplicated appendectomy may be given a 2-day LOS. Books of LOS are broken down by regions in the country and by diagnoses. They are further delineated by age and other factors such as surgical procedures. The estimated LOS for each category is given in percentiles—10%, 25%, 50%, 75%, 90%, 95%, and 99%. For example, a patient 65 years of age or older with paroxysmal supraventricular tachycardia may be given an LOS of 1 day (10th percentile) to 7 days (99th percentile). Most insurance companies use the 10 to 50% range for assignment of LOS.

A landmark legal case developed around an assignment of an LOS in *Wickline v. State of California* in the late 1980s (Saue, 1988). This case involved a Medi-Cal (California's Medicaid plan) patient, Mrs. Wickline, with peripheral vascular disease and occlusion of the abdominal aorta. Mrs. Wickline was admitted to a California hospital, where an artery was removed and replaced with a synthetic graft. The postoperative course was described as "stormy" with several complications, so the attending physician asked the state agency for 8 additional days after the LOS was established. The LOS was extended for only 4 more days, at which time the patient was discharged in stable condition. Home health nursing was provided, but within days after discharge, the patient's leg became more painful and started to change color. At about 9 days after discharge, the leg pain became unbearable. It was determined that at some point Mrs. Wickline developed a clot in her leg and a graft infection. Antibiotics, anticoagulants, and bed rest failed to save the leg, and a below-knee amputation was deemed necessary and performed. Nine days later, the patient needed an additional above-knee amputation.

Subsequently, Mrs. Wickline filed a multimillion dollar lawsuit against the state of California, stating that Medi-Cal forced her out of the hospital prematurely and that the physician was intimidated by the Medi-Cal program and complied with their LOS. This case went to the California Supreme Court, which ruled in favor of the state. In its judgment, the Court stated that the attending physician—not Medi-Cal—was ultimately responsible for treatment decisions concerning the care of patients and that the physician cannot abdicate that responsibility for any reason. It is important then for case managers to know that physicians are legally responsible for the treatment plan. As the court warned in the Wickline Case, "a physician could not shift legal responsibility for his patient's welfare to a third party by complying with a cost containment program" (Saue, 1988, p. 83).

At the time of this case, Medi-Cal did not have an appeals process; it is now law that beneficiaries must be provided with an appeals process. Physicians, case managers, and the treatment team must put the patient before the payment. Appeals are frequently won on the side of the hospital and in the patient's best interests.

Insurance companies frequently give short LOS—24 to 48 hours—for admission diagnoses that are more symptomatic than diagnostic (e.g., chest pain, abdominal pain). As the case develops, additional LOS days can usually be negotiated. If a patient is stable after several days and care can be given at a less cost-intensive setting (a lesser level of care), the company may not extend the LOS further but may agree to pay for an alternative plan. (More on LOS can be found in "Utilization Management Modalities" in Chapter 4.)

PER DIEM REIMBURSEMENT

Per diem reimbursement is based on a fixed dollar amount per day for services provided to a patient regardless of actual costs, rather than on charges or patient acuity. Cost-based reimbursement is based on the actual costs of a patient's care. Many insurance companies favor the per diem method of payment. They often pay for the day of admission, but not the day of discharge. Occasionally, certain expensive items can be billed separately. Per diem reimbursement may be a different dollar amount for different service lines. Intensive care services have a higher per diem rate than surgical service lines; a medical patient may be reimbursed more than a behavioral health patient in a per diem system.

CAPITATION

Capitation is a fixed monthly payment to a provider, paid in advance of services and regardless of whether services were needed and provided; a full range of medical services may be expected for each member capitated (Kongstvedt, 2003). The amount paid to a provider is based on a per member per month negotiated rate. Capitation started out as a popular method for reimbursing primary care physicians (PCPs)/gatekeepers and became more common with increased use of managed care health plans. Now capitated contracts can be seen in every area of healthcare.

Here is a simplified fictitious example of how capitation works for a PCP. Dr. Jones has 100 members from Managed Care Insurance Company A. The capitated rate is $15 per member per month, so Dr. Jones will receive $1,500 per month from Insurance Company A to manage its 100 members.

Capitation rates vary widely across the country and even among counties in one state. Also variable is what the PCP, hospital, or other capitated facility/

agency includes in the capitation rate. For example, a capitation for office visits would be less costly than a capitation that includes office visits and all laboratory tests. The capitation rate will be higher still if the PCP agrees to see these members in the event that they are hospitalized. From the managed care standpoint, capitation allows a health plan to budget for medical costs. For years, capitation was used essentially as a budget tool for outpatient services such as physician office visits. Now that capitation has moved into all managed care settings, case managers will need to manage the use of all resources.

Capitation provides a powerful incentive to contain costs, but balances in this system are delicate; underutilization of services can have far-reaching consequences through compromised quality of care. Some feel that the capitation system is unfair to those PCPs with sicker patients who require more office visits per month; conversely, a healthy member is a profitable member. Physician incentives to not refer to specialists or provide various procedures have visited the legal arena in the past several years; in response, many laws and accreditation organizations require that financial "incentives" be provided openly.

FEE-FOR-SERVICE

Fee-for-service is the old method of reimbursement, in which a healthcare provider sends a bill (referred to as a claim) to the insurance company and then the insurance company pays it. The bill is determined based on the services provided and reflective of the actual costs. With this form of reimbursement, healthcare costs go up as more services are provided. Some feel that fee-for-service was a major reason for the healthcare crisis, and at this time most insurance companies are agreeing to pay only "reasonable" charges. PPOs use a variation of fee-for-service: the physician gets paid each time the member requires services (in contrast to capitated physicians) but at contracted rates agreed on in advance. High-level specialists may be paid fee-for-service by some insurance plans.

There is an interesting dilemma that occurs if, for example, a hospital is paid by an HMO by the capitated method, and yet the physicians in the network are reimbursed on a fee-for-service basis. The hospital case manager may have his or her hands full with these cases; the hospital is at financial risk, but the physicians are "encouraged" to provide more services. Add to the equation that the physician incentives/actions also strengthen the patient's resolve to demand more resources. Patient benefit books prescribing what is allowed are vague at best and therefore are of little assistance in this scenario. The good news is that phrases like "appropriate utilization of services" and "medical necessity" are becoming more concrete with the evolution of utilization protocols, medical guidelines and pathways, and more precisely written benefit designs.

DISCOUNTED FEE-FOR-SERVICES

In the discounted fee-for-services reimbursement schedule, healthcare providers are reimbursed similar to the fee-for-service schedule, however, the reimbursements are discounted. The percentage discount is usually agreed on between the insurance company and the provider in advance of the provision of services.

PAY-FOR-PERFORMANCE

Pay-for-performance (P4P) structures have been implemented recently as incentive structures by some commercial insurance companies, and over the past few years have infiltrated the governmental health benefit programs, including Medicare and Medicaid. In the commercial insurance arena, P4P is being paid in the form of incentives for providers who meet certain predetermined outcomes criteria such as reduction in the need for acute care admissions, emergency department visits, or other clinical outcomes that are disease specific in nature. Examples of clinical outcomes are patient's knowledge of medication (including compliance with use), and mortality and morbidity rates.

Governmental health benefit programs are currently moving away from the incentive approach of P4P and are implementing reimbursement approaches that are based on performance. Examples of the measures used to assess performance and determine reimbursement include mortality rates, morbidity rates, medical errors, nosocomial infections, pressure ulcers, and patient satisfaction with care.

BUNDLING AND UNBUNDLING

Bundling case rates indicate that the facility charges and the physician charges are all bundled together and reimbursed based on one bill/claim. This is also known as package pricing or global payment. For example, a plan may negotiate a rate of $30,000 for a cardiac bypass. This would include everything from the surgeon and anesthesiologist to postoperative hospital care (Kongstvedt, 2003).

Unbundling is a term that explains the practice of billing separately for items that were once bundled together in a single bill (Kongstvedt, 2003). For example, a minor surgical procedure was once a single charge. When unbundled, it may include fees for the

procedure, physician services, instruments, hospital room, and dressings.

▶ Enrollment Terms and Qualification for Special Insurance

ENROLLEE

An enrollee, also known as a beneficiary, member, or participant, is an individual eligible for health benefits under a health plan contract. HMO beneficiaries are usually referred to as members, while PPOs may refer to these individuals as enrollees.

ENROLLMENT

Enrollment in a health plan may require specific qualifications. Medicaid, for example, requires the patient to be financially impoverished; Medicare Part A requires a specified number of work hours into which Social Security is paid and may have age restrictions or a disabled health condition. Private insurance plans may (although rare today) refuse enrollment for persons with preexisting medical conditions or they may accept a chronically ill member for a high monthly premium. The following three definitions explain aspects of a member's enrollment.

OPEN ENROLLMENT PERIOD. Open enrollment is a time period, usually during a specified month of the year, when a member may change health plans (Kongstvedt, 2003). As a rule, most managed care plans (specifically HMOs) have their open enrollment period in the fall; the changes become effective January 1. In Arizona, for example, open enrollment for the state's Medicaid plan is in August and goes into effect October 1. For members unhappy with their health plan, it is important to know when open enrollment periods come around, because it is the one time of year that a plan change can be made without financial penalty to the member, regardless of health status.

DISENROLLMENT. Disenrollment is the process of terminating insurance coverage (Kongstvedt, 2003). Voluntary termination involves a member quitting simply out of personal desire. Involuntary termination can include reasons such as losing or changing jobs (see "CONSOLIDATED OMNIBUS BUDGET RECONCILIATION ACT" [COBRA], below). A serious form of involuntary disenrollment can be for reasons such as fraud, abuse, nonpayment of agreed-on copayments or premiums, or a demonstrated inability to comply with recommended treatment plans. Disenrollment for some of these reasons may be very difficult to prove and is therefore rare.

SPEND DOWN. Spend down is the process by which a patient or family can financially qualify for welfare medicine, most commonly known as Medicaid. In essence, the patient must impoverish him- or herself with medical bills. These medical expenses are subtracted from the patient's annual income until the income eligibility limits for Medicaid benefits are met. This yearly financial income allotted depends on such factors as family size and personal property ownership.

Following is a simplified example with no extra variables of a spend down in a patient. Mrs. Barrett receives $12,000 per year income. To qualify for Medicaid, it had been assessed that Mrs. Barrett must not earn over $5,000 per year. Therefore, she must incur $7,000 in medical expenses or, in other words, spend down $7,000 to qualify for Medicaid benefits. Mrs. Barrett was in the hospital in February and was billed $4,500. She spent $1,000 in medications and outpatient doctor bills. It is May and she is currently in the hospital again as an inpatient. Her hospital bill has exceeded the remaining $1,500 charge, so she has met her spend down amount. Mrs. Barrett can now qualify for Medicaid coverage.

CONSOLIDATED OMNIBUS BUDGET RECONCILIATION ACT

Under the Consolidated Omnibus Budget Reconciliation Act (COBRA), employers with 20 or more employees are required to offer terminated employees an opportunity to continue health coverage under the present medical plan in exchange for a monthly premium. This premium may cost up to 102% of the actual cost of the premium, with 2% being administrative expenses (Williams & Torrens, 1993). The former employee has 60 days to decide if he or she desires to purchase insurance under COBRA. If a COBRA policy is desired and the person is eligible, the employee can pay for it for 18 to 36 months. The length of time a person is allowed to maintain COBRA insurance depends on several variables, ranging from reason for eligibility (e.g., termination versus disability) to whether the person is the primary beneficiary or a family member.

❱ TYPES OF INSURANCE MODELS/ SYSTEMS

The following section discusses various types of insurance strategies. Matching needed services for patients with available resources is a primary case management responsibility. Few people can afford medical services without the benefit of some form of insurance. A basic understanding of insurance types is essential for the case manager: what the benefits are, what is covered, how the services are reimbursed, what the patient's fiscal responsibility is, what the care provider's responsibility is, with whom the patient is allowed to follow up, where the patient must fill prescriptions—these and many other questions must be assessed with the insurance company for effective care planning and reimbursement.

It is a well-known fact that managing healthcare came about because of the tremendous price tag of this care; the price is still escalating. Managed care can be defined as an organization that provides and/or finances medical care using provider payment mechanisms that encourage cost containment, involves selective contracting with networks of care providers (individuals and organizations), and imposes controls on the utilization of healthcare services. More than 130 million Americans are enrolled in managed care, and it is the predominant mode of healthcare delivery and financing for privately insured populations in the United States. In addition, many states have shifted their Medicaid and Medicare beneficiaries into managed care programs, and some states have chosen managed care as the mode for the state children's health insurance program, which was included in the Balanced Budget Act of 1997 (BBA).

Managed care has infiltrated nearly every insurance strategy: even the last great indemnity plan—traditional Medicare. Although Medicare is separated into the "traditional" (fee-for-service) track and the managed Medicare track for clarification purposes in this book, the extensive changes in Medicare reimbursement today (as described in Chapter 5) have most definitely changed Medicare forever. Both traditional Medicare and managed Medicare are now intensely "managed."

❱ Coordination of Benefits

Many families possess health plans from more than one health insurance company. Multiple coverage can occur in such instances when both parents are working and each has insurance as an employee benefit, when a child has a catastrophic condition or is developmentally disabled, or when automobile insurance or workers' compensation is involved. State laws have been written to deter fraud by standardizing coordination of benefits (COB) for holders of multiple insurance plans.

When a patient has more than one insurance plan, it is important to first determine who is the primary payor. If the case manager is working on a case with health plans from two or more insurance companies, then the tertiary payor must also be determined. The "rules" can be quite interesting. One group we worked with uses the birthdays of the married couple as the gauge; the health plan of the person with the first birthday in the year becomes the primary plan. In general, if there is a private insurance and Medicaid coverage, Medicaid is usually the payor of last resort. However, because there are no absolutes in healthcare, the case manager must determine the rank order on a case-by-case basis. Plans covered under the Employee Retirement Income Security Act (ERISA) rules, for example, are exempt from traditional COB regulation.

To ensure healthcare coverage for dependent children, special rules apply when parents are divorced or separated. Divorced parents and their dependent children may follow a sequence such as this (Newell, 1996):

1. The plan of the parent in custody of the child(ren).
2. The plan of the spouse of the parent in custody of the child(ren).
3. The plan of the parent without custody of the child(ren).
4. The plan of the spouse without custody of the child(ren).

❱ Medicare

Perhaps the most well-known of all insurance plans in the United States, Medicare is a federally funded program under Title XIX of the Social Security Act, enacted in 1964. Medical services are provided to U.S. citizens older than 65 years of age who have worked at least 10 years (40 quarters, considered work credits), to those who qualify for SSD for at least 24 months, to those under 65 and with certain disabilities, and to persons with permanent kidney failure/end-stage renal disease and requiring either dialysis or kidney transplant. This federal health insurance program is overseen by the Centers for Medicare & Medicaid Services (CMS).

Not all citizens automatically receive Medicare in their 65th birthday month. They often need to file an application. For a patient who is 65 years old or older with a reliable work history and who does not show coverage under Medicare, social services may be able to help get the person on Medicare; the case manager and/or social worker could be of value in this case and in guiding the person through the application process. Persons with renal failure may also apply (CMS, 2008a). Renal patients are eligible for Medicare after

3 months of hemodialysis; if private group health insurance is in effect, that policy must cover hemodialysis for 30 months before Medicare takes over. No age limits are imposed in this case. Benefits will continue until 1 year after hemodialysis stops or a kidney transplantation is performed.

The care of Medicare patients is monitored by quality improvement organizations (QIOs) in each state. These are independent groups of physicians and other healthcare professionals, including nurses and social workers, hired by the federal government to assess whether the care Medicare beneficiaries receive meets standards of quality, is reasonable and necessary, and is provided at the most appropriate level of care. They also review any complaints from Medicare members; these range from poor care to premature discharge. QIOs are also involved in auditing care rendered by healthcare organizations and individual providers for the purpose of reviewing not only quality of care, but acts of fraud and abuse as well. QIOs also provide quality improvement consultation through state projects.

NOTE

Two important Web sites for Medicare information include:

www.cms.hhs.gov: the official Centers for Medicare & Medicaid Services Web site
www.medicare.gov: a Web site that offers useful information to Medicare beneficiaries and case managers working with this population. Among other important information, this site includes the *Medicare and You Handbook* (online) and has a section entitled *Medicare Compare,* which displays comparisons of various Medicare health plans.

MEDICARE PART A

Medicare is divided into two distinct and separately financed parts. Part A is known as hospital insurance and includes coverage for hospital care, including critical access hospitals, inpatient rehabilitation facilities, inpatient stays at an SNF, home healthcare, hospice care, and inpatient care in a religious nonmedical health care institution. Part A is usually premium free and is earned based on a person's or spouse's employment credits. It is financed through a portion of the Social Security (FICA) tax that all employees and employers pay.

Part A may be purchased by those who are 65 years of age or older and who are not eligible for premium-free benefits. Examples include those who did not work or did not pay enough Medicare taxes while working, and those who are disabled and have returned to work. In 2008, the monthly premium for those who desired to buy Part A benefits was $423. In most cases those who buy Part A must also have or purchase Part B benefits. If a person has limited income or resources, state government may be able to help.

Medicare benefit periods are also known as "spells of illness." They measure the beneficiary's use of Part A or inpatient care. The dollar amounts change yearly for Medicare. The following is based on the year 2008.

- A benefit period begins on admission to an inpatient facility.
- A benefit period ends when the member has been out of a hospital, SNF, or rehabilitation facility for 60 consecutive days (including the day of discharge).
- There is no limit to the number of benefit periods the member can have for hospital and other SNF care.
- Each time a benefit period is begun, a $1,024 hospital deductible charge is incurred. There is no coinsurance for days 1 to 60 for each benefit period.
- Medicare will pay for 100% of the beneficiary's hospitalization (minus the above deductible) for the first 60 days of any benefit period.
- From the 61st day until the 90th day in the hospital, the member is responsible for $256 per day. This $256 charge is called the coinsurance.
- If more than 90 inpatient days are needed in a benefit period, lifetime reserve days help offset medical expenses.
- Only 60 lifetime reserve days are given per beneficiary. These may be used up in one, two, or any number of benefit periods. If 10 reserve days are used up in 1 year, the member has 50 left to use any time that a benefit period exceeds 90 days. They are not renewable.
- Lifetime reserve days pay all hospital expenses except for $512 per day. This $512 per day is the responsibility of the member.
- Members can opt out of using the reserve days by telling the hospital in writing of their wishes.

Long or frequent inpatient admissions can cause eventual loss of Part A benefits. To lose these benefits, the patient would have to be in the hospital or a SNF for 150 days (using up 90 days plus the 60 lifetime reserve days), without a reprieve of 60 consecutive days out of the hospital or SNF. Although this rarely happens, case managers need to be aware of this possibility. Medigap plans cover an additional 365 hospital days after the lifetime reserve is used up. If the patient does not have a Medigap plan, that patient will most likely have to spend down to become eligible for a Medicaid plan.

Medicare Part A also pays for some posthospital SNF care. The patient must have been in the hospital under an acute admit (not observation status) for 3 nights at the minimum. The patient may be discharged directly into a Medicare-certified SNF or can go home and, if a skilled SNF need is discovered, can be admitted to a SNF within 30 days of the hospital discharge date.

Medicare Part A helps pay for a maximum of 100 days in each benefit period for skilled care in a SNF (Table 3.1). The member pays nothing for the first 20 days; Medicare pays 100%. If the patient still needs additional skilled care at a SNF level, 80 additional days will be paid for, but the coinsurance to the member is $128 per day (CMS, 2008a). After 100 days in each benefit period, Medicare will not be financially responsible. See Chapter 5 for further reimbursement changes in the SNF level of care.

Medicare Part A also pays for home healthcare provided in lieu of hospitalization if certain criteria are met. Essentially, the member must be homebound, have a physician-ordered home healthcare treatment plan, and must require intermittent (rather than intensive) skilled nursing or skilled rehabilitation services. As long as the above criteria are met, the Catastrophic Coverage Act of 1988 ensures that home health services can be covered for a maximum of 38 consecutive days. If the services are deemed appropriate, they will be reimbursed at 100%. However, dramatic changes are shifting the provision of home health services to Medicare beneficiaries in the reimbursement of Medicare home health services (see Chapter 5 for detailed discussion).

Durable medical equipment (DME) has a coinsurance payment of 20%; Medicare will pay for 80% of covered DME. Hospice care is also covered under certain conditions. Inpatient psychiatric care is reimbursed for up to 190 days, if needed. Detailed requirements for SNF, home health services, rehabilitation care, and hospice coverage are discussed in Chapter 5.

MEDICARE PART B

Part B is also known as medical insurance and includes coverage for medically necessary services including physician's services, outpatient hospital services, DME, other

▶ TABLE 3.1   Payment According to Level of Care in Each Benefit Period (2008)

	MEMBER PAYS	MEDICARE PAYS
Hospital		
Day 1–60	Deductible $1,024	All other qualified expenses
Day 61–90	$256/day coinsurance	All other qualified expenses
Day 91–150	$512/day	All other qualified expenses
Lifetime reserve days[a]		
Skilled Nursing Facility		
Day 1–20	$0	All qualified expenses
Day 21–100	$128/day	All other qualified expenses
Day 101 and over	All cost	$0
Home Health Care		
Home care services	$0	All qualified expenses
Durable medical equipment	20% of Medicare-approved amount	80% of approved amount

From the Centers for Medicare & Medicaid Services (CMS). *Medicare and you, 2008.* Available for free online at www.medicare.gov

Note: Medicare Advantage Plans cover these services. However, costs vary by plan and may be higher or lower than those stated above.

[a] Unlike other benefit periods, lifetime reserve days are not renewable and can be used only once in a member's lifetime.

miscellaneous services, or those not covered by Part A. The monthly premium for Part B in 2008 for a single individual started at $96.40.

Medicare Part B can be purchased even if Part A requirements have not been met. Some Medicaid plans purchase Medicare Part B for their ineligible (Part A) members as a cost-saving method. Part B has an annual deductible of $135, and any Part B service can be used to fulfill that deductible. The member also owes a 20% coinsurance payment for many Part B services. In general, Part B helps cover physician services, outpatient hospital care, diagnostic tests, radiology and pathology services (inpatient or outpatient), DME, home health services, physical/occupational/speech therapies, and limited chiropractic, podiatry, dentistry, and optometry services.

Like Medicare Part A, Part B will pay for 100% of approved home health services and 80% of DME, but not until after the $135 annual deductible is met. Kidney dialysis and kidney, liver, and heart transplantations may be partially covered under Part B when strict criteria are met.

Both Part A and Part B cover blood components such as red blood cells, platelets, and fresh-frozen plasma. Both sections of Medicare require the recipient to pay for any replacement costs on the first three units. This replacement fee is the amount charged for blood that is not replaced. The replacement fee criteria can be satisfied with use of either the Part A or Part B side.

Part A pays all costs from the fourth pint each calendar year. Part B pays for 80% starting with the fourth pint. The annual Part B deductible must also be met.

Tables 3.2 and 3.3 summarize the detailed list of insurance covered services in both Part A and Part B. These tables are based on 2008 figures. The Medicare system is not only complicated, but subject to changes in any year. Case managers may benefit from the most recent CMS publications accessible on their Web site at www.cms.hhs.gov.

NOTE

Centers for Medicare & Medicaid Services
6325 Security Boulevard
Baltimore, MD 21207-5187
Telephone: (410) 786-3000
Web site: www.cms.hhs.gov

MEDICATIONS AND HOME INFUSION PUMPS

Under certain circumstances, Medicare Part B pays for or helps to pay for:

▶ Antigens if they are ordered by a physician and administered by a properly instructed person (who could be the patient/family) under the supervision of a physician.

▶ **TABLE 3.2 Medicare (Part A): Hospital Insurance-Covered Services for 2008**

SERVICES	BENEFIT	MEDICARE PAYS	MEMBER PAYS
Hospitalization			
Semiprivate room and board, general nursing and other hospital services and supplies	First 60 days	All but $1,024/benefit period	$1,024
	Day 61 to 90	All but $256/day	$256/day
	Day 91 to 150[a]	All but $512/day	$512/day
	Beyond 150 days	Nothing	All costs
Skilled Nursing Facility Care			
Semiprivate room and board, general nursing, skilled nursing and rehabilitative services, and other services and supplies[b]	First 20 days	100% of approved amount	Nothing
	21–100 days	All but $128/day	Up to $128/day
	Beyond 100 days	Nothing	All costs
Hospice Care			
Part-time or intermittent skilled care, home health aid services, durable medical equipment, and supplies and other services	Unlimited as long as Medicare conditions are met	100% of approved amount; 80% of approved amount for durable medical equipment	Nothing for 20% of approved amount for durable medical equipment
Hospice Care			
Pain relief, symptom management, and services for the terminally ill	For as long as physician certifies need	All but limited costs for outpatient drugs and inpatient respite care	$5 copay per prescription for outpatient drugs and 5% of approved amount for inpatient respite care
Blood	Unlimited if medically necessary	80% of all but first 3 pints per calendar year	First 3 pints and 20% of all other pints[c]

From the Centers for Medicare & Medicaid Services (CMS). *Medicare and you, 2008.* [Online]. Available: www.medicare.gov.

Note: Medicare Advantage Plans cover these services. However, costs vary by plan and may be higher or lower than those stated above.

Most people do not pay Part A monthly premiums because they paid Medicare taxes while working. If not eligible for premium-free Medicare Part A hospital insurance, premium is $423/month, or more for those who must pay a surcharge for late enrollment.

[a] This 60-reserve-days benefit may be used only once in a lifetime.

[b] Neither Medicare nor private Medigap insurance will pay for most custodial care.

[c] Blood paid for or replaced under Part B of Medicare during the calendar year does not have to be paid for or replaced under Part A

▶ Erythropoietin if the patient has end-stage renal disease and is on dialysis, and requires it for treatment of anemia.
▶ Hemophilia clotting factors.
▶ Hepatitis B vaccine.
▶ Immunosuppressive drugs within 1 year of organ transplantations.
▶ Flu and pneumococcal pneumonia vaccines.
▶ Oral chemotherapy for cancer, if the same drug is available in injectable form.

In the 1990s, traditional Medicare approved a limited number of intravenous (IV) medications to be administered in the home setting, where previously no IV medications were covered in the home. Because the cost of the medications is so high, many otherwise independent patients had to be transferred to nursing homes, where IV medications are covered for long-term IV antibiotic regimens.

According to the Medicare Durable Medical Equipment Regional Center (DMERC) Guide, the criteria for home IV medications include use of an infusion pump and a prolonged infusion of at least 8 hours or infusion of the drug at a controlled rate to avoid toxicity. Another means of accomplishing the infusion is not acceptable or safe. The DME portion of the home health benefit covers approved supplies, drugs, and biologicals. These claims are subject to review on a case-by-case basis.

▶ **TABLE 3.3   MEDICARE (PART B): MEDICAL INSURANCE-COVERED SERVICES FOR 2008**

SERVICES	BENEFIT	MEDICARE PAYS	MEMBER PAYS
Medical Expenses			
Doctors' services, inpatient and outpatient medical and surgical services and supplies, physical and speech therapy, diagnostic tests, durable medical equipment, and other services	Unlimited if medically necessary	80% of approved amount (after $135 deductible); 50% of approved charges for most outpatient mental health services	$135 deductible,[a] plus 20% of approved amount and limited charges above approved amount
Clinical Laboratory Services			
Blood tests, urinalyses, and more	Unlimited if medically necessary	Generally 100% of approved amount	Nothing for services
Home Health Care			
Part-time or intermittent skilled care, home health aide services, durable medical equipment, and supplies and other services	Unlimited as long as you meet Medicare conditions	100% of approved amount; 80% of approved amount for durable medical equipment	Nothing for services; 20% of approved amount for durable medical equipment
Outpatient Hospital Treatment			
Services for the diagnosis or treatment of illness or injury	Unlimited if medically necessary	Medicare payment to hospital based on hospital cost	Copayment or coinsurance that varies by service (after $135 deductible)[a]
Ambulatory surgery	Unlimited if approved	100% of approved amount after deductible	Coinsurance applies as well as $135 deductible if was not yet satisfied
Blood	Unlimited if medically necessary	80% of approved amount (after $135 deductible and amount starting with 4th pint)	First 3 pints plus 20% of amount approved for additional pints (after $135 deductible[b])
Mental health	Unlimited if medically necessary	50% of approved amount (after $135 deductible[b])	50% of approved amount (after $135 deductible[b])
Ambulance services	If medically necessary	Approved amounts after $135 deductible	Coinsurance and $135 deductible apply

From the Centers for Medicare & Medicaid Services (CMS). *Medicare and you, 2008.* [Online]. Available: www.medicare.gov.

Note: Medicare Advantage Plans cover these services. However, costs vary by plan and may be higher or lower than those stated above.

In 2008, there were limits on physical therapy, occupational therapy, and speech-language pathology services. There also were exceptions to these limits. 2008 Part B monthly premium for a single individual starts at $96.40 (premium might be higher if you enrolled late).

[a] Once $135 of expenses for covered services in 2008 is spent, the Part B deductible does not apply to any further covered services received for the rest of the year.

[b] Blood paid for or replaced under Part A of Medicare during the calendar year does not have to be paid for or replaced under Part B.

External infusion pumps are covered for the following indications:

▶ Deferoxamine for the treatment of chronic iron overload.
▶ When treating primary hepatocellular carcinoma or colorectal cancer in cases in which this disease is unresectable or in which the patient refuses surgical excision of the tumor.

▶ For morphine when used in the treatment of intractable pain caused by cancer.

Some approved medications (with the above criteria) include:

▶ Administration of fluorouracil, cytarabine, bleomycin, doxorubicin, vincristine, or vinblastine by continuous infusion over at least 24 hours when the regimen is proven or generally accepted to have significant advantages over intermittent administration regimens.

▶ Administration of selected narcotic analgesics (in addition to morphine) for intractable pain not responding to, or if the patient cannot tolerate, other forms of pain control.

▶ The following antibiotics/antivirals: acyclovir, foscarnet, amphotericin B, vancomycin, and ganciclovir.

▶ Dobutamine if the individual meets *all* the following criteria:
 1. The individual is an accepted cardiac transplant candidate on an active status;
 2. Even with treatment of maximum doses of diuretics and angiotensin-converting enzyme inhibitor, along with a simultaneous administration of a vasodilator, the individual remains dyspneic on minimal exertion or at rest;
 3. Physiological response readings demonstrate an increase in cardiac output, an increase in left ventricular ejection fraction, and a decrease in the pulmonary wedge pressure;
 4. The documentation supports the deterioration in the client's condition when dobutamine is discontinued under observation in the hospital; *and*
 5. There is no need for intensive electrocardiograph monitoring in the patient's home and any life-threatening arrhythmia is controlled.

Note: The above information was obtained from the *Federal Medicare Intermediary* in Oxnard, California.

The home health agency called in to care for the patient can help the case manager in assessing which home IV medications are covered under Medicare. Most prescription medications are not covered under either part of Medicare. This is a real hardship for chronically ill persons on fixed incomes. Frequent readmissions should be assessed for "noncompliant patients" who are not taking their prescribed medications. The following reasons for noncompliance should be assessed:

▶ Can the patient afford the prescribed medications?

▶ Is the patient carefully doling out the medications, cutting the dose so the bottle will last longer?

▶ Some patients hoard old prescriptions for "emergency" use; the medications may be expired or the dosage may be too low or too high.

People with no pharmacologic insurance coverage should be assessed and possibly helped to acquire needed medicines.

MEDICARE ADVANTAGE PLANS (PART C)/ MEDICARE HEALTH PLAN CHOICES— TRADITIONAL AND MEDICARE MANAGED CARE

Medicare Advantage Plans (MAPs or MAs) are health plan options (like HMOs and PPOs), approved by Medicare and run by private companies. MAPs are not supplemental insurance and must follow rules set by Medicare. For several years Medicare risk contracts have offered prepaid, comprehensive health coverage to Medicare beneficiaries. Instead of paying hospitals the traditional DRG payment, these risk contracts are actually commercial, private, or managed care plans that contract with the CMS to provide services to Medicare beneficiaries for a fixed monthly payment paid by Medicare on behalf of the beneficiaries who opt to enroll in a MAP. The plan is "at risk" if the services needed are more costly than the fixed payment. From a member perspective, the out-of-pocket costs (coinsurance, copayment, and deductibles) may be different than traditional Medicare.

Services provided to enrollees include all of those offered under Medicare Part A and Part B; however, MAPs may offer additional services such as preventive and wellness care, dental care, hearing aids, and eyeglasses. They also include Medicare prescription drug coverage, usually for an extra cost. As in all managed care plans, MAPs have provider networks, services must be preapproved, and authorized care providers (individuals and facilities) must be used which may include a referral from a PCP to a specialist. If urgent care is required, it can be provided outside the plan's service area. Gatekeeper-style PCPs are generally required.

Case managers often have to coordinate care with the Medicare plan's case manager to coordinate for necessary services and discharge planning including posthospital services. These plans offer less freedom of choice in that the case manager must match the home health agency or SNF (for example) to the Medicare-contracted networks. Some advantages include more home IV medication coverage and added pharmacy and ancillary coverage for the patient.

The BBA required many stipulations that protect Medicare beneficiaries and changed Medicare forever. MAPs are intended to provide Medicare beneficiaries with a range of options for the financing and delivery of their healthcare. Under the MAP choices, beneficiaries may be able to choose from one of the following:

▶ Managed care plan, specifically an HMO, with or without a point of service (POS) option.

▶ PPO.

▶ Provider-sponsored organization (PSO).

▶ Medical savings account (MSA).

▶ Private fee-for-service (PFFS) insurance plan.

▶ Original "traditional" Medicare.

Generally and as a rule of thumb, the case manager must remember that under the MAP arrangement, beneficiaries are expected to receive at a minimum the same services they would otherwise have received under the original Medicare benefits program; they also have the same rights. The main case management/patient advocate role will be to assure the Medicare beneficiaries that CMS will work with them; the traditional fee-for-service plan is always an option, so they will not be left without healthcare services.

The BBA also provides Medicare beneficiaries with other benefits, including screening mammograms, screening Pap smears and pelvic examinations, colorectal cancer screening tests, prostate cancer screening tests, coverage for diabetic supplies and diabetic education (whether the beneficiary is insulin dependent or not), and procedures to identify bone mass/density or bone quality in certain at-risk patients. Flu and pneumococcal vaccine benefits will continue to be covered as well.

Emergency department care has come under scrutiny because many insurance plans have denied payment for emergency care when the medical problem turned out to be nonemergent. The BBA stipulates that under any chosen plan, coverage for care that a "prudent lay person" would consider to be an emergency must be considered and paid. In other words, if a patient was admitted to the emergency department with complaints of chest pain and it turned out to be a hiatal hernia (nonemergent), a prudent lay person would not have known that—the emergency department claim must be paid.

Medicare has paid managed care companies a fixed monthly amount per beneficiary, adjusted only by geographical area. To "level the playing field" for those health plans that care for frail and elderly Medicare beneficiaries, CMS has implemented a new payment method. Known as risk adjustment, this method reflects the health status of Medicare beneficiaries. It is hoped that this will lessen the incentive to enroll only the healthiest of the Medicare population. Risk adjustment looks at a person's diagnosis in 1 year and predicts how much, if any, additional cost there will be for that person the next year. If a Medicare beneficiary has an appendectomy one year, that will not likely increase costs; however, if the person has a major stroke, the plan would receive a larger payment-per-

month to cover expected expenses. These risk-adjusted payments began in January 2000 with a 10% incremental increase; they came into full effect in 2004. There are rules for this method of payment. For example, CMS is excluding hospital admission diagnoses that are rarely the principal reason for inpatient hospital care or that are vague or ambiguous; one-day hospitalizations are also excluded to reduce the incentive to increase marginal admissions.

MEDICARE PART D

Medicare offers prescription drug coverage for everyone with Medicare. This coverage is called Medicare Part D. A beneficiary is eligible to receive this benefit after joining a Medicare drug plan; such plans are usually run by insurance companies approved by Medicare. Plans vary in cost, based on options and drugs covered. If one does not take a lot of prescription drugs and opts not to join this benefit, he or she can join later on when drug expenses have increased and pay a required late-enrollment penalty fee.

There are two ways for a Medicare beneficiary to join a prescription drug plan: (1) join a Medicare Prescription Drug Plan, known as PDP, or (2) join a MAP, known as MA-PD. Everyone with Medicare benefits is eligible to join a Medicare drug plan. When a beneficiary joins a Medicare drug plan, he or she pays a separate monthly premium in addition to the original Medicare fees. Monthly premiums vary by plan; on average the 2008 premium was $27.93 per month. Late penalty fees are also charged if one does not join the drug plan during the annual enrollment period. However, if a person's needs change after joining a plan, one can switch to another plan that better meets his or her needs. MAPs that offer prescription drug coverage do not require additional monthly premiums for prescription drugs.

Medicare drug plans have a list of drugs covered by the plan, known as a "formulary." To access these, the patient's condition and need must always meet Medicare's requirement. There may be special rules for filling a prescription even if a drug is included in the formulary. The list of drugs may change at any time because of changes in therapies, the addition of new drugs, and the removal of others. If the formulary stops including a drug a person is taking, the drug plan must notify the individual at least 60 days in advance. In this case the individual may either change the drug to another on the list or may be required to pay more into the plan to continue taking the same drug.

Those who join Medicare drug plans also are responsible for a deductible and coinsurance or a copayment. These amounts are determined based on the tiers of drugs covered in the plan. An example of a plan's tiers is available in Table 3.4. After a person spends a certain amount of money for covered drugs (called the limit) he or she will have to pay all costs out of pocket. The amount varies by plan. This situation is called "coverage gap." The beneficiary will continue to pay the monthly premium even during the coverage gap. Each state offers at least one plan with some type of coverage during the gap. Plans with gap coverage may charge a higher monthly premium. Some may cover brand-name drugs only and may offer generic drug coverage during the gap. Some, even when they offer gap coverage, may not cover all the drugs.

Once a person reaches the limit set by the plan, he or she may get "catastrophic coverage." This is offered for persons with extremely high drug costs. Under such arrangements, the individual pays a coinsurance or copayment after spending no more than $4,050 for drugs covered. This amount is based on 2008 information and varies by plan. The coinsurance is about 5% of the drug cost and the copayment is between $2.25 and $5.60 for each prescription.

MEDIGAP PLANS

In July 1992, the federal government approved a list of 10 standardized insurance policies designed to supplement, or fill in the gaps of, original Medicare coverage. Today, there are 12 Medigap plans in use. These plans pay the deductibles, coinsurance, and other out-of-pocket expenses for healthcare services and supplies not covered by Medicare. Some Medigap policies cover extra benefits for an additional cost. Before these plans were standardized, Medicare beneficiaries had to choose among so many vague Medicare supplemental policies that often case managers would find that their patients had supplements that were both inadequate and duplicative; in some instances, patients

were unaware they had supplements. Although the federal government does not offer these policies (because they are private insurance policies), it does require strict adherence to guidelines. Both federal and state laws govern the sales of Medigap insurance. Insurers may not sell a policy that duplicates the member's present health plan or sell a policy that is not one of the approved standard policies. The premiums for these policies have increased tremendously over the past several years; for example, the 1998 premium went up as high as 13% over the 1997 amount. This is very difficult for beneficiaries with fixed incomes, and the consequence is that they are enrolling in the managed Medicare plans.

The 12 plans are identified by the letters A through L (Table 3.5). In Massachusetts, Minnesota, and Wisconsin, they are standardized in a different way. Each plan must include a core package of benefits. All 12 plans cover an additional 365 days of approved inpatient hospitalization after the long-term reserve days have been used (see "Medicare" section). These plans only work with the original Medicare plan and cannot be used to pay the copayments or deductibles for MAPs. In addition, all must be clearly identified as Medicare Supplemental Insurance.

The core benefits include the following:

▶ Part A hospital coinsurance, which equals $256 per day for days 61 to 90 and $512 per day for days 91 to 150 while using the 60 lifetime reserve days (CMS, 2008b).
▶ Part B coinsurance, which is 20% of Medicare approved charges after meeting the $135 yearly Part B deductible. Copayment is also in effect.
▶ First 3 pints of blood each year.
▶ Hospice care: $5 copay for each prescription drug while in the home setting and 5% of approved Medicare amount for each day of inpatient hospice care, up to certain limits.

▶ **TABLE 3.4 Tiers or Categories on a Medicare Drug Plan/Formulary (2008)**

TIER (FORMULARY)	YOU PAY	WHAT IS COVERED?
1	Lowest Copayment	Most Generic Prescription Drugs
2	Medium Copayment	Preferred,[a] Brand-name Prescription Drugs
3	Higher Copayment	Nonpreferred, Brand-name Prescription Drugs
Specialty Tier	Highest Copayment or Coinsurance	Unique, Very High-Cost

From the Centers for Medicare & Medicaid Services (CMS). *Medicare and you, 2008.* [Online]. Available: www.medicare.gov.

Note: Medicare Drug Plans place drugs into different tiers called formularies. Drugs in each tier have different costs. Some plans may have more tiers, some may have fewer.

[a] Preferred brand-name prescription drug is a drug that has been determined by the plan to be less costly, but as effective as other drugs.

▶ TABLE 3.5 Standard Medigap Policies (Plan A–L, 2008)

BENEFITS	PLANS											
	A	B	C	D	E	F[a]	G	H	I	J[a]	K[b]	L[c]
Core benefit (Basic)	X	X	X	X	X	X	X	X	X	X	X	X
Skilled nursing coinsurance			X	X	X	X	X	X	X	X	50%	75%
Hospice care											50%	75%
Coinsurance or copayment												
Blood (first 3 pints)	X	X	X	X	X	X	X	X	X	X	50%	75%
Part A Deductible		X	X	X	X	X	X	X	X	X	50%	75%
Part B Deductible			X			X				X		
Part A Coinsurance or copayment	X	X	X	X	X	X	X	X	X	X	X	X
Part B Coinsurance or copayment	X	X	X	X	X	X	X	X	X	X	50%	75%
Part B Excess charges						X	80%		X	X		
Foreign travel emergency[d]			X	X	X	X	X	X	X	X		
At-home recovery				X			X		X	X		
Preventive care coinsurance (included in Part B)	X	X	X	X	X	X	X	X	X	X	X	X
Preventive care not covered by Medicare (up to $120)					X					X		

From the Centers for Medicare & Medicaid Services (CMS). (2008). 2008 Choosing a Medigap policy: a guide to health insurance for people with Medicare. Baltimore, MD: Author.

a Medigap plans F and J also offer a high deductible option; $1,900 in 2008 before Medigap policy pays anything.
b Plan pays 100% of covered services after one meets out-of-pocket yearly limit ($4,440 in 2008) and yearly Part B deductible ($135 in 2008).
c Plan pays 100% of covered services after one meets out-of-pocket yearly limit ($2,220 in 2008) and yearly Part B deductible ($135 in 2008).
d Separate foreign travel emergency deductible applies ($250 per year in 2008).

The core benefits do not include such basics as the Part A inpatient deductible ($1,024 per benefit period in 2008) or the Part B deductible ($135 annually in 2008).

Medigap's Plan A covers only the core benefits. Plans B through L include the core benefits plus a menu of variable coverage. Of course, the more coverage, the higher the premium rate. Plan J includes eight benefits, which are as follows:

1. Basic (core) benefits.
2. Skilled nursing coinsurance—Nothing for first 20 days and up to $128 per day (in 2008) while in a SNF from day 21 to day 100.
3. Part A deductible—$1,024 per benefit period in 2008.
4. Part B deductible—$135 annually in 2008.
5. Part B excess charges: No more than 15% above the Medicare approved amount (for doctor's fees and other assigned Part B services).
6. Foreign travel emergencies.
7. At-home recovery—provides short-term assistance with various activities of daily living (ADLs) for members who are recovering from an episode of illness, injury, or surgery. Services may include a personal care aide, $0 for Medicare-approved home health services, and 100% coverage for services not covered by Medicare.
8. Preventive care—includes such services as vaccines, hearing tests, urinalysis, occult stool testing, serum cholesterol, thyroid function testing, and mammogram. A $135 Part B deductible for some benefits and all coinsurance; and all costs for preventive care not covered by Medicare.

The monthly premium for Medigap policies is set or rated in one of three ways:

1. Community-rated (also called no-age rated): The same monthly premium is charged to everyone who has the Medigap policy regardless of age. Premiums may go up because of inflation and other factors.
2. Issue-age-rated: The monthly premium is set based on the age the beneficiary is at the time a policy is purchased. Premiums are lower for people who buy a policy at a younger age, and will not change as the person gets older. However, premiums may go up because of inflation and other factors.
3. Attained-age-rated: The monthly premium is set based on the beneficiary's age at the time the policy is purchased; however, the premium increases as the person gets older. Premiums are low for younger buyers. This policy type may be least expensive at first, but may become the most expensive in later years. The premiums may also go up because of inflation and other factors.

In most cases, a beneficiary may not have the right under federal law to switch Medigap policies unless he or she is within the 6-month open enrollment period. Beneficiaries may switch between policies for reasons that include the following:

▶ You are paying for benefits you do not need.
▶ You need more benefits compared to your needs at the time you signed up.
▶ Your current Medigap policy has the right benefits, but you are unhappy with the insurance company.
▶ Your current Medigap policy has the right benefits, but you would like to find one that is less expensive.

MEDICARE SELECT

In some states, one may be able to buy another type of Medigap plan called Medicare SELECT. Medicare SELECT is a plan that supplements traditional Medicare; it allows the same choice of the 12 plans as any Medigap insurance supplement. The only difference is that Medicare SELECT requires the use of specific providers (hospitals and, in some cases, specific doctors) to receive full benefits. Emergent care may be out-of-network. The premiums are generally lower than the standard Medigap policies.

▶ Medicaid

Medicaid, like Medicare, is a federally funded healthcare program under Title XIX of the Social Security Act. Medicaid was enacted into law on July 20, 1964 and is part of the federal and state welfare systems. Before 1965, physicians and hospitals often gave out charity care or billed on a sliding-scale basis. Eligibility for Medicaid is based on income and/or various welfare categories such as AFDC. Generally speaking, Medicaid provides medical benefits to groups of low-income people and some who may have no or inadequate medical insurance. Although the federal government establishes the general guidelines for the program, Medicaid requirements are actually established by each state. Whether a person is eligible for Medicaid depends on the state where he or she lives. Some states may include people in the Medicaid program other than those specified in the federal guidelines.

Many Medicare recipients also financially qualify for Medicaid. If a patient has both Medicare and Medicaid, a supplemental policy may be redundant. The Medicaid portion will cover all Medicare deductibles, coinsurance, medically necessary care, and prescription medications. Home IV medications may also be covered under this insurance arrangement.

The member with only Medicaid generally has no premiums, deductibles, or coinsurance costs. Prescription drugs are paid for, although some states have a "negative formulary list," which excludes some medications and substitutes others. Some states may also require a small out-of-pocket charge for doctor visits or prescriptions; this is rarely enforced.

Medicaid programs are subject to state regulatory agencies; therefore, wide variations in coverage and eligibility exist among the different states. Title XIX of the Social Security Act mandates certain basic health services. Each state, however, may determine the scope of services offered or may offer optional services such as clinic services and dental or optometry services.

MEDICAID ELIGIBILITY

The following are some of the categories that allow Medicaid eligibility. To be categorically eligible, individuals must fit into a category that makes them eligible according to Title XIX (Medicaid) of the Social Security Act. Recipients of Social Security Income (SSI) and those who qualify for AFDC are automatically eligible for Medicaid.

▶ Medical assistance only (MAO): a special category of Medicaid recipients under AFDC or SSI who receive only Medicaid benefits and not financial assistance.
▶ Medically needy/medically indigent (MN/MI): a category of Medicaid recipients in which Medicaid receives funds only from country and state treasuries. Other categories may also receive matched federal funds.
▶ Sixth Omnibus Budget Reconciliation Act (SOBRA): one of Medicaid's maternal and child health reforms that was passed by Congress and became effective in 1987. Pregnant women and children with family incomes at or below the poverty level become eligible for Medicaid.
▶ Persons with specific medical conditions that states may include under Medicaid plans: one is a time-limited eligibility group for women who have breast or cervical cancer; the other is for people with tuberculosis (TB) who are

uninsured. The first group receives all services; TB patients receive only services related to the treatment of TB.

Blind and disabled persons who also receive SSI, and persons in certain other specifically defined categories, are also eligible for Medicaid. If a case manager has a patient who may qualify for Medicaid, he or she will work with the patient to complete a Medicaid application and coordinate the process for seeking eligibility for Medicaid benefits. Most large hospitals and Department of Economic Security (DES) or Social Security Administration offices have eligibility workers that assist in the processing and review of such applications. These are employees of a county, DES, or Social Security, whose job is to determine eligibility for Medicaid through interviews and assessment of medical and financial data. Social workers are another valuable source with whom case managers can work closely to coordinate the application process.

Some core Medicaid benefits include the following:

▶ Hospital inpatient care.
▶ Hospital outpatient services.
▶ Pregnancy-related services including prenatal care and services for other conditions that might complicate pregnancy. This also includes 60 days of postpartum pregnancy-related services.
▶ Laboratory and radiography services.
▶ SNF care for persons 21 years of age and older.
▶ Home health services for those who meet home care criteria. This includes home health aides, medical supplies, and appliances for use in the home.
▶ Physician services.
▶ Family planning services and supplies.
▶ Certified pediatric and family nurse practitioners (when licensed to practice under state law).
▶ Rural health clinic services.
▶ Medical and surgical services of a dentist.
▶ Early and periodic screening, diagnosis, and treatment (EPSDT) for persons younger than 21 years of age.
▶ Nurse-midwife services.
▶ Certain federally qualified ambulatory and health center services.

The vagueness of some covered Medicaid services means that the case manager may be able to negotiate resources for the patient. If services requested are in lieu of hospitalization or an SNF placement or are necessary for patient safety, the Medicaid plan may choose to accommodate the request. Because of budget cuts, however, fewer nonemergent services are being provided. This makes the patient advocacy role of the case manager even more critical when it comes to planning safe and adequate discharges.

Some Medicaid plans do not cover services such as inpatient drug or alcohol programs. The case manager and social worker may be limited to community programs, which might be free or may charge on a sliding-fee scale. A baseline knowledge of what your state's Medicaid coverage includes can save the case manager, from assessment of time-consuming plans that will not be approved.

Medicaid began as a fee-for-service program in the 1960s. Currently, all states have changed to some form of Medicaid managed care, using capitated payments or per diem rates as a primary method of reimbursement. In Arizona, for example, the state's Medicaid plan (Arizona Health Care Cost Containment System; AHCCCS) pays hospitals on a per diem basis. As an example, the medical patient receives approximately $750 per day for care in the hospital. Magnetic resonance imaging (MRI) uses up most of that, but also included in the per diem rate is all care from laboratory tests to radiology to nurses. Because hospital patients are so ill, it is easy to see that for many multi-system-failure patients who need resource-intensive care, this rate will be inadequate. Tight utilization of resources is important. The challenge is providing medically necessary care to ill patients while striving for a fiscally healthy institution—all within the confines of a Medicaid per diem rate.

▶ Tricare

Tricare, formerly known as the Civilian Health and Medical Program of the Uniformed Services (CHAMPUS), is a program of medical benefits for covered military personnel and eligible family members or survivors. By strict definition, Tricare is not an insurance program. It does not involve a contract guaranteeing medical coverage in exchange for a premium, and it is not subject to the state regulatory agencies that cover most insurance plans. Tricare is provided for by U.S. governmental funds, which are appropriated through Congress. Medically necessary and certain psychologically necessary services are covered and are detailed in the U.S. Department of Defense directive (Kongstvedt, 2003). Benefits under Tricare are equivalent to high-option plans of the public sector.

Because of Tricare's historical generosity to its members, expenditures and claims have doubled since 1985. Reform initiatives are changing the face of Tricare, and now some Tricare programs strongly resemble HMOs and PPOs; like Medicare, they reimburse

hospitals at a DRG rate. Tricare reform has created two major channels:

1. The indemnity option: TRICARE standard is most expensive to the beneficiary but provides the most freedom.
2. The managed care options: TRICARE Extra (the PPO option) and TRICARE Prime (the HMO option).

▶ Workers' Compensation

Workers' compensation laws began in 1908 by federal statute. The first state to enact the law was New York in 1914, in response to a factory fire in which 146 women died. Mississippi was the last state to enact the law, doing so in 1950. Workers' compensation is compulsory in most states and is designed to provide compensation and medical benefits if an employee is hurt or becomes disabled while on the job. Workers' compensation laws and programs have been implemented not only in all states, but in U.S. territories as well.

Three types of benefits are provided, although the scope is mandated by individual states.

1. Indemnity cash benefits in lieu of lost wages.
2. Reimbursement for necessary medical expenses.
3. Survivors' death benefits.

Workers' compensation, like all facets of the healthcare industry, is a victim of a system out of control. In 1992, workers' compensation claims reached an estimated $70 billion. That is triple the benefit figure of 1980 (InterQual, Inc., 1993). In 2000, workers' compensation programs incurred costs in claims for 126.5 million workers (NASI, 2002). It is reported that, on average, each claim costs about $19,000. To offset the spiraling costs, recent changes have been implemented, including adaptations of PPOs, HMOs, hospital utilization review, and case management. These types of managed care modalities will continue to grow rapidly; they have already proven effective in reducing LOS and even avoiding medically unnecessary acute care admissions.

Workers' compensation claims frequently involve trauma, repetitive motion, or neuromuscular impairment. There is a growing trend toward alleged soft tissue claims with nonspecific diagnoses. These claims pose a challenge from the utilization review perspective because they often lack objective physical findings. From a patient advocate perspective, an admitting diagnosis of severe back pain (especially without positive test results) often opens up these patients to denials of insurance-covered hospitalizations and even judgmental attitudes among hospital staff. Yet, as healthcare providers such as nurses (who are especially prone to back injuries) know, the most painful sprains, muscle spasms, and pinched nerves do not show up on scans, but can lead to inability to work and frequent reinjuries. Often the patient needs reassurance that care is necessary and that it can be provided for at a different level of care (i.e., it does not always need to be done in the hospital). The primary goal of workers' compensation is for the patient to return to work.

▶ Indemnity Plans

Indemnity plans are the traditional plans used before the days of managed care. Although they now use some managed care concepts such as prehospital certification and catastrophic case management, indemnity plans still offer the most flexibility (Kongstvedt, 2003); virtually any hospital or doctor can be chosen by the member. Monthly premiums are generally higher for this freedom, and other out-of-pocket expenses may include deductibles and a percentage of the bills (usually 20%) up to a ceiling of $500 to $5,000 per year. As with all insurance companies, the case manager needs to know the specific types of allowable coverage and possible patient costs to formulate a workable discharge plan. Indemnity plans often cover behavioral health and alcohol and drug detoxification treatment, both inpatient and outpatient, within certain limited time frames and dollar amounts. Indemnity plans, by their very nature, do not require tight control of utilization. In fact, the incentive may be to use up services and resources; it is this type of insurance planning that has been blamed for the necessity for managed care.

▶ Managed Indemnity Plans

As an evolution of the old indemnity plans, managed indemnity plans (MIPs) use utilization management strategies such as hospital preadmission screening, authorization for services to be rendered, concurrent review, second surgical opinions, outpatient procedure services review, and case management. They keep the traditional indemnity approach of members' freedom of choice of physicians/providers and fee-for-service payment to these providers.

▶ Managed Care Organization

Managed care organization (MCO) is a generic term that applies to managed care health plans. These plans have programs that include utilization management modalities: authorization for services, preadmission, concurrent and retrospective review programs, case management, referral management, utilization reporting and evaluation programs, and provider incentive programs. MCOs also focus on quality assurance activities, such as credentialing, quality assessment studies, and peer review. The evolution of healthcare is toward some variation of MCO, such as HMOs, PPOs, and POS plans (Kongstvedt, 2003).

▶ Health Maintenance Organizations

In its purest form, an HMO is nearly synonymous with managed care; a member must go through the chosen PCP who acts as a gatekeeper for any needed services (Kongstvedt, 2003). Only HMO-contracted facilities and physicians are allowed. Members who use unauthorized doctors or facilities are usually placing themselves at risk for being required to pay for services rendered. Limited psychiatric and dental care and limited coverage when traveling are other disadvantages.

HMOs have potentially the least expensive premiums, often with no or low deductibles, coinsurance, or claim forms. Some copayments at the time of service may be expected. Physicians and other healthcare professionals are paid for through capitation, thereby sharing the risk of financing the healthcare services for the enrolled population. If the provider incurs expenses exceeding budgeted cost, they would be required to absorb those excesses, not the member.

HMO MODELS

There are five models of HMOs: staff model, group model, independent practice association (IPA), network model, and the direct contract model. The relationship between the HMO and the physicians distinguishes the various models.

1. Staff model: In this model, the HMO employs the physicians who work in HMO clinic-type settings (exclusively) for salaries. This model is considered the most cost-effective but also the most restrictive.
2. Group model: Here, the HMO contracts with multispecialty physician groups. These groups provide all services to the HMO's members. The members' choice of providers is wider in this model.
3. IPA: IPA model HMOs recruit physicians from all specialties to care for their HMO members. These physicians are also free to service non-HMO patients, if desired. The IPA is paid on a capitation (per member per month) basis by the HMO, and the physicians are in turn paid in either a fee-for-service or capitated manner.
4. Network model: This model combines elements of the staff, group, and IPA styles. The HMO

contracts with more than one group practice. The group practices tend to be located in various locations to allow access to services in the various regions where the members reside.

5. Direct contract model: In this model, the HMO contracts directly with the physician, rather than through an intermediary such as an IPA. The gatekeeper approach is common in this model. Fee-for-service or capitation is the reimbursement method, although capitation is the preferred method because it limits financial risk for the HMO and places it on the care provider side.

PRIMARY CARE PHYSICIAN

The PCP is the main physician assigned to a member of a healthcare plan. This physician tends to be a generalist, a family practitioner, or a pediatrician. HMO-style insurance companies use PCPs in a gatekeeper role (see below). Members of these types of health plans are expected to go through the PCP before accessing other providers of care such as specialists; that is, require a referral from the PCP.

SPECIALIST CARE PROVIDER

The specialist care provider (SCP) is a physician specializing in a particular area of health care such as cardiology, digestive diseases, or neurology. Health plan members may not be able to access the SCP without a referral from the PCP.

GATEKEEPER

The gatekeeper concept is an important one in the world of managed care. *Gatekeeper* is an informal term used to define the role of the PCP. Essentially, the PCP stands at the gate of available medical services and decides which services each member requires. The gatekeeper is responsible for the basic medical care of the patient and also determines when that member needs laboratory tests, radiographs, a specialist, or virtually anything medicine has to offer including referral to a SCP. True emergencies are excluded when members may be served in emergency departments. The gatekeeper concept is a predominant characteristic of HMOs.

Although the gatekeeper concept can be an excellent method to manage escalating healthcare costs, it can also become a barrier to access of specialty services. Depending on a physician's practice patterns and financial incentives, the PCP may under-refer or over-refer to various specialists or services.

❱ Preferred Provider Organizations (PPO)/ Preferred Provider Arrangements (PPA)

The PPO/PPA model falls somewhere between an HMO and an indemnity plan. PPOs use a preferred panel of physicians who have been selected because of their cost-efficient and quality care (Kongstvedt, 2003). The member has a monthly premium, a deductible, and often a 10% to 20% coinsurance up to a specific ceiling of about $500 to $2,000 per year. The premium is higher than that in HMO arrangements. A major advantage for some members is the ability to use doctors who are not in the plan, but reimbursement is at a lower rate (i.e., more out-of-pocket for the member). This is important to some people who hesitate to choose an HMO because HMOs do not pay at all if outside facilities or physicians are used. In many PPOs, members are encouraged, but not obligated, to use the gatekeeper PCP concept. Medicare beneficiaries are being offered HMO and PPO options. Medicare pays more for contracted providers; however, noncontracted providers may be used although a higher out-of-pocket expense is incurred.

❱ Point of Service (POS)

POS plans combine elements of an HMO model and an indemnity plan. The member does not have to choose how to receive services up front; when a service is needed, the member may choose to stay in the plan or use outside providers (Kongstvedt, 2003). Significant differences in out-of-pocket expenses for the member may apply (e.g., 100% compared with 60%). The physicians may be reimbursed through capitation or performance-based methods and may act as gatekeepers. POS plans were hybrids of HMOs mainly in response to a market that clearly wanted freedom of choice to pick a well-known specialist if the need should arise.

❱ Provider-Sponsored Organizations (PSO)

PSOs are a form of managed care and are similar to HMOs. The difference is that PSOs are formed by a group of hospitals and physicians who directly take on the financial risk of providing comprehensive health benefits for Medicare (and other) beneficiaries. These types of arrangements are less common today than in the 1990s.

❱ Private Fee-for-Service

Private fee-for-service is an option for Medicare beneficiaries that was established in 1999. Beneficiaries may elect a private indemnity-type insurance plan. The insurance plan, rather than the Medicare program, decides how much to reimburse for services provided. Medicare pays the private plan a premium to cover traditional Medicare benefits. Providers are allowed to bill beyond what the plan pays (up to a limit), and the beneficiary is responsible for paying whatever the plan does not cover. The beneficiary may also be responsible for additional premiums.

❱ Physician Hospital Organizations (PHO)

The PHO model bonds a hospital with the attending physician staff for the purpose of linking with a managed care plan (Kongstvedt, 2003). Like IPAs, PHOs have their own internal political structure and therefore can define on their own terms what is high quality or cost effective. Some PHOs use outside utilization review firms; such arrangements allow some degree of objectivity. Similar to PSOs, PHOs were more popular in the 1990s.

❱ Medical Savings Accounts

In the late 1990s, the U.S. Congress authorized up to 390,000 Medicare beneficiaries to participate in an MSA demonstration project. This option is not as popular today. The plan works in the following manner. The beneficiary chooses a Medicare MSA plan—a health insurance policy with a high deductible. Medicare pays the premium for the MSA plan and makes a deposit into the Medicare MSA that is established by the beneficiary. The beneficiary uses the money in the Medicare MSA to pay for services provided before the deductible is met and for other services not covered by the MSA plan. Unlike other Medicare plans, there are no limits on what providers can charge above the amount paid by the Medicare MSA plan. In addition, individuals who enroll in MSAs are locked in for the entire year.

❱ Long-Term Care (LTC)

In some ways, long-term care becomes one of the biggest challenges for the case manager. Although an increasing number of people are buying private LTC insurance policies, and most states have coverage for poor, chronically ill patients, there are often waiting periods of up to 3 months for all the paperwork to be approved and placement in LTC facilities to commence. Sometimes families can manage in the interim. Often, this is a time of frequent readmissions into the acute care setting. Medicare, Medicaid, and most private insurance will pay for short stays in a nursing home for skilled care. A case manager can assess patients for a possible need of greater than 3 weeks of nursing home care or a probable deterioration of the

patient's condition with little chance of recovery. It is vital to start LTC paperwork quickly; early, careful assessment of postdischarge needs (sometimes with a "plan B" in mind) is also essential. Custodial care needs, as well as skilled needs, are assessed. Many LTC programs have home-based and SNF-based support. Family support and available respite can be assessed for possible home-based LTC placement. A case manager who is familiar with the eligibility requirements and enrollment process of their state's LTC program will be better prepared to meet these challenging situations.

Some types of private LTC insurance policies are referred to as "tax qualified long-term care insurance contracts." They provide federal income tax advantages. Patients should contact their state insurance counseling office and tax advisor if considering one of these policies. Another consideration is that not all nursing facilities accept all types of contracts. The contract must be matched to the desired placement.

❱ Other Weird Arrangement

The acronym OWA (for other weird arrangement) applies to any new, nonconforming, or hybrid managed care plan that provides a new twist (Kongstvedt, 2003).

NOTE

Two good resources for long-term care and nursing home placement are:

A Shopper's Guide to Long-Term Care Insurance
National Association of Insurance Commissioners (NAIC)
120 W. 12th Street, Suite 1100
Kansas City, MO 64105-1925
Guide to Choosing a Nursing Home
Centers for Medicare & Medicaid Services
Medicare Hotline: (800) 638-6833

❱ Self-Funded Employer Health Insurance Plans

In 1974, the **Employee Retirement Income Security Act (ERISA)** created laws that govern the health plans of employees. The intent was that when a large employer or union group crossed state lines, they would not have to comply with conflicting individual state laws; rather, ERISA laws would apply. For example, ERISA plans cannot be forced to comply with various state rules that cover COB; they must comply with federal regulations instead.

In self-funded plans, the organization often hires a third-party administrator to handle claims, utilization management, and case management activities. Claims are often handled by a separate company than the one handling utilization and case management. This lends an extra level of protection to the employees, with the independent opinion of the utilization and case managers. These independent utilization/case management firms hire and train expert personnel and retain large panels of specialists for second opinions, determinations of medical necessity in tough circumstances, and during the appeals process. Case managers may also be internally hired by the self-funded plan; however, if the employee is well-known to the company, the element of objectivity may be threatened. Self-funded plans usually have stop loss carriers that protect the fund in catastrophic cases. These stop loss amounts can range from $25,000 to $100,000 or more depending on the fund amount, number of employers, past claims, and other factors.

▶ Viatical Settlements

Viatical settlements, or living benefits, are not classified as an insurance product. Rather, they involve selling one's life insurance policy to a third party before one's death. The funds can then be used to improve the quality of the last weeks, months, or even years of the individual's life. This process can be better explained by an example.

> Mr. A had a rare type of aggressive cancer and a rare type of health insurance coverage, whereby he must work at least 30 hours per week or lose his benefits. Another option would be to pay approximately $370 per month for continued coverage. His financial situation did not allow Mr. A the luxury of quitting work; his basic food and rent needs would not be met, and he certainly did not have an extra $370 per month. Although in hospice care, he continued to go to work and put in 30 hours per week. There came a time when he was so weak and exhausted that family and friends had to drive him to and from his job. His last days were being spent working to pay bills and continue to qualify for health insurance coverage. He had a small life insurance policy that was sold as a viatical settlement; that act helped him to die with dignity.

Viatical settlements allow the policy holder, rather than the beneficiary(s), to benefit from life insurance policies. The term comes from the Latin word, *viaticum,* which means "provisions for a journey." To *viaticate* means to sell a life insurance policy; the *viator* is the seller of the life insurance policy. There are some serious considerations that case managers should be aware of if viatical settlements are a potential option for a patient.

▶ When the seller of the policy accepts an offer, all persons listed as beneficiaries must sign a release to waive any current and future rights to the policy. In reality, there are obvious reasons that this may be a touchy subject, ranging from greed to need.

▶ Viatical settlements take at least 4 to 6 weeks for completion. There must be time or the effort will be wasted.

▶ There may be tax ramifications. The Health Insurance Portability and Accountability Act (HIPAA) of 1996 allows that individuals with a life expectancy of 24 months or less can sell their life insurance policy tax free if the viatical settlement company complies with specific licensing and regulatory requirements; however, the settlement may be subject to state and local taxes.

▶ Additional funds can sometimes jeopardize the patient's current assistance, such as Medicaid or other public assistance programs. The settlement may cause the patient to lose important benefits.

▶ The policy is usually sold for between 40% and 90% of the face value, depending on several circumstances. Life expectancy is the main issue; if a patient is expected to live less than 6 months, the settlement will be closer to the 90% range.

NOTE

Viatical Settlement Resources:

Viatical Association of America
1200 19th Street, NW—Suite 300
Washington, DC 20036
Telephone: (800) 842-9811 or (202) 429-5129
Web site: www.viatical.org\viatical

National Viatical Association
1200 G Street, NW—Suite 760
Washington, DC 20005
Telephone: (800) 741-9465
Fax: (202) 393-0336
Web site: www.nationalviatical.org

▌ The case manager should suggest a financial planner for assistance. There are often other options such as accelerated death benefits on selected plans.

▌ Not all states have licensing requirements at this time for viatical settlement companies. The case manager should call the Viatical Association of America or the National Viatical Association for licensed companies.

▌ Some policies contain a rescission clause of 15 to 30 days, to allow for a change of mind.

▌ INSURANCE PLAYERS

▌ Third-Party Payor

In this arrangement, the two primary parties are the patient and the payor. The third party is the payor of the medical care that is provided to the patient. This is usually a private insurance carrier, prepayment plan, employer, or government agency.

▌ Claims Administrators

This group reviews insurance claims to determine whether to pay claims to enrollees, physicians, hospitals, or others on behalf of the health benefit plan. Many case managers must work with claims personnel to determine what benefits a patient is allowed and how much of the benefit the patient has used. However, claims data are usually not current, so the case manager may get only a general idea of how much of the benefit has been exhausted.

▌ Reinsurance/Stop Loss Personnel

Case managers may work with carriers for reinsurance (previously discussed in this chapter). Experience has determined that once a patient reaches stop loss, some companies want the stop loss carrier case manager to take over the case. However, this is not always the situation, especially if the current case manager has a good relationship with the patient/family and especially if there may be legal ramifications in the case. Understanding of the procedures of stop loss insurance by the case manager is essential for effective management of benefits and coordination of care and services.

▌ Employer Groups

When an employer group self-funds its insurance benefits, the case manager may be working with a benefits specialist in the group. This contact is crucial for the case manager, as everything from authorization for case management services to special benefits may be obtained through this person. One other "level" of contact may be the healthcare consultant that the employer group uses to develop the self-funded plan. For very tough situations, the case manager may have to go "all the way up" to the consultant for answers. These people may, in turn, have to consult the company's board for the answer.

▌ BILLING-RELATED TERMS

▌ Current Procedural Terminology

Current Procedural Terminology (CPT) codes list procedures and services and differentiate them with a five-digit number. These codes function as a record of physician utilization practices by HMOs (and other insurance companies/benefit programs) and are useful for billing purposes. The American Medical Association revises and publishes *CPT* annually.

▌ International Classification of Diseases

International Classification of Diseases, 9th revision–*Clinical Modifications* (ICD–9) (formerly called ICD–9–CM) and ICD–10 are the most widely used classifications of diseases in the world. These alphanumeric codes are used by hospitals and other providers when reporting diagnostic and treatment information about members of federally funded programs such as Medicare, Medicaid, and Maternal and Child Health. All third-party payors are required to submit ICD codes for billing purposes. When a claim is submitted, it usually includes primary and secondary ICD codes reflective of diagnostic and treatment categories/procedures.

▌ Fee Schedule

A fee schedule consists of a listing of fee allowances for specific procedures or services that a health plan will reimburse.

▌ Global Fee

Global fee is a predetermined all-inclusive fee for a specific set of related services, treated as a single unit for billing or reimbursement purposes.

▌ Withhold

Withhold is a portion of payments to a provider held by the managed care company until year end. This amount is not returned to the provider unless certain targets are achieved. Typically, withhold is used by managed care companies to curtail costs such as utilization of services rates including referrals to SCPs, use of ancillary services (e.g., lab and radiology expenses), and emergency department visits.

▶ IMPORTANT MISCELLANEOUS ORGANIZATIONS AND TERMS

▶ The Joint Commission

The Joint Commission (TJC), formerly known as the Joint Commission on Accreditation of Healthcare Organizations (JCAHO), is a private organization founded in 1951. It establishes quality standards and surveys hospitals, nursing homes, home care agencies, and other outpatient facilities to accredit the facilities. Accredited facilities are deemed to meet the U.S. Department of Health and Human Services certification requirements. It is hoped that the accreditation process encourages the facility to maintain the highest quality, safety, and performance levels. TJC accreditation is necessary for hospitals and other facilities to be eligible to receive reimbursement from Medicare and other health plans.

▶ Grievance

Grievance is a term that refers to the complaint process that can occur when an adverse action, outcome, decision, or policy is challenged. A member can file a grievance for any number of reasons, such as a physician complaint, denial of a medical claim or service, denial of a piece of equipment, or a poor hospital outcome. A hospital or other facility may file a grievance for a denial of a claim it felt was medically justified.

▶ Management Information System

Management information system (MIS) is the computer term for hardware and software that provides support for managing health plans, including case management.

▶ Office of Prepaid Health Care Operations and Oversight

The Office of Prepaid Health Care Operations and Oversight (OPCOO), a federal agency that is part of the CMS, oversees eligibility and compliance of HMOs and competitive medical plans (CMPs).

▶ Clinical Data Abstraction Centers

Clinical data abstraction centers (CDACs) are data collection firms contracted by CMS. These centers are expected to collect clinical data from medical record reviews of a large national sample of patients' records; millions of records are reviewed. The data gathered are then analyzed by the Medicare QIOs to identify areas of care for quality improvement projects.

▶ Notch Group

The term *notch group* refers to the portion of the U.S. population whose annual income is too low to afford medical insurance premiums but too high to be eligible for Medicaid programs. This concept seems innocuous enough, but a staggering statistic is attached to it: according to the Census Bureau in 2007, more than 45 million Americans are uninsured.

▶ Days per Thousand

Days per thousand is a measurement commonly used by insurance companies that states the average number of hospital days used per year for each 1,000 members (Kongstvedt, 2003). This is a measure of healthcare utilization that MCOs tend to track over time. Other measures include average cost per case and average number of visits to the emergency department per 1,000 members.

▶ MANAGED CARE CONTRACTS

Healthcare providers (individuals and organizations) have been engaging in managed care contracts (MCCs) since the inception of MCOs. The impetus for establishing a managed care contract may originate from either the MCO or the provider. Such arrangements assist the MCO in reducing the costs of healthcare services and the provider in securing new or maintaining old business. Issues that are negotiated in an MCC are numerous. Display 3-1 lists the major issues that

---

display 3-1

▼ GENERAL ISSUES FOR NEGOTIATION IN A MANAGED CARE CONTRACT

1. Scope of services to be provided to the covered population.
2. Services to be excluded or carved out from the contract.
3. Agreements with other providers, especially those across the continuum of care and settings.
4. Payment methodology and reimbursement rates including withhold and incentives.
5. Administrative procedures.
6. Claims filing and management process.
7. Marketing arrangements.
8. Legal issues such as settlement of disputes.
9. Denials and appeal rights and procedures for handling these.
10. Utilization review and management procedures including referrals and areas of noncoverage.
11. Quality management and reporting procedures.

are discussed and agreed on in the contract. Some of these issues have a direct impact on the provider's case management program including the role of the case manager; others impact the MCO's case management program and the payor-based case manager.

The team involved in negotiating a MCC consists of representatives from both sides: the provider and the MCO. These include senior administrators/executives, finance, case management, quality, accounts payable, marketing, and legal counsel. Some organizations include clinicians on an ad hoc basis; others may exclude case management. In any case, consulting with clinicians and including case management as a permanent member of the negotiation team is essential, especially because most of the procedures to be agreed on impact the role of the case manager. Examples are utilization review and management procedures and denials and appeals management processes. Clinicians' feedback on the scope of services being agreed on in the MCC is also important to make sure that the provider will be able to meet the scope of services expectations and that what is agreed on does not place the provider at risk for noncompliance or any cost inefficiencies. Examples of issues that impact the practice of clinicians are the pattern of referrals by primary care providers to specialist care providers and noncoverage of certain treatments or procedures. A rule of thumb for the effective management of MCCs is "approach the negotiation as a system; that is, include representatives from administration, finance, quality, and clinicians."

During the negotiation period (usually occurring over a series of meetings) both parties share important information about themselves. This exchange of information tends to be covered under HIPAA agreements. Privacy and confidentiality are maintained and a HIPAA agreement is executed before such exchange takes place. Information the provider of care shares includes a general description of the organization, availability and type of services, costs of care, discharge planning, utilization review and case management procedures, staffing, and quality of care and patient safety programs.

Information shared by the MCO also includes a description of the organization, the number of the enrollees or covered lives (the population being contracted), demographics of the population and its historical healthcare utilization data, costs of care, desired goals of the MCC, utilization review procedures including denials and appeals processes, reimbursement arrangement, and measures of quality of care. Once the exchange of information has occurred, negotiation commences. During the negotiation process, issues are identified, prioritized, and discussed, and resolutions are achieved.

▶ Implications for Case Management Practice

There are certain areas in the MCC that have a direct impact on the case management department and the role of the case manager. These include the scope of services to be provided to the population, agreements with other providers across the continuum of care and settings, utilization review procedures including denials and appeals, compensation for case management services, and quality/outcomes measurement. These issues have a great impact on the daily operations of case managers. For example, knowing the services to be furnished to the covered lives informs the case manager whether outpatient and ancillary services are included and allows the case manager to manage the follow-up visits and cost of services more effectively.

Arrangements with other providers across the continuum of care provides the case manager with information about how to manage referrals between one provider and another and how to arrange for posthospital discharge services (e.g., home care, rehabilitation, and transportation services). Lack of such arrangements may impact negatively on the provider's performance; that is, the provider may incur increased costs due to prolonged length of hospital stay and overutilization of acute care services.

Information about the utilization review procedures allows the case manager to better meet the MCO's expectations in the areas of preadmission reviews, authorization of services, concurrent and care progress reviews, and the appeal process in case of denial or services. As for compensation for case management services, if offered, it helps the provider to offset the expense needed to enhance its case management program to meet the demands of the negotiated managed care contract. Not every MCO or MCC offers compensation for case management services. If offered, it is usually a specific amount per month, calculated based on the size of the population.

In the area of quality and outcomes measurement, knowledge of the metrics the MCO uses to measure provider's performance is important for proactive management of these outcomes. Some of these metrics may directly impact the role of the case manager. For example, timeliness of preadmission reviews, authorization of services, and referral patterns are measures the case managers can impact greatly and influence not only adherence to procedures, but achievement of desired performance as well.

Every MCC includes provisions and stipulations that impact the role of the case manager, including decision making (whether clinical or operations in nature) and daily case management activities (whether utilization review or resource allocation related). Involving the case management department in contract negotiation allows a provider to negotiate more desirable contract, reduce risk, and increase its chances to meet the demands of the contract successfully. After all, the case manager is the key member in an organization that will allow the provider organization to meet the demands of the negotiated contract.

❭ THE FUTURE

Future changes to the face of healthcare leave the possibility of wide revisions on many types of medical insurance. Even Medicare—almost a part of American tradition—is dramatically changing in an effort to lower its budget by several million dollars. Many visions of future healthcare have been proposed. Although the first major attempt at national health reform in the 1990s was unsuccessful, one thing is certain: the cost of healthcare is high and rising rapidly, and change is still sorely needed to cover the needs of millions of uninsured Americans. The crystal ball has not revealed the final answer, but one probability looms large: that case managers, in grass roots fashion and on a case-by-case basis, will continue to make an impact on the high cost of health services and to help ensure quality, cost-effective care in the bargain.

STUDY QUESTIONS

1. What health insurance plan do you personally have? What type is it? How does it compare to those cited in this chapter?

2. How do Medicare and Medicaid benefits compare and contrast?

3. How many reimbursement structures for healthcare services are there? What are they? Are they available in every state? Which one presents more risk for the payor? For the provider? For the patient?

4. Is a Medicare beneficiary better off enrolling in a Medicare Advantage Plan or a Medigap plan? What are some of the reasons for your decision?

5. Under what circumstances should someone be advised to switch his or her Medigap policy?

6. What do you think of the withhold concept? Who benefits the most from it? How does it affect the consumer of healthcare services?

7. What can a case manager do to assist a patient in understanding his or her health benefits?

8. What role can a case manager play in effectively implementing the managed care contract in which the healthcare institution is participating? What is the rationale of each of these activities?

❭ REFERENCES

Centers for Medicare & Medicaid Services (CMS). (2008a). *Medicare and you 2008.* Baltimore, MD: Author.

Centers for Medicare & Medicaid Services (CMS). (2008b). *2008 Choosing a Medigap policy: a guide to health insurance for people with Medicare.* Baltimore, MD: Author.

InterQual, Inc. (1993). *Utilization review and management training manual.* North Hampton, NH: Author.

Kongstvedt, P.R. (2003). *Essentials of managed health care* (4th ed.) Gaithersburg, MD: Aspen Publishers.

Milliman & Robertson. (1992). *Health care management guidelines.* Seattle, WA: Author.

National Academy of Social Insurance (NASI). (2002). *Workers' compensation benefits, costs, and coverage, 2000 new estimates.* Available online, www.nasi.org.

Newell, M. (1996). *Using nursing case management to improve health outcomes.* Gaithersburg, MD: Aspen Publishers.

Saue, J.M. (1988, August).Legal issues related to case management. *Quality Review Bulletin, 14*(8), 239–244.

Williams, S. & Torrens, P.R. (1993). *Introduction to health services.* New York: Delmar.

PART 2

Case Management Processes and Activities

"You ought not attempt to cure the eyes without the head, or head without body; so you should not treat body without soul."

SOCRATES

Utilization Management

Case managers who came from the ranks of the utilization review (UR) nurses feel at home with the utilization management (UM) role. Many case managers who came straight in through the clinical doorway (intensive care unit [ICU] nurses, staff nurses) find UR and UM overwhelming and challenging. This chapter breaks down the concepts into clear and usable pieces. It is not difficult, so relax! However, it is sometimes frustrating. Not all patients fit neatly into the allotted categories, and the criteria are constantly changing, getting stricter, and becoming more demanding each year.

Good UR or UM includes the use of medical instincts or nursing intuition. Often a patient does not meet official criteria to be hospitalized, but the case manager senses something unstable about the patient. Within 24 hours, the patient "crashes" and is admitted to an ICU. Perhaps the case manager spoke to the insurance UR/UM department earlier and received a denial notice; a second telephone call would rescind the denial and substantiate why the case manager was hesitant to push for a discharge or transfer to a lesser level of care or setting. Occasionally, an insurance reviewer is very set on using the company's chosen utilization management modality as though it were law. Cookbook UR and UM is very frustrating and probably accounts for the number one reason why many case managers prefer root canals to UR and UM responsibilities.

▶ HISTORICAL BACKGROUND

Utilization management is not new to the healthcare industry; it has been in existence since the 1970s. It began with the professional standards review organizations, previously known as peer review organizations (PROs), and known today as quality improvement organizations (QIOs). These review organizations were created to evaluate the healthcare services rendered to Medicare and Medicaid beneficiaries. Initially, the main focus of UM was review of hospital-based services provided to Medicare and Medicaid beneficiaries. This review entailed matching patients' needs to necessary care interventions with the goal of reducing waste and overutilization of services. Such review was coordinated through independent but state-related agencies (e.g., QIOs).

To maintain compliance with resource utilization standards, hospitals employed nurses to assume UR functions. The UR nurse reviewed the patients' record and if a patient did not meet acute care criteria, the nurse rectified the situation with the physician and instituted appropriate action. Gradually these functions expanded to outpatient services and by the mid-1980s to commercial insurance companies. As a result of this expansion, UR shifted from being merely a review function to utilization management activities that impacted not only quality of care and resource utilization, but reimbursement as well. Today UM is an integral aspect of case management and is applied to the care of every patient regardless of the type of health insurance plan (private or governmental) he or she carries.

Health maintenance organizations (HMOs), preferred provider organizations (PPOs), workers' compensation (WC), and QIOs all use UM today. This resulted in the evolution of case management programs employed by a healthcare organization from being focused on nursing/clinical care management to having clinical care, transitional planning, and UM functions all integrated into one program; often these functions also are integrated in the role of one key healthcare professional—the case manager. This evolution increased the complexity of the case manager's role and at the same time raised its importance for the organization.

Utilization management allows an organization to review its compliance with healthcare-related laws and regulations (e.g., provision of care in the appropriate level of care/setting) and managed care organizations' (MCOs) utilization procedures and practices (e.g., authorizations for care and services). UM functions have direct impact on reimbursement for care rendered. The case manager ensures that patients meet pre-established criteria to support the level of care being delivered, including the setting where patients are cared for. Therefore, reimbursement is dependent on a match between the patient's health/clinical condition (acuity or severity), the treatment plan and options (intensity of resources), and the level of service (care setting/physical location across the healthcare continuum).

▶ THE RELATIONSHIP AMONG UR, UM, AND CASE MANAGEMENT

▶ Definitions

▶ UR is the process in which medical review determinations are made based on clinical guidelines and structured processes. UR modalities use established criteria to evaluate medical services for necessity, level of care for appropriateness, quality, and the timeliness of discharge (Sederer, 1987).

▶ UM is the management and "evaluation of the medical necessity, appropriateness, and efficiency of the use of healthcare services, procedures, and facilities under the auspices of the applicable health benefit plan" (Carneal, 1998). The goal is to use the healthcare resources to provide the highest quality of patient care in the most cost-effective and efficient setting.

▶ Case management is a "collaborative process of assessment, planning, facilitation, and advocacy for options and services to meet an individual's health needs through communication and available resources to promote quality and cost-effective outcomes" (Case Management Society of America [CMSA], 2002).

There do not appear to be significant differences in the definitions between UR in the late-1980s and UM in the late-1990s. However, there are important evolutionary changes that have moved UR closer to case management. The more appropriate term in use today is *utilization management*, because utilization/case managers are managing the utilization of healthcare resources and no longer merely reviewing them. In fact, today it is more common to see UM integrated in case management programs rather than as an independent function.

Case managers must be clear about the subtle differences between UM and UR. Cesta and Tahan (2003) differentiate these two concepts based on certain categories and in an easy-to-understand way. They state that UM is practiced across all settings of the healthcare continuum and entails:

1. Prospective and concurrent review of patients' medical records.
2. Use of criteria for the determination of medical necessity.
3. Patient and family contact.
4. Monitoring of resource utilization for appropriateness.
5. Transitional planning functions.
6. Direct contact with the interdisciplinary healthcare team.
7. Interaction with representatives from all types of health insurance agencies.
8. Appeals of denials.
9. Case conferencing with patients and families to resolve issues or clarify certain aspects of care.

UR, on the other hand, although similar to UM in certain areas, remains different and of a narrower focus. Cesta and Tahan (2003) note that UM is practiced mainly in acute care settings and some outpatient services, and entails:

1. Retrospective review of patients' medical records.
2. Use of criteria for the determination of medical necessity.
3. No patient or family contact.
4. Monitoring of the allocation of resources.
5. Minimal transitional planning function.
6. Indirect contact with the interdisciplinary healthcare team.
7. Minimal interaction with representatives from health insurance agencies.
8. Limited to no appeals of denials.
9. No case conferencing with patients and families.

UM is one of the components of case management and is within the scope of the case management responsibilities; case management enhances all aspects of patient care—financial and psychosocial as well as medical. As stated in the CMSA case management definition, the case management role is wider, encompassing responsibilities such as collaboration as well as planning, coordinating, monitoring, and evaluating cases. Whereas UM responds to one event, case management coordinates the needs of the patient by looking at the patient's whole universe of care—past, present, and future utilization of services and needs. Both must provide the provision of the right healthcare, at the right time, in the right setting, by the right provider, and utilizing the right amount of services.

Many companies and third-party administrators provide both UM and case management services. The UM division often detects and substantiates patient triggers that require a referral to case management. These cases are complex and require more than UM services typically provide. It is no longer enough to merely use clinical UM modalities. With the advent of many best practice clinical guidelines, new changes in the use of medications, and advancing technology, case managers must be up-to-date clinically. Further, they must also know about the patient's use of complementary and alternative medicine (CAM) to assess any contraindications. The patient must be looked at from a broader perspective.

Utilization managers, or concurrent review nurses, can be a support or a challenge to case managers. UM is primarily a cost-containment activity; therefore, it is essential for the case manager to focus on the patient advocacy role. Astute UM professionals and case managers assess the whole clinical picture to ensure that services are neither underutilized nor overutilized. If the two disagree, and an insurance company's UM professional comes in with inappropriate threats of denied stays, the case manager may let the company know that it will be challenged for reasons of patient safety or medical necessity. This requires thorough knowledge of UM modalities and criteria and a thorough assessment of the patient. Bear in mind that UM nurses are constantly asking themselves, "What is it about this case that makes it impossible for the patient to be safely cared for at a lesser level of care, or at home?" The case manager must be prepared to answer this question and to back up the answer with clinical and objective facts.

UM is important. It allows services to be authorized by insurance companies; simply put, providers must get paid for services to survive. Utilization modalities also encourage fiscally responsible length of stay (LOS) and offer the case manager an efficient template for determining medical necessity as the patient moves through the healthcare maze. However, in a real sense, UR is reactive to medical criteria, whereas nursing case management is proactive. Cookbook UR (i.e., poor UR) has the goal of removing the patient from cost-intensive settings as quickly as possible. Good case management may have the same end point, but it uses patient advocacy and a multidisciplinary team approach to planning and implementing care to achieve that end point.

One of the finest testaments to the profession of case management came from Garry Carneal, JD, MA, Past President and CEO of the American Accreditation HealthCare Commission/Utilization Review Accreditation

Commission (The Commission/URAC), the premiere accreditation organization for UM activities and case management programs. Between the lines, this story demonstrates the connection of, and the distinction between, UM and case management:

> One of my senior accreditation reviewers arrived in my office one day and told me something I will never forget. The reviewer had just completed an accreditation review of an HMO pursuant to the American Accreditation HealthCare Commission/URAC's Health Utilization Management Standards. She shared with me that during the review she could not detect any instances where the HMO had made denials for health care services based upon medical necessity. I immediately questioned if this was true. How could a managed care organization (MCO) be running an efficient company without a utilization review system that periodically makes denials?
>
> The reviewer looked at me with a smile and said yes, it was true. She even had the audacity to tell me that they don't practice traditional utilization management (UM). Now I was getting even more skeptical. I asked her, how could an HMO not practice UM in a state that mandates that all managed care companies have URAC Health UM accreditation?
>
> Finally, she let the cat out of the bag. She reported that the HMO had a more integrated approach to the delivery of care. She called this system case management (Carneal, 1998, p. 18).

▶ UM Services

The following are the main types of UM services. Each one reflects management of the utilization of resources in various stages of the delivery of healthcare services.

PREADMISSLON REVIEW OR PROSPECTIVE REVIEW

Also called precertification, prospective review or preadmission review is completed by a representative from the healthcare provider agency to ensure that the decision to admit a patient to an inpatient facility is appropriate or justified and that an authorization for the provision of specific aspects of care will be obtained from the insurer. This review takes place before ("pre") services are rendered. Here the reviewer determines whether admission to the facility (i.e., hospital, rehabilitation unit, surgicenter, skilled nursing facility [SNF]) is reasonable and medically necessary. Because the attending physician has the ultimate responsibility for the patient, this physician will determine admitting status, regardless of authorization. A compromise may be a 24-hour authorization to see whether the patient needs that particular level of care or a pending review status.

Most managed care organizations require this type of review. The advantage to such review is that utilization of resources or quality issues can often be found before the delivery of patient care; the major disadvantage is that necessary services may be delayed or denied.

Prospective review addresses that:

- ▶ Insurance coverage and benefits are verified.
- ▶ Managed care program requirements/procedures are met.
- ▶ Quality of care issues are identified, addressed, and resolved when possible.
- ▶ Alternatives to care are identified before admission.
- ▶ Care is medically necessary.
- ▶ Care is rendered at the most appropriate level of care and setting.
- ▶ Selection of the provider is appropriate and within the preferred network if possible.
- ▶ Assessment of needs/discharge planning is initiated.
- ▶ Initial LOS is determined if the patient is an inpatient.

CONCURRENT REVIEW

A concurrent review is performed while the patient is in the healthcare facility and being cared for. The reviewer from the insurance company sometimes visits the facility for this role, but with more UM firms cropping up, other modes of reviews (e.g., telephone, fax, or electronic mail reviews) are equally as common. When the review is not completed on site, a representative from the care provider agency completes the review and communicates with the insurance company. Here, the UM professional would be assessing the appropriateness of the level of care such as ICU, step down, telemetry, floor care, extended care, rehabilitation care, or home with home health. Medical appropriateness is gauged by monitoring and evaluating the medical condition of the patient against the services performed. Concurrent review has two parameters:

1. Admission review—performed within 24 hours of admission to a facility.
2. Continued stay review—performed at specific points during the patient's stay to determine that each day of a hospital stay is necessary and that care is rendered at the appropriate level and in the right setting. If the patient is critical, a review every 2 to 3 days may be an acceptable time frame. If the patient is nearing a change in level of care, daily reviews are

necessary. Continued stay reviews focus on monitoring the patient's health condition and healthcare resources utilized during the inpatient stay.

Concurrent review is intended to ensure that (InterQual, Inc., 1997):

▶ Accurate patient information is captured in a timely fashion.
▶ Care continues to be provided at an appropriate level of care, setting, and with the appropriate utilization of resources (avoiding over- or underutilization).
▶ Care is coordinated; for example, no delays occur.
▶ Complex clinical and psychosocial situations are referred to case management.
▶ Insurance coverage and benefits still match the patient's requirements.
▶ Quality issues are monitored and, if triggered, appropriate notification is made.
▶ Discharge criteria are met.

RETROSPECTIVE REVIEW

A retrospective review is performed after a patient's discharge. Reviewers from insurance companies typically come to the healthcare facility, request patient charts from medical records, and perform the review. They may authorize the whole hospital or SNF admission or deny payment in whole or in part. Although concurrent review feels more honest and up front, retrospective review is a reality that case managers need to be aware of. Retrospective review is less common than in the past, because more payors require precertification for most services, except those that are "low tech" or emergently necessary.

Retrospective review is a useful tool for looking at quality control. Monday morning quarterbacking can often prevent similar quality issues from repeating themselves if a preventive plan is assessed and imple-

mented. However, a major disadvantage is that when the review is done after the fact, it does not allow intervention to change and improve a course of events.

TELEPHONIC REVIEW

Telephonic review is UM that is performed via telephone, usually concurrently. Telephone triage and telephonic UM will continue to grow in use because more health insurance companies use demand management strategies and 24-hour coverage. Telephonic reviews are a less expensive way for insurance companies to perform UM, but the reviews are only as good as the information elicited. Poor or inadequate information can result from the reviewer's not knowing medically important questions to ask for a particular admitting diagnosis. The information must be elicited systematically; the reviewer must ask the questions that will efficiently demonstrate whether the patient needs continued stay at the present level of care. The staff nurses should know what intravenous (IV) medications the patient is receiving, some laboratory test results, and the patient's response to treatment. However, their time is limited, and many staff nurses resent speaking to insurance companies or feel they cannot give out information over the telephone because of confidentiality issues.

Telephonics without a good UM nurse or case manager on the patient end is the least effective means of UM; further, it can result in case management actions fraught with liability. Yet a good case manager or UM nurse combined with insurance telephonics may be good for everyone. Such arrangements keep hundreds of UM nurses out of a facility and still maintain that the institution is user-friendly. For insurance companies, use of telephonics is the least expensive method of acquiring the information they require.

Your voice is your tool and it can relay a message that can cause cooperation or a problem. Display 4-1 describes some telephone tips for those engaged in telephonic UM reviews.

---

display 4-1 ▼ **TIPS FOR TELEPHONIC UTILIZATION MANAGEMENT AND REVIEW**

▶ Listen to your tone of voice. The voice is your connection to the patient; sincerity, frustration, hurriedness, or kindness does come through.
▶ Be clear on your reasons for the call. Your words can give you away if you are not clear on the reason for the call. Take a minute before reaching for the telephone to gather your thoughts and objectives for the call.
▶ Name-drop. Use the name of the person you are talking to; make it a point to at least use the name while

saying good-bye. However, using a person's name too often has been a worn-out tactic in the sales industry, so do not overdo it.
▶ Use active listening. No one can hear you nod your head, so use verbal forms of active listening.
▶ Be focused and answer the necessary questions. If you have additional important information, volunteer that information as long as you think it will enhance a positive/affirmative decision.

TELEPHONIC CASE MANAGEMENT. Telephonics is not just for UM purposes. Many case managers use telephonics almost exclusively, especially those who manage patients in other cities or states. Telephonic case management is no hardship when dealing with claims payors, providers, payors, or company contact personnel. Nevertheless, it is not always the easiest way to make a patient-centered decision, and certainly telephonic case managers have wished they could see their patients on occasion. Telephonic case management is a reality many must work around; however, there are times when an on-site examination cannot be avoided, and many case managers have that option as well. Initial examinations, for example, may need to be on site, especially for specific case types such as workers' compensation or automobile accident patients. Sometimes, physician summaries give a clear patient picture. Sometimes, additional therapy notes increase the clarity. And sometimes, nothing but an on-site view of the patient reflects what is needed for the case manager to accurately perform his or her duties. This is especially true for litigious or angry patients or families. It takes longer to build a rapport by telephone than in person, and sometimes time is of the essence. The point is that the case (within the constraints of the case management contract) will dictate if on-site versus telephonic case management will better serve the patient.

INSURANCE AUTHORIZATIONS

Types of insurance authorization follow logically from the types of UM.

ADMISSION CERTIFICATION. A form of authorization that indicates the approval of a patient's admission to a hospital or other inpatient facility (for example, an acute or subacute rehabilitation). The decision is made based on criteria such as medical necessity and intensity of services.

PROSPECTIVE OR PRECERTIFICATION AUTHORIZATION. This is authorization given before services are rendered. Prospective authorization is not interchangeable with prospective payment. Prospective authorization is a concept specific to commercial insurance, while prospective payment is mainly used in Medicare and Medicaid benefit programs. Prospective payment usually refers to a diagnosis-related group (DRG) payment, in which one amount is given for all services needed based on a specific diagnosis (see Chapter 3: Reimbursement Concepts).

CONCURRENT AUTHORIZATION. This authorization is generated at the time the service is rendered.

Often it is pursued in cases where patients may require continued hospital stays.

RETROSPECTIVE AUTHORIZATION. This authorization is approved after services have been performed. Often the patient has already been discharged from the hospital.

PENDED (FOR REVIEW). Here the hospital keeps its fingers crossed in hopes of a real authorization. Pending review has been described as a state of authorization purgatory because the institution is unsure if an authorization will be given regardless of the pressing situation that the patient is still in the hospital receiving care. This state may lead to retrospective review and authorization or a denial of services in whole or in part.

DENIAL. Denial is also called noncertification, lack of certification, or adverse determination. In this situation, no authorization is given for all or part of the services, for an admission to a hospital setting, or for continued stay in a hospital. Other denials are of the "reimbursement" type, that is, lack of payment. Often denial decisions are made based on lack of medical necessity. Grievance procedures may commence and are often won, especially with good physician, case manager, and UM documentation. Appeals have been elevated to legal status and often require assistance from case managers (see Chapter 8, Legal Issues in Case Management, for a detailed discussion). The following are some of the reasons for denials:

- Information not shared within reasonable or requested time frame.
- Procedures performed in the wrong level of care/setting.
- Weekend-related lack of services resulting in additional 1 to 2 inpatient/hospital days.
- Services not covered by the health plan, such as dental or cosmetic surgery.
- Untimely billing.
- Lack of prior authorizations/certifications.
- Clinical condition not requiring continued inpatient stay.
- Condition not meeting inpatient admission criteria.

SUBAUTHORIZATION. One authorization number allows other services to piggyback on it. For example, a single authorization number is given for a cholecystectomy. This number can be used by the surgeon, radiologist, pathologist, anesthesiologist, and for laboratory tests or radiographs.

APPEAL. This is the formal process or request to reconsider a decision made not to approve an admission or a particular aspect of care and services, reimbursement of services rendered, or a patient's request to postpone the date of discharge from a hospital. Usually appeals are managed by the case manager or the UM nurse on behalf of the care provider (e.g., hospital) and/or the patient.

An appeal should be filed based on the contractual agreement between the care provider or agency and the insurance company. It also should comply with insurance and public health laws. One generally has between 30 and 60 days to file an appeal and the insurance company is obligated to review the appeal and respond within 30 to 60 days of the date it is filed. When the review is completed, it may result in the appeal being upheld in its entirety, the denial being amended to a portion of the care/services, or a complete reversal.

When writing an appeal letter, it is best to involve the attending physician of record. It is also important to reference any authorization numbers obtained during UM interactions with the representative of the insurance company. In addition, it is advisable to reference in the appeal letter the UM criteria/guidelines used by the insurance company such as InterQual or Milliman Care Guidelines (described later in this chapter). The appeal letter must reflect how the criteria match the patient's condition, including the interventions applied and the outcomes achieved.

▶ UM Skills

The most important skills that a UM professional—or case manager with UM responsibilities—needs are a first-rate clinical databank and excellent communication techniques. Many physicians believe that UM nurses are "nurses telling doctors how to practice medicine." They resist reviewers (feeling that their toes are being stepped on), yet UM nurses should not necessarily be looked on as adversaries during this questioning process; their documentation can often prevent the insurance denial process. Some doctors inadequately document assessments or plans in the medical record; this often leads to insurance denials. Physicians who are poor documenters often have acceptable plans, but it takes time and communication skills to elicit them. Display 4-2 presents some practical ideas to help in UM responsibilities. Case managers and UM nurses should use these tactics to enhance their communication with physicians, especially when engaged in utilization review and management activities.

▶ UM Documentation

As in all aspects of medical care, documentation for UM activity is vitally important. If, for example, you are working with a physician who is a poor documenter, your documented conversations with the physician(s) and insurance reviewer may make the difference between an insurance authorization or a denial of inpatient days, services, or reimbursement. Some insurance companies demand that physician documentation be evident in the patients' charts, so the case manager's responsibility will be to attempt to obtain that documentation or make sure that it is completed if it is found to be lacking.

UM documentation does not have to be lengthy, but proper documentation of facts is necessary to validate the patient's diagnosis and support the necessity of the treatment plan. Most insurance plans will not pay for services if a doctor's order is missing or if they

---

display 4-2

PRACTICAL TACTICS FOR EFFECTIVE COMMUNICATION WITH PHYSICIANS ABOUT UM

▶ Focus on the patient. The patient-centered approach diffuses suspicion and allows the reviewer and the physician to focus on the same goal.

▶ Be colloquial and not adversarial in your approach to physicians. Gain a reputation for solving problems, not becoming one.

▶ Be succinct and to the point about your needs and concerns. Physicians are busy and often have a low tolerance for rambling conversations with reviewers.

▶ Make sure you have an accurate and thorough clinical assessment of the situation before your conversation with the physician.

▶ When discussing discharge or transfer plans, make sure you have the patient's/family's cooperation in a plan before you discuss it with the physician; this

saves wasted steps. On the other hand, some physicians have known their patients and families for many years and can provide preliminary information that will be very helpful when assessing the plan.

▶ Be assertive, not aggressive.

▶ Keep lines of communication open and follow through on what is discussed. More trust will be gained because of good follow-through than any other approach you may use.

▶ Make sure in your conversation that the physician understands UM and its procedures.

could not find documentation that the service was necessary and in fact performed.

The use of utilization modalities is not a substitute for thorough and accurate documentation. For example, if in a court of law, a healthcare provider claims to have followed a clinical pathway, the documentation must support that declaration. When documenting from a UM perspective, the case manager should perform the following:

▶ Record all clinically pertinent data. Objective data should be exact. For example, record a patient's temperature as 39.2° C, rather than "high temp." Other clinical data may include results of laboratory work, radiographs, scans, vital signs, biopsies, cultures, and so on. Subjective data may support the facts. All data should validate the diagnosis and necessity of the treatment plan.

▶ Document any time a patient deviates from the UM modality or critical pathway implemented. It is not enough to show that a patient deviated from the critical pathway; document why the patient went "off the path" and what was done to address any problems.

▶ Record the patient's response or lack of response to the treatments and services.

▶ As stated earlier, accurately document conversations with physicians, insurance reviewers, and all other people pertinent to the services needed and treatment plans. We all can remember situations where documentation could not support the plan because it was lacking and the patient was at risk for denial of treatment of continued hospital stay. For example, one novice UM nurse denied a patient with a persistent high fever continued hospital stay because all IV antibiotics had been discontinued (this patient had been given three antibiotics). What was lacking in the chart was the plan to discontinue the antibiotics and pan-culture the patient in the hopes of "catching" the offending bug. The reviewer missed the order to pan-culture, and the documentation lacked a clear picture and a black-and-white plan. After explaining to the reviewer that this was an approved standard of treatment for a fever of unknown origin, she rescinded the denial but required physician documentation of the medical plan.

▶ Include times and dates of conversations. Many insurance companies (not all) give the facility 24 hours to supply requested data before the denial goes into effect. Other companies simply end the

LOS. If the case manager or physician can provide pertinent data, the insurance companies will also approve the day of the conversation (usually until midnight).

▶ Demonstrate the patient's status at any given point in time. If another reviewer picks up the case, no backtracking should be needed.

▶ Make careful documentation of discharge or transfer planning. If a discharge or transfer plan needs to be changed, include reasons for the changes in the report. Also include the level of care that is planned, home health nursing services, durable medical equipment needed, transportation and all other arrangements made, and the reasons for medical necessity. It is also important to reveal the name and title of the insurance company representative who approved payment of these discharge services.

▶ Document outcomes of care, especially those that are tied to the goals of care, the treatment plan, or the critical pathway if one is in use. Documenting progression, or lack of it, allows a better concurrent review process between the hospital-based case manager (or those in other inpatient facilities) and those in the insurance company. Lack of progression, when well-documented, enhances the argument a case manager makes to obtain approval for continued/extended hospital stay.

▶ Document authorization or certification numbers as you obtain them. All insurance companies provide certification numbers for services that are approved for a particular patient. Documenting the number is important for reimbursement or for following up with the insurance company in certain situations such as the case of retrospective claim denial. The case manager or UM nurse can use the certification number when attempting an appeal.

The Centers for Medicare & Medicaid Services (CMS) services requires specific documentation to ensure Medicare reimbursement for care rendered. These requirements pertain to patients and care providers in the acute care setting.

1. Physician orders that clearly designate admission status (inpatient, outpatient, or observation), including date and time.
2. History and physical (H & P) that justifies the admission and treatment. This must be performed within 30 days prior to or within 24 hours of the admission. The H & P must include the patient's chief complaint, history of

present illness, past medical history, allergies, medication intake, family and social history, and complete systems exam, with special focus on the reason for a procedure if applicable.

3. Daily progress notes that should include the patient's current health condition and progress; any revisions made to the diagnostic impressions, especially in the case of new evidence/findings; conditions or possible diagnoses that have been ruled out; conditions that verify or support the reason for admission to an inpatient setting; and rationale for change in admission status (e.g., change from inpatient to observation status).

4. Discharge summary that includes the principal and secondary diagnoses as well as the principal and secondary procedures; brief description of the hospitalization, disposition and follow-up care arrangements; and results of diagnostic findings, especially those that confirm the principal diagnosis. If there were any surgical procedures performed, these must be included as well. Secondary diagnoses are as important as the primary diagnosis because they provide evidence of comorbidities at the time of admission to the hospital.

5. Discharge summary addendum if any. This may consist of clarifications requested by medical record personnel after the patient's discharge concerning the principal or secondary diagnoses and procedures. This may also include the addition of test results or other information obtained post discharge.

LAG DAYS AND VARIANCES

Inappropriate acute inpatient days, also known as lag days, may occur at the beginning of a hospital stay (on admission), during the stay, or at the end of a hospitalization when a patient could have been discharged or transferred sooner than was actually done. These days are considered nonacute by insurance companies; here overutilization of resources becomes apparent. It is not uncommon for insurance companies to deny portions of a hospitalization (on admission, during, or at the end of a stay) if they feel these portions were due to avoidable delays. Good case management can minimize these lag days, and hospitals are seeing an encouraging impact in this area. At times, unavoidable lag days still occur; when this happens, the case manager should help to get the case back on track as quickly as possible.

Given all the people involved and factors that make up each case, it is not surprising that lag days occur with monotonous consistency. The reasons for lag days are varied, and closely related to these nonacute days is the issue of variation or variances. Variances are deviations from normal, quality care. Unexpected or worrisome occurrences that affect the course of illness can be identified through analysis of variance data (Anonymous, 1989). These data, in turn, can identify possible opportunities for performance improvement. In fact, one of the primary goals of tracking and analyzing variance data through the use of case management plans (CMPs), clinical pathways, or other UM tools, is to aid in early identification and resolution of healthcare issues. In continuous quality improvement (CQI) circles, a variance, or variation, is considered a basic cause of instability in a process. Stability in a process depicts a process that is well-defined and consistent in methods used and application. Variability in a process is just the opposite; variable processes are inconsistent and changeable. It is difficult to attribute outcomes to processes that are unstable. Case managers who perform outcomes studies based on such tools as clinical pathways often use variance data to draw conclusions and improve care processes.

Sources for variance identification used by case managers include nurses and physician documentation, verbal communication with the multidisciplinary healthcare team, and variances found on clinical pathways. The patient or family members are another source (and sometimes a cause) of variances.

The causes of variances, which may lead to lag days and undesired outcomes, are generally assigned to four categories: (1) patient/family reasons, (2) practitioner reasons, (3) institution/systems reasons, and (4) community reasons. Variances can be caused by social factors, financial factors, environmental factors, patient or family responses or lack of responses, physician-induced reasons, or hospital (institution) responsibilities. Display 4-3 lists some examples of variances that may lead to lag days. The list is by no means complete, as very creative and interesting circumstances can (and do) pop up unexpectedly!

The causes of variances are seemingly endless. The more complicated the discharge, the more opportunities for variances and lag days to occur and the more a detailed social evaluation is needed. We heard of one case in which the case manager worked very hard putting together a complicated discharge with various pieces of durable medical equipment. On the day of discharge, someone in the family happened to mention that there was no electricity at home! Assessment had missed this crucial fact. This, of course, delayed the patient's discharge. The case manager should always be alert for possible changes and be prepared with a "plan B."

VARIANCES REQUIRING CASE MANAGER AWARENESS

Characteristics of Variance

▶ Occurs when what is supposed to happen does not take place or is delayed.
▶ Deviates from a standard, norm, goal/target, or threshold.
▶ Omits an activity.
▶ Does not meet expectations or expectations are met too soon.

Patient/Family Variances

▶ Unsafe home environment.
▶ Refusal to leave the hospital.
▶ Lack of family support (i.e., no caregiver at home).
▶ Refusal of procedure and/or treatment regimen as prescribed by physician.
▶ Indecision regarding treatment or discharge plan.
▶ Indecision about a test, procedure, or surgery.
▶ Insistence that the patient is too ill to be discharged.
▶ No family shows up to pick up the patient after arrangements were made.
▶ Inability of family member responsible for at-home care to arrive from out of state on the day the patient is ready for discharge.
▶ Lack of patient cooperation with the medical program, causing delayed diagnosis and treatment.
▶ The patient suffering an intraoperative myocardial infarction (MI) or other medical complication (e.g., hemorrhage, shock, ileus, postoperative infection, or pneumonia).
▶ Although educational needs were attended to early in the admission, significant knowledge deficit exists and additional teaching needed for patient or family.
▶ Delayed transfer or discharge because of inadequate discharge planning details.
▶ Family members changing their minds about the discharge plan at the last minute (e.g., the case manager's suggestion that an extended care facility may be appropriate suddenly sounds good!).
▶ Chronically ill patient with inadequate (or no) insurance support and poor social support, causing a difficult discharge dilemma (if available, charity care may be needed).
▶ Inability to reach family members.
▶ Pressure ulcer present on admission that requires treatment.
▶ No clothes or key to apartment; therefore cannot discharge yet.
▶ Inability to self-care or administer insulin injections.
▶ Poor historian or withholding important information.

Practitioner Variances

▶ Physician is late in providing service, scheduling procedures, writing prescriptions, and/or ordering laboratory tests.
▶ Discharge order is not written by the physician in a timely manner.
▶ Primary physician is inaccessible.
▶ Specialist is inaccessible.
▶ Physician insists on an inappropriate level of care.
▶ All SNFs in which the patient's physician will follow are full; the physician will not go to other suggested SNFs; or the patient refuses care by a "strange" physician. This variance can be attributed to the patient/family or physician, depending on how one looks at it.
▶ The doctor writes the discharge order at 10:00 PM, when visiting hours are over and patients and their families are usually asleep!
▶ The physician comes in early—before the day's laboratory test results are back and before the patient's progress for the day can be assessed—and writes "will discharge tomorrow if the patient is stable today."
▶ The patient was admitted for a problem outside the expertise of the attending physician. Delays occurred getting specialist consultations.
▶ The physician's practice pattern is such that only one test is ordered at a time, and the results must be back before any other diagnostic action is taken.
▶ Tests are ordered in poor sequence, causing delays because of extensive preparation.
▶ Poor practitioner's techniques cause complications.
▶ There are delays in ordering needed services (i.e., social service, physical therapy, rehabilitation consultation).
▶ There is a failure to conduct proper financial screening.
▶ There is inappropriate use of medical equipment.
▶ Miscommunication occurs among healthcare team members or with patient/family.
▶ There is a delay in checking results of tests and therefore delay in progressing the treatment plan.
▶ There is a failure to obtain certifications for services.

Institution/Systems Variances

▶ Orders are not transcribed in a timely manner.
▶ Equipment malfunctions or break downs.
▶ Delay occurs in services, tests, and/or procedures.
▶ No beds are available (all levels of care).
▶ There is refusal to accept patient in next level of care.
▶ There are transportation problems.

(continued)

VARIANCES REQUIRING CASE MANAGER AWARENESS (*Continued*)

▶ Scheduling delay for tests, procedures, or surgery may be the result of full operating rooms or tests that are run only on specific days.

▶ Test or biopsy results are delayed, which postpones further procedures or discharge.

▶ A lower level of care would have adequately met the needs of the patient, but traditional Medicare requires 72 hours in acute care before transfer to a SNF level.

▶ The institution does not have the necessary equipment, so that transfer to another hospital is necessary for a test or procedure.

▶ Beds are unavailable for new admissions.

▶ Weekend coverage is lacking in certain services.

Community Variances

▶ Private insurance causes delay (authorization, transfer problems, finding contracted providers).

▶ Durable medical equipment is unavailable or delivered late.

▶ SNF is unavailable (no beds) or refuses patient at last minute.

▶ Regional natural disasters back up all healthcare services and beds.

▶ Child protective services are late to arrive.

▶ Shelter will not take patient after certain hours or on the weekend.

▶ Utilization Management

A comprehensive survey of the nation's UR laws completed by URAC in the late 1990s demonstrates that state policymakers continue to focus on UM issues, including emerging issues such as external review and specific state licensure. UR regulation continues to evolve; the role of URAC (and other case management professional societies such as CMSA) in formulating case management agendas, including accreditation in managed care organizations, will further propel this evolutionary change. (See Chapter 10 for further information about The Commission/URAC.)

Survey findings include the following:

1. Approximately 95% of Americans enrolled in private health plans are subject to some level of UR.

2. States currently regulate UR:
   ▶ Prohibitions against financial incentives based on numbers or on rate of UR adverse determinations.
   ▶ Stipulations that only physicians (or clinical peers) may render adverse determinations.
   ▶ Requirement of appeal processes; some have access to external appeals (see Chapter 8 for detailed appeals information).
   ▶ Some states require the reviewers to be licensed in the state where the review is conducted.
   ▶ Some states incorporate URAC accreditation into the regulatory process.

3. Although state utilization laws share many common elements, they vary enough to present *a significant compliance challenge to multistate UR organizations.*

▶ UM Modalities

The out-of-control economics of healthcare have been apparent since the 1980s. Various ways and modalities

> **NOTE**
>
> Utilization Review Accreditation Commission (URAC)
> Address: 1220 L Street, NW, Suite 400
> Washington, DC, 20005
> Telephone: 202-216-9101
> Web site: www.urac.org.
> E-mail: info@urac.org

of managing the utilization of healthcare resources have come and gone; more will likely emerge. The staggering dollar amounts being spent for healthcare are forcing this search for better management of resources. Some UM tools have changed and become more efficient. Still others are in their adolescence—raw, but with good potential. There are many UM tools. The four modalities discussed here are the most commonly used UM tools at this time: length of stay (LOS), InterQual, clinical pathways, and Milliman Care Guidelines (MCGs).

As a UM modality, LOS assigns a number of days' allowance to a particular episode of illness. InterQual is a criteria-based system that includes objective and measurable symptoms and services. These criteria should guide the UM reviewer in assessing medical necessity and appropriateness of the level of care. Clinical pathways give a daily plan of care for a particular illness; they also sequence all aspects of that care for optimal quality and efficiency. MCGs are a combination of clinical pathways and length-of-stay modalities.

When using UM tools, it should be kept in mind that they are just that—tools. They are not mandatory. More importantly, they are only a part of total case management. They do, however, speak a language that insurance companies understand, and insurance companies pay the bills. Criteria are intended to be used by physician personnel when caring for patients, and by case managers or nurse reviewers when engaged in UM activities. It is common practice that nurse reviewers may authorize appropriate services. However, they may not deny services; that can only be done by a physician reviewer.

Sometimes merging the roles of UM and patient advocacy seems to cause conflict (see Chapter 9). This conflict may signal the need for discussion between a physician and a case manager, or even a full conference with the multidisciplinary team on the case. There have been times when case managers have felt sandwiched between an insurance company's threat to deny payment unless the physician moves the patient to a lesser level of care and a physician angry over the insurance company's decision. At these times it helps to get everyone's focus back on the patient and what that patient needs to receive proper and safe care. At other times, the physician is grateful for the added "support" of an insurance denial if the patient or family is adept at manipulating or malingering. In either case, knowledge of utilization modalities will aid the case manager; impending insurance denials will not be a surprise because the case manager already predicted the possibility and therefore the discharge plan was already in place well into the case management process.

LOS

Length of stay is perhaps the most fundamental attempt at controlling costs of healthcare. An LOS is essentially a number of days that a patient should stay in the hospital for a specific diagnosis or procedure. Many factors have affected LOS over the past two decades, including:

▶ The Prospective Payment System.
▶ The type and prevalence of managed care strategies in different geographical regions.
▶ The quality of utilization managers.
▶ New technology that allows less invasiveness and earlier recovery.
▶ More postacute capabilities at all levels of care.
▶ Community resources.
▶ Accreditation agencies and new standards requiring closer attention to patient safety and patient flow.
▶ Focus of inpatient facilities (e.g., hospitals) on efficiency and patient flow.
▶ Attention given to outpatient and observation status versus inpatient status.
▶ Case management's skillful coordination of complex and catastrophic cases.

Healthcare organizations subscribe to regional and/or national databases to which they contribute their own organization-based data; in return, they are given the opportunity to benchmark against performance of other organizations. An organization has the choice to benchmark against the other organizations in its region or in the nation, or against a select group of organizations that participate in the same database. The benchmark data usually are reported in averages, with the opportunity for an organization to see its variance from the average and the percentile in which it falls. The benchmark data include other metrics beside the LOS, such as volume, demographics (gender, age, socioeconomic class), case mix index, health plan distribution (Medicare, Medicaid, commercial insurance), distribution by diagnosis and procedure, and others. Data are calculated based on reviews of millions of actual patient discharge records from the hospitals that participate in the database. From a case management perspective, those who compile these statistics believe that the data assist in the following aspects of managed care:

▶ Preadmission authorization.
▶ Concurrent review and discharge planning.
▶ Benefit plan evaluations.
▶ Reimbursement review, determination, and adjudication.
▶ Establishment of baselines and benchmarks.

Healthcare professionals use the databases to generate LOS guidelines that can be reported as national data or broken down by region/state in the United States. Custom reports can also be generated, such as choosing a select group of hospitals for benchmarking purposes; in this latter case data are reported based on the medical records submitted from the select set of hospitals. In addition to the previously mentioned metrics, the guidelines can also be displayed by year, cause of hospitalization (i.e., primarily diagnostic or surgical), age (eight or more categories), *International Classification of Diseases*, 9th revision-*Clinical Modifications* (ICD-9-CM) coding, single versus multiple diagnoses, operation status, and percentile. Percentiles may include 10th, 25th, 50th, 75th, 90th, 95th, and 99th. The 10th percentile perhaps demonstrates the lowest realistic LOS; the upper ranges may demonstrate potential overutilization of resources or a lack of case management coordination. HCIA's LOSs are not subjective goal lengths of stay (GLOS) but are based on empiric data from actual discharges; therefore, they help to set benchmarks in the industry. The LOS guidelines for *Diagnosis and Operation, Psychiatric LOS by Diagnosis,* and *DRG and Payment Source* are divided by geographical area. There are also special editions of *Diagnosis and Operation* LOS for geriatric and pediatric patients. See Appendix 4.A for a template example of LOS guidelines.

A GLOS is used within the MCGs' *Optimal Treatment Guidelines* (OTGs) and is perhaps stricter than even the 10th percentile. MCGs include this cautionary note about LOS: "Length of stay assignment has an overassignment problem because it is usually based on retrospective data, assigns number of days without explicit references to expected clinical care, and is often viewed by physicians as an uninformed negotiating stance." The empirical data are retrospective; however, unlike the late 1980s and early- to mid-1990s, LOSs have gotten extremely tight, and even retrospective data are likely to be "in the ballpark." Therefore, using the most recent statistics available is highly recommended. Benchmark data used by an organization should be updated annually so that the most recent benchmarks are used to maintain good reputation, competitiveness, and efficiency.

Although benchmark data are rarely used by insurance companies as the sole consideration for authorization of hospital stays, they are a useful tool for case managers to grasp an average length of time a patient should stay in the hospital for a specific diagnosis or procedure. If a patient is admitted, and the case manager is not familiar with the illness or procedure, knowing the usual LOS (average based on national or regional benchmark data) may be a comforting place to start. It is suggested that case managers (especially those without clinical pathways to guide them) make a cheat sheet of 10%, 25%, and 50% for common problems encountered on the service they are mostly involved in. For case managers who perform case management duties telephonically in different geographical areas of the country, it is a helpful guide because there is a difference in LOSs in various regions.

INTERQUAL

InterQual was first introduced in 1978 and has experienced many revisions and additions (InterQual, Inc., 1993a, 1993b). It is perhaps the most well-known and commonly used of all UR criteria. InterQual criteria are primarily used in utilization review and management for patients with Medicare and Medicaid benefits. InterQual provides UM tools through its CareEnhance products that consist of evidence-based and clinically validated content that is organized into different books or software applications for use by hospitals, health plans, government agencies, and other care/case management providers.

InterQual products and criteria focus on proactive care management, improvement of patient care delivery and safety, resource management, fostering collaborative relationships among healthcare providers and agencies, and enhancing quality of care. They are organized into six clinical decision support products that can be used either proactively, concurrently, or retrospectively for UM. These include the following:

1. Care Planning Criteria: help healthcare organizations determine the suitability of care-related interventions prospectively to manage resource utilization, or retrospectively as a quality assurance tool. They can also serve as an educational tool to help promote sound and efficient use of resources, as well as foster communications between physicians and health plans.

2. Level of Care Criteria: cover the continuum of care, from acute settings through home care and outpatient treatment. They consider the patient's severity of illness, comorbidities, and complications. They also include sets of criteria for inpatient rehabilitation, subacute, and skilled nursing facilities. In addition, they contain objective endpoints for service, allowing healthcare professionals to perform reviews of discharge or transfer readiness based on the individual's clinical needs. The clinical review process guides the reviewer toward the safest and most efficient level of care.

3. Behavioral Health Criteria: assist in making initial and concurrent level-of-care decisions based on each patient's presentation and allow for movement up and down the continuum of care. Content is tailored to the needs of seniors, adults, adolescents, and children. The criteria allow reviewers to consider the severity of illness as well as other episode-specific variables, and match the level of care to the patient's current condition.

4. Workers' Compensation and Disability Management Criteria: support case and care management decisions for safe, timely return-to-work and increased operational efficiency. These tools provide clinical evidence that works for a range of organizations—workers' compensation, auto injury, and disability management—and professionals—utilization managers, case managers, adjusters, and physician advisors.

5. Retrospective Monitoring Criteria: help healthcare organizations evaluate the appropriateness of surgical and nonsurgical invasive procedures for retrospective

justification and validation. With this criteria set, one can check for pathology test results when applicable, document whether the procedure in question was performed adequately, and record whether evidence of significant pathology was present, and the expected preoperative or preprocedure criteria were met.

6. Clinical Evidence Summaries: synthesize medical research on complex and controversial diagnoses to foster physician-to-physician communication. Case managers also use these clinically rich narratives as an effective evidence-based management learning aide. This collection of concise and current "white papers" can also serve as a foundation for the development of evidence-based clinical pathways or case management plans. This product includes a library of than 100 clinical evidence summaries which focus on specific diagnoses and conditions ranging from chronic pain to sleep apnea. The papers include discussions of the latest medical practices and technologies as well as complementary/alternative therapies.

This section focuses on the use of the InterQual criteria in the hospital setting. It breaks down the intensity of service (IS), severity of illness (SI), and discharge screen (DS) criteria into user-friendly pieces, and dispels some of the anxiety associated with use of this modality. Together, IS, SI, and DS are referred to as ISD. Presented here is a brief and basic overview of InterQual's main points. ISD criteria sets have been included in this chapter as an example so that the reader can be more familiar with the ISD format.

INTERQUAL'S CRITERIA. ISD stands for:

I—intensity (of service)

S—severity (of illness)

D—discharge screens (how stable the patient is for discharge).

The ISD criteria address critical and acute care levels. The acute criteria are broken down into classifications that are clinically divided as follows:

▶ Blood/lymph/immune.
▶ Cardiovascular.
▶ Central nervous system/head.
▶ Endocrine/metabolic.
▶ Eye, ear, nose, and throat.
▶ Gastrointestinal tract and abdomen.
▶ Genitourinary.
▶ Gynecology.
▶ Mental health.
▶ Musculoskeletal/spine.
▶ Obstetrics—preterm.
▶ Obstetrics—term.
▶ Peripheral vascular.
▶ Respiratory/chest.
▶ Skin/connective tissue.

Companion sets to ISD cover admission, continued stay, discharge readiness for subacute care (ISD-SAC), rehabilitation (ISD-RHB), and home care (ISD-HC), and are designed to be adjunctive to the acute care ISD sets and to facilitate transfers/discharges to the appropriate levels of care. InterQual also provides other clinical support systems such as indications for surgery and procedures (ISP), indications for imaging studies and x-rays (ISX), indications for workers' compensation clinical management (IWC), and indications for primary and specialty care management (IPS). The systems previously listed are intended for concurrent, prospective use. Surgical indications and invasive procedure monitoring (SIMS *plus*) is for retrospective clinical support (Inter Qual, Inc., 1997).

ISD categories are divided into three criteria subsections: severity of illness, intensity of service, and discharge screens.

Severity of Illness (SI). SI criteria are objective and measurable clinical indicators of a patient's condition. How sick is the patient? Do the patient's clinical findings indicate that this level of care is appropriate? What treatments and services are the patient receiving? The data are gathered from a thorough patient assessment and include any signs or symptoms the patient is exhibiting that reflect a need for acute hospitalization. Some SI criteria use time of onset of the symptoms as part of the definition. These criteria are:

Acute/sudden onset = with 24 hours.

Recent onset = within 1 week.

Recently or newly discovered = greater than 1 week.

Newly discovered = new findings during this episode of illness.

So that the reader may get a feel for how ill a patient must be for an acute hospital authorization, Display 4-4 lists some examples of SI criteria. Time of onset is not listed, but this might further prevent some patients from meeting SI criteria. In addition, if a patient almost meets an aggregate of three SI criteria,

EXAMPLES OF INTERQUAL'S SEVERITY OF ILLNESS CRITERIA

display 4-4

Oral temperature 104°F (40°C) (Note: Other temperature criteria are offered but with further delineating factors)

Sustained pulse ≥ 60 bpm

Repsiratory rate ≥26 with a pulse oximeter reading ≥ 85% on room air

Blood pressure systolic ≥ 250 or < 80 mm Hg

Blood pressure diastolic ≥ 120 or < 40 mm HG

Hgb < 7 g

HCT < 21 g (Note: Hgb and HCT criteria may change in future revisions)

Pneumothorax/hemothorax

Acute myocardial infarction

Gross blood in vomitus, stool, or gastric aspirant

Open wound to bone

Sudden loss of vision

Block or filling defect of major blood vessel

Gross and persistant hemoptysis

Adapted from InterQual, Inc., 1993a, 1993b.

clinical rationale for hospital admission may be approved (InterQual, Inc., 1993a, 1993b).

Intensity of Service (IS). IS criteria define the diagnostic and therapeutic services for each category. Essentially, IS constitutes the physician orders. What is being done for this patient in terms of diagnosis identification and treatment? Should the patient be in this level of care to receive the ordered treatments and medications? What resources does the patient require?

Some IS criteria may be preceded by an asterisk. This is to alert the reviewer to be mindful that these criteria may reflect a treatment that can be safely accomplished at a nonacute level of care. This would be the expected plan of care if the patient is not meeting SI screens but is demonstrating discharge readiness. Display 4-5 lists some examples of IS criteria.

Discharge Screens. Discharge screens are objective, clinical, and functional parameters indicating the patient's readiness and stability for either discharge home or transfer to another level of care. They facili-

tate the answer to the questions: Is the patient clinically and functionally ready for discharge/transfer? Is the patient stable and ready for discharge? All criteria include explanatory notes to assist in their use and application. This addition has made ISD criteria more concrete and user-friendly. Examples of notes are included in this section.

THE ISD REVIEW PROCESS. There are four potential types of review in InterQual's review process: preadmission review, admission review, subsequent reviews, and discharge reviews.

Preadmission Review. Preadmission review is initiated before the patient's admission to the inpatient facility. The reviewer determines whether the diagnostic services and therapeutic modalities are appropriate and match the level of care.

Admission Review. Admission review may often be the initial chart review on a patient. If a patient is admitted directly from a physician's office or from the

EXAMPLES OF INTERQUAL'S INTENSITY OF SERVICE CRITERIA

display 4-5

IV fluids requiring ≥ 30 mL/kg of body weight in 24 hours (72 hours postoperatively)

IV/IM analgesics at least 4 × per 24 hours or a continuous IV analgesic drip

Ventilator assistance

Initial tracheostomy care

Chest tube suction/drainage

IV antibiotics, antifungals, antidiuretics, steroids

IV cardiac glycosides (e.g., digitalis)

IV insulin

IV anticoagulants

Protective isolation

Skin care requiring professional nursing care at least 6 × per 24 hours (e.g., major burn care)

Intermittent bladder irrigation

Initial training for functional mobility with prosthesis, orthosis, assistive device, and/or splint

Adapted from InterQual, Inc., 1993a.

emergency department, no reviewer may have seen the chart. More progressive hospitals are placing social workers and UM nurses or case managers in the emergency department level of care. In general, admission reviews, also known as initial reviews, are done within 24 hours of admission. This review also determines medical necessity and appropriateness of the level of care.

Subsequent Reviews. Subsequent reviews are done intermittently throughout the hospitalization, with a 3-day interval between reviews considered maximum. The frequency is determined by the level of care, the severity of the patient's illness, and other factors. An experienced reviewer has a feel for when the next review needs attention. As a patient nears discharge or transfer to another level of care, these reviews become more frequent, usually daily.

Discharge Reviews. Discharge reviews use the discharge screens from the same category as were used to assess IS and SI. These reviews are used to determine stability for treatment and services at a lesser level of care. Documentation of discussions of why a patient does not meet discharge screens is important; documentation of discharge planning is equally important.

If a patient is not meeting discharge screens and a discharge is initiated, and that patient is readmitted to an acute care facility within 30 days, Medicare may look at the first hospitalization for quality of care issues or premature discharge indications. If the patient was discharged without documentation of passing discharge screens and had a bad outcome connected to the discharge, it could mean a risk management issue for the hospital. Discharge documentation should also include improvements noted from previous reviews. If the patient was initially admitted with a temperature of 39.8°C, a chest radiograph showing a right middle lobe infiltrate, and a white blood cell count of 25.5 TH/UL, and is receiving IV antibiotics every 4 hours, then discharge documentation might reflect that the patient is afebrile, no longer receiving IV antibiotic therapy (i.e., taking oral antibiotics) for 24 hours, the white blood cell count is 9.6 TH/UL or lower, and the chest radiograph is now clear.

Appendix 4-B presents an overview of InterQual's ISD criteria, which will provide the case manager with a basic understanding of the criteria. Examples of other InterQual ISD criteria follow. If your facility or agency does not have an InterQual manual or review system to examine, call or write one of the main branches for information about materials and seminars.

NOTE

InterQual, Inc.
Address: McKesson Health Solutions
275 Grove Street, Suite 1-110
Newton, MA 02466-2273
Telephone: 800-522-6780
Web site: www.interqual.com

CASE MANAGEMENT PLANS AND CLINICAL PATHWAYS

Of all utilization modalities, Case Management Plans (CMPs) and clinical pathways most completely take into account the total multidisciplinary aspects of the patient's care. Various names and formats for these pathways have been used: clinical pathways, critical pathways, practice parameters, clinical protocols/guidelines, Care MAP (Zander, 1992), progress pathway, and progress map. Although we look at pathways as a medical tool, the methodologies have been around for decades in the construction and engineering fields. The healthcare field researched them as early as the 1970s, but the environment was unreceptive to their use at that time (Coffey et al., 1992). Clinical pathways have become popular standard tools in case management programs, and case managers use them to monitor a patient's care progression. Generally, these tools have come to be known as case management plans.

Clinical pathways are a multidisciplinary management tool that proactively depicts important events that should take place in a day-by-day sequence. Throughout the entire episode of illness, the key events change daily and move the patient and the healthcare team toward discharge. The overall goal is to achieve optimal quality of care while minimizing delays and unnecessary resource utilization (Coffey et al., 1992); they are also written to stay within the DRG-allotted LOS. Pathways can be used by all team members to coordinate, plan, deliver, and monitor care, and document and perform UM activities concurrently. Clinical pathways have been written for various patient populations. Some are based on DRG-related diagnoses such as pneumonia or acute coronary syndrome. Other pathways were written for patient conditions such as ventilator dependency weaning. Surgical procedures such as total knee replacements or lumbar laminectomies comprise many pathways. Some pathways are used for more chronic conditions. Patients with end-stage renal disease (ESRD), chronic obstructive pulmonary disease (COPD), benign prostatic hypertrophy (BPH), or Crohn's disease could benefit from these pathways in the ambulatory setting. Clinical pathways can also be written for various timelines of care. The first and most common scope of care was the inpatient hospital pathway; however, that is changing and pathways now can be found from SNFs to home health agencies, and connecting through the continuum.

With the proliferation of clinical guidelines, clinical protocols, and clinical pathways, some confusion exists. The following define the three (Mateo et al., 1998, p. 3):

▶ Clinical pathways are outlines of the optimal sequencing and timing of interventions to provide resource-efficient, high-quality care by reducing practice variation. They are often developed by multidisciplinary teams that consist of clinicians and experts from various specialties. A timeline for providing interventions is included. Pathways usually apply to disease-specific populations of patients with a single uncomplicated diagnosis or procedure.

▶ Clinical guidelines are algorithms that represent a resource-efficient, evidence-based approach to the diagnosis and management of a clinical condition, either a diagnostic entity or a symptom. They are usually developed by multidisciplinary teams that consist of appropriate clinicians from multiple specialties, including experts in the field. Guidelines usually do not follow strict timelines.

▶ Clinical protocols are orders that prescribe diagnosis or procedure-specific activities that have traditionally required a written order in the medical record. They do not have a sequencing timeline or an outcome assessment.

Visually, many pathway formats are set up very similarly. An inpatient clinical pathway will be used as an example. In chart form, the patient days stretch across horizontally, and the key categories align vertically (Display 4-6). The medical events are cross-referenced by category and hospital day; these events may differ (e.g., a clinical path for a total hip replacement alters from that for congestive heart failure). Clinical pathways have four basic components (Strassner, 1996):

1. Aspects of care:. The following categories are addressed in this component: assessment, monitoring, treatments, medication, activity, diet, patient teaching, discharge planning, and outcomes evaluation. These categories follow the flow of patient care (i.e., starting with assessment and ending with outcomes evaluation). The aspects of care will change depending on the setting of the clinical pathway and the disease-specific type of clinical pathway.

2. Phases of care: These depict the time intervals for the treatments or care; they must be meaningful and based on best practices. When has outcomes research determined the best time to change to oral antibiotics for a particular illness? What is the best time to begin physical therapy? What are the medications that must be addressed before discharge (e.g., beta blockers and ACE inhibitors after MI)? The intervals depend on the clinical setting. For example, a home health clinical pathway may be in intervals of weeks; an ED clinical pathway may be 15-minute intervals to hours; a hospital clinical pathway is usually in intervals of days.

CRITICAL PATHWAY CHART

display 4-6

	Day 1	Day 2	Day 3	Day 4	Day 5
Treatments					
Consults/referrals					
Diagnostic tests					
Medications					
Activities/safety-mobility					
Diet/nutrition					
Transitional/discharge planning					
Teaching/education					
Outcomes					

3. Clinical pathway functions: These are the activities, processes, or interventions implemented by the multidisciplinary staff. Here is where the disclaimer is important: no clinical guideline must preempt the medical judgment of a professional. Consider how the pathway will be used in areas such as documentation and communication purposes. Also consider if it is a permanent part of the medical record; take into consideration the legal aspects of a clinical pathway. Determine all the disciplines that must use the pathway. Is it adequate to meet their documentation requirements or is it just another piece of paper?

4. Outcomes: Clinical pathways must be updated as best practices change and new evidence is discovered; they must also be changed when the outcomes determine that there is a better method or time frame to address a clinical issue. Both cost and quality issues must be measured and evaluated, but to do that, the organization must first determine its goals. Outcomes measurement and management for clinical pathways and for all aspects of care requires knowledge of quality improvement principles, process improvement tools, and project management.

In Display 4-6 the following may be filled in:

▶ Treatments include interventions that must be performed by the healthcare team, such as tube/catheter and site care, telemetry, daily weights, Foley catheter care, vital and neurological sign checks, suture removal, IV site changes, and small volume nebulizer treatments.
▶ Consults/referrals bring in other members of the healthcare team, such as those in ostomy care, social service, diabetic education, rehabilitation, physical therapy, or dietary services.
▶ Diagnostic tests include measurable data, such as radiology, radiography, laboratory tests, electrocardiography (ECG), urine or stool studies, and blood sugar monitoring.
▶ Medications include the drugs ordered with dosage, times, and route. IV antibiotics may be ordered on days 1 and 2, whereas oral antibiotics may be charted for the following hospital days. Medications may include anything from anticoagulants to stool softeners. Pain control is also documented, along with route of medications (oral, intramuscular, IV, or epidural).
▶ Activities/mobility outlines the patient's allowable activities. Across the days, this may progress from bed rest to chair to ambulation,

or sitting up in a chair or head-of-bed elevations. The length of time that the patient sat in the chair or how far he or she ambulated should be documented.
▶ Diet/nutrition defines the patient's dietary needs and may advance from nothing by mouth (NPO) to a regular or specialty diet, depending on the patient's requirements. Chart the percentage of diet taken and how well the patient tolerated it. Discharge planning optimally starts before admission. Because this is not always possible, a social service referral may be charted for day 1 or 2. Insurance eligibility or SNF placement referrals may be recommended.
▶ Transitional/discharge planning defines the activities that will need to take place to move a patient from one level of care to another, less intense level, in preparation for discharge to home or another less acute facility. These may include UR and UM review and other activities that focus on ensuring safe discharge plan.
▶ Teaching/education interactions are necessary to help the patient/family become more independent and self-sufficient. Teaching may include physical therapy safety modalities, proper administration of medications (with possible side effects), insurance explanations, tube-feeding administration, diet, exercise, post-transplantation necessary lifestyle modifications, or disease process. All events are tailored to the needs of the diagnosis and hospital day.
▶ Outcomes define the intermediate and discharge outcomes. Intermediate outcomes are the milestones that will need to be achieved to ensure that a patient is progressing well toward discharge to a lesser acute setting (home or SNF), which is indicative of improvement in the patient's condition. These outcomes can be designed based on InterQual or MCGs criteria.

Depending on the level of care and diagnosis, each clinical pathway has its own unique features. A home health clinical pathway for a coronary artery bypass graft (CABG) or valve replacement patient may be delineated by weeks: week 1 may include 3 visits, week 2 may include 2 visits, and week 3 may include 1 to 2 visits. Each week consists of different goals: patient goals, knowledge goals, physical reconditioning goals, nutritional goals, incision healing, pain control, medication response and compliance, symptoms, vital sign stability—all the components of good nursing care.

Clinical pathways for *subacute care* have been published by the National Association of Subacute/

Postacute Care (NASPAC) and are entitled *Clinical Guidelines for Subacute Units.* For more information, call NASPAC at 410-882-0143. Essentially, subacute clinical pathways incorporate five core areas (Madigan, 1997):

1. Include all important disciplines with appropriate benchmarks and interventions.
2. Include adequate education information that would encourage patient/family participation.
3. Integrate admission criteria.
4. Integrate discharge criteria.
5. Address measurement and analysis of outcomes.

Clinical pathways leave unanswered questions and signal limitations. They are not ideally suited to patients with multiple concurrent medical problems, although many healthcare professionals are working on solutions to this problem. In general, it is recommended that the staff use the clinical pathway matching the most immediate problem the patient presents with, which is usually the primary driver for care decisions. For example, if a postoperative patient is having a difficult time weaning from ventilator assistance, change the pathway to a ventilator pathway until the patient can get back on the original path. In less extreme circumstances, the patient may deviate from the pathway and smaller adjustments may need to be made; pathways are an outline and a tool, and it may not always be possible to follow them exactly. Other problems may arise if one patient has multiple physicians with multiple practice patterns. If an agreement cannot be reached, the pathway may cause additional stress and defeat its purpose.

Although not a limitation per se, the event changes are not standing orders; rather, these are clinical protocols as defined above. If an attending physician has already visited the patient that day, and the nurse has been prompted by the clinical pathway that a change to oral (from IV) medication may be recommended, the nurse can call the physician for clarification. Perhaps the physician had a reason to continue the IV medication (e.g., the patient is NPO); perhaps it was an oversight and the telephone call could save resources and possibly an extra day in the hospital. More facilities are writing concurrent standing orders that coincide with each day's events.

Many organizations and professionals have created clinical pathways for patients using lay, rather than technical, terminology. They have proved to be a support to both patients/families and medical staff. Patients who can "see" that what they are experiencing is common are not as anxious as those who do not understand what is happening to them. Many physicians appreciate the at-a-glance multidisciplinary chart-ing. They have also received positive feedback from their patients. Patient-focused pathways are an important tool for patient teaching and for encouraging a patient to assume an active role in his or her care.

Reactions to clinical pathways have been mixed, especially from physicians. Although physicians have been essential to their development, underlying fears include increased liability and loss of autonomy, especially in the area of decision making and judgment about a patient's treatment plan. Some physicians believe that clinical pathways are a road map for a plaintiff's attorney; certainly they are sometimes used as a sword—and sometimes used as a shield—in court. Physicians also state that pathways represent a loss of their own autonomy, usually referred to as cookbook medicine. To remedy this, some hospitals have used more than one pathway for the same DRG diagnoses to accommodate the different practice patterns of various physicians. However, this was found to be cumbersome, expensive, and has fallen out of favor. Legal recommendations in the literature state that a disclaimer should be on the clinical pathway, because it is a guideline and does not preempt the clinical judgment of a physician. A disclaimer should include that the pathway is only a representation of a common pattern of treatment and that all patients are different; acceptable medical practice includes a variety of responses to a particular clinical problem.

When a patient's care does not meet the changes as outlined in the clinical pathway, a variance has occurred, that is, a detour off the path. These detours can be positive or negative, avoidable or unavoidable. A positive variance may show a patient progressing quicker than the pathway anticipated. Negative variances usually result in an extended LOS, and the patient takes longer to reach desired outcomes (see "Lag Days and Variances" earlier in this chapter).

Proponents of clinical pathways say that because a variance can be sighted almost immediately (through the prompting inherent in the clinical pathways system), lag days can be reduced. The goal is to recognize and resolve the variance as quickly as possible and get the care back on the path in a timely manner. Variance sheets are filled out and the causes of the deviation are explored immediately, allowing corrective action to be taken. Analysis of variance data is directly related to quality improvement activities, allowing less fragmentation of hospital systems.

BENEFITS AND GOALS OF CASE MANAGEMENT PLANS AND CLINICAL PATHWAYS. A summation follows of some of the benefits and goals of clinical pathways.

▶ The UM and quality improvement activities, as well as the multidisciplinary activities, are supportive and all-inclusive.

▶ Of all the various utilization modalities, the patient (not only symptoms or physician's orders) is the primary focus in clinical pathways. Therefore, the patient is the common denominator of all activities, and the patient/family satisfaction is improved. It has been noted that patients who have been made aware of the day-by-day changes in their clinical pathway have a decreased level of anxiety—they know approximately what to expect—and an increased sense of involvement and control. Hence, the patients use the changes as goals to attain.

▶ Clinical pathways are an effective tool for decreasing LOS and resource utilization, because they efficiently move the patient toward discharge goals. Last-minute oversights are avoided.

▶ Quality of care is enhanced with continuous, concurrent attention to variances.

▶ Satisfaction and communication among the multidisciplinary team members are enhanced. It is case management at a glance.

▶ Clinical pathways are compatible with other utilization modalities.

▶ Clinical pathways are easy to use.

▶ When clinical pathways are used as a documentation tool, nurses report less time spent on charting and improved shift reports.

▶ Clinical pathways serve as excellent guidelines for novice nurses who may be unsure of the course a patient should be taking for a particular DRG or diagnosis. They can be used as education tools and orientation models, delineating expected outcomes. One case manager commented that what had taken her 2 years to know and understand through constant experience with a case type, a new clinician could now master within 6 weeks (Etheredge, 1987).

▶ Clinical pathways provide cues to the staff for all aspects of care.

▶ Clinical pathways lend themselves as a tool for an applied research process, whereby algorithms are embedded within the pathway itself (Zander, 1992).

▶ Clinical pathways written for patients support the healthcare process and lessen anxiety.

DEVELOPMENT OF A CASE MANAGEMENT PLAN AND CLINICAL PATHWAY. Crozer-Keystone Health

System in Pennsylvania has introduced an 11-step process for the development of extended-care clinical pathways used in disease management programs (Anonymous, 1997). The changes in the SNF level of care necessitate the use of disease management and UM strategies; clinical pathways are the connection between the two. However, this process can be used in any level of care when development of a clinical pathway is required. The 11 steps include the following (Anonymous, 1997):

1. Select a target population. This is based on the individual needs of the SNF; clinical and cost issues must be examined. With the advent of the new discharge/transfer rules in acute care, one of the 10 DRGs may be a cost-effective selection to make. This rule is discussed in more detail in "Incentives of Change" in Chapter 5.

2. Create a core working group. One of the most important tasks before undertaking a change such as use of clinical pathways is the choice of a "physician champion"—one of the most important success factors in any healthcare project. Physician input at the beginning will lessen physician resistance at the implementation stage. The rest of the work group can consist of adjunctive specialists who have knowledge of the disease state and comorbidities, case managers who understand UM and discharge planning strategies, computer systems personnel if the pathway is going to be computerized, and any other pertinent persons with knowledge of the process.

3. Create a written vision and goals statement. The group must share a common vision and common goals to be successful.

4. Assess existing programs and services for the targeted population or disease. Reinvention of the wheel is not necessary. Keep the processes that are working, change the processes that require modification, reduce or discard any processes that are redundant, and create new processes to blend or improve the foundation.

5. Assess the care and service needs of this population. Existing services are matched to the population's needs. Gaps are filled in through creative approaches. If additional knowledge is required at this stage, bring other experts into the working group.

6. Determine the pathway format. Research the literature for various pathway formats and come to a consensus on one that will work for your culture and organization.

7. Develop high-level flowcharts that define the process flow for all steps in the delivery of care. The flowchart is one of the simplest and most useful tools for process improvement. Become familiar with how they are formatted and how to use them. Processes such as handing off patients often have never been flowcharted or made into a formal process; this process is also a common cause of problems. When developing a clinical pathway, consider how it will flow to all parts of the continuum and with all members of the multidisciplinary team. When creating flowcharts, it is essential to include all pertinent people in the brainstorming session who have knowledge of the process (from unit secretaries to nursing assistants to maintenance personnel).

8. Develop quality improvement feedback loops to track and report the selected indicators. Reporting of outcomes is expected in healthcare today. Developing quality indicators and using them to target areas of improvement is one excellent use of clinical pathways. This step may necessitate inclusion in the planning team of information systems and quality management experts.

9. Implement the pathway. Quality improvement strategies recommend initially implementing any new process on a small scale. It is a test drive rather than the long haul. If something in the pathway causes problems, the small scale effort may involve tweaking rather than a full-blown organizational change.

10. Establish benchmarks. A benchmark is essentially a goal to be achieved and is derived from the best in the field. When a facility implements a change in a process, it wants to know if that change has caused a good result or a negative situation. Benchmarks are one method to measure the effect of the process; they demonstrate if goals have been met. Crozer-Keystone uses two approaches for benchmarking (Anonymous, 1997):

   a. Establish clear benchmarks for measured quality indicators, based on the most recent data available on the target population. The goal is to determine if the use of the pathway improves care to your patients, at least to the point of the benchmark.

   b. Use a concurrent control group methodology where two similar groups are in the test: one is managed with the clinical pathway, and the other group uses the old process of care without the clinical pathway.

11. Evaluate and manage the program. This is a basic tenet of quality improvement. Anything that can be done, can be done better.

Appendix 4-C provides several examples of clinical pathways. Five pathways for acute care were written in the mid-1990s (pneumonia, total hip replacement, total knee replacement, laminectomy, CABG). Many hospitals, including the Phoenix, Arizona-based hospital that provided the examples, have expanded their clinical pathways, which often begin in the emergency department. These were created with constant input from respected cardiologists practicing at the hospital; therefore, there was little physician resistance. The MI example includes:

▶ An ED protocol for chest pain/acute MI.
▶ Physician orders for admission, acute MI after emergency department care.
▶ Physician transfer orders—acute MI after stabilization of the patient.
▶ The actual uncomplicated MI clinical pathway.
▶ A patient information summary for uncomplicated acute MI. This sheet walks the acute MI patient through a typical hospital stay for the diagnosis; it is aligned with the professional's clinical pathway.

Many of the quality improvement concepts involved in the development of a clinical pathway are not commonly taught to case management professionals. However, healthcare has changed and case managers will be required to participate in or administer healthcare developmental and improvement programs.

MILLIMAN CARE GUIDELINES

Milliman Care Guidelines (MCGs), previously known as Milliman & Robertson Healthcare Management Guidelines (HMGs), consist of a set of optimal clinical practice benchmarks for treating common conditions for patients who generally have no complications; they resemble a combination of LOS criteria and mini-clinical pathways. MCGs are written based on diagnoses or diseases; unlike InterQual criteria, which are written based on body systems. First developed in 1984, HMGs were created as a tool to support the desire of providers and healthcare managers to deliver care more efficiently—that is, to achieve desired patient care outcomes using an optimal level of resources. Their purpose is not to ration or reduce care but rather to help minimize waste and inefficiency in the healthcare system, thereby making the best use of the limited healthcare resources available.

The guidelines have been continuously updated and expanded since 1984 and are based on observed best practices of actively practicing physicians and published research. To date, Milliman Care Guidelines, Inc. has published seven sets of guidelines that emphasize the continuum of care. These publications have been expanded to include easier online access to the guidelines and updates to each of the volumes. The current seven volumes address ambulatory care, inpatient and surgical care, general recovery, recovery facility care, home care, chronic care, and behavioral health. The guidelines are described below.

NOTE

Milliman Care Guidelines, Inc.
Address: 719 Second Avenue, Suite 300
Seattle, WA 98104
Telephone: (888) 464-4746
Technical support: (800) 598-2292
Web site: www.careguidelines.com

---

1. *Ambulatory Care Guidelines* (ACGs) enable access to evidence-based criteria for imaging, diagnostic testing, rehabilitative services, ambulatory surgery, injectable drugs, immunizations, referrals, and transplantation. Healthcare professionals can find the authorization criteria they need when caring for patients in the ambulatory care setting, as well as access to over 70 OTGs for comprehensive background, scope, diagnosis, and treatment information.

2. *Inpatient and Surgical Care Guidelines* (ISCGs) offer benchmarks for patients with uncomplicated courses of recovery. Used in conjunction with professional medical judgment, the OTGs detail the practices that make good use of available resources, while leading to optimal health outcomes for each patient. The OTGs are categorized into five groups (medical, surgical, pediatric, mental health, and psychoactive substance abuse) and also contain GLOS and inpatient care and utilization models. See Appendix 4-D for sample OTGs. The inpatient and surgical care guidelines include actionable admission/procedure and discharge criteria; detailed, day-by-day care pathway tables that assess level of care, clinical status, activity, interventions, and medications; comprehensive observation care

admission/discharge criteria for over 80 topics, including abdominal pain, syncope, and chest pain; quality measures that are incorporated within workflow; and case management activities. Each OTG is organized as follows:
   a. OTG description;
   b. ICD-9-CM and/or Current Procedural Terminology (CPT) codes;
   c. Case management actions;
   d. Adequate reasons for admission;
   e. Inadequate reasons for admission;
   f. Alternatives to admission;
   g. Day 1 expected patient progress;
   h. Day 2;
   i. Day 3; and
   j. Goal length of stay in days.

3. *General Recovery Guidelines* (GRGs) provide expanded decision support for management of comorbidities, multiple illnesses, or unclear diagnoses. They also provide reliable guidance for clinically complex situations where another guideline cannot easily be applied. The GRGs are ideal for those circumstances in which there are no other care guidelines to address a specific diagnosis. Some of the main benefits of using the GRGs are efficient management of multiple diagnoses, handling comorbidities and complex health conditions, and access to long-term acute care guidelines.

4. *Recovery Facility Care Guidelines* (RFCGs) describe a well-coordinated plan for the successful transition of more complex patients to recovery facilities such as SNFs and subacute care—and their subsequent discharge to the appropriate setting. RFCGs provide criteria for admission and discharge, and quick reference charts to identify appropriate care settings and complete discharge plans. They also allow the healthcare team to establish a care path strategy in the initial phases of case management, with main focus on the needs of the individual patient, and to more effectively manage the quality of healthcare delivery. These guidelines are closely correlated with the Inpatient and Surgical Care and Home Care Guidelines to direct care across the continuum.

5. *Home Care Guidelines* (HCGs) play a vital role in prompt hospital discharge and avoidance of rehospitalization. A well-defined, well-coordinated plan is essential, particularly for successful transition of more complex patients. HCGs facilitate a multidisciplinary approach to support patients through an episode of care at

home. They are closely correlated with Inpatient and Surgical Care and Recovery Facility Care guidelines to guide healthcare professionals through the continuum of patient care. Treatment plans for many specific conditions are included in this volume, as well as a general approach appropriate for more complex or unusually severe cases. HCGs include traditional nursing care and home care plans, clinical indications that make a patient a candidate for early discharge with home health support, types and descriptions of home health encounters (telephonic versus on-site), number of encounters for specific services, and discharge goals.

6. *Chronic Care Guidelines* (CCGs) provide a robust framework for disease or care management of patients with chronic, complex, or multidiagnosis health conditions. Each of the 24 chronic conditions covered in the CCGs include a set of patient education materials that are written at a fourth-grade level, designed to be sent to a member as part of an intervention. The educational materials are available in both English and Spanish. The CCGs can be used by healthcare professionals to help meet chronic care management goals and to ensure the provision of evidence-based care. Some of the benefits of the CCGs are facilitation of outpatient care for patients with chronic/complex health conditions; patient and family education through the use of fourth-grade level education materials; management of secondary prevention, posttransplant care, and end-of-life care; promotion of quality through consistent care and integrated outcome measures; development of case management plans for 24 chronic conditions; and provision of care that is evidence-based.

7. *Behavioral Health Guidelines* (BHGs) provide indications at five different levels of care, and the appropriateness of specific psychological, behavioral, and pharmacologic therapies is addressed. BHGs include tools and criteria that can aid in developing outpatient alternatives to higher levels of care, facilitating the progress of patients whose recovery is delayed, and developing comprehensive case management plans for transition from one level of care to another. The BHGs consist of 15 guideline groups that cover the full spectrum of behavioral health diagnoses. They are known to integrate behavioral health with other UM activities, include relevant and latest evidence,

reduce inappropriate care, address chronic comorbidities, and facilitate proactive care.

The various volumes assist case managers and other healthcare professionals to understand where the recovery process fits into the continuum of care. Home care, for example, requires planning early in the care delivery process. The guidelines provide clinical indications that make a patient a candidate for early discharge and include a description of the goals that should be met before discharge. They also describe the role of recovery facilities as an alternative to a prolonged stay in acute care facilities, or to direct admission to other types of facilities that may not have been necessary. Five levels of care are described, and patients may move from one level to another as they progress.

1. Acute rehabilitation: appropriate if multidisciplinary therapies are required and the patient's medical stability, physical endurance, and cognitive capability allow cooperation for at least 3 hours per day.
2. Subacute rehabilitation: if multidisciplinary therapies are not required or capacities are limited to cooperation for less than 3 hours per day.
3. Skilled rehabilitation: if the patient's needs are limited to physical therapy for gait training.
4. Subacute medical/nursing: if the patient is less stable than the typical skilled nursing care patient and requires a greater IS for safety.
5. Skilled medical/nursing: the most common reason for use of a recovery facility; suitable for patients with skilled needs at least 3 times per day and whose activities of daily living cannot be supported temporarily by an adequate caregiver at home.

The *Inpatient and Surgical Care Guidelines* provide a list of procedures and/or diagnoses and recommended GLOS for different types of procedures. Many users find the classification by *Current Procedural Terminology*, 4th edition (CPT-4), ICD-9, and *Diagnostic and Statistical Manual of Mental Disorders*, 4th edition (DSM-IV) codes to be helpful. In addition, information about the appropriate settings for the various GLOS is also included. "A" indicates conditions that generally should be treated on an ambulatory basis. However, admission may be appropriate depending on the severity of the condition. "1," "2," etc., indicate conditions that ordinarily require hospitalization. The number indicates the recommended first review point or GLOS. UR is a collaborative and proactive process that should begin well before surgery, rather than on the day of surgery.

Examples of GLOS are as follows:

▶ CABG = 3 days postoperative.
▶ Hip arthroplasty = 3 days postoperative.
▶ Radical prostatectomy = 1 to 2 days postoperative.
▶ Pneumonia, community-acquired = 2 days.
▶ Septicemia with ICU admission = 2 days.
▶ Asthma = 1 day.
▶ Seizures including new onset = A.
▶ Pleural biopsy, closed = A.

Critics have charged that the OTGs are unrealistic or that they are an excuse for insurance companies to attempt to squeeze more-complex patients into inappropriate treatments. However, the guidelines are meant to be used under optimal conditions, always to support the judgment of the providers who are delivering care and not as a substitute for clinicians' judgment. Achieving the GLOS requires improvement in the process of care, such as preoperative education, preemptive analgesia, earlier ambulation, and earlier feeding.

ORGs that are included for preview include:

▶ S-390 CABG.
▶ S-560 hip arthroplasty (total).
▶ S-960 radical prostatectomy, not transurethral.
▶ M-281 pneumonia, community acquired.
▶ M-330 septicemia, with ICU admission.
▶ M-55 asthma.
▶ M-327 seizures.

ADMISSION AS PER CASE MANAGEMENT PROTOCOL

The admission as per case management protocol, developed by the Florida QIO, is a fairly new phenomenon that is implemented by hospitals in certain states (e.g., Arizona, Florida, Nebraska) in an attempt to decrease unnecessary admissions to the hospital setting. It primarily focuses on reducing the number of patients who are admitted to the hospital setting and who stay as inpatients for 2 days or less. In many of the cases, the status could have been "observation." Under Medicare and Medicaid benefits, if these patients were billed by hospitals as inpatient admissions, these claims would often experience high reimbursement denial rates. Commonly seen diagnoses in the 2-days-or-less admissions are chest pain, abdominal pain, and esophagitis.

A decision that an admission to the hospital is unnecessary is made primarily based on documentation that is inappropriate or that lacks support for medical necessity and the acute inpatient level of care. This is often attributed to a physician's lack of knowledge of medical necessity and hospital admission criteria.

When lack of knowledge is not the issue, lack of documentation usually is. Case managers involved in documentation improvement or UM activities are the best individuals to prevent such determinations from happening and they can enhance reimbursement or reduce the risk for reimbursement denials because of billing for inappropriate status, that is, an inpatient admission instead of an observation status.

The use of admission as per case management protocol aims to increase the number of hospitalized patients assigned the correct inpatient versus observation status; to decrease unnecessary hospital admissions; and to further decrease Medicare payment/reimbursement error and denial rates. The protocol addresses incorrect billing issues and does not affect the quality of care patients receive. Hospitals that implement such a protocol have it approved prior to implementation by case management and UM departments, medical staff, compliance officers, and other business departments.

When a patient is admitted as per case management protocol, the case manager/UM nurse would then assign the patient to the appropriate status (i.e., observation or inpatient) based on the hospital's admission criteria. The decision would be binding and upheld by the physician writing the order. If the assignment of a particular patient was to an observation status, conversion to an inpatient status could be done at any time up to 48 hours post initial assignment. However, during the 48 hours, the patient is monitored and assessed on an ongoing basis to allow better determination of admission status, appropriate level of care and, ultimately, appropriate Medicare billing. The decision to convert a patient status is best done at or before 23 hours.

Hospitals adopting the admit as per case management protocol must:

1. Have a well thought-out process whereby the admitting or case management department creates a hold status for these patients until a decision of observation or admission status is made.
2. Determine, and clearly communicate, the hold status time frame; commonly 2 to 6 hours and not exceeding 23 hours.
3. As a default mechanism, place a patient on observation status and convert status later when new findings and information support the conversion.
4. Notify the attending/admitting physician when a conversion in status occurs. The physician must then write an order confirming the conversion.

5. Have a process of handling such protocol on off shifts, the weekends, and holidays. If a process does not exist, it is advisable to implement the protocol during weekdays and regular business hours, or when it is feasible, for example, during case managers' hours of operation.

The admission as per case management protocol is an important, evolving tool that helps a hospital to maintain compliance with Medicare reimbursement standards. QIOs usually review or audit medical records of Medicare patients on a regular basis. During such reviews, quality of care and appropriateness of hospital admissions are evaluated. If an admission to a hospital setting is found to be inappropriate, the hospital would be either denied reimbursement or asked to refund the payment received from Medicare. CMS monitors payments through its Hospital Payment Monitoring Program (HPMP). Billions of dollars are paid by Medicare annually for unnecessary admissions to hospitals. Case managers can assist hospitals in reducing their risk of refunding Medicare payments they inappropriately receive.

CONDITION CODE 44

Condition Code 44 is a term that refers to changing an inpatient admission to an outpatient status after care has been rendered, the patient has not been discharged from the hospital, and the claim has not yet been submitted to Medicare for reimbursement. This occurs when a physician admits a patient to an inpatient bed (the hospital); however, after a case manager or UM nurse later reviews the case, he or she determines that the patient level of care does not meet the hospital admission criteria; as a result of the review the patient's admission status is changed.

Condition Code 44 has been in use since April 1, 2004 on outpatient claims only. This rule allows a hospital to bill for inpatient services ordered by a physician and performed by the hospital, but on internal review before the claim was initially submitted to Medicare, the hospital found the services did not meet its inpatient admission criteria. The services are then billed under the Outpatient Prospective Payment System (OPPS) (CMS, 2004).

A hospital may change a Medicare beneficiary's status from inpatient to outpatient and submit an outpatient claim for medically necessary Medicare Part B services that were furnished to the beneficiary, provided all of the following conditions are met:

1. The change in status was made prior to the patient's discharge or release from the hospital.
2. The hospital has not submitted a claim to Medicare for the inpatient admission.

3. A physician concurs with the utilization review determination.
4. The physician's concurrence with the determination is documented in the patient's chart.

In these situations, the entire episode of the hospital admission must be treated as an outpatient encounter. The claim should clearly reflect the change and should always adhere to the required paperwork; that is, using the exact forms as designated by Medicare. Case managers and UM nurses can play an effective role in reviewing such events and in ensuring that hospitals submit appropriate claims to Medicare. Such careful reviews allow a hospital to maintain compliance with the Medicare Conditions of Participation and to reduce reimbursement errors and denial rates.

MEDICARE OBSERVATION STATUS GUIDELINES

Observation status is an administrative classification of patients, seen in hospital emergency rooms or outpatient clinics, who have uncertain conditions that are potentially serious enough to warrant close observation, but usually not so serious to warrant admission to the hospital (AHRQ, 2002). Healthcare providers and hospitals tend to place these patients in beds, usually for less than 24 hours, without formal admissions to the hospital as inpatients. During this time frame, the patient is monitored and frequently assessed until a final determination is reached whether to admit or discharge.

CMS defines observation services as those that are furnished by a hospital on its premises, including the use of a bed; at the least, they include periodic monitoring by a hospital's nursing or other staff. These services must be reasonable and necessary to evaluate an outpatient's condition or determine the need for a possible inpatient admission. The purpose of observation status is to evaluate and treat a patient's medical condition to determine if there is a need for further treatment in an inpatient setting. The time period for an observation status may extend until a decision is confidently made either to admit the patient to the hospital with an "inpatient status" or to discharge. The most common time period for observation status is 24 hours; it may extend to 48 hours. Under special circumstances, however, sometimes the observation period may be as long as 72 hours.

Observation status is common in outpatient clinics, emergency departments, and ambulatory surgery centers. Patients with "observation status" may receive care in any setting including telemetry, ICU, etc., although it is most common in the following three areas:

1. Emergency department/treatment units: designated areas within and under the direction

of the emergency department physicians and other clinical staff for patients who require further treatment or evaluation.

2. Holding units: designated areas within the outpatient settings that may or may not be under the control of the emergency department where a patient is held pending prearranged actions such as admission or transfer.

3. Observation status beds: designated beds in the inpatient areas of a hospital in which a patient may be evaluated or treated until a decision about disposition is needed or made.

In these settings, a patient is assessed, monitored, evaluated, and treated. He or she is placed on observation status, discharged, or admitted to an inpatient setting. If placed on observation status, he or she is then evaluated at a later time (usually less than 24 hours) and a decision is made to either admit to an inpatient setting or discharge. Figure 4.1 includes a decision tree hospitals may implement as part of its observation status guidelines. Display 4-7 is another helpful tool that can aid case managers and physicians in effectively determining if a patient's condition warrants an inpatient admission or observation status.

Payment/reimbursement for observation status varies by state and payor. Payment issues such as fee schedules, prospective payment systems, private insurance, or other arrangements, and limits on payments such as hours of observation status, affect reimbursement. From a case management or UM perspective, documentation of medical necessity is essential for appropriate payment/reimbursement. A physician's order must specify "admit to observation" and must be signed and dated. A physician's order that states only "Admit" will be considered

an inpatient admission. When a change in status occurs, physician notes and orders must also specify such change.

When a patient has been in observation status, documentation of progress must include the need to continue observation. The patient's medical record must include documentation at certain intervals during the 24 hours. If documentation of progress includes the conversion in status to an inpatient admission, the record must reflect the presence of evidence that the patient's condition meets admission and medical necessity criteria. If documentation of progress indicates the decision to discharge the patient, the record must reflect evidence of medical stability and a plan for follow-up care as needed.

PRESENT ON ADMISSION

CMS was mandated under Section 5001(c) of the Deficit Reduction Act (DRA) of 2005 to implement a requirement that hospitals report Present on Admission (POA) information for inpatient acute care hospital claims to Medicare effective October 1, 2007. After April 1, 2008 hospitals submitting inpatient claims that lack the POA indicator had their claims returned unpaid. POA is defined as a condition present at the time the order is written for inpatient admission. Conditions that develop during an outpatient encounter, emergency department event, observation, or outpatient surgery, are considered as POA.

Present on Admission makes a distinction between a patient's condition at the time the order is written for inpatient admission (including comorbidities) and complications acquired during the course of treatment while in the inpatient/hospital setting. The use of POA

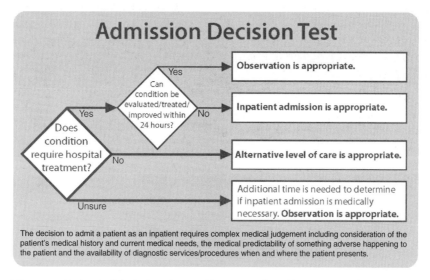

Figure 4.1 Deciding on a Patient's Admission Status. (Courtesy of Health Services Advisory Group, Phoenix, AZ.)

INPATIENT VS. OUTPATIENT OBSERVATION—8 KEY QUESTIONS FOR PHYSICIANS TO ASK

1. In what condition will the patient most likely be tomorrow?

   "Better" = Consider observation

2. Is it risky to send the patient home today?

   "Yes" = Consider observation

3. Is it likely I will know whether to admit or send the patient home by tomorrow?

   "Yes" = Consider observation

4. Are vital signs stable?

   "Yes" = Consider observation

5. Will a diagnosis likely be made in 24 hours?

   "Yes" = Consider observation

6. Will treatment, such as IV fluids, require standard monitoring and be complete within 24 hours?

   "Yes" = Consider observation

7. Is the patient being admitted with symptom(s) (e.g., chest pain, abdominal pain, TIA)?

   "Yes" = Consider observation

8. Is the patient having an unusually long recovery period following an outpatient procedure (e.g., pain management issues, cardiopulmonary concerns, urinary retention)?

   "Yes" = Consider observation

(Reprinted with permission. Richards, F., Pitluk, H., Collier, P., Powell, S., Dion, C., Struchen-Shellhorn, W., and Plunkett, M. (2008). Reducing Unnecessary Medicare Hospital Admissions for Chest Pain in Arizona and Florida. *Professional Case Management, 15*(2).

on claims will impact reimbursement. Those conditions acquired during the course of a hospital treatment such as falls-related injuries, nosocomial infections (e.g., urinary tract infection, hospital-acquired pneumonia), pneumothorax as a result of central line or chest tube insertion, and other "never events" may not be reimbursed. An example of "never events" is wrong site surgery. Therefore, hospitals will be penalized for poor care and medical errors. CMS identified five reporting options for POA conditions:

1. Y—present at the time of inpatient admission.
2. N—not present at the time of inpatient admission.
3. U—documentation is insufficient to determine if condition is POA.
4. W—provider is unable to clinically determine whether condition was POA or not.
5. Exempt from POA—left blank if condition is unreported or is not applicable.

According to the guidelines, medical record coders may apply the following rules. Case managers and UM nurses must be familiar with these rules to enforce compliance with standards and regulations and to answer questions when asked to clarify vague or questionable situations.

▶ Y & N: Must be explicitly documented; i.e., hypertension, diabetes mellitus, or asthma.
▶ U: Assign when medical record documentation is unclear; should not be routinely assigned; used in very limited circumstances. Coders encouraged to query providers when

documentation is unclear before coding has been completed.

▶ W: Assign when medical record documentation indicates that it cannot be clinically determined whether or not condition was POA.
▶ Y: Assign for conditions that were clearly present, but not diagnosed, until after admission occurred—diagnoses subsequently confirmed *after* admission are considered POA if, at the time of admission, they are documented as suspected, possible, ruled in or ruled out, differential diagnoses, or constituting an underlying cause of a symptom that is POA.

RECOVERY AUDIT CONTRACTORS

On January 11, 2005, CMS announced a 3-year demonstration project called the Recovery Audit Contractors (RACs), mandated by the Medicare Prescription Drug Improvement and Modernization Act of 2003. The demonstration project intended to use RACs to search for improper Medicare payments that might have been made to healthcare providers and that were not detected through existing program integrity efforts. The states that participated in this project included California, Florida, and New York; before the project concluded, CMS extended the RACs to three other states: Arizona, Massachusetts, and South Carolina. RACs were successful in allowing CMS to recoup Medicare overpayments. Due to their success, CMS expects to implement the RAC program in all 50 states by 2010. The expansion will be as follows (AHA, 2009):

1. **Region A** through Diversified Collection Services, Inc. of Livermore, California: initially working in Maine, New Hampshire, Vermont, Massachusetts, Rhode Island, and New York.
2. **Region B** through CGI Technologies and Solutions, Inc. of Fairfax, Virginia: initially working in Michigan, Indiana, and Minnesota.
3. **Region C** through Connolly Consulting Associates, Inc. of Wilton, Connecticut: initially working in South Carolina, Florida, Colorado, and New Mexico.
4. **Region D** through HealthDataInsights, Inc. of Las Vegas, Nevada: initially working in Montana, Wyoming, North Dakota, South Dakota, Utah, and Arizona.

RACs employ certain mechanisms to detect and respond to inappropriate billing. They use a careful review process that entails requesting Medicare claims history and medical records from hospitals. The review may include looking at specific DRGs, durable medical equipment, high-cost injectable drugs, renal dialysis, outpatient services such as physical therapy or psychiatric encounters, and physician services. DRGs most commonly reviewed included are those of chest pain, heart failure, gastroenteritis, and back pain. These tend to have a shorter LOS which makes them susceptible to conversion to observation status. The RACs focus primarily on these DRGs because of the likelihood that patient encounters were billed as inpatient stays when an appropriate and careful review of medical necessity may have placed them in the observation status or outpatient category. Therefore, the opportunity to find Medicare overpayment is greater in these DRGs.

After completing a thorough review, RACs are able to determine if over- or underpayments exist. If an overpayment is detected, the contractor will pursue payment and will be reimbursed a percentage of those recoveries. For underpayments, RACs will provide the necessary documentation to the Medicare contractors for processing payment to the provider. The financial ramifications of the RACs to healthcare organizations (particularly hospitals) are enormous especially in the areas of case management and UM. Employing case managers or UM nurses to primarily focus on patients' eligibility for inpatient admissions, medical necessity reviews, and evaluation of the appropriateness of observation status and outpatient care is of great value. Case mangers and UM nurses will ensure compliance with Medicare payment procedures, and provision of services in the appropriate setting and at the right level of care.

STUDY QUESTIONS

1. What is the difference between prior, concurrent, and retrospective review? Authorization or certification?

2. Under what circumstances is a case manager able to achieve certification/authorization for continued or extended length of stay?

3. Compare and contrast InterQual criteria and Milliman Care Guidelines. For which populations is each commonly used?

4. How can a case manager best apply the criteria or guidelines in the UM activities? Discuss the application differentiating admission, from continued stay, from discharge.

5. What makes case management plans/clinical pathways effective? What makes them ineffective?

6. What conditions are considered inappropriate for a hospital to claim reimbursement from Medicare? Differentiate present on admission from hospital-acquired conditions.

7. What is observation status? Discuss the benefits and disadvantages of observation status.

8. What documentation is required when changing a patient's status from observation to inpatient?

9. Why does CMS focus on reviewing payments/reimbursement? How will RACs benefit CMS? How will RACs benefit the care providers/hospitals?

▶ REFERENCES

Agency for Healthcare Research and Quality (AHRQ). (2002). *Healthcare cost and utilization methods series: Observation status related to US hospital records.* Report # 2002-3. Washington, DC: U.S. Department of Health and Human Services, AHRQ.

American Hospital Association. (2009). (accessed 4/13/2009). *Recovery audit contractor program.* [Online]. Available: http://www.aha.org/aha/issues/RAC/index.html.

Anonymous. (1989). Managed care: integrating "Q.A." in everyday practice. *Definition,* 4(3), 1–2.

Anonymous. (1997). Extended care pathway development process can help manage disease across the continuum. *Post Acute Care Strategy Report,* 2(11), 9–12.

Carneal, G. (1998). Getting accredited. *Continuing Care,* 17(10), 18–24, 42.

Case Management Society of America (CMSA). (2002). *Standards of practice for case management.* Little Rock, AR: Author.

Centers for Medicare & Medicaid Services (CMS). (2004, September 10). Inpatient admission changed to outpatient. *CMS manual system: Use of condition code 44.* Publication number 100-04, Medicare Claims Processing. Baltimore, MD: U.S. Department of Health and Human Services, CMS.

Cesta, T., & Tahan, H. (2003). *The case manager's survival guide: winning strategies for clinical practice* (2nd ed.). St Louis, MO: Mosby.

Coffey, R.J., Richards, J.S., Remmert, C.S., LeRoy S.S., Schoville, R.R., & Baldwin, P.J. (1992). An introduction to critical paths. *Quality Management in Healthcare, 1*(1), 45–54.

Etheredge, M.L. (1987). Critical paths: marking the course. *Definition, 2*(3), 1–4.

InterQual, Inc. (1993a). *Utilization review and management training manual.* North Hampton, NH: Author.

InterQual, Inc. (1993b). *The ISD-A (TM) review system with adult ISD (TM) criteria.* North Hampton, NH: Author.

InterQual, Inc. (1997). *Certified professional utilization review study guide* (5th ed.). North Hampton, NH: Author.

InterQual, Inc. (1998). *Clinical decision support criteria.* North Hampton, NH: Author.

Madigan, P. (1977). Clinical guidelines for subacute units. *Case Review, 3*(1), 61–63.

Mateo, M., Matzke, K., & Newton, C. (1998). Designing measurements to assess case management outcomes. *Nursing Care Management,* (3), 1, 2–6).

Sederer, L.I. (1987). Utilization review and quality assurance: staying in the black and working with the blues. *General Hospital Psychiatry, 9,* 210–219.

Strassner, L. (1996). Evaluating critical pathways. *Continuing Care, 15*(4), 24–28, 33.

Zander, K. (1992). Physicians, Care Maps™, and collaboration. *Definition, 7*(1), 1–4.

APPENDIX 4-A Generic Template LOS Data Reported Based on Participation in a National Database

Region: UNITED STATES   Date Period: From ___/___/___ to ___/___/___

ICD-9 Code:_____   Description:_____

TYPE OF PATIENTS	NUMBER OF PATIENTS	ACTUAL ALOS	EXPECTED LOS	VARIANCE LOS	PERCENTILES						
					10TH	25TH	50TH	75TH	90TH	95TH	99TH

1. SINGLE DX
A. Medical

0–1 Year											
>1–3											
4–10											
10–19											
20–34											
35–49											
50–64											
> 64											

B. Surgical

0–1 Year											
>1–3											
4–10											
10–19											
20–34											
35–49											
50–64											
> 64											

TYPE OF PATIENTS	NUMBER OF PATIENTS	ACTUAL ALOS	EXPECTED LOS	VARIANCE LOS	PERCENTILES						
					10TH	25TH	50TH	75TH	90TH	95TH	99TH
2. MULTIPLE DX											
A. Medical											
0–1 Year											
>1–3											
4–10											
10–19											
20–34											
35–49											
50–64											
> 64											
B. Surgical											
0–1 Year											
>1–3											
4–10											
10–19											
20–34											
35–49											
50–64											
> 64											

SUBTOTALS:

1. SINGLE DX

	NUMBER OF PATIENTS	ACTUAL ALOS	EXPECTED LOS	VARIANCE LOS	10TH	25TH	50TH	75TH	90TH	95TH	99TH
A. Medical											
B. Surgical											

2. MULTIPLE DX

	NUMBER OF PATIENTS	ACTUAL ALOS	EXPECTED LOS	VARIANCE LOS	10TH	25TH	50TH	75TH	90TH	95TH	99TH
A. Medical											
B. Surgical											
TOTAL											

	NUMBER OF PATIENTS	ACTUAL ALOS	EXPECTED LOS	VARIANCE LOS	10TH	25TH	50TH	75TH	90TH	95TH	99TH
0–1 Year											
>1–3											
4–10											
10–19											
20–34											
35–49											
50–64											
> 64											
GRAND TOTAL											

Central Nervous System/Head (Adult, Acute)

SEVERITY OF ILLNESS	INTENSITY OF SERVICE

SEVERITY OF ILLNESS
Rule

ONE:
- Elective surgery/Invasive procedure, **both:**
  ▶ Scheduled same day as admission
  ▶ Designated inpatient setting
- $\geq$ **One SI** *or* $\geq$ **Three** marginal **SI**

Clinical Findings
(Onset within 1 wk)

...
Multiple seizure episodes over **24h**
Change in seizure pattern[1]
Severe headache *and* one:
- Syncope/Presyncope[3]
...

IMAGING FINDINGS
(New Finding This Episode)

Brain abscess
Block of ventricular system (intracranial/...

LABORATORY FINDINGS
(New Finding This Episode)

Cerebrospinal Fluid
RBC $\geq$ **100**/*cu.mm (100 $\times$ 10^6/L)* (nontraumatic tap)
...

Hematology
Platelets $\leq$ **60,000**/*cc.mm (60 $\times$ 10^9/L)* **and** bleeding
...

Chemistry
Na $\leq$ **115** *mEq/L (115 mmol/L)*
Na $\leq$ **120** *mEq/L (120 mmol/L)* **and** one:
- Seizures
- Change in mental status[8]
...

INTENSITY OF SERVICE
Rule

ONE:
- $\geq$ **One IS**
- $\geq$ **Three *IS**

TREATMENTS/MEDICATIONS
(At Least Daily)

Post surgery/procedure care $\leq$ **2d** *and* $\geq$ **two:**
- IV fluids $\geq$ **50** *mL/h*
- IV/IM/ED analgesics
- IV/IM antiemetics
- IV/IM corticosteroids
- IV/IM diuretics

Post critical care craniotomy $\leq$ **2d**

...
Neurologic assessment $\geq$ **1x/h**[11]
Isolation $\leq$ **3d** (Dx: CNS infection/meningitis)
IV anticoagulants[12]
IV anticonvulsants

...
* **Blood/Blood products**
* **Volume expanders**
* **Cervical skeletal traction (continuous/cyclic)**
* **IV fluids $\geq$ 75 *mL/h***
* **Mechanical ventilation**
* **Neurologic assessment $\geq$ 6x/24h**[11]
* **IV/IM corticosteroids $\geq$ 3x/24h**
* **IV/IM diuretics $\geq$ 2x/24h**
* **IV/NaCl 3% *(0.03)* (hypertonic)**
...

DISCHARGE SCREENS

RULE

BOTH:
- **Clinical, one:**
  ▶ Acute episode (**SI**) resolving/stabilized (apply related clinical discharge indicators)
  ▶ End stage disease[17]

Functional, one:
  ▶ Care needs (***IS***) could be met at alternate level (apply related functional discharge indicators)
  ▶ Treatment refused

DISCHARGE INDICATORS
Clinical

$\geq$ **One:**
- Vital signs stable last **8h**[13]
- Neurologically stable last **24h**[14]
- Seizures controlled/Unchanged seizure pattern last **12h**[15]

...

Functional

One:
- Patient/Primary caregiver able to verbalize understanding of, **all:**
  ▶ Diagnosis(es) **and** medical treatment plan[18]
...

(continued)

APPENDIX 4-B—*CONTINUED*

Central Nervous System/Head (Adult, Acute)

NOTES

1: Change in seizure pattern (e.g., frequency/type) of a patient with a known history of epilepsy or a first seizure in a patient with no history of epilepsy.

2: ...

3: Syncope is the transient loss of consciousness and postural tone caused by diminished cerebral blood flow.

Presyncope (near-syncope) is an episode of near-fainting/passing out to include, but not limited to, lightheadedness, dizziness, and blurred vision that may precede a syncopal episode.

4: ...

8: Change in mental status includes coma, stupor, or increasing lethargy. This excludes chronic coma or stupor.

9: ...

11: The neurologic assessment is a serial assessment of all of the following: level of consciousness, pupillary response, reflexes (biceps/Achilles/patellar), and known focal neurologic deficits including:
- Aphasia = impaired comprehension or communication by speech, writing, or signs
- Ataxia = inability to coordinate voluntary muscle activity
- Dysarthria = disturbance of speech and language
- Paresis = partial paralysis of voluntary muscles
- Paralysis = loss of power of voluntary muscle.

12: Most anticoagulants can be given at a lower level of care than the acute level, and are usually given the *IS designation. However, when the disease being treated requires the acute level of care, InterQual's medical consultants recommend an IS designation. When a thrombosis is caused by errors of the blood clotting system (e.g., DIC), the acute level of monitoring justifies the IS assignment.

13: In general, the stability of vital signs considered adequate to leave the acute level of care meets the following ranges: heart rate 50–100/minute, respiratory rate 12–18/minute, systolic BP 90–180, diastolic BP 60–90, temperature 94.0° F–100.5° F (34.5° C–38.1° C), and postural systolic BP drop < 30 (*Current Critical Care Diagnosis & Treatment*, ©1994, pp. 1–12).

14: A finding of neurologic stability includes:
- No significant change in the mental status exam or level of consciousness.
- Seizures controlled.
- No new neurologic deficits including aphasia (impaired comprehension or communication by speech, writing, or signs), ataxia (inability to coordinate voluntary muscle activity), dysarthria (disturbance of speech and language), paresis (partial paralysis of voluntary muscles), paralysis (loss of power of voluntary muscle), visual field loss, or blindness.

15: Seizures controlled is either the absence of generalized seizures (e.g., grand mal) or the improved/unchanged focal seizure pattern.

16: ...

17: End stage disease is an irreversible, chronic disease incapable of achieving stability of vital signs, clinical and/or laboratory findings (SI).

18: Care and use of specialized equipment/assessment of change in seizure pattern/other warning signs/potential complications.

(continued)

APPENDIX 4-B—*CONTINUED*

Neuromuscular (Adult, Rehabilitation)

PREREQUISITES

CLINICAL	OPERATIONAL

CLINICAL

ALL:
- Illness/injury **with** recent/progressive functional disability
  and ≥ **one:**
  - ▶ Physical impairment
  - ▶ Cognitive impairment
- Clinically stable

...

OPERATIONAL

ALL:
- Physician(s) providing, **all:**
  - ▶ Rehabilitation services[3]
  - ▶ Medical services[4]
  - ▶ Active direction of multidisciplinary team[5]

...

SEVERITY OF ILLNESS RULE

BOTH:

CLINICAL FINDINGS

Recent illness/exacerbation/injury/surgery, **one:**
- Anoxic brain injury
- CVA
- Traumatic brain injury

...

Impairment, ≥ **one:**
- Respiratory impairment/Ventilator dependency
- Cognition/Communication deficit

...

INTENSITY OF SERVICE RULE

ONE:
- ≥ **One IS**
- ≥ **Three *IS**

REHABILITATION PROGRAM
(At Least Daily)

Progressive activity program[1]
Self care independence program[2]
Swallowing training

...

- * **TPN/Enteral feeding**
- * **Pain management**[5]
- * **Speech/Language training**
- * **Prosthetic management**
- * **Bowel/Bladder management**[6,7]

...

DISCHARGE SCREENS

RULE

ONE:
- Clinical/Functional plateau reached[9]
- Care needs exceed rehabilitation level
- Treatment refused
- Clinical **and** functional goals achieved (apply related discharge indicators)

DISCHARGE INDICATORS
Clinical

≥ **One:** (relevant to admission SI)
- Ventilator D/C'd/dependence modified

...

Functional

All:
- Patient/Primary caregiver able to **both:**
  - ▶ Perform/Assist in performing ADLs
  - ▶ Verbalize understanding of ≥ **one:** (relevant to SI)
    - ■ Progressive activity program[1]
    - ■ Respiratory management[3]
    - ■ Communication adaptive techniques
    ...
- Follow up care arranged[12]

...

(continued)

APPENDIX 4-B—*CONTINUED*

Neuromuscular (Adult, Rehabilitation)

PREREQUISITES–NOTES

1: ...

3: Physician trained/board certified in a rehabilitation related specialty (e.g., physical medicine, and rehabilitation (psychiatry), orthopedics, neurology) who provides direct rehabilitation services/rehabilitation oversight of professional services, and who demonstrates current clinical competence as credentialed by provider agency(ies).

CARF... Rehabilitation Accreditation Commission (formerly The Commission on Accreditation of Rehabilitation Facilities) considers the following qualifications necessary for medical directorship of inpatient rehabilitation programs for Category One patients (potentially medically unstable with multiple medical and nursing needs) requiring $\geq$ 3h of professional services daily, $\geq$ 5d/wk:
- Board certification in the area of specialty
- Appropriate experience and training necessary to provide rehabilitation physician services through formal residency in physical medicine and rehabilitation, or $\geq$ 2 years of experience in providing rehabilitation services for patients typically seen in all comprehensive inpatient categories.

The requirement necessary for provision of direct physician rehabilitation services for Category One patients is that the physician be qualified in rehabilitation (e.g., physiatrist or physician qualified by virtue of training and experience).

4: Physician trained/board certified in a medical specialty (e.g., internal medicine, family medicine, pulmonary, neurology, or physician extender) per state law who provides direct medical services/medical oversight of professional services, and who demonstrates current clinical competence as credentialed by provider agency(ies).

5: A multidisciplinary team includes licensed professionals representing various specialty areas (e.g., nursing, physical therapy, occupational therapy, respiratory therapy, nutritional services, clinical social services).

NOTES

1: A progressive activity program is an incremental exercise program designed to promote gradual improvement in physical endurance/functioning.

2: A self-care independence program includes assessment and intervention to maximize self-care independence by education, use of appliances and devices, strength and endurance/exercise training and recommendations for home and community reintegration.

3: Respiratory management includes the assessment and intervention necessary to maximize respiratory function. Examples of these include energy conservation and breathing techniques, pulmonary toilet, medical gas management, management of appliances, education in disease process(es), and development of self-care skills.

4: ...

6: Bowel management is a group of assessments and interventions that result in the elimination of, or reduction in, episodes of fecal impaction/incontinence (e.g., evaluation of hydration, nutritional status, and bowel pattern), and the establishment of bowel regime including diet/exercise/medications/mechanical disimpaction.

7: Bladder management is a group of assessments and interventions that result in the elimination or reduction in episodes of incontinence (e.g., assessment of hydration and voiding patterns, catheter insertion, establishment of voiding schedule and education in the intermittent self-catheterization).

8: ....

9: A plateau is a stage in the rehabilitation process whereupon no further progress in functional improvement is expected and rehabilitation goals are unlikely to be met.

10: ...

12: Follow-up care can include physician visit(s), out-patient care, home care, or community-based care (e.g., community-based rehabilitation program).

(continued)

APPENDIX 4-B—*CONTINUED*

Cardiovascular (Adult, Subacute)

PREREQUISITES

CLINICAL	OPERATIONAL
ALL:	**ALL:**
• Diagnosis *and* treatment plan established, **one:**[1]	• Physician assessment ≥ **1x/wk**
▶ Recovery from acute illness/injury	• Professional services ≥ **4h/24h**[3]
▶ Recovery from major surgery/procedure	• Treatment plan developed by physician directed
...	multidisciplinary team[4]
• Clinically stable	
...	

SEVERITY OF ILLNESS RULE

BOTH:

CLINICAL FINDINGS

Recent illness/exacerbation/surgery, **one:**
- MI[1]
- CHF[2]
- Cardiomyopathy[3]

...

Compromised physical endurance/
Post cardiovascular surgery *and* ≥ **one:**[4]
- Angina[5]
- Arrhythmia(s)[6]
- Dyspnea
- Uncontrolled/Labile hypertension
- Nutritional deficit[7]
- Postoperative pain uncontrolled

...

INTENSITY OF SERVICE RULE

ONE:
- ≥ **One IS**
- ≥ **Three *IS**

TREATMENTS/MEDICATIONS
(At Least Daily)

Cardiac monitoring
Cardiac rehabilitation[10]
Pre-heart/Heart-lung transplant per protocol[11]
Post-heart/Heart-lung transplant per protocol[11]
IV antihypertensives

...

* **Respiratory management**[12]

...

* **TPN/Enteral feeding**
* **IV/IM anti-infectives**

...

DISCHARGE SCREENS

RULE

ONE:
- Clinical/Functional plateau reached[15]
- Care needs exceed subacute level
- Treatment refused
- Clinical *and* functional goals achieved (apply related discharge indicators)

DISCHARGE INDICATORS
Clinical

≥ **One:** (relevant to admission SI)
- Angina controlled/manageable
- Dyspnea improved/O$_2$ SAT at baseline
- Arrhythmia(s) controlled/manageable

...

Functional

Both:
- Patient/Primary caregiver able to verbalize understanding of ≥ **one:** (relevant to IS)
  - ▶ Cardiac exercise program[16]
  ...
- Follow-up care arranged[22]

...

(continued)

APPENDIX 4-B—*CONTINUED*

Cardiovascular (Adult, Subacute)

PREREQUISITES—NOTES

1: In general, the stability of vital signs considered adequate to leave the acute level of care meets the following ranges: heart rate 50–100/minute, respiratory rate 12–18/minute, systolic BP 90–180, diastolic BP 60–90, temperature 94.0° F–100.5° F (34.5° C–38.1° C), and postural systolic BP drop <30 (*Current Critical Care Diagnosis & Treatment*, ©1994, pp. 10–12).

3: Professional services refers to those services provided by a licensed individual who has acquired proficiency in technical skills and training and who conforms to the ethical standards of that profession (e.g., nursing, physical therapy, occupational therapy, speech therapy).
   . . .

NOTES

1: . . .

3: Cardiomyopathy (dilated) is characterized by decreased function of the left ventricle (LV) associated with its dilatation. CHF is caused by impaired biventricular systolic function usually from LV hypokinesis.

Cardiomyopathy (hypertrophic) is characterized by thickening of the ventricular septum and the walls of the LM. Initial symptoms may include dyspnea, angina, palpitations, syncope, and even unexpected death.

Cardiomyopathy (restrictive) is characterized by impaired diastolic function (poor compliance) similar to that seen in constrictive pericarditis but usually limited to the LV. Clinically, . . .

4: Patients with compromised physical endurance requiring monitoring or treatment outside the home environment have symptoms (e.g., fatigue, palpitations, dyspnea, or anginal pain) at rest or with < ordinary physical activity. Ordinary physical activities include: walking 1–2 blocks; climbing one flight of stairs; non-stop showering; stripping and making a bed; cleaning one set of windows; walking at 2.5 mph; bowling; golf; or dressing without stopping.

5: . . .

10: A cardiac rehabilitation program includes assessment and interventions to prevent or minimize disability/complications of cardiac diseases and increase physical endurance and ability to manage self-care and prescribed therapeutic regime (e.g., angina control with medication(s) management); arrhythmias management using telemetry monitoring and medication(s); physical/occupational therapy to maximize oxygen consumption and increase exercise endurance; and mental health management, which may include counseling and medication(s).

11: Protocol refers to locally defined written operational protocols or accepted facility standards.

12: Respiratory management includes the assessment and intervention necessary to maximize respiratory function. Examples of these include energy conservation and breathing techniques, pulmonary toilet, medical gas management, management of appliances, education in disease process(es), and development of self-care skills.

13: . . .

15: A plateau is a stage in the rehabilitation process whereupon no further progress in functional improvement is expected and rehabilitation goals are unlikely to be met.

16: A cardiac exercise program consists of an individualized exercise prescription, energy conservation techniques, pulse assessment, and cardiac warning signs education.

22: Follow-up care can include physician visit(s), outpatient care, home care, or community-based care (e.g., community-based rehabilitation program).

(continued)

APPENDIX 4-B—CONTINUED

Cardiovascular (Adult, Home Care)

PREREQUISITES—HOME CARE

CLINICAL

ALL:
- Diagnosis established *and* medical plan of care developed, **one:**
  - ▶ High risk of complications
  - ▶ High risk for injury due to physical/cognitive deficit
...

OPERATIONAL

ALL:
- Clinical services are, **all:**
  - ▶ Under direction of a physician
  - ▶ Managed *and* administered by nursing staff/interdisciplinary professionals
...

SEVERITY OF ILLNESS
RULE

BOTH:

CLINICAL FINDINGS

Recent illness/exacerbation/surgery, **one:**
- CHF[1]
- CAD
- Hypertensive heart disease
- MI[2]
...

Actual/Potential impairment, ≥ **one:**
- Dyspnea
- Recurrent angina[5]
- Labile hypertension (actual)
- Immobility (actual)[6]
- Infection
...

INTENSITY OF SERVICE
RULE

≥ **One IS**

TREATMENTS/MEDICATIONS

(Professional Services)
Clinical assessment[7]
Periodic reassessment[8]
Clinical social work services[9]
Infusion therapy[10]
Venipuncture *and* lab values assessment
Venous access site management[11]
Compliance *with* home care program[12]
Therapeutic exercises for strength/ROM/endurance/energy conservation techniques/nonpharmacological pain management[13]
...

DISCHARGE SCREENS

RULE

ONE:
- Clinical/Functional plateau reached[18]
- Clinical/Technical needs exceed home care level
- Continuing care not required
- Clinical *and* functional goals achieved (see related discharge indicators)

DISCHARGE INDICATORS

Clinical

≥ **One:** (relevant to admission SI)
- Dyspnea relieved
- O$_2$ SAT stabilized
- Breath sounds improved
...

Functional

All, patient/primary caregiver:
- Manages ADLs *and* IADLs
- Verbalizes understanding of, **all:**
  - ▶ Condition
  - ▶ Complications *and* signs/symptoms to report (self-monitoring)[19]
...

(continued)

APPENDIX 4-B—*CONTINUED*

Cardiovascular (Adult, Home Care)

NOTES

1: . . .

5: Angina is defined as a pressing or squeezing type of chest pain radiating into the neck, shoulders, or arms. Symptoms vary from patient to patient and include sensations of pain, choking, pressure, squeezing, tightness, heaviness, and burning. Characteristically it is brought on by exertion, stress, or cold and lasts from 2–15 minutes, it is relieved promptly by rest or nitroglycerin (*Current Medical Diagnosis & Treatment*, ©1996, pp. 321, 331).

6: Immobility is the condition which results when a patient has an illness, injury, or surgery that restricts their ability to leave their place of residence except with the aid of supportive devices, special transportation, assistance of another person, or when this activity is medically contraindicated.

7: The clinical assessment of the patient at the home care level will normally include an evaluation of most of the following: vital signs, lung sounds, dyspnea, pain, weight, edema, hydration/nutritional status, mental status, elimination, skin color and integrity, surgical incision site (if applicable), medication effectiveness, functional ability, signs of domestic abuse, coping skills, and understanding of the disease process.

8: Periodic reassessment refers to intermittent patient assessment/intervention by a professional for compliance/follow-up teaching after clinical stability has been achieved (e.g., catheter change for patient with a neurogenic bladder).

9: Clinical social work services include psychological, social, and spiritual support for the patient/primary caregiver, individual/family counseling, psychosocial assessment, community service referrals, information about and assistance in accessing financial resources, coordination of services, long-term planning, legal referral, and support of the plan of care.

10: Infusion therapy includes the initiation and teaching of the prescribed therapy and related safety precautions pertaining to IV administration of medications. It also includes evaluation of medication effectiveness. Examples of IV medications that can be given at this level of care include adrenergics (per local medical policy), analgesics, antiemetics, anti-infectives, chemotherapy (per local medical policy), corticosteroids, diuretics, electrolytes, IV hydration, immunosuppressants (per local medical policy), and SC tocolytic pump (per local medical policy). Infusion therapy requires 24h availability of physician, home care staff, laboratory, pharmacists, and suppliers of fluids, medications, and medical equipment.

11: Venous access site management includes inspection of the site for the presence of extravasation, of equipment for integrity, and for infusion technique/complications.

12: Compliance with the home care program requires adherence to all prescribed treatment and procedures of care including, but not limited to, medications, diet, activity, and services.

13: . . .

18: A plateau is a stage in the rehabilitation process whereupon no further progress in functional improvement is expected and rehabilitation goals are unlikely to be met.

19: Self-monitoring means the patient/primary caregiver is able to adequately monitor the patient's conditions (e.g., vital signs, diet/fluid intake, pain tolerance, wound healing, side effects of drug therapy, complications to report, and safety precautions).

20: . . .

(continued)

DRG <u>89</u>   Estimated LOS: <u>4 days</u>

Admit Date _____

Payer _____

(for DC planning purposes)

Interdisciplinary Clinical Pathway: Simple Pneumonia & Pleurisy with Comorbidity (≥ 17 yr)

	DAY 1	DAY 2
Assessment	TPR; resp system; O$_2$ sat; baseline mental status; psycho/social needs; consider TB screen	Mental status; O$_2$ sat; TPR; resp system
Diagnostic Studies	Sputum by RT (RT sputum induction policy); GS; C&S; *ABG; CXR-PA&LAT; Smac; *BCx2; UA; *C&S; *EKG; CBC with diff	Stool for C. diff if diarrhea; CBC; CXR-PA&LAT if condition warrants (evaluate for pleural effusion)
Treatments	I/O; saline lock/IV; O$_2$ as indicated; encourage po fluids; turn, deep breathe; suction prn; activity as tolerated in room.	Ambulate TID
Key Medications and IV Therapy	IV ABX; saline flushes as indicated; consider adrenergic beta-2 (bronchodilator) via SVN/MDI; Prns: antipyretic; NSAID/narcotic prn pleuritic pain; antacid; antiemetic BCOC; hypnotic	
Nutrition and Fluids	Advance DAT; encourage po fluids.	
Consults/ Multidisciplinary Education	*Pulmonary; Case Management; *Dietary consult; assess educational needs	Discuss postdischarge options with family/S.O.
Key Outcomes/Goals	IV ABX started in ED or within 2 hrs if direct admit; sputum collected	Patient afebrile; tolerates ambulation without respiratory complications; note GS result

---

* = if indicated
Date Adopted Medical Department/Committee _____ Date to MEC _____
Clinical Pathways are guidelines only and do not preempt the independent judgment of the physician.

DAY 3	DAY 4	DAY 5
Same as Day 2	Same as Day 3	Same as Day 4
*CBC		
D/C saline lock/IV, evaluate need for O_2 by spot check O_2 sat (RT O_2 Therapy Policy)	D/C I&O (evaluate need for O_2)	Discharge
Consider switch to MDI; consider D/C IV ABX after 24-hour afebrile period and start po ABX; D/C saline flushes	Consider switch to MDI	D/C on po ABX; consider adrenergic beta-2 INH; NSAID/narcotic prn pleuritic pain
Contact: Primary Home Caregiver, Home Health, ECF; MDI Instruction	Initiate transfer form if applicable; disease process education	Home care management/discharge instruction
Sputum cult report in patient record; po ABX started if criteria met; normal rate, rhythm and depth of resp	Independent ADLs; afebrile	Discharge

APPENDIX 4-C—*CONTINUED*

DRG <u>209</u>   Estimated LOS: <u>4 days</u>

Admit Date _____

Payer _____

   (for DC planning purposes)

Interdisciplinary Clinical Pathway: Total Hip Replacement

	DAY 1 (SURGERY)	DAY 2 (POD 1)
Assessment	Neurovascular checks q 2 hrs, vital signs and hemovac checks q 4 hrs	Neurovascular checks and vital signs q 4 hours if stable, hemovac check q 8 hrs
Diagnostic Studies	Post-op x-ray	H/H, protime if on coumadin
Treatments	Hemovac, antiembolic hose, cough and deep breathe, I&O, abduction pillow, straight cath/foley,* bedrest, HOB up 30°, turn q 2 hrs	Hemovac, up in chair × 30 min × 1, HOB up 60° maximum, ambulate 10′× 1
Key Medications and IV Therapy	IVF as ordered, IV antibiotics, PCA/epidural/IM pain medication, anticoagulants, routine medications as ordered	IV–saline lock, discontinue IV antibiotics, PCA/IM/epidural/pain meds, stool softeners, BCOC
Nutrition and Fluids	Regular diet, clear liquid if no bowel sounds or N/V	Diet as tolerated
Consults/Multidisciplinary Education	Respiratory Therapy,* Internal Medicine/Family Practice physician*	Social Services*, Physical Therapy
Key Outcomes/Goals	Pain Management, stabilize post-op	Begin activity, afebrile

* = if indicated
Date Adopted Medical Department/Committee _____ Date to MEC _____
Clinical Pathways are guidelines only and do not preempt the independent judgment of the physician.

DAY 3 (POD 2)	DAY 4 (POD 3)	DAY 5 (POD 4)
Routine vital signs	Assess bowel function	System discharge assessment
H/H, protime if on coumadin	Protime if on coumadin	
Hemovac discontinued, dressing changed, Foley discontinued,* straight cath,* up in chair × 2 × 30 min, HOB up 75° maximum, ambulate 20' × 2, bedside commode	Dressing change per orders, up in chair × 2 × 45 min, ambulate 40'/BRP, minimum assist & OOB	Enema/suppository if no BM
Saline lock discontinued, IM/PO pain medication, anticoagulants	PO analgesics	PO pain meds/instructions
I&O discontinued		
HHC/ECF liaisons/DME, OT for ADL training		Follow-up Social Services/HHC/DME, physician as needed, review home exercise protocol, dislocation precautions, discharge medications
Increase activity level, switch to PO pain meds	Establish plan for discharge needs, bowel movement	Discharge

APPENDIX 4-C—*CONTINUED*

DRG <u>209</u>   Estimated LOS: <u>4 days</u>

Admit Date _____

Payer _____

  (for DC planning purposes)

Interdisciplinary Clinical Pathway: Total Knee Replacement

	DAY 1 (SURGERY)	DAY 2 (POD 1)
Assessment	Hemovac checks q 4 hrs, vital signs q 4 hrs, neurovascular checks q 4 hrs	Vital signs/neurovascular checks q 4 hrs
Diagnostic Studies	Post-op x-ray	H/H, Protime if on coumadin
Treatments	Antiembolic device, dressing and neurovascular checks q 2 hrs, cough and deep breathe, I&O, hemovac, straight cath/Foley,, turn q 2 hrs, HOB up for comfort, CPM machine if ordered, advance per orders	Up in chair × 2 × 30 min, stand, ambulate 10′ × 1, CPM
Key Medications and IV Therapy	IVF per orders, IV antibiotics, epidural/PCA/IM pain meds, anticoagulants, routine medications as ordered	Anticoagulants, IV−saline lock, IV antibiotics discontinued, PCA/IM/PO pain meds,[*] stool softeners, BCOC
Nutrition and Fluids	Regular diet−clear liquids if no bowel sounds or N/V	Diet as tolerated
Consults/Multidisciplinary Education	Internal Medicine/Family Practice physician,[*] Respiratory Therapy[*]	Social Services,[*] Physical Therapy
Key Outcomes/Goals	Pain management, stabilize post-op	Begin activity, afebrile

[*] = if indicated
Date Adopted Medical Department/Committee _____ Date to MEC _____
Clinical Pathways are guidelines only and do not preempt the independent judgment of the physician.

DAY 3 (POD 2)	DAY 4 (POD 3)	DAY 5 (POD 4)
Routine vital signs	Assess bowel function	System discharge assessment
H/H, protime if on coumadin	Protime if on coumadin	
Hemovac discontinued, dressing changed, up in chair × 2 ×45 min, ambulate 25′ × 2, CPM 0–50°	Dressing change per orders, up in chair × 1 hr × 3/BRP, ambulate 50′ × 2, minimum assist I & OOB	Assure BM prior to discharge, minimum assist needed for BRP, COPM
PO pain meds, anticoagulants as ordered	Anticoagulants as ordered	PO pain meds/instructions
Discontinue I&O		
HHC/ECF liaison, DME		Follow-up with Social Services, HHC, DME, physician,* review exercise protocol for home, discharge medications
Switch to PO pain meds, increase activity level	Established plan for discharge needs	Discharge

APPENDIX 4-C—*CONTINUED*

DRG <u>80.51</u>   Estimated LOS: <u>4 days</u>

Admit Date _____

Payer _____

   (for DC planning purposes)

Interdisciplinary Clinical Pathway: Post-op Lumbar Laminectomy Without Fusion, Without Complications, Nontraumatic, Non-CA

	DAY 1	
	PREOP/SURGERY	POSTOP
Assessment	H&P; initial anesthesia assessment; VS; neuro exam (LOC, motor & sensory); systems assessment	VS and neuro exam q 4 hr; assess lumbar drsg q 4 hr; systems assessment
Diagnostic Studies	CBC, CMAC, coags, EKG, CXR, type and screen	
Treatments	Activity as tolerated; refer to standard surgical protocol; Teds	Up OOB to chair/commode in evening; Teds; PAS*; inc spirometer*; Foley*; TCDB q 2 hr
Key Medications and IV Therapy	Preop meds	IVF as ordered; pain meds IV/IM*; antibiotics IV × 24 hrs; steroids*; antimetics*; muscle relaxers*
Nutrition and Fluids	NPO except for meds	NPO until fully awake and bowel sounds active; clear liquids then ADAT
Consults/Multidisciplinary Education	BNI Education Guide; preop teaching; informed consent; special consents (i.e., blood); medical consults*	Resp Therapy*; Social Services*; Case Manager*
Key Outcomes/Goals	Verbalize understanding of preop teaching; discharge planning initiated	Stabilize patient

* = if indicated
Date Adopted Medical Department/Committee _____ Date to MEC _____
Clinical Pathways are guidelines only and do not preempt the independent judgment of the physician.

DAY 2	DAY 3	DISCHARGE DAY
VS and neuro exam q shift; assess drsg/ incision line q shift; assess last bowel movement; systems assessment	VS and neuro exam q shift; incision line q shift; assess last BM; systems assessment q shift	VS and neuro exam q shift; assess incision line q shift; assess ability to care for self
CBC*; CP*		
Up in chair TID; ambulate in hall w/help; D/C Foley; straight cath if unable to void; bowel care; temp >38°C; start inc spirometer; Teds	Ambulate in halls TID; ADLs with minimal assist (i.e., shower); remove drsg if not done already	Ambulate independent; bowel care (i.e., BM prior to discharge); ADLs done independently; Discharge
S.L. IV until completion of antibiotics, if no nausea and tolerating PO; bowel care meds; switch to PO pain meds	D/C S.L.; PO pain meds*; steroid taper*	PO pain med Rx; other Rx* (i.e., steroids, muscle relaxers, stool softeners)
ADAT	Regular diet	Regular diet
PT/OT C/S* if patient reluctant or weak; teach patient bed mobility and proper body mechanics; Home Health*		"Laminectomy discharge instruction sheet"; follow-up with Social Services, contact output therapies for any necessary arrangements for home; follow-up with neurosurgeon for suture/staple removal; review prescriptions; review proper body mechanics and activities allowed
Continue discharge planning; patient will ambulate in halls with assistance	Patient prepared for discharge	Meet discharge criteria; patient will verbalize understanding of discharge instructions and teaching

APPENDIX 4-C—*CONTINUED*

DRG <u>107</u>   Estimated LOS: <u>4 days</u>

Admit Date _____

Payer _____

   (for DC planning purposes)

Interdisciplinary Clinical Pathway: CABG

	DAY 1		
	PRE-OP TESTING	ADMISSION-DAY 1- SURGERY	DAY 2 (POD 1)
Assessment	Admission assessment	Complete assessment; H&P on chart	Vital signs q 1–2 hrs; complete assessment q 2 hrs
Diagnostic Studies	CBC, CXR, EKG, CP-SMAC, T&C, Coag profile, ABG-RA, bedside PFT	H&H, K +, EKG, ABG, CXR, cardiac output, PTT*	CPK–MB × 1, H&H, chem panel, EKG, CXR, ABG
Treatments	Daily weight; permit signed; surgical shower; up ad lib	IV, art line, PA cath; pace-maker/wires; Foley, chest tubes; NGT ETT-ventilator, pulse oximetry, end-tidal; wean → extubated; I.S.; SVN*; bedrest	Dressing change; D/C; CT; D/C PA cath; I.S.; daily weight; heplock; evaluate for transfer; SVN*; dangle A.M., chair P.M, ROM × 5
Key Medications and IV Therapy	Continue present meds; bowel prep	Antibiotic–pre & post; KCl, analgesic, heparin, ASA, O$_2$, Inotrope,* anti-arrhythmic,* vasopressors,* MgSo4*	Antibiotic, analgesic, O$_2$, ASA, stool softener
Nutrition and Fluids	Regular; NPO following MN	NPO	Clear liquids → advance to soft
Consults/Multidisciplinary Education	Pre-op teach, Cardiac Rehab, Anesthesia, Case Management		
Key Outcomes/Goals	Ready for surgery	Stabilized post-op, extubate 12 hrs post-op	Hemodynamically stable, initiate activity, pain management

* = if indicated
Date Adopted Medical Department/Committee _____ Date to MEC _____
Clinical Pathways are guidelines only and do not preempt the independent judgment of the physician.

DAY 3 (POD 2)	DAY 4 (POD 3)	DAY 5 (POD 4)	DAY 6 (POD 5)
Vital signs q 4 hrs	Routine vital signs	Routine vital signs	Routine vital signs
CPK–MB × 1, H&H*; chem panel*, EKG*, CXR*, ABG*		CBC, CP, CXR, EKG, check RA O$_2$ sat–if > 92, D/C O$_2$	
Transfer to tele; D/C art line; D/C Foley; restart heplock; I.S.; daily weight; dressing change; SVN*; ambulate up to 100' × 1, ROM × 5	Telemetry; I.S.; daily weight; dressings off; ambulate 100–300' BID; active ROM	Telemetry; daily weight; I.S.; up ad lib; ambulate 1–2 laps TID, O$_2$	Daily weight; I.S.; up ad lib; ambulate 2–3 laps QID
Analgesic–PO, ASA, stool softener, O$_2$	Stool softener, ASA, routine home meds, analgesic, laxative, O$_2$	ASA, routine home meds, analgesic	ASA, home meds, analgesic
Regular diet	Regular diet	Regular diet	Regular diet
	Discharge teaching, Cardiac Rehab	Attend Cardiac Rehab class	
Transfer to tele floor, switch to PO pain meds	Increased activity	Established plan for discharge needs	Discharge

APPENDIX 4-C—*CONTINUED*

**St. Joseph's Hospital
and Medical Center**
Mercy Healthcare Arizona

CHEST PAIN/ACUTE MI PATHWAY

LABORATORY		ER STAT LAB		
☐ ABG	☐ PELVIC BATTERY	☑ CHEM 5	☐ ANKLE L R	☐ IVP
☐ AMYLASE	☑ PT, PTT	☑ EKG	☐ C-SPINE	☐ KNEE L R
☐ BLOOD CULT x 1 x 2	☐ QUANT. HCG	☑ HEME - 8	☐ CT SCAN B OR E	☐ L-SPINE
☑ CARDIAC ENZ	☐ TOX. ED	☐ MED PROFILE (ABG,	☐ CXR	☐ PELVIS
☐ CHEM 15	☐ TRAUMA PROFILE	CHEM 5, HEME - 8)	☑ PCXR	☐ SHOULDER L R
☐ CREATININE	☐ TRAUMA PROFILE (PED)	☐ UA DIP	☐ ELBOW L R	☐ T-SPINE
☐ ETOH	☐ TYPE & SCREEN	☐ URINE PREG (+) (-)	☐ FOOT L R	☐ WRIST L R
☐ LIPASE	☐ URINE	**X-RAY**	☐ HAND L R	☐ US_____
☐ MAG	☐ URINE C & S	☐ AAS	☐ HIP L R	

Check Where Applicable and Time Your Orders

Date Ordered	TIME LAB DONE	UNIT SEC SIGNATURE	✓	Time Done	Signature
	Phase I: First 15 Minutes				
	1. Stat EKG - Obtain previous EKG and records stat - Notify E.R. MD. stat				
	Triage Assessment (Determine if Cardiac Etiology)				
	Nursing and Pain Scale Assessment				
	2. O2: Nasal prongs/face mask at 2-4 liters/min or 40-60%				
	3. IV: 0.9% NaCl TKO, 2NC IV pre				
	4. Page primary care physician:				
	5. Page cardiologist:				
	6. Allergies:				
	7. ASA 160 mg, chewed				
	8. NTG 0.4 mg SL, repeat q 5 minutes pre chest pain x3				
	9. M.S. 2-4 mg. IV q 10 minutes pre chest pain				
	10. Portable upright CXR to be taken to ICU with patient upon admission				
	11. CPK-MB2 or troponin levels				
	ED Physician Assessment: Cardiac vs. Non Cardiac:				
	Phase II: First 15-30 Minutes				
	Physician/Nursing Reassessment				
	Patient/Family Education - Reassurance				
	12. **Decision for additional MI treatment modality:**				
	Angioplasty (strongly consider for Large MI) see Emergent PTCA Orders				
	Thrombolysis - see Acute MI thrombolysis orders				
	Study protocol - see special study orders				
	13. **Heparin 5000 unit IV bolus**, then 25.000 units in 250 cc at 1000 units per hr.				
	14. **Arterial line** for hypotension not responsive to IV fluids				
	15. **Emergency treatment:** RN to initiate treatment, then physician to be notified immediately				
	Bradycardia: HR < 50 with SBP < 90 and symptomatic, give:				
	Atropine 0.5 mg - 1.0 mg IV q 5 minutes x 3 pre				
	Ventricular fibrillation: Defibrillate at 200 joules, repeat at 300 joules, then at 360 joules				
	if necessary. If defibrillation ineffective, begin CPR, give Epinephrine 1 mg IV and				
	defibrillate at 360 joules.				
	Asystole: Begin CPR, Epinephrine 1mg IV, Initiate transcutaneous pacing				
	Sustained ventricular tachycardia: Notify MD STAT. If SBP < 70, cardiovert at 100 joules.				
	Repeat at 200 joules, 300 joules, then 360 joules if necessary.				
	Non-sustained Ventricular tachycardia (>5 beats in a row) or frequent PVC's: notify M.D.				
	16. **Notify Chaplain Services**				
	Phase III: First 30-60 Minutes				
	Physician/Nursing Reassessment: Admit Diagnosis: ☐ AMI ☐ Unstable Angina ☐ Acute Chest Pain ☐ Critical Care Unit		☐ Telemetry ☐ Step-Down Unit	
	17. **Call Report/Print Monitor Report/Send X-Rays**				
TIME	NURSE'S SIGNATURE	RESIDENT SIGNATURE	PHYSICIAN SIGNATURE		

X-MR-3455   (02/96)   **EMERGENCY DEPARTMENT PATHWAY, CHEST PAIN**

Authorization is given for dispensing non-proprietary name unless checked here. ☐

APPENDIX 4-C—*CONTINUED*

**St. Joseph's Hospital
and Medical Center**
Mercy Healthcare Arizona

Authorization is given for dispensing non-proprietary name unless checked here.

Date Ordered	PHYSICIAN'S ORDERS - ADMISSION, ACUTE MI
	1. Admit to: ☐ ICU
	☐ Telemetry
	2. Heparin 5000 units SQ q. 12 hours if no IV heparin given
	3. ASA 160 mg. PO QD
	4. O2: _____
	5. IV: _____
	6. Beta-Blocker treatment: (If no contraindications: Heart Block, Bradycardia, Hypotension, Asthma)
	☐ Atenolol 5 mg. IV over 5 minutes x 2, waiting 5 minutes between doses; then Atenolol 50 mg.
	PO 15 minutes after 2nd IV dose.
	☐ Atenolol 50 mg. PO q. 12 hours - hold for SBP < 100, HR < 60
	OR
	☐ Metoprolol 5 mg. IV bolus at 2 minute intervals x 3, then Metoprolol 50 mg. PO 15 minutes after
	3rd IV dose.
	☐ Metoprolol 50 mg. PO q. 8 hours - hold for SBP < 100, HR < 60
	7. Diet:
	8. Labwork: CPK with Isoenzymes q. 8 hours x 3, SMAC and CBC in AM
	9. Portable upright CXR in AM
	10. EKG q. AM x 2
	11. Activity: Bedrest with commode privileges
	12. Recurrent angina after MI:
	NTG 0.4 mg. SL q. 5 minutes x 3 prn
	☐ Notify House Staff
	☐ Notify Attending Physician
	13. PRN Medications:
	Tylenol ii tabs q. 4 hours prn non-anginal pain
	MS 2-4 mg. IV q. 15 minutes prn severe pain
	Sleep: _____
	Apprehension: _____
	Nausea/Vomiting: _____
	Bowel care: _____
	14. Other orders including regular medications:
	15. Dietician to see
	16. Cardiac Rehab
	Signature

MR-3489 (12/94)

PHYSICIAN'S ORDERS - ADMISSION, ACUTE MI

APPENDIX 4-C—*CONTINUED*

St. Joseph's Hospital and Medical Center
Mercy Healthcare Arizona

Authorization is given for dispensing non-proprietary name unless checked here. ☐

Date Ordered	PHYSICIAN'S TRANSFER ORDERS - ACUTE MI
	1. Transfer to Telemetry
	2. IV: Saline Lock with Flush every 8 hours
	3. O$_2$: _____
	4. Lab: _____
	5. Diet: _____
	6. Activity: Up in chair, bathroom privileges
	7. Beta-Blocker Therapy: _____
	8. ACE-Inhibitor: (If desired. Consider for large MI and/or significant LV dysfunction.)
	_____
	Begin on: _____
	9. ASA 160 mg. PO QD
	10. Recurrent angina after MI:
	NTG 0.4 mg SL q. 5 minutes x 3 prn
	☐ Notify House Staff
	☐ Notify Attending Physician
	11. PRN Medications:
	Tylenol ii tabs q. 4 hours, prn for non-anginal pain
	MS 2-4 mg. IV q. 15 minutes prn severe pain
	Sleep: _____
	Apprehension: _____
	Nausea/Vomiting: _____
	Bowel Care: _____
	12. Other orders including regular medications
	_____
	_____
	_____
	_____
	_____
	_____
	13. Cardiac Rehab
	Signature _____

MR-3568 (6/95) **PHYSICIAN'S TRANSFER ORDERS-ACUTE MI**

APPENDIX 4-C—*CONTINUED*

Estimated LOS: <u>4 days</u>

Admit Date _____

Payor _____
(for DC planning purposes)

Interdisciplinary
CLINICAL PATHWAY
UNCOMPLICATED MYO CARDIAL INFARCTION
Page 1 of 2

* = if indicated

	ADMISSION	CICU/TELE
KEY PATIENT GOALS/ OUTCOMES	Chest pain is relieved ___ Advance directives confirmed ___ Pt. verbalizes understanding of pt. rights and responsibilities ___ Conditions of admissions signed Lungs clear s̄ crackles/rales Resolution of ST/T wave Δ's, pulse ox > 90%	Chest pain relieved O2 sat >90% ___ Initiate cardiac rehab ___ MI continue pathway, if R/O'd dc pathway No arrhythmia Hemodynamics stable
ASSESSMENT	___ Risk/Falls assessment completed ___ H&P on chart ___ Nursing systems assessment completed per unit standard Chest pain assessment q̄ 1-2° prn S/S of bleeding (if given thrombolytics) ___ TB screening completed	Chest pain assessment q̄ 4° if stable S/S of heart failure S/S of bleeding (if given thrombolytics) Site of sheath* c̄ distal pulses ___ Eval. pt. stability to transfer to telemetry*
TESTS / DIAGNOSTICS	___ EKG ___ SMAC ___ *ABG's ___ CXR ___ CPK c̄ isoenzymes q̄ 8° x3 ___ PT/PTT/INR ___ *Cardiac cath ___ CBC	___ EKG ___ PT*/PTT*/INR* ___ H/H ___ CXR* if day 1 shows s/s CHF ___ SMAC ___ Echocardiogram/MUGA*
TREATMENTS	___ NS lock ___ Cardiac monitor ___ O2 2-4l min N.C. (maintain O2 sat > 90%) ___ Daily wt. ___ *Thrombolytic therapy ___ *PTCA ___ Medical therapy ___ I&O ___ IV *prn	___ NS lock/IV prn* ___ Cardiac monitor ___ Daily wt. ___ I&O
MEDICATIONS	___ MS0₄ IV prn chest pain ___ Beta blocker ___ ASA ___ Ntg sl ___ IV ntg ___ IV heparin* ___ Ace inhibitor ___ Stool softener ___ O₂ ___ Antiarrhythmics as indicated* ___ Inotropes* ___ Coumadin*	___ MS0₄ IV prn chest pain ___ Beta blocker ___ ASA ___ Ntg sl ___ IV ntg ___ IV heparin* ___ Ace inhibitor ___ Stool softener ___ O₂ ___ Antiarrhythmics as indicated* ___ Inotropes* ___ Coumadin*
NUTRITION	2-4 gm na ↓ fat if ↑ serum lipids, cardiac or NPO*	___ Same
ACTIVITY	___ Bedrest c̄ BSC* (unless sheath in place) ___ Assist c̄ ADL's prn	___ Bedrest c̄ BSC ___ Assist c̄ ADL's ___ OOB to chair x30* TID
CONSULTS	___ Cardiologist* ___ Cardiac rehab* ___ CNS*	___ Same
EDUCATION	___ Review c̄ pt & family S/S of chest pain or any unusual sensations ___ Review clinical pathway ___ Orient to room ___ Review AM tx's & procedures ___ Offer "After your heart attack" booklet	___ Assess barriers to learning ___ Review MI diagnosis if applicable ___ Activity restriction ___ Basic A&P of heart & cause of C/P ___ Energy conservation ___ Review risk factors
EMOTIONAL/CULTURAL NEEDS/CONCERNS	___ Pt needs to verbalize fears & feeling about having an MI Spousal support & future fears of MI Evaluate coping mechanisms of pt./family	___ Spouse/pt. family support group available ___ Spousal support & future fears of MI
DISCHARGE PLANNING	___ Initial discharge planning Case manager*	___ Referral to home care* prn

Date Adopted Medical Department / Committee _____ Date to MEC _____

Clinical Pathways are guidelines only and do not preempt the independent judgement of the physician.

MR-3561 3/96

APPENDIX 4-C—CONTINUED

Estimated LOS: <u>4 days</u>

Admit Date _____

Payor _____
(for DC planning purposes)

Interdisciplinary
CLINICAL PATHWAY
<u>UNCOMPLICATED MYO CARDIAL INFARCTION</u>
Page 2 of 2

* = if indicated

	DAY 3	DAY 4	DAY 5
KEY PATIENT GOALS / OUTCOMES	Chest pain relieved ___ Transfer to telemetry unit No arrhythmias Increase ambulation	___ D/C plan is completed, order written ___ Rx written for pt. Pain free No arrhythmias c̄ ↑ activity	___ Discharge ___ Pt. able to verbalize physical limitations at home; ___ understands progressive ↑ in activity level
ASSESSMENT	Chest pain assessment Assess S/S of heart failure Assess arrhythmias c̄ ↑ activity	Chest pain assessment Assess arrhythmias	___ No arrhythmias ___ Pain free Lungs clear / ⊖ S/S of edema Wt WNL for pt.
TESTS/DIAGNOSTICS	___ EKG PTT* / PT* / INR* ___ Chem panel ___ Cardiac cath *prn	___ EKG *EST *prn *Cardiac cath prn	EKG, EST *prn
TREATMENTS	___ NS lock ___ Cardiac monitor ___ Daily wt. I&O ___ O2* Pulse oximeter	___ NS lock ___ Cardiac monitor ___ O2*	___ NS lock Dc'd ___ Cardiac monitor dc'd
MEDICATIONS	___ ASA ___ Ace inhibitor* ___ Heparin* ___ Beta blocker ___ Ntg sl prn* ___ Stool softener ___ MSO₄ prn chest pain	___ ASA ___ MSO₄ *prn ___ Beta blocker ___ Ace inhibitor* ___ Stool softener	D/C rx given to pt.
NUTRITION	Same	Same	Same
ACTIVITY	Ambulate in room, BRP, amb c̄ assistance 25-75' ft bid	Amb 50-150' bid (up ad lib in room)	Amb 150-250' TID (up ad lib)
CONSULTS	Cardiac rehab* Dietitian* Physical therapy* if more extensive gait training required CNS*	Cardiac rehab* Dietitian* CNS*	Cardiac rehab* review d/c progressive activity plan

EDUCATION	___ Orient to telemetry unit
	___ Teach re: meds/diet/↓ risk factors
	  ___ Sexual activity
	  ___ Progressive physical activity
	  ___ Limitations of physical activity
	  ___ Who to call when you are home if C/P reoccurs
	Pt. understanding of diagnosis & Rx plan.
		___ Review "After your H.A." booklet
		  ___ S/S of chest pain
		  ___ Diet ___ Meds
		  ___ Activity
		  ___ Sexual functioning
		  ___ Weight monitoring (*S/S of ___ CHF)
		  ___ Reduction of risk factors
		___ Pt./family understanding of dx of MI
		___ If going home on coumadin:
		___ Tx book ___ Coumadin
		___ Tape ___ Lab values to know
			Review D/C plan
			  Understand by pt./family & able to verbalize understanding
			Review self-management strategies:
			  ___*Who to call in case of emergency
			  ___Stress reduction techniques
			  ___Physician appointments made.

EMOTIONAL/CULTURAL NEEDS/CONCERNS	Eval pt. & spouse feeling of impact of diagnosis on their relationship ___ Support groups (inpt.)	Continue c̄ emotional support ___ Who to call & what to do in case of C/P	___ Referrals* in hospital & or MD's to contact for questions or concerns
DISCHARGING PLANNING	___ Referral to home care* prn	___ Home care referral/eval completed* equipment ordered etc.	Discharge

Date Adopted Medical Department / Committee _____   Date to MEC _____

Clinical Pathways are guidelines only and do not preempt the independent judgement of the physician.

MR-3561 3/96

APPENDIX 4-C—*CONTINUED*

PATIENT INFORMATION SUMMARY

Uncomplicated Acute Myocardial Infarction

ADMISSION - DAY 1

The following will help you and your family understand the plan of your hospital stay. Your physician, your patient care team caring for you and the case manager will keep you informed of how you are doing. Please feel free to ask any questions that you have regarding your progress

- You will be admitted to Intensive Care Unit (ICU) or Telemetry Unit
- An electrocardiogram (ECG), blood work and chest x-rays will be done
- You will have an intravenous line (IV) started so that you may be given medications as needed
- You doctor may order oxygen
- You may be asked not to eat or drink anything at this time because your doctor may order further tests
- You may be asked to stay in bed and give your heart a rest
- You may be started on medications to relieve pain and improve your heart function
- It's very important to tell your patient care team if you are having any pain so that they can help to relieve it before any further heart damage is done

DAY 2

- You will continue to be monitored frequently
- More blood work and ECG will be done to be compared to yesterday's tests

- If you are in the ICU, you may be transferred to the Telemetry unit today
- Your activity may be increased today if approved by your physician
- You will meet with staff to help with discharge needs
- If you have no complications you may go home two or three days from now

DAY 3

- Another ECG and more blood work will be done for comparison
- Your heart will continue to be monitored on a portable telemetry monitor
- You will increase your activities
- The cardiac rehab nurse may visit to help you with exercise and education

DAY 4

- You will continue to be monitored
- You will continue to increase your activity
- The cardiac rehab nurse will discuss home exercise guidelines
- You might go home today or tomorrow

DAY 5

- Your intravenous line and telemetry monitor will be discontinued
- Reveiw of discharge information

Mercy Healthcare Arizona
St. Joseph's Hospital and Medical Center

S-390 CORONARY ARTERY BYPASS GRAFT (CABG)
CPT-4: 33510, 33511, 33512, 33513, 33514, 33516, 33517, 33518, 33519, 33521, 33522, 33523, 33530, 33533, 33534, 33535, 33536, 33572
ICD-9: 36.10, 36.11, 36.12, 36.13, 36.14, 36.15, 36.16, 36.19
ICD-9: 410.XX, 411.1, 411.8X, 413.X, 414.0X

Case Management: Coordinate Care & Anticipate Needs

1. *Preoperative:* Coronary artery bypass graft surgery is an acceptable alternative to coronary angioplasty. Diabetics have better outcomes with surgery. Surgery results in more complete revascularization, fewer subsequent procedures, and possibly long-term survival. Angioplasty avoids major surgery in approximately 70% of patients and is associated with shorter hospitalizations, lower initial costs, and possibly fewer periprocedural infarctions.
Ensures patient education about postoperative rehabilitation and recognition of complications. Coordinates medical evaluation of any surgical risk factors which may include diabetes, cerebrovascular disease, or renal disease.
Assesses home safety, needs, and capabilities.

2. *Acute:* For emergency presentation, including unstable angina or myocardial infarction, facilitates scheduling of diagnostic services and surgery, monitors daily progress; continues patient education; coordinates multiple professional caregivers as appropriate; coordinates decision about home care or recovery facility. Most patients will be discharged home. Hemodynamically stable patients who require ventilator weaning can be transferred to a recovery facility. Other candidates for recovery facility include patients with complex active or potential medical problems, debilitated and/or deconditioned state, or lack of an adequate home caregiver. For rehabilitation of postoperative CVA, see ORGs M81-84.

3. *Recovery Facility:* Coordinates development of treatment goals and treatment plan which includes recognition of recurrent myocardial ischemia, arrhythmias, and congestive heart failure; rounds at the facility or communicates with professional caregiver, facility nursing staff, patient and/or family daily; facilitates transition home or to a residential or custodial setting as appropriate; ensures timely referral to appropriate community resources and applications for public funding.

4. *Home:* May require skilled assessment, IV antibiotics, therapies, and oversight of wound. Continues patient education for activity allowances and limitations, compliance with medication, diet, and energy conservation techniques; helps develop long-term program of risk factor reduction.

5. *Risk Factor Reduction:* The progression of coronary artery disease can be retarded or reversed with low-fat diet, cholesterol-lowering drugs if diet alone insufficient to achieve LDL < 100 and HDL > 35, control of hypertension, exercise, stress reductions, cessation of smoking, and tight control of diabetes. Cardiac rehabilitation programs are an effective means of implementing risk reduction.

Day 1: Operating room, ICU, intubated, chest tube, central lines, pacer wires, parenteral fluid, medication, and antibiotics. Possible PCA or epidural analgesia. Possible extubation.

Day 2: Extubated, hemodynamically stable. Discontinue chest tube and central lines. Stepdown unit for monitoring, oxygen, parenteral fluid, parenteral or oral medication, light diet, chair and minimal ambulatory activity. Possible PCA or epidural analgesia.

Day 3: Step-down unit with monitoring, oxygen, parenteral fluid. Oral medication, increased ambulation and diet. Rhythm stable. Discontinue pacer wires. Possible PCA or epidural analgesia.

Day 4: Discontinue PCA or epidural analgesia. Oral medication, advanced diet and increased activity. Discharge.
Goal Length-of-Stay: 3 days postoperative

(continued)

APPENDIX 4-D—*CONTINUED*

S-560 HIP: ARTHROPLASTY (TOTAL)
CPT-4: 27130, 27132, 27134, 27137, 27138
ICD-9: 81.51, 81.53
ICD-9: 711.05, 714.0, 715.15, 715.25, 715.35, 716.15, 733.42

Case Management: Coordinate Care & Anticipate Needs

1. *Preoperative:* Patient education, assessment of home care capabilities and needs, medical evaluation of surgical risk factors, upper body strengthening, walker or crutch training, and collection of autologous blood.
2. *Acute:* Monitors daily progress; coordinates multiple professional caregivers as appropriate; coordinates decision about home care or recovery facility. Home health care is preferred for the majority of patients if medical conditions have stabilized and they are ambulatory with an assistive device. Recovery facility may be used for patients with complex acute or potentially unstable medical problems, a debilitated and/or deconditioned state, or lack of an adequate home caregiver. Acute and subacute rehabilitation are rarely indicated for this procedure.
3. *Recovery Facility:* Coordinates development of treatment goals and treatment plan; rounds at the facility or communicates with professional caregiver, facility nursing staff, patient and/or family daily; facilitates transition home or to a residential or custodial setting as appropriate; ensures timely referral to appropriate community resources and applications for public funding.
4. *Home:* May continue to require skilled assessment, home safety evaluation, additional therapies, oversight of wound, and management of medical comorbidities and anticoagulation.

Day 1: Operating room, parenteral fluid, medication, and antibiotics. Possible PCA or epidural analgesia and/or nonsteroidal analgesia. Anticoagulation.

Day 2: Parenteral fluid, medication, and antibiotics. Physical therapy for transfer training and gait training with crutches or walker. Diet as tolerated. Possible PCA or epidural analgesia and/or nonsteroidal analgesia.

Day 3: Discontinue IV, PCA or epidural analgesia. Parenteral or oral medication. Physical therapy. Regular diet.

Day 4: Afebrile, oral medication, regular diet. Physical therapy stand-by. Discharge, with possible home healthcare and physical therapy for gait training with crutches or walker.

Goal Length-of-Stay: 3 days postoperative

N.B. Patients in whom a slower recovery is anticipated may be transferred to a skilled nursing facility on day 3 to continue physical therapy for gait training with crutches or walker.

(continued)

APPENDIX 4-D—*CONTINUED*

S-960 PROSTATECTOMY, NOT TRANSURETHRAL, INCLUDING RADICAL
CPT-4: 55801, 55810, 55812, 55815, 55821, 55831, 55840, 55842
ICD-9: 60.3, 60.4, 60.5, 60.62
ICD-9: 185, 233.4

Case Management: Coordinate Care & Anticipate Needs

1. *Preoperative:* Provides education about management of Foley catheter, pain control, and recognition of complications including infection, bleeding, and deep venous thrombosis. Coordinates medical evaluation of any surgical risk factors which may include cardiac, respiratory, or renal disease. Assesses home care capabilities, needs, and safety.
2. *Acute:* Monitors daily progress; continues patient education; coordinates multiple consultants as appropriate. Most patients will be discharged home, possibly with home healthcare support. Recovery facility is utilized for patients with complex comorbidities, debilitated and/or deconditioned state, or lack of an adequate home caregiver.
3. *Recovery Facility:* Coordinates development of treatment goals and treatment plan; rounds at the facility or communicates with professional caregiver, facility nursing staff, patient and/or family daily; facilitates transition home or to a residential or custodial setting as appropriate; ensures timely referral to appropriate community resources and applications for public funding.
4. *Home:* May require home nursing contact for skilled assessment, pain control, management of complications, supervision of medications, administration of antibiotics, or reinforcement of education.
5. Prevention/Early Detection. Digital rectal examination should be performed annually for men over 40 years of age who are at increased risk for prostate cancer (family history and African-American males). All men should be examined yearly after age 50. Prostate Specific Antigen should be done annually for men over 40 who are at increased risk and for men over 50 with symptoms of prostatic obstruction (nocturia or hesitancy).

Day 1: Operating room. Parenteral fluid and medication. Epidural anesthetic catheter removed. Foley catheter or suprapublic tube with possible drain. Subcutaneous heparin. Up in chair. Oral or parenteral nonsteroidal anti-inflammatory analgesia.

Day 2: Ambulatory. Clear liquids to regular diet, discontinue IV. Oral analgesia. Possible discharge.

Day 3: Regular diet. Oral analgesia. Discharge with Foley catheter or suprapubic tube, possible drain, and possible home healthcare services.

Goal Length-of-Stay: 1–2 days postoperative

(continued)

APPENDIX 4-D—*CONTINUED*

M-281 PNEUMONIA, COMMUNITY ACQUIRED
ICD-9: 480.X, 481, 482.XX, 483.X, 484.X, 485, 486, 487.0

Case Management: Coordinate Care & Anticipate Needs
1. *Office or Rapid Treatment Site:* Coordinates decision about home care or recovery facility for those patients incapable of self-care at home. Patients who do not require acute care but who have comorbid conditions, a debilitated and/or deconditioned state, or lack of adequate home caregiver can be admitted directly to a recovery facility from the ambulatory setting or rapid treatment site.
2. *Recovery Facility:* Coordinates development of treatment goals and treatment plan; rounds at the facility or communicates with professional caregiver, facility nursing staff, patient and/or family daily; facilitates transition home or to a residential or custodial setting as appropriate; ensures timely referral to appropriate community resources and applications for public funding.
3. *Home:* Provides skilled assessment with emphasis on patients in whom pneumonia may resolve slowly such as those with chronic obstructive pulmonary disease, alcoholism, or heart failure; may continue to require IV antibiotics, oxygen, and respiratory therapy.
4. *Prevention:* Pneumococcal vaccine is recommended for all individuals who are age 65 or older or otherwise at risk for pneumococcal disease. Yearly influenza vaccination is given in the autumn to a similar population.

Adequate Reasons for Admission
• Hemodynamic instability
• Respiratory failure
• Empyema
• Extensive involvement with hypoxia
• Inability to clear respiratory secretions
• Failure of appropriate outpatient treatment
• Severe neutropenia under 1,000/cu. mm.
• Severe coexisting illness
• Altered mental status

Inadequate Reasons for Admission
• Pleurisy
• Consolidation
• Cough, bloody sputum
• Fever, toxicity (depending on underlying health status)

Alternatives
• Outpatient care in an emergency room, rapid treatment site, urgent care, clinic, or office
  ◦ Sputum gram stain, culture and begin therapeutic trial
  ◦ Re-evaluate exam, hemodynamics, gases after 8 hours
• Home Care
  ◦ House call by physician
  ◦ Nursing visits for assessment, laboratory work
  ◦ Parenteral antibiotics if indicated
  ◦ Respiratory therapy, oxygen
• Recovery Facility
  ◦ Skilled Care
    ■ Parenteral fluid and medication
    ■ Respiratory treatment, oxygen
    ■ Management of stable comorbidities
  ◦ Subacute Care
    ■ Frequent assessment and treatment
    ■ Management of unstable comorbidities

Goal Length-of-Stay: Alternatives rather than acute care

(continued)

APPENDIX 4-D—*CONTINUED*

M-330 SEPTICEMIA
ICD-9: 038.XX, 998.59, 999.3

Case Management: Coordinate Care & Anticipate Needs

1. *Office or Rapid Treatment Site:* Early appropriate antibiotic therapy is associated with significantly improved survival; therefore, prompt recognition is vital. Usually, the patient will first manifest symptoms and signs related to the primary focus of infection such as pneumonia or pyelonephritis. In debilitated and/or deconditioned elderly or immunocompromised patients, the only signs may be confusion and rapid respiration.
2. *Acute:* In the complex ICU patient, ensures communication between the patient, family and multiple physician consultants. As recovery begins, coordinates decision about home care or recovery facility. Selected hemodynamically stable patients are candidates for ventilation weaning, hemodialysis, or chest tube/surgical drain management in a recovery facility. Home care may provide parenteral antibiotics and other services.
3. *Recovery Facility:* Coordinates development of treatment goals and treatment plans; rounds at the facility or communicates with professional caregiver, facility nursing staff, patient and/or family daily; facilitates transition home or to a residential or custodial setting as appropriate; ensures timely referral to appropriate community resources and applications for public funding.
4. *Home:* Requires skilled assessment of manifestations of reemergence of infection or superinfection; ensures adequate nutritional intake which may require parenteral nutrition; may require coordination of transportation to an outpatient dialysis facility; may continue to require IV antibiotics, IV fluid, respiratory care, and oxygen.
5. *Risk Factor Reduction:* Pneumococcal and influenza vaccination in patients who are elderly, immunocompromised, or have chronic medical disease. Prompt removal of Foley catheters and intravascular lines.

Day 1: Admitted to ICU for hypotension or to routine floor care for fever, toxicity. Cultures, lab work, imaging or possible surgical consultation as appropriate, parenteral fluid, and antibiotics. Diet as tolerated. Discharge planning.

Day 2: Temperature declining, hemodynamically stable. Routine floor care. Positive blood culture and perhaps other cultures. Imaging has not shown a cause requiring surgical drainage. Parenteral fluid and antibiotics. Activity and diet as tolerated.

Day 3: Afebrile. Infectious organism and antibiotic sensitivities identified. No need for surgical drainage. Discontinue parenteral fluid. Discharge on parenteral or oral antibiotic, possibly to a recovery facility or home care.

Goal Length-of-Stay: 2 days

(continued)

APPENDIX 4-D—*CONTINUED*

M-55 ASTHMA
ICD-9: 493.X0
Case Management: Coordinate Care & Anticipate Needs
1. *Office or Rapid Treatment Site:* Early intervention in the ambulatory setting frequently reduces the severity of airways obstruction and shortens the hospitalization. Home will suffice for most patients who require care extended beyond the rapid treatment site. Patients who do not require acute care but who have complex potentially unstable medical problems, or patients who lack an adequate home caregiver can be admitted directly to a recovery facility from the office or rapid treatment site.
2. *Recovery Facility:* Coordinates development of treatment goals and treatment plan; rounds at the facility or communicates with professional caregiver, facility nursing staff, patient and/or family daily; facilitates transition home or to a residential or custodial setting as appropriate; ensures timely referral to appropriate community resources and applications for public funding.
3. *Home:* May continue to require skilled assessment of respiratory status; ensures medication knowledge and compliance, utilization of peak-flow meter, and removal of environmental allergens; may continue to require respiratory therapy and oxygen.
4. *Prevention/Education:* Recognition and avoidance of precipitating stimuli, proper use of medication especially metered-dose inhalers, self-monitoring of peak expiratory flow rates, influenza and pneumococcal vaccinations.

Adequate Reasons for Admission
• Respiratory failure (CO_2 retention)
• Failure to respond to 4 to 8 hours of intensive outpatient treatment with persistent dyspnea, use of accessory muscles, and peak expiratory flow rate below 60% predicted

Inadequate Reasons for Admission
• Frequent attacks
• Severe dyspnea on presentation to office or ER
• Coexistent infection

Alternatives
• Outpatient care in an emergency room, rapid treatment site, urgent care, clinic, or office
  ◦ Parenteral fluid and medication for hours
  ◦ Parenteral corticosteroids
  ◦ Aggressive inhaled beta-agonists, inhaled, injected, or orally
• Home Care
  ◦ House call by physician
  ◦ Nursing visit with assessment, parenteral treatment including medication and intravenous parenteral fluid, instruction and observation of peak flow rate measurements
  ◦ Laboratory testing
  ◦ Respiratory treatment and training
• Recovery Facility
  ◦ Skilled care
  ◦ Parenteral fluid and medication
  ◦ Respiratory treatment, education, possible oxygen
  ◦ Management of stable comorbidities
  ◦ Subacute care
  ◦ Frequent assessment and respiratory treatment
  ◦ Management of unstable comorbidities
  ◦ Possible cardiac monitoring

Goal Length-of-Stay: Alternatives rather than acute care

(continued)

M-327 SEIZURE
ICD-9: 345.1X, 345.3, 345.4X, 345.9X

Case Management: Coordinate Care & Anticipate Needs

1. *Office or Rapid Treatment Site:* Patients with status epilepticus, increased intracranial pressure, meningitis, or newly diagnosed structural lesion (tumor, stroke, abscess, trauma) are admitted to acute care. Patients with a first seizure who lack an adequate home caregiver for observation, a readily reversible metabolic defect, or mild sedative-hypnotic withdrawal are candidates for direct admission to a recovery facility from the rapid treatment site. These patients often have complex potentially unstable medical conditions or debilitated and/or deconditioned state. Home care can provide appropriate care for patients with lesser needs. Ensure appropriate notification of governmental agencies.
2. *Recovery Facility:* Coordinates development of treatment goals and treatment plan; rounds at the facility or communicates with professional caregiver, facility nursing staff, patient and/or family daily, facilitates transition home or to a residential or custodial setting as appropriate; ensures timely referral to appropriate community resources and applications for public funding.
3. *Home:* May require skilled assessment including neurologic signs and symptoms; assesses safety of the home environment.

Adequate Reasons for Admission
- Status epilepticus
- Increased intracranial pressure
- Meningitis
- Sedative, hypnotic, anxiolytic agent withdrawal
- Metabolic predisposition, e.g., prolonged hypoglycemia

Inadequate Reasons for Admission
- First seizure
- Focal neurological finding
- Fever, if lumbar puncture negative
- Inadequate control by medication unless status epilepticus is present
- Neurodiagnostic workup

Alternatives
- Outpatient care in an emergency room, rapid treatment site, urgent care, clinic, or office
  - Neurological consultation and evaluation including EEG and imaging
  - Lumbar puncture, if indicated
  - Observe with change in medication
- Home Care
  - Nursing visit
  - Outpatient workup
- Recovery Facility
  - Skilled Care
- Parenteral fluid and medication
- Management of stable comorbidities
  - Subacute Care
- Management of unstable comorbidities

Goal Length-of-Stay: Alternatives rather than acute care

CHAPTER 5

Transitional Planning: Understanding Levels and Transitions of Care

LEARNING OBJECTIVES

Upon completion of this chapter, the reader will be able to:

1. Define the terms discharge planning, transitions of care, and levels of care.
2. Discuss the relationships between transitions of care and levels of care.
3. Differentiate between the various care settings across the healthcare continuum.
4. Differentiate skilled from nonskilled care.
5. Explain the relationships among transitional planning, utilization management, and reimbursement.
6. Describe the role of the case manager in the various practice settings.
7. Report the impact of case management on care quality and patient safety during transitions of care.

ESSENTIAL TERMS

Air Ambulance • Advanced Life Support (ALS) Ambulance • Basic Life Support (BLS) Ambulance • Custodial Care • Discharge Planning • Extended Care Facility • Grievance Process • Home Health Services • Hospice • Hospital-Issued Notice of Noncoverage (HINN) • Intermediate Care • Long-Term Care (LTC) • Nonskilled Services • Notice of Noncoverage (NONC) • Notice of Discharge and Medicare Appeal Rights (NODMAR) • Quality Improvement Organization (QIO) • Rehabilitation Services • Skilled Care • Skilled Nursing Facility (SNF) • Specialty Pharmacy Providers • Subacute Care • Three Nights Rule • Transfer DRGs • Transitions of Care • Transitional Planning

Transitional planning, discharge planning, and safe transfers of patients to alternative levels of care are a major case management responsibility. These require a basic understanding of levels of care, reimbursement, and health insurance coverage. Case managers have earned the reputation of being transitional and discharge planning experts; therefore, their roles in safe discharge and transitional planning are significant.

Transitional planning is defined as a dynamic, interactive, collaborative, and interdisciplinary process of assessment and evaluation of the healthcare needs of patients and their families or caregivers during or after a phase/episode of illness. It aims to transition patients from one level of care to another. It also includes assessment of the patient's and family's needs and planning and brokering of necessary services identified based on the patient's condition (Cesta & Tahan, 2003). In addition, the process ensures that services are provided at the

appropriate level of care—at the right time, in the right amount, by the right provider, and in the right setting.

In contrast, discharge planning is integral to and subsumed in transitional planning. It basically focuses on discharging patients from an inpatient hospital setting to another facility or home (Cesta & Tahan, 2003). The use of the term *transitional planning* became more common with the advent of managed care and the need for utilization management/review, where criteria for care provision in each of the various levels of care (e.g., acute care hospital, subacute, SNF, home care, and so on) were reinforced through the authorization/certification process.

Despite the difference in the use of the terms *transitional planning* and *discharge planning*, regulatory and accreditation standards continue to focus mainly on discharge planning. For example, The Joint Commission (TJC) requires hospital policies and procedures on discharge planning. It also requires policies and procedures on patient flow that indirectly implies standards around transitional planning despite the lack of use of such term. In January 1995, the Centers for Medicare & Medicaid Services (CMS), known then as the Health Care Financing Administration (HCFA), gave more power to TJC (also known then as the Joint Commission on Accreditation of Healthcare Organizations [JCAHO]) requirements when the CMS *Conditions of Participation for Hospitals—Discharge Planning Regulations* stated that "the hospital must arrange for the initial implementation of the patient's discharge plan" (CMS, 2009). Today, TJC's guidelines for the provision of care and services including discharge planning consist of the following standards (TJC, 2008).

▶ The hospital accepts for care, treatment, and services only those patients whose identified care, treatment, and services it can meet.

▶ Development of a plan for care, treatment, and services is individualized and appropriate to the patient's needs, strengths, limitations, and goals.

▶ Care provision and services must be according to the plan for care.

▶ Coordination of care, treatment, and services provided to a patient as part of the plan for care, treatment, and services must be consistent with the hospital's scope of care, treatment, and services.

▶ The patient receives education and training specific to his or her needs and as appropriate to the care, treatment, and services provided. Education and training are specific to the patient's abilities. For patients who are children and youth, academic education must be provided as needed.

▶ Patients may be discharged home from the hospital or transferred to another level of care, treatment, and services, to different health professionals, or to other settings for continued services. The process of transfer or discharge must be based on the patient's assessed needs.

▶ To facilitate a discharge or transfer, the hospital assesses the patient's needs, plans for discharge or transfer, facilitates the discharge or transfer process, and helps to ensure that continuity of care, treatment, and services is maintained.

▶ The discharge planning process must address the need for coordination of care and continuing care, treatment, and services after discharge or transfer from the hospital. An ideal process is one that employs case management concepts and addresses the following:
  ○ The reasons for transfer or discharge.
  ○ The conditions under which transfer or discharge can occur.
  ○ Shifting responsibility for the patient's care from one clinician/provider of care, organization, clinical program, or service to another.
  ○ A mechanism for appropriate and safe transfer: internally within an organization (e.g., from one patient care unit to another or from a generalist provider to a specialist) and externally from one organization to another (e.g., from a hospital to a skilled nursing facility [SNF] or from a hospital to a subacute care rehabilitation facility).
  ○ The accountability and responsibility for the patient's safety during transfer of both the organization/provider initiating the transfer and the one receiving the patient.

For a hospital to ensure an effective discharge planning process is in place, the following standards and expectations must be carefully considered. Case managers can play an essential role in making sure that the provision of care adheres to the standards described above as well as the nine listed below, described based on the Medicare's Conditions of Participation.

1. Hospitals must identify, at an early stage of hospitalization (preferably at time of admission and no more than 24 hours), patients who are likely to suffer adverse health consequences if discharged without adequate discharge planning.

2. Hospitals must provide a discharge planning evaluation for patients identified under the requirement listed above and for other patients on the request of the patient or his or her representative.

3. Any discharge planning evaluation must be made on a timely basis to ensure that appropriate arrangements for posthospital care will be made before discharge and to avoid unnecessary delays in discharge.

4. This discharge planning evaluation must include the patient's likely need for and availability of appropriate posthospital services. It also must be included in the patient's medical record for use in establishing an appropriate discharge plan, and the results of the evaluation must be discussed with the multidisciplinary team involved in the care, the patient, and/or his or her representative.

5. The discharge planning evaluation must include an assessment of the patient's capacity for self-care or of the possibility of the patient being cared for in the environment from which he or she entered the hospital.

6. Hospitals must reassess the discharge plan if there are factors that may affect continuing care needs or the appropriateness of the discharge plan.
7. Hospitals must provide the patient with a list of agencies and/or facilities that are appropriate to the identified care needs and are Medicare participating. In the case of Medicare managed care plans, a list of those contracted with the plan must be provided.
8. If a transfer or referral is needed, hospitals must transfer or refer the patient along with necessary medical information to the appropriate facility, agency, or outpatient services as needed for follow-up and ancillary care.
9. A registered professional nurse, social worker, or other appropriately qualified staff member must develop or supervise the development of the discharge planning evaluation or discharge plan.

Number 9 is interesting in that most (although not all) case managers who perform this function at the acute level of care have one of the two licensures listed. The law supports what nurses, case managers, and social workers do. The responsibility for discharge planning, then, based on the Medicare's Conditions of Participation, should be multidisciplinary; it should not be restricted to a one specific discipline or professional. A case manager may play a primary role in discharge planning, but he or she should work collaboratively with the rest of the multidisciplinary team.

As utilization management criteria continue to tighten, patients with increased physiologic needs are more than ever being moved to lower levels of care. The sooner the case manager can start the assessment process for a patient's actual and potential discharge needs, the more time can be spent matching appropriate services to these needs. When considering discharge planning, all levels of care options should be explored. Discharging a patient home with family support is preferable in most cases. If family is unavailable, friends, neighbors, religious affiliation volunteers, or community referrals can sometimes provide the needed link between the patient's independence and his or her having to go to a supervisory or foster care setting. Social services can be an invaluable asset in care planning with this type of patient.

If more skilled care is required than can be provided by family or volunteers, perhaps the patient is safe to go home with the addition of home nursing services. Consider the use of home RN visits for care, teaching, or assessments; home physical therapy (PT); occupational therapy (OT) and speech/language therapy (ST); home aides (restrictions apply); home psychiatric nursing; or home social services. Many insurance plans provide home health services only if the patient's condition and needs meet certain criteria such as being homebound; this is an important point to assess. Also, determine just what the patient's health insurance plan provides; many plans allow only a few intermittent visits, which do not always meet the patient's total needs.

If a patient is not homebound or can easily be transported by family or volunteers, consider the use of outpatient services such as outpatient rehabilitation departments, which provide physical, speech, and occupational therapies. Freestanding clinics may provide a wide range of services from wound care to the administration of intravenous antibiotics or chemotherapy. When sending patients home, one needs to assess outpatient pharmaceutical benefits, especially prior to, or close to, the time of discharge. This is necessary because one of the primary causes for readmission to the acute care hospital setting is improper medication regimen and administration. Educational deficits may contribute to this problem; reviewing the medication reconciliation process and assessing knowledge deficits relating to medications are important case management responsibilities. Another underlying contributor to the problem may be financial; not all insurance plans have adequate prescription coverage and some people cannot afford the prescriptions. For example, patients with traditional Medicare have few pharmaceutical benefits. Detective work may be needed to see whether the patient's plan covers medications.

Until recently, traditional Medicare did not cover home intravenous antibiotics. Sending a Medicare patient home with intravenous antibiotics was nearly impossible unless the patient could personally finance the medications. This has changed. If the Medicare plan is one of the "risk" contracts that pays for hospitalizations on a per-diem or capitated basis (instead of the case rate applied in the diagnosis-related groups [DRGs] prospective payment system (PPS)), it is financially beneficial to the plan to send the patient home with intravenous medications. Therefore, the health insurance company (i.e., the insurance-based case manager) often works with the provider-based case manager on the discharge plan to make sure it is cost effective, safe, and meets the patient's discharge needs. Under the traditional Medicare DRG reimbursement, only the hospital is financially penalized for keeping a patient in-house for a long time for antibiotic administration, which is why traditional Medicare has little incentive to change this benefit.

If the insurance company does not pay for home intravenous antibiotics and the patient is otherwise stable for discharge, assess whether the patient can receive the antibiotics at a freestanding clinic or at the doctor's office. It may be necessary to set up an observation admission or an outpatient admission on weekends for the dosage. Sometimes emergency departments can be used, although this should be discouraged, be a last resort, and done with the facility's approval. Traditional Medicare will pay for the nurse to administer the medication, so if the patient can afford the drug, this plan sometimes works (refer to Chapter 3, Reimbursement Concepts, for more information on drug benefits).

Medicaid plans generally pay for most prescriptive needs. It often has a "negative formulary" disallowing certain prescriptions. Some newer, expensive medications may need prior approval. No over-the-counter medications are covered (this also applies to most of the other insurance plans). Managed care pharmacy benefits may vary from the member paying 100% to the insurance company paying 100% (rare). Some members must purchase prescription riders on their policies to receive the benefit. Usually, the benefits require a copayment of $3 to $50 per prescription, an annual deductible, or a 20% coinsurance fee. The patient may also be reimbursed only at a generic rate if a generic equivalent is available (Kongstvedt, 2003). Another consideration is that many insurance plans with pharmaceutical benefits require the member to fill the prescription at designated contracted pharmacies. The case manager may need to find out where these pharmacies are if the patient does not know.

Discharging patients home is often the best plan of care for the patient and is also the least resource-intensive plan for the health insurance company. However, this is not always safe or possible. Discussions about the alternatives—nursing homes, rehabilitation, long-term care (LTC), and hospice—along with more details on home coverage follow. In all discharge plans, insurance verification of coverage is essential. Occasionally, nonbenefit options can be negotiated, but in all cases prior authorization should be obtained.

Early discharge planning, even in the preadmission phase, has been emphasized several times. Even with a good plan and prior authorization, the discharge plan may fall through or may require certain modifications. The patient's medical stability may change; family members may change their minds 30 minutes before transfer or discharge time; and various other surprises may pop up. Sometimes the case manager already had a nagging feeling that something was going to delay the discharge and therefore had an alternative plan in mind. A case manager's intuition is a useful skill and it prepares us for sudden stops and detours.

If a mentally competent patient decides to go home refusing all available services, documentation may be all that is needed. If there is a question of mental competency and the patient would be unsafe with his or her chosen discharge plan, a psychiatric consultation may be necessary to assess the patient's mental capacity.

▶ NOTICES OF NONCOVERAGE

Medicare beneficiaries are granted exceptional rights under the Medicare statutes. All Medicare beneficiaries enrolled in any of the Medicare health plans, including fee-for-service, health maintenance organizations (HMOs), and other Medicare options, must receive the "Important Message from Medicare" at the time of admission to an acute care hospital (Display 5-1). The message outlines beneficiaries' rights to discharge planning and their right to pursue a grievance process if they feel that they are being discharged too soon or without adequate posthospital care arrangements. The message must include details on how a patient or family member could request a review or an appeal by the relevant Quality Improvement Organization (QIO).

In reality, unfortunately, the day of admission is not the best time for patients or their families to read long legal notices, so they may not fully understand their rights. The hospital is responsible for informing patients of their rights and implementing those rights; as a patient advocate, the case manager should make sure that the patient understands these documents. Notices of Noncoverage (NONCs) deny coverage in hospitals, rehabilitation facilities, SNFs, or for various special services. Within acute hospitals, there can be preadmission/admission notices, continued stay notices, or notices for days at the end of the stay. These are called Hospital-Issued Notices of Noncoverage (HINNs) for traditional Medicare beneficiaries. They used to be called Notice of Discharge and Medicare Appeal Rights (NODMAR) for patients covered by Medicare Advantage Plans or Medicare managed care plans. Today the same notice is used for all Medicare beneficiaries regardless of the type of plan to which the beneficiary belongs.

In 1998, CMS, known then as HCFA, reinterpreted the regulations on NONCs. Beneficiary advocates were concerned that patients did not know their rights and were not sufficiently informed of those rights at the time of hospital discharge. In the past, notices were issued only if a dispute arose or when one

display 5-1

IMPORTANT MESSAGE FROM MEDICARE

Patient Name:_____

Patient ID Number:_____

    Name of Physician:_____

Department of Health and Human Services
Centers for Medicare & Medicaid Services
OMB Approval No. 0938-0692

AN IMPORTANT MESSAGE FROM MEDICARE ABOUT YOUR RIGHTS

AS A HOSPITAL PATIENT YOU HAVE THE RIGHT TO:

▶ Receive Medicare covered services. This includes medically necessary hospital services and services you may need after you are discharged, if ordered by your doctor. You have a right to know about these services, who will pay for them, and when you can get them.

▶ Be involved in any decisions about your hospital stay, and know who will pay for it.

▶ Report any concerns you have about the quality of care you receive to the Quality Improvement Organization (QIO) listed here

    Name of QIO: _____

    Telephone Number of QIO: _____

YOUR MEDICARE DISCHARGE RIGHTS

Planning for Your Discharge: During your hospital stay, the hospital staff will be working with you to prepare for your safe discharge and arrange for services you may need after you leave the hospital. When you no longer need inpatient hospital care, your doctor or hospital staff will inform you of your planned discharge date.

If You Think You Are Being Discharged Too Soon:

▶ You can talk to the hospital staff, your doctor and your managed care plan (if you belong to one) about your concerns.

▶ You also have the right to an appeal, that is, a review of your case by a Quality Improvement Organization (QIO). The QIO is an outside reviewer hired by Medicare to look at your case to decide whether you are ready to leave the hospital.

  ○ **If you want to appeal, you must contact the QIO no later than your planned discharge date and before you leave the hospital.**

  ○ If you do this, you will not have to pay for services you receive during the appeal (except for charges like copays and deductibles).

▶ If you do not appeal, but decide to stay in the hospital past your planned discharge date, you may have to pay for services you receive after that date.

▶ **Step by step instructions for calling the QIO and filing an appeal are on page 2.**

To speak with someone at the hospital about this notice, call:_____

Please sign and date here to show you received this notice and understand your rights.

Signature of Patient of Representative:_____ Date:_____

Form CMS-R-193

According to the Paperwork Reduction Act of 1995, no persons are required to respond to a collection of information unless it displays a valid OMB control number. The valid OMB control number for this information collection is 0938-1019. The time required to complete this information collection is estimated to average 60 minutes per response, including the time to review instructions, search existing data resources, gather the data needed, and complete and review the information collection. If you have comments concerning the accuracy of the time estimate(s) or suggestions for improving this form, please write to: CMS, 7500 Security Boulevard, Attn: PRA Reports Clearance Officer, Mail Stop C4-26-05, Baltimore, Maryland 21244-1850. *CMS 10066 (approved 5/2007)*

(continued)

IMPORTANT MESSAGE FROM MEDICARE (*Continued*)

STEPS TO APPEAL YOUR DISCHARGE

▶ **STEP 1:** You must contact the QIO no later than your planned discharge date before you leave the hospital. If you do this, you will not have to pay for the services you receive during the appeal (except for charges like copays and deductibles).

○ Here is the contact information for your QIO

Name of QIO (in Bold): _____ Telephone Number: _____

_____

○ You can file a request for an appeal any day of the week. Once you speak to someone or leave a message, your appeal has begun.

○ Ask the hospital if you need help contacting the QIO.

○ The name of this hospital is: _____ Provider ID Number: _____

_____

▶ **STEP 2:** You will receive a detailed notice from the hospital or your Medicare Advantage or other Medicare managed care plan (if you belong to one) that explains the reason they think you are ready to be discharged.

▶ **STEP 3:** The QIO will ask for your opinion. You or your representative need to be available to speak with the QIO, if requested. You or your representative may give the QIO a written statement, but you are not required to do so.

▶ **STEP 4:** The QIO will review your medical records and other important information about your case.

▶ **STEP 5:** The QIO will notify you of its decision within 1 day after it receives all necessary information.

○ If the QIO finds that you are not ready to be discharged, Medicare will continue to cover your hospital services.

○ If the QIO finds you are ready to be discharged, Medicare will continue to cover your services until noon of the day after QIO notifies you of its decision.

IF YOU MISS THE DEADLINE TO APPEAL, YOU HAVE OTHER APPEAL RIGHTS:

▶ You can still ask the QIO or your plan (if you belong to one) for a review of your case:

○ If you have Original Medicare: Call the QIO listed above.

○ If you belong to a Medicare Advantage Plan or other Medicare managed care plan: Call your plan.

▶ If you stay in the hospital, the hospital may charge you for any services you receive after your planned discharge date.

For more information, call 1-800-XXX-XXXX

ADDITIONAL INFORMATION: _____

_____

_____

Adapted from CMC <annual System, Pub 100-04 Medicare Claims Processing. Available online at http://www.cms.hhs.gov/Transmittals/downloads/R1257CP.pdf

was anticipated. Recently, the new interpretation of the regulations required that every Medicare HMO enrollee admitted to the hospital receive a NODMAR at least 24 hours prior to discharge. Today, however, CMS has extended this rule to HINNs for all Medicare beneficiaries (not just those in HMOs).

Implementation of these rules has created problems for HMOs and their enrollees and for providers of care to Medicare beneficiaries. Because of short lengths of hospital stays, many enrollees do not receive the notice in a timely fashion or prior to discharge as was intended; some do not receive one at all. The documents were written by expert lawyers and are not easily understood by ill and recovering Medicare beneficiaries; all they read is that their Medicare benefits have been

cut off or denied. Worried Medicare beneficiaries tend to sit on the QIOs' doorsteps on Monday mornings after having spent a weekend upset over these legal documents. Therefore, as a service to their patients, case managers can prepare patients by informing them of their rights to receive necessary hospital services, discharge plans, and the impending notice.

The most common conflict leading to a QIO review of an NONC occurs when the Medicare beneficiary requires custodial care, which Medicare does not cover. The family may not be able to take care of the patient's medical and activities of daily living (ADLs) needs, but they do not understand the difference between skilled and nonskilled care. As a case manager, you can avoid possible conflict by educating patients and families early in the hospital stay about Medicare coverage, benefits, and possible patient needs.

Medicare mandates that discharge planning begin at the time of admission. From the case manager's perspective, careful documentation of the patient's medical, financial, psychosocial status, and adequate discharge planning are needed; in fact, the HINN may be denied if the discharge plan is not clearly documented in the patient's record and in place. This documentation should show good faith and evidence that the patient is medically stable, aware of the plan of care (including the discharge plan) and that the discharge is based solely on medical status and not related to a DRG payment. The discharge plan should be the result of collaboration with the patient, family, and physician. If the patient or family is uncooperative or unrealistic, the case manager should document in the record the attempts to make a reasonable discharge plan. Medicare expects that every reasonable effort be made to ensure a safe, comprehensive plan for continuity of care. If that is not possible due to financial or social reasons, document, document, document. Occasionally, the Medicare beneficiary will refuse to sign the NONC. The NONC is still valid even without a signature. However, back-up documentation is imperative to show the notice was issued and the patient refused to sign. The case manager may also want to call the QIO if the patient refuses to sign as additional good faith; the QIOs can then immediately start the review process so that all parties are given coverage and attention.

▶ Highlights of the Important Message from Medicare

The Important Message (IM) from Medicare has been around for many years; however, CMS revised the IM and a new version went into effect as of July 2, 2007. The revisions grew out of a ruling on a lawsuit filed against Medicare (*Weichardt v. Leavitt*, C-03-5490 VRW). The revised IM streamlined the information to be communicated to patients and their families regarding their right for services and the process that can be followed if they disagree with the discharge plan or the date/time of discharge. The revised IM (Display 5-1) clearly highlights the following (Powell, 2007):

▶ The Medicare beneficiary's right to services as a hospital inpatient and for posthospitalization (discharge). Hospital in this case refers to any inpatient facility.
▶ The Medicare beneficiary's right to request an expedited review and determination of the discharge decision. The IM also includes

a detailed description of the QIO's review and appeal process to be followed, and the availability of other appeals processes if the beneficiary fails to meet the deadline for an expedited review/determination. This also includes contact information of the QIO to whom the patient must report the concerns.
▶ The circumstances under which a beneficiary will or will not be financially liable for charges for continued hospital stay.
▶ The Medicare beneficiary's right to receive additional detailed information and as needed.
▶ The Medicare beneficiary's signature requirement to indicate that he or she has received the notice and comprehends its contents.

The Medicare beneficiary's rights as a hospital patient include receipt of necessary hospital services covered by Medicare; information about any decisions made by the hospital, his or her doctor, the health plan, or any one else involved about the hospital stay; and who will pay for it. The rights also include the hospital's obligation to arrange for services the patient will receive postdischarge such as home care or transfer to a subacute care facility or SNF. In addition, the patient also has the right to be informed in advance about the name of the agency to provide the services and who will be paying for these services. Although patients always had these rights in the past, the rights were not consistently placed in front of patients the way they are now.

Today, CMS dictates that hospitals provide the patient, in writing (i.e., the IM from Medicare Notice), with the information about their rights for services within 2 calendar days of the day of admission to the hospital, obtain the patient's signature, and keep a copy of the IM in the patient's record. Hospitals are also required to inform the patient in writing of his or her discharge plan, again as soon as possible prior to the patient's discharge, but no more than 2 calendar days before discharge. In cases where the delivery of the initial IM occurs within less than 2 days of the date of discharge, the hospital is not required to issue a new IM. For Medicare beneficiaries who request an appeal, the hospital is obligated to deliver a detailed notice to the patient. To clarify the timeline of this process, let us consider a situation where a patient is admitted to the hospital on Monday, given the initial IM notice on Wednesday and discharged on Friday; the second IM notice will not be required. However, if the patient was admitted to the hospital on the 10th of the month, received the initial IM notice on the

12th of the month and was discharged on the 16th, the patient would require a second IM notice be given no earlier than the 14th of the same month.

Timing of the initial IM notice can be prior to the hospital admission date in elective admissions. In such cases, the notice can be given during the preadmission or preregistration visit but not more than 7 calendar days prior to admission. However, one should avoid routine delivery of the second/follow-up IM notice to the patient on the day of discharge. The IM notice that a hospital should deliver to a patient should be the standardized notice available on the CMS's Web site. The form is known as CMS-R-193. Hospitals are not allowed to modify the notice; however, they are allowed to add their names, logos, and address/contact information. CMS requires that the patient sign the notice; however, if he or she refuses, the date of refusal should be documented as date of receipt of the notice. A copy is usually given to the patient and another is kept in the patient's medical record.

The IM from Medicare does not apply in the case of swing beds, outpatient departments such as emergency services, observation status, and changes in a patient's status from inpatient to outpatient. Medicare beneficiaries where the IM rule applies include enrollees in the original Medicare and Medicare Advantage plans, dual eligible Medicare and Medicaid individuals, and other beneficiaries where Medicare is a secondary payor.

▶ The Review Process

The Medicare beneficiary is guaranteed the right to an independent review by the QIO in the event the beneficiary or his or her family believes he or she is being asked to leave the hospital too soon or that the postdischarge services are inadequate. The grievance process starts when the attending physician and the case management department (or utilization review department if separate from case management) believe the patient no longer meets medical criteria for the acute hospital level of care. If the patient or family disagrees with the discharge decision/notice, they can appeal it with a prompt telephone call to the QIO by noon of the next business day after receiving the IM from Medicare Notice. This call starts the grievance (review and appeal) process (Display 5-1). The QIO's decision of the appeal is communicated to the patient or family using another Medicare form called the "Detailed Notice of Discharge." The hospital uses this form as a patient letter to communicate the QIO's decision (Display 5-2). Without the telephone call to the QIO, the patient or family may be liable for hospital charges, starting on the third day after receiving the NONC. If the QIO agrees with the

original NONC, the patient may be billed for all charges beginning on the day after he or she received the QIO's final decision. If the patient/family continues to disagree with the discharge provisions, a request for reconsideration can be made. Hospitals are obligated to communicate to the patient the QIO's decision about the review/appeal filed by the patient. Display 5-2 includes the letter given to patients describing the QIO's decision about the discharge appeal.

If the patient feels that the NONC is in error, the case manager must be able to articulate the review/grievance process. This is no easy task, as many specific details apply according to the person who gives the NONC, who receives it, and when it is received. It is recommended that the case management department find a contact person in the QIO in their state for such situations.

The QIO can be a resource for Medicare information for you and your patients. If Medicare beneficiaries do not accept information from you, then the QIO, the fiscal intermediary (Part A), or other Medicare organizations may be able to educate the beneficiary. Educate yourself about Medicare information sources and materials. The Medicare (www.medicare.gov) and CMS (www.cms.hhs.gov) Web sites are a good source of information; and *The Medicare Handbook* is a valuable resource for patients and professionals. The *Handbook* can be obtained from Social Security, your state's QIO, your Area Agency on Aging, or other organizations; it is also available on the CMS Web site.

The IM from Medicare includes information about the process a Medicare beneficiary would use in case of a review or appeal. The information must use the specific language as mandated by CMS. (Refer to Display 5-1 for more information.) The notice also must include directions a beneficiary would follow if he or she desires to file an appeal with the QIO. The IM from Medicare notice contains additional information about the patient's other appeal rights; for example, missing an appeal deadline but still wishing to file an appeal. Patients can still appeal as long as the request for review and appeal is made within 30 calendar days of the discharge date.

The four Hospital Issued Notices of Noncoverage include the following:

1. The Preadmission/Admission HINN is used to notify the patient that Medicare is not likely to pay for the admission because it is not considered medically necessary or it could be furnished safely in another setting.
2. The HINN 11, Notice for Noncovered Services in a Covered Stay, is used to notify patients that their physician has ordered specific services

display 5-2

IMPORTANT MESSAGE FROM MEDICARE: PATIENT LETTER ON DECISION OF DISCHARGE APPEAL

Patient Name:_____

Patient ID Number:_____

Name of Physician:_____

Department of Health and Human Services
Centers for Medicare & Medicaid Services
OMB Approval No. 0938-1019

DETAILED NOTICE OF DISCHARGE

You have asked for a review by the Quality Improvement Organization (QIO), an independent reviewer hired by Medicare to review your case. This notice gives you a detailed explanation about why your hospital and your managed care plan (if you belong to one), in agreement with your doctor, believe that your inpatient hospital services should end on ____/_____/_____. This is based on Medicare coverage policies listed below and your medical condition.

This is not an official Medicare decision. The decision on your appeal will come from your Quality Improvement Organization (QIO).

Medicare Coverage Policies:

_____Medicare does not cover inpatient hospital services that are not medically necessary or could be safely furnished in another setting. (Refer to 42 Code of Federal Regulations, 411.15 (g) and (k)).

_____Medicare Managed Care policies, if applicable: (insert specific managed care policies)

_____ Other _____{insert other applicable policies}_____

Specific information about your current medical condition:

▶ If you would like a copy of the documents sent to the QIO, or copies of the specific policies or criteria used to make this decision, please call {insert hospital and/or plan telephone number:

▶ Telephone Number: _____

According to the Paperwork Reduction Act of 1995, no persons are required to respond to a collection of information unless it displays a valid OMB control number. The valid OMB control number for this information collection is 0938-1019. The time required to complete this information collection is estimated to average 60 minutes per response, including the time to review instructions, search existing data resources, gather the data needed, and complete and review the information collection. If you have comments concerning the accuracy of the time estimate(s) or suggestions for improving this form, please write to: CMS, 7500 Security Boulevard, Attn: PRA Reports Clearance Officer, Mail Stop C4-26-05, Baltimore, Maryland 21244-1850. CMS 10066 (approved 5/2007)

Adapted from CMC <annual System, Pub 100-04 Medicare Claims Processing. Available online at http://www.cms.hhs.gov/Transmittals/downloads/R1257CP.pdf

that are potentially not covered during a hospital stay even if the hospital stay is covered. For example, this notice is issued in the event the physician ordered a diagnostic or therapeutic procedure or service that is not part of the care of the condition for which the patient is admitted to hospital. In this case the procedure cannot be bundled into payment or treatment for the diagnosis that justifies the inpatient stay. HINN 11 certifies the patient's consent to accept financial liability for the noncovered procedure.

3. The HINN 12, Notice for Noncovered Continued Stay, is used to notify patients that the hospital believes Medicare may not pay for their continued stay in the hospital beginning on a certain date. The notice would include the estimated cost of the continued stay.

4. The Notice of Hospital Requested Review (NHRR) is used when a hospital requests a

QIO review for a discharge decision when the attending physician does not concur with the hospital's opinion that the patient is ready for discharge. NHRR notifies patients that the hospital has requested a medical opinion from the QIO because it had determined that the patient's condition no longer meets Medicare criteria for continued hospital stay; that is, the hospital stay is no longer medically necessary but the physician disagrees. This notice alerts patients that the QIO may contact them and that the QIO will be reviewing the facts and determine whether there is a need for continued stay.

▶ LEVELS OF CARE

Interpretations vary about what constitutes skilled, subacute, intermediate, or custodial levels of care, causing confusion that at times extends to reimbursement issues. A definition of skilled care in one SNF may constitute the subacute level in another facility. Hospice benefits are interpreted differently among hospice companies. Home health may be provided by one agency, whereas another agency may feel the care is too technical. Appropriate assessment of a patient's needs is essential and may provide clues to the case manager as to whether insurance will pay for the planned level of care. These definitions and criteria may vary from facility to facility, so clarification may be needed. For explanation purposes, this chapter separates the levels of care into two phases: acute and subacute care.

I. Acute care. This level includes:
   a. Acute care hospitals.
   b. Inpatient acute rehabilitation hospitals.
   c. All services within these hospitals (such as emergency department care).
II. Postacute care. This includes the following services:
   a. SNFs (freestanding and hospital-based).
   b. Hospice (freestanding and hospital-based).
   c. Rehabilitation units (freestanding and hospital-based) that are not considered acute.
   d. Home health agencies.
   e. Specialty pharmacy providers.

Within the two phases, various types of services can be provided; there are no definite lines separating the real care of patients. This is why case management that focuses on the patient rather than on the level of care provides the greatest benefits. A home health patient may require acute care; an acute care patient may require hospice care; or an LTC patient may require

hospitalization, custodial care, or home health and assisted living. However, a basic understanding of what constitutes custodial care, intermediate care, skilled nursing care, and LTC are important when matching a patient to a potential next level of care; it is also imperative to understand these levels when dealing with reimbursement issues. It is essential to understand health insurance coverage of various medical levels of care; however, many insurance plans have their own customized rendition of what is covered or excluded. Some coverage is disappointing, whereas other coverage may be surprisingly generous. Medicare insurance criteria have been used as an example in most cases in this chapter for the following three reasons:

1. Medicare is the largest supplier of medical coverage in the United States.
2. Medicare criteria are often used as a basis for private coverage.
3. Medicare reimbursement changes usually precede reimbursement changes in other health plans (See "The Incentives of Change" below).

Medicare coverage rules are usually taken from the traditional form of Medicare. The managed Medicare plans provide wide variations in their coverage. At all times, obtain verification of coverage and authorization for services; all insurance plans have their own rules for coverage.

NOTE

All insurance plans have their own rules for coverage. At all times obtain verification of coverage and authorization for services because:
▶ The insurance coverage may not have the specific benefit that the case manager, multidisciplinary team, or patient requests.
▶ The insurance coverage may not be adequate to cover the medical needs of the patient.
▶ A patient may have already exhausted, or partially exhausted, the needed benefit(s).

▶ Custodial Care

Custodial care may also be referred to as personal care, supervisory care, or assisted living. Group homes and foster homes may also be included at this level of care. The CMS definition of custodial care is care that is primarily for the purpose of helping patients with their personal care needs such as ADLs; this care could safely and reasonably be supplied by persons without professional skills or training. Examples include helping patients get out of bed, eating, and bathing.

Custodial care requires the least skilled personnel of all the levels of extended care. We have never had an insurance company pay for a patient who needed only custodial care (LTC patients may be an exception). The rule of thumb for Medicare and most insurance companies is as follows:

- ▶ If custodial care is the only kind of care needed, Medicare will not pay.
- ▶ If skilled care is required, custodial care can be included in the services.

This level of care is generally characterized by patients who can:

- ▶ Ambulate independently with or without assistive devices such as walkers, wheelchairs, or canes.
- ▶ Transfer from the bed to a chair or toilet with standby assistance.
- ▶ Accomplish ADLs such as eating, dressing, grooming, or bathing with only minimal assistance. Food preparation may be needed.
- ▶ Be considered continent of bowel and bladder although may require minimal assistance in caring for indwelling urinary catheters or colostomy appliances.
- ▶ Take own medications with general staff monitoring; no sliding scale or adjusted dosages.
- ▶ Able to interact socially. These patients may have intermittent episodes of confusion, impaired judgment, or agitation but do not require restraints to control behavior.

Sometimes home health nursing and an assisted living arrangement can be provided if, for example, an otherwise custodial care patient needs help only with sliding scale insulin or PT. Call the home's main caretaker or owner. Many of these patients are considered family in their group homes, and the staff will work with the case manager in discharge planning.

▶ Intermediate Care

The patient needing intermediate care requires moderate assistance with ADLs and restorative nursing supervision for some activities. These persons are not as independent as those classified under custodial care, and in some facilities the distinction between the two levels of care is blurred. Health insurance companies usually do not pay for this level of care unless skilled care is also required. The intermediate level of care is generally characterized by a patient who:

- ▶ Needs no more than one staff person for transferring from a bed to a chair or toilet.
- ▶ Needs assistance with ambulation but can self-propel a wheelchair.
- ▶ Requires a moderate amount of assistance in bathing, grooming, eating, and dressing.
- ▶ May need restraints.
- ▶ Has routine medications and treatments that can be provided for with general staff monitoring.
- ▶ May be intermittently incontinent of bowel or bladder and may need help with an indwelling Foley catheter or colostomy.
- ▶ Can socially interact but may have periods of confusion, agitation, or emotional outbursts that can be controlled with moderate staff intervention.

▶ Skilled Nursing

In some SNFs, the delineation between skilled nursing care and subacute care is one of progressing complexity of the patient's medical and functional needs. This level of care is considered the most intensive in the SNF system. Patients may require maximum assistance with ADLs, may be totally incontinent of bowel and bladder, and may be disoriented, confused, combative, or even obtunded. Yet these characteristics alone will not qualify a patient for health insurance coverage. For an insurance company to pay for care at a SNF level, a need from a skilled licensed professional provided on a daily basis and the assessment that this care must take place at the SNF level for reasons of patient safety and economy are also required. The skilled services below represent some services covered under many insurance plans. A patient with injections, more frequent or complex dressing changes, or more invasive tubes may be considered to need subacute rather than skilled care.

Even if a patient is medically stable, SNFs may not be able to provide the level of care needed (due to staffing restraints) if the care is too complex. A transitional hospital should be considered in these complex cases.

Skilled nursing services may include (but are not limited to):

- ▶ Daily injections: intravenous fluids, intravenous medications, intramuscular injections, subcutaneous injections (such as sliding scale insulin or heparin).
- ▶ Daily wound care requiring aseptic technique.
- ▶ Tube feedings or tube care: nasogastric tube, duodenostomy tube, gastrostomy tube,

jejunostomy tube, tracheostomy care (initial teaching and care).

▶ Frequent observation and assessment by licensed personnel to prevent deterioration of the patient's condition or complications; this change would require prompt nursing response.

▶ Treatment of decubitus ulcers (severity of grade 3 or worse) or severe skin conditions.

▶ Initial phases of a regimen that involves administration of medical gases such as bronchodilator therapy.

▶ Early postoperative care and teaching for colostomies, ileostomies, Hickman catheters, and other tubes.

▶ PT and possibly adjunctive ST or OT.

▶ Teaching a newly diagnosed diabetic patient about diet, sliding scale insulin injections, and foot care.

▶ LONG-TERM CARE

The expression *long-term care* used to be synonymous with nursing home placement. This is no longer the case; chronically impaired people who are dependent on others to care for them can be found in homes, foster homes, day care centers, and a variety of other institutional and noninstitutional settings.

There is no single regulatory definition of LTC, but most emphasize the dependence and chronicity of the patient. In general, LTC is targeted at persons with functional disabilities that may present as a physical or mental problem. The goal of LTC is to promote or maintain as much independence and quality of life as possible. If the patient is terminally ill, the goal is to maintain comfort and dignity. A broad spectrum of services is provided, depending on the unique needs of the individual and family. Private LTC coverage is available, and the number of individual LTC policies grew exponentially in the 1990s. It is rarely financed with company insurance policies, and the consumer must usually pay for the entire, somewhat expensive premium (Kongstvedt, 2003). State coffers provide LTC to persons who can pass the strict medical and financial requirements. Consider the changing demographics of the United States: chronically ill patients are living longer and the number of elderly people and younger people with chronic diseases such as end-stage renal disease (ESRD) is increasing. These factors are making a significant impact on the LTC budget. With the advent of aging baby boomers, this trend is likely to continue. This is also why LTC policies are being sold in increasing numbers.

Candidates qualifying under the definition of LTC generally fall into one of two groups: (1) those requiring complex care and extensive convalescence, such as a major trauma victim, and (2) those with chronic and multiple medical, mental health, and social problems who are unable to care for themselves (Williams & Torrens, 1993). Some patients with diagnoses such as severe mental retardation, cerebral palsy, or spastic quadriplegia fall into the chronic category. They live in group homes where all of their needs are met. If these patients need hospitalization, insurance authorization is not usually required to return them to that facility. In many cases, LTC patients have fairly stable discharge dispositions. There is no inherent limit to the number of medical or custodial resources that a LTC patient can consume.

Many patients have acute medical insurance and short-term extended care benefits. The case manager needs to see beyond these benefits and assess the need for LTC. Even if the patient meets the strict state requirements, the process to qualify for state LTC coverage can take up to 90 days; again, early assessment and planning can avoid future problems.

▶ ACUTE CARE

Acute care services are self-explanatory, with the exception of various rehabilitation services and transitional hospitals, which are explained in more detail below.

▶ Rehabilitation Services

Rehabilitation services, PT, OT, and ST can be provided at various levels of care depending on the patient's functional ability and support system. Home PT/OT/ST can be provided on an intermittent basis. For daily rehabilitation needs, a SNF level may be required. Inpatient acute rehabilitation facilities generally require that the patient can tolerate 3 hours of combined rehabilitative services daily and follow at least one- to two-step commands. Transitional hospitals can take patients at any level of rehabilitation needed and can generally move them within the hospital structure to the appropriate therapies.

A trauma or stroke patient in an acute hospital often requires an inpatient rehabilitation consultant. If the patient is said to be at "too high a level" for inpatient rehabilitation, it means that he or she does not require the intense focus of this level of care. An SNF level or even home care with home therapy services may be more appropriate. If the patient is said to be at "too low a level" for inpatient rehabilitation, it may mean that the patient cannot follow commands or cannot yet tolerate 3 hours of intense rehabilitation. Again, a SNF level may be more appropriate, with the hope and intention of the patient improving enough to graduate to an inpatient facility.

Again, health insurance coverage is the key in most cases. Some companies cover their members at varying degrees of dysfunction in the different rehabilitative levels.

There is a Medicare exception to the 3 hours of rehabilitation daily. If the patient has a complicating condition that prevents him or her from participating for 3 hours, but inpatient rehabilitation is the only reasonable means by which even a low-intensity rehabilitation program can be safely carried out, it may be authorized. Documentation must support the claim.

❱ Inpatient Rehabilitation Centers

Inpatient rehabilitation care is covered under many major insurance plans, but strict criteria must be met because this is a cost-intensive setting. The criteria listed below follow reimbursement guidelines under Medicare. As in any discharge plan, consult the patient's insurance coverage or request that the rehabilitation hospital/unit of the patient's choice look into coverage. Most admission departments can let the case manager know about coverage within 24 hours of a request. It is also beneficial to contact the insurance-based case manager or other representatives and discuss the patient's situation. Some insurance plans use stricter guidelines than the Medicare criteria. If the provider-based case manager and rehabilitation physician feel strongly that the patient is an excellent rehabilitation candidate but the insurance company is reluctant to cover services, try negotiation. Sometimes a short stay can be agreed on, with frequent monitoring of the patient's progress toward self-care.

INSURANCE CRITERIA

Four main categories of criteria reflect Medicare requirements for authorization in an inpatient rehabilitation facility. Other insurance companies may use the same general criteria.

1. Admitting diagnosis must include at least one of the following conditions:
   ❱ Amputation.
   ❱ Arthritis.
   ❱ Cardiac conditions.
   ❱ Chronic pain.
   ❱ Congenital disorder.
   ❱ Cerebral vascular accident (CVA).
   ❱ Diabetes mellitus.
   ❱ Fracture.
   ❱ Head trauma/brain injury.
   ❱ Multiple trauma.
   ❱ Musculoskeletal disorder.
   ❱ Neurologic disorder.

❱ Orthopedic condition.
❱ Pulmonary condition.
❱ Spinal cord injury.

2. The primary problem must include a recent functional loss, whereas before the illness or accident, the patient was independent in that function. There also must be dependence on the assistance of another person to carry out that function. Some functional categories include the following:
   ❱ Bladder dysfunction—incontinence, use of external catheter.
   ❱ Bowel dysfunction—incontinence, maintenance of an excretory pattern.
   ❱ Communication—major receptive or expressive aphasia.
   ❱ Cognitive dysfunction—change in patient's attention span, memory, or intelligence.
   ❱ Medical monitoring—patient's medical status requiring intensive medical monitoring or nursing attention at least once daily because of a cardiovascular, gastrointestinal, urologic, endocrine, or neurologic disorder. This is in addition to the primary diagnosis as stated in number 1 above.
   ❱ Medical safety—patient either exhibits or is at risk for secondary complications such as decubitus ulcers, contractures, urinary tract infections, or major spasticity.
   ❱ Mobility dysfunction—patient must learn safe transfers to chair/bed/toilet/shower, walking (usually with appliances), negotiating stairs, wheelchairs, and so on.
   ❱ Pain control—pain severely prohibits active motion or functional use.
   ❱ Personal safety—the patient is physically unsafe alone.
   ❱ Self-care activities—ADLs must be renegotiated, such as feeding, drinking, dressing, grooming, brace and prosthesis care, bathing, toileting, and perineal care.
3. The physician must document the expectation of significant improvement in functional ability within a reasonable time frame.
4. If a patient was previously in a rehabilitative program with an unsuccessful outcome, this patient must have some change in condition or circumstances that would indicate that progress is now possible; otherwise, he or she will not be eligible.

Other important criteria for admission to an inpatient rehabilitation unit include medical stability, mental ability to follow one- to two-step commands, and ability to withstand at least 3 hours of therapies daily and five times per week. The 3 hours can consist of any combination of PT, OT, and ST.

A patient may be discharged from a rehabilitation unit for several reasons, including:

▶ The stated goals of rehabilitation have all been met.
▶ There has been no progress toward stated goals after an adequate trial (usually 1 week without any appreciable headway).
▶ A severe complication develops necessitating a transfer to acute care.
▶ A complication develops that inhibits the multidisciplinary approach for more than 1 week. In this case, it is sometimes necessary and reasonable to transfer the patient to a SNF level of care until the rehabilitation treatment modalities can be reinstated.

▶ Transitional Hospitals

Although uncommon today, it is still important for the case manager to be aware of them and understand their characteristics. Transitional hospitals are acute care hospitals for medically stable patients with long rehabilitative needs and care that is too complex for SNFs to handle/meet.

These hospitals usually have a lower price structure than traditional acute care hospitals, mainly because fewer specialists are on staff and the facilities contain only basic diagnostic or surgical equipment. They usually do not have expensive and sophisticated equipment such as computed tomography (CT) scanners or magnetic resonance imaging (MRI), but do have the basics such as x-ray capabilities. Major surgeries are not done on site, but surgical procedures such as surgical feeding tube placement or tracheostomies can be performed. Registered nurse staffing is reported to be the same as at other acute care hospitals; that is, it is dependent on the patients' acuity levels and care needs.

These hospitals can handle patients just below the intensive care unit (ICU) level with multiple complex medication regimens and treatments, which may include:

▶ Ventilator-dependent patients, including weaning patients.
▶ Use of total parenteral nutrition (TPN) or hyperalimentation.
▶ Extensive wound care.
▶ Infectious disease management.
▶ Intravenous medication therapies.
▶ Burn care.

▶ All rehabilitative modalities (OT/PT/ST).
▶ Hemodialysis patients.
▶ Prehospice patients—pain control therapies.
▶ Coma recovery, cognitive rehabilitation, neurobehavioral rehabilitation.
▶ Most other treatments that can be done at other acute hospitals or levels of care.

In the early-1990s, one patient with AIDS also developed Guillain-Barré syndrome and became ventilator-dependent for many months. It took almost 1 month to obtain placement in a SNF that handled ventilators because of the long waiting periods. A Gallup poll in 1991 revealed that there was an average waiting period of 35 days between the time that a chronic ventilator-dependent patient could be discharged and the availability of an appropriate bed (Anonymous, 1991). It now takes less time to place a complex patient in an SNF.

If a patient's condition is very complex but "too low a level" for inpatient rehabilitation, transitional hospitals should be considered. For example, a patient came in for a coronary catheterization, suffered a stroke and a cardiac arrest during the procedure, and required a tracheostomy. Eventually, this patient was weaned from the ventilator. She was alert and oriented but too weak to tolerate intensive rehabilitation modalities. She also required more frequent tracheal suctioning than SNFs can usually handle. The transitional hospital further stabilized the respiratory function and strengthened her. Later this woman was placed in an inpatient rehabilitation unit, where she did very well.

▶ POSTACUTE CARE
▶ Definitions of Subacute Care

Subacute care fills in the gap between acute hospitalization and LTC. Patients who are eligible for subacute care may also require intense care. However, they do not require the complex diagnostic work-ups and are considered medically stable with a fairly constant treatment plan. Sometimes the term *postacute care* is used; this includes all levels of care below acute hospitalization, including home healthcare. Subacute care has received an enormous amount of attention as a cost-saving level of care, yet few will agree on what it is or even where it is. The delivery of care may be in either inpatient settings (as in the definitions below) or outpatient settings. Some feel subacute care is a transitional phase between the acute stage and the rehabilitation stage, or a service that fills the gap between acute care and skilled home care (Table 5.1). TJC and the Commission on Accreditation of Rehabilitation Facilities (CARF) have developed subacute accreditation standards for inpatient facilities.

TJC (2008, Glossary) has defined subacute care as:

Care that is rendered immediately after, or instead of, acute hospitalization to treat one or more specific, active, complex medical conditions or to administer one or more technically complex treatments in the context of an individual's underlying long-term conditions and overall situation.

The National Association of Subacute/Postacute Care (NASPAC) emphasizes the following definition:

Subacute care is a comprehensive, cost-effective inpatient level of care for patients who:

▶ have had an acute event from injury, illness, or exacerbation of a disease process.
▶ have a determined course of treatment.
▶ though stable, require diagnostics or invasive procedures, but not intensive procedures requiring an acute level of care (NASPAC, 2009).

The severity of the patient's condition requires:

▶ active physician direction with frequent on-site visits.
▶ professional nursing care.
▶ significant ancillary services.
▶ an outcomes-focused interdisciplinary approach utilizing a professional team.
▶ complex medical and/or rehabilitation care (NASPAC, 2009).

The American Health Care Association (AHCA), a national organization representing nursing and residential care facilities, defines subacute care as:

A comprehensive inpatient program designed for the individual who has had an acute event as a result of illness, injury, or exacerbation of a disease process; has a determined course of treatment; and does not require intensive diagnostic and/or invasive procedures.

The severity of an individual's condition requires an outcome focused interdisciplinary approach utilizing a professional team to deliver complex clinical intervention (medical and/or rehabilitation). These highly specialized programs promote quality care by utilizing health care resources efficiently and effectively.

Subacute care requires the coordinated services of a multidisciplinary team of care providers such as a physician, case manager, nurse, physical therapist, occupational therapist, social worker, and others. It is generally more intensive than traditional care provided in a SNF and less intensive than care provided in an acute care/hospital setting. Moreover, it requires frequent patient assessments that could vary from daily to weekly depending on the condition being treated. In addition, it involves a review of the clinical course of treatment and plan for care for the time period until the condition being treated is stabilized or the predetermined treatment course is completed (TJC, 2008). Integral to the provision of care in a subacute care facility TJC identified seven characteristics that are described in Display 5-3.

There are four general categories of subacute patients classified based on their projected length of stay and intensity of service (Newell, 1996).

1. **Transitional subacute.** The estimated length of stay is 3 to 30 days. The intensity of rehabilitation and/or nursing care is 5 to 8 hours per day. These patients' conditions are rather intense, such as those requiring chemotherapy, postsurgical interventions, and intravenous antibiotics. The care can be rendered in a hospital-based or a freestanding SNF.
2. **General subacute.** The estimated length of stay is 10 to 40 days. The intensity of rehabilitation and/or nursing care is 3 to 5 hours per day. A stroke patient may require this level of care. Care can be rendered in a freestanding SNF.
3. **Chronic subacute.** The estimated length of stay is 60 to 90 days. The intensity of rehabilitation and/or nursing care is 3 to 5 hours per day. These patients may have intensive but chronic conditions, such as a stable ventilator patient or one with a medical plus a cognitive deficit such as Alzheimer's disease and a total hip replacement. These facilities will require careful choice; not all skilled care environments are staffed for this level of care.
4. **Long-term transitional subacute.** The estimated length of stay is 25 days or more. The intensity of rehabilitation and/or nursing care is 6 to 9 hours per day. It is most likely that this type of subacute care will end in placing the patient in an LTC facility. Here the care is more intensive than LTC as patients may be developmentally impaired with head trauma or birth defects.

Subacute rehabilitation services can be divided into three general categories according to Carr (2000). These are:

1. Short-term rehabilitation for patients with significant medical and nursing needs but too ill to tolerate rigorous rehabilitation therapy in an acute care setting. These patients also require high use of PT, OT, and ST services. Common medical problems include orthopedics such as

▶ **TABLE 5.1** Subacute Levels of Care

LEVELS OF CARE	SUBACUTE AND REHABILITATION	SKILLED NURSING	INTERMEDIATE CARE	ASSISTED LIVING/ CUSTODIAL CARE
Medical stability	Can be complex and unstable; requires ongoing monitoring by RNs; complex care for multi-medical problems may be provided	Can be complex and generally stable; requires skilled nursing observation and modification of care plan to prevent further deterioration	Client medically stable; intermittent nursing and medical services needed to maintain medical stability	Client medically stable
Injections	Complex IV therapy regimen; multiple IV medications requiring infusion pumps	IV push therapy; simple IV therapy; central line care	IM and SC injections	No IV, IM, SC injections; may retain home health nurses to provide these services
Medication regimen	Complex medication regimen due to unstable conditions; at least five medication changes per week by the attending physician may be required to meet this level of care	Medication regimen requiring some adjustments in dosages or frequency of medication; done through observation and assessment of vital signs or laboratory data	Administration of routine medication; RN or LPN monitoring may be necessary with occasional dose or frequency changes when ordered by attending physician	Stable regimen of oral medications; home health nurses may be hired to monitor more complex medications such as sliding scale insulin
Respiratory treatments	Some facilities care for patients on respirators. including frequent suction and SVN PRN treatments	May have oxygen, SVN treatments, inhaler therapies	Routine oxygen administration and a stable respiratory therapy regimen	May have home oxygen, simple oxygen, simple inhalers
Suctioning	Frequent (more than every 4 hours) tracheal suctioning allowed; new tracheostomy care	Nonsterile suctioning or intermittent sterile suctioning	Simple, routine nonsterile suctioning	No suctioning
Invasive tube care	Can handle complex tube care including tracheostomy tube, gastrostomy tubes, ijejunostomy tubes, ileostomies, colostomies, indwelling tubes, T tubes, catheters; may include irrigation, monitoring, replacement PRN, site care, and self-care instructions	Same as subacute, but patient and care must be fairly stable; patients at this level with several types of tubes not accepted at some facilities	Routine maintenance and care of uncomplicated catheters, tubes, ostomies; may do intermittent irrigations	Empty drainage tubes and do simple, routine care (more complex care may require intermittent home health nursing visits)
Wound care/ dressings	Complex treatments and wound care; Criteria: treatment over 20 minutes, performed by RN level nurse, 2 or more times per 8-hour shift	Will perform complex, sterile, and frequent dressing changes or wound cases needing close monitoring (wounds can be infected and acute)	Will perform routine care for non-infected, chronic wounds and skin conditions	May perform simple care such as salves and simple dry dressing; may call in a home health RN for further care
Rehabilitation	Usually require minimum of two therapies (physical, occupational, or speech) and patient's ability to tolerate at least 3 hours of therapy daily	Rehabilitation therapy needed on a daily basis and performed by a licensed therapist	May be supervised by a licensed therapist (restorative nursing); may include assistance with ambulation. range of motion, positioning, and so on	Not a safe level of care if patient requires rehabilitation, unless home health is involved in non-complex case

▶ **TABLE 5.1 Subacute Levels of Care** (*Continued*)

LEVELS OF CARE	SUBACUTE AND REHABILITATION	SKILLED NURSING	INTERMEDIATE CARE	ASSISTED LIVING/ CUSTODIAL CARE
Mobility	Requires complex assistance from licensed personnel	Usually requires assistance of more than one person in mobility, transfers to chair, bed, toilet, or bath; unable to help very much in these activities; assistive devices may be used	Patient possibly able to participate in mobility and transfers to chair, bed, toilet. or bath; assistive devices may or may not be needed	Often allows wheelchair-bound clients, but must be independent in getting to and from bathroom and eating areas and independent in getting in and out of bed
Patient education	Teaching needs identified and taught by licensed professional staff; administration of medications, self-care of tubes, wounds, use of equipment is taught on ongoing basis in preparation for discharge to a lesser level of care	Teaching needs identified and taught by licensed professional staff; administration of medications, self-care of tubes, wounds, use of equipment, and other needs taught on an ongoing basis in preparation for discharge to a lesser level of care	Simple teaching done by nonlicensed professionals but under the supervision of licensed staff; may teach basic ADL support, feeding techniques, use of assistive devices, and so on	No teaching skills at this level of care; home health nurses may be retained if needed
Nutrition	Can accommodate TPN, IV fluids, use of infusion pumps, tube feedings with residual checks	TPN and IV fluids accommodated at some facilities; tube feeding with or without infusion pump and maximum assistance with oral feeding accommodated	Requires some assistance with self-feeding	Most require client to be able to get to dining room and feed self
Personal hygiene and toileting	Can accommodate total care of personal hygiene and toileting including disimpaction when needed and perineal care	Can accommodate total care of personal hygiene and toileting, including disimpaction when needed and perineal care	Assists with toileting, perineal care, bathing, and grooming	Most require client to be continent; some accept indwelling catheters and assist with dressing and grooming efforts
Behavioral/ mental		May be confused, disoriented, combative; may need physical or chemical restraints for safety of patient or others; patients with active, serious psychological disorders are not legally allowed at this level of care in many states	May be intermittently confused or disoriented, requiring staff intervention and possibly restraints for protective purposes; patients with active, serious psychological disorders not legally allowed at this level of care in many states	May be slightly forgetful; not a safe level of care for confused, disoriented clients

ADL, activities of daily living; *IM*, intramuscular; *PRN*, as needed; *SC*, subcutaneous; *SVN*, small volume nebulizer; *TPN*, total parenteral nutrition.

display 5-3

CHARACTERISTICS OF THE PROVISION OF SUBACUTE CARE ACCORDING TO THE JOINT COMMISSION

1. Time: Care is rendered immediately after, or instead of, an acute care hospital stay.

2. Reason: Treatment of one or more specific, active, complex, or unusual medical conditions or administration of one or more technically complex treatments in the context of the patient's underlying long-term conditions and overall situation.

3. Caregivers: Requirement of the services of an interdisciplinary team of healthcare professionals who are trained and knowledgeable in the assessment and management of the specific conditions and performance of the necessary procedures.

4. Site: Care is provided in an inpatient setting.

5. Frequency: Care requires frequent patient assessment and review of the clinical course and treatment plan.

6. Intensity: Care is provided at a level that is generally more intensive than a traditional SNF/nursing home and less intensive than that provided in an acute inpatient care unit/hospital.

7. Duration: Care may last for a limited time or until a condition is stabilized or a predetermined treatment course is completed (e.g., intravenous antibiotics course). Time period may vary from several days to several months depending on the course of treatment and patient's progress.

Adapted from The Joint Commission. (2008). *Comprehensive accreditation manual for hospitals.* Oakbrook Terrace, Ill: Joint Commission Resources.

total hip or knee replacements and neurology such as stroke, brain, or spinal cord injury.

2. Short-term rehabilitation for patients with complex medical conditions. These patients require intense medical and nursing management. These patients require high use of respiratory, laboratory, and pharmacy services as well as medical supplies. Common medical problems include cardiology, oncology, pulmonary, dialysis, complex wounds, intravenous fluid therapy, and parenteral nutrition.

3. Long-term or chronic rehabilitation for patients who have experienced extended acute care stays, are medically stable but have relatively high nursing needs and ancillary services. Common medical conditions include head injuries, coma, multiple trauma, and mechanical ventilation dependency.

▶ Skilled Nursing Facilities

SNFs offer a level of care below acute hospitalization, in which the patient still requires ongoing skilled care from licensed personnel (e.g., nurses, social workers, OT, PT, ST) on a daily basis. Other names include nursing home (NH), nursing home placement (NHP), intermediate care facility (ICF), or extended care facility (ECF).

The use of acronyms is fine for medical personnel, but it is best to use the entire term when talking to patients or their families. We sometimes use the term "extended care facility" and explain that this is an extension of the hospital care the patient is now receiving but at a less intense pace. We do not like using the term "nursing home" or "convalescent center." These terms often bring up unfavorable images or frightening memories of neglect or of loved ones dying.

Most communities have books listing their SNFs, along with names, addresses, and telephone numbers. Other information such as ratings, level of care offered, and Medicare certification is usually provided. Not all facilities provide the same levels of care or even quality of care. It is worth a visit to these sites for a thorough understanding of the level of skilled care each one can provide. These visits can be real eye openers. We learned about a SNF in which a licensed nurse was on duty only from 6:00 AM until 10 PM; the case manager, therefore, could not send to that facility anyone with even a "to keep open (TKO)" intravenous line, in case it needed attention at 2:00 AM. However, this SNF had a good PT department; if that was the patient's sole need, this facility would be a good match.

Keep the following factors in mind when choosing a SNF:

▶ Does the facility's skill level meet the assessed needs of the patient?

▶ Will the patient/family agree to this facility? Is it an acceptable location for visiting purposes?

▶ Does the patient's primary physician go to this facility? If not, would the physician prefer another SNF that is also acceptable to the patient/family? Perhaps the physician, family, and patient would agree to have another physician follow up on the patient while at the SNF of choice.

▶ Is the chosen SNF a contracted facility with the payor?

▶ Will the services that the patient needs be covered at the SNF level of care by the payor?

INSURANCE CRITERIA

Traditional Medicare patients (those reimbursed under the DRG system) may enter a SNF level of care when certain criteria have been met:

▶ The patient must be in the hospital for 3 consecutive days. (This criterion is not required for the Medicare Advantage Plans); refer to section on the 3-Midnight Rule below for more information.

▶ The 3-day stay must have been medically necessary;

▶ The SNF reason for admission must also be congruent with the reason the patient was in the hospital; or

▶ Posthospital SNF placement may take place within 30 days of hospital discharge. The 3-day rule applies.

The 3-day hospital stay is for an inpatient status only; patients admitted under observation status do not qualify. If it appears that the patient will need SNF placement and meets acute inpatient medical criteria, ask the physician for an order to change the patient to inpatient status.

In addition, Medicare and other insurance plans also mandate the following criteria before a patient can be admitted to a SNF:

▶ The medical condition requires daily, skilled services of a licensed professional.

▶ Those services cannot be provided at a lesser level of care or it would be impractical, uneconomical, or inefficient to do so.

▶ The care provided must be based on physician orders.

COVERAGE OPTIONS

The following SNF coverage options are specifically for Medicare-reimbursed patients, but many insurance companies have the same or similar provisions. Major SNF services covered under Medicare Parts A and B include:

▶ A semiprivate room.

▶ Meals, which may include special diets.

▶ Nursing services.

▶ PT, OT, and ST.

▶ Blood transfusions (nonreplacement fees may be required).

▶ All medications furnished by the SNF during the admission and prescribed by the attending physician.

▶ Medical supplies such as splints, casts, and dressings.

▶ Use of durable medical equipment (DME) such as walkers or wheelchairs.

Some SNF services not covered by Medicare include:

▶ Personal convenience items such as televisions and telephones (not all SNFs provide them unless the patient requests them and rents them).

▶ Private duty nurses.

▶ The extra charge necessary for a private room, unless the private room is deemed to be medically necessary.

▶ Hospice

Hospice programs began in Great Britain many decades ago. The concept reached the United States in the 1970s and has recently gained much respect and popularity. The philosophy of hospice is that terminally ill patients should be allowed to maintain their final days of life comfortably, with respect and dignity. Ideally, these last days take place at home with family and loved ones present, if desired. Hospice may be the plan of care of choice when nothing further can be done medically for the patient, the patient and family agree that death is imminent, and the patient and family want only palliative and comfort measures taken, not aggressive curative measures. Hospice does not hasten or postpone death but allows nature to take its course. The hospice philosophy reminds case managers that this dying person is a living person.

Often families and medical staff are confused about the difference in services between home health services and hospice. Although hospice is similar to home health services in many ways, it differs in some important aspects. Following are some differences between Medicare home health coverage and Medicare hospice coverage services as the standard guideline. Be aware that insurance companies other than Medicare may or may not include hospice benefits; if they do have the hospice benefit, they may include different covered services.

In 1995, a new revision was added to the Medicare hospice regulations. It states that "A discharge planning evaluation must include an evaluation of a patient's likely need for appropriate post-hospital services, including hospice services and the availability of those services" (Hamilton & Thomsen, 1998).

Payment for hospice services under Medicare is based on four levels of care. Depending on the intensity of services, the per diem rate is adjusted. The four levels include the following (Hamilton & Thomsen, 1998):

1. Routine home care;
2. Continuous home care (24 hours in a crisis situation);
3. Inpatient respite care (not to exceed 5 consecutive days at a time); or
4. General inpatient care (for pain control or other symptom management that would be difficult to control in lesser settings).

COMPARISON BETWEEN HOSPICE COVERAGE AND HOME HEALTH COVERAGE

▸ *Skilled nursing services are provided on an intermittent basis.* Both home health and hospice provide this, but hospice covers these services on a 24-hour, 7-day-a-week, on-call basis.
▸ *Nonskilled services.* Most home health agencies do not provide nonskilled nursing services because they are rarely covered under insurance agreements. Nurse aides may be covered under Medicare for two to three 1-hour visits per week for personal care, but only under strict criteria. Hospice can provide 12 to 16 hours of personal aides per week if needed, including some homemaker services.
▸ *Physician services.* Both home health and hospice care must be under the guidance of an ordering physician.
▸ *Bereavement services and counseling (including spiritual counseling).* This is perhaps the most important distinction between home health services and hospice services. Bereavement and counseling services are often offered to the family for several months after the death of the patient. More importantly, if hospice is called in early enough, these trained persons help to prepare the family for the impending death, often averting shock and crisis situations.
▸ *Social services and volunteers.* With hospice, social service personnel and volunteers are part of the multidisciplinary staff. Home health agencies are allowed very limited social service attention at home.
▸ *Homebound requirement.* Under home health criteria, the patient must be homebound or must need to undergo an unusual hardship to get care through outpatient facilities. Although terminal hospice patients are often homebound, this is not a mandatory requirement for hospice care.

▸ *Prescription drugs for symptom management and pain control.* Traditional Medicare rarely pays for prescription medications at home (exceptions are noted in "Medicare" in Chapter 3). Under the hospice benefit, prescription medications to manage symptoms and control pain are covered. There is a 5% or $5 charge toward each prescription, whichever is less.
▸ *DME and home oxygen.* Medicare has strict criteria for many types of DME including oxygen (see home oxygen criteria in "Home Care Services"). Hospice guidelines for various types of DME are more lax and can be provided for the comfort of the patient.
▸ *Respite care.* This is not a covered service under home health. With hospice, limited respite care in a SNF allows the family to take care of needed business or take a break so that they do not get overwhelmed with the extensive care that most terminal patients require. The respite is limited to 5 consecutive days per benefit quarter.
▸ *Physical, occupational, and speech-language therapy.* These therapies are carried out for the purpose of symptom control or to allow the patient to maintain basic ADL function. Both home health and hospice benefits cover this service.
▸ *Continuous care during periods of medical crisis.* Only hospice carries this benefit. For some families, continuous care during this period is the key benefit that allows the patient to die at home with dignity.
▸ *Deductibles.* There are no deductibles under the hospice benefit.

MEDICARE HOSPICE CRITERIA

The hospice benefit may be used by a Medicare beneficiary if all three criteria are met:

1. A physician certifies that the patient is terminally ill.
2. The patient (or family) chooses to use the hospice benefit.
3. The hospice agency is Medicare certified.

If these three criteria are met and the patient is in the hospital, a physician order for hospice will be needed. After a call is made to refer this patient to hospice, a representative will come to the hospital, meet the patient and family, and answer questions. A hospice referral can also be made while a patient is at home, but also with the above criteria.

Although a patient chooses to forego standard Medicare benefits in lieu of hospice benefits, standard benefits begin if treatment for a problem unrelated to the hospice condition is needed. For example, if a patient with terminal AIDS falls and breaks a leg, then the necessary care for this accident will be paid for by standard Medicare.

HOSPICE BENEFIT PERIODS

Special benefit periods apply to the hospice portion of Medicare. When a patient opts for the hospice benefit, the benefit periods define the extent of his or her coverage (see "Medicare" in Chapter 3 for standard Medicare benefit periods). Part A will pay for two 90-day benefit periods and unlimited 60-day benefit periods. Extension periods of indefinite duration protect the patient in case of long terminal stages of illness (Hamilton & Thomsen, 1998).

Patients can choose to cancel hospice and return to Medicare benefits or vice versa as long as there are remaining benefit periods; when someone cancels the hospice benefit, the remaining days in the benefit period are lost. If any benefit periods remain, they may still return to hospice and use those remaining periods.

MYTHS AND REALITIES

Perhaps because hospice is so similar to home health or because it is simply misunderstood, myths about hospice abound. These are some myths that are commonly heard from patients and families.

Myth: Hospice is only for terminal cancer patients.

Reality: Hospice is for any terminal condition: chronic obstructive pulmonary disease (COPD), AIDS, cystic fibrosis, and any end-stage disease (cardiac, liver, renal, Alzheimer's disease to name a few terminal conditions).

Myth: The patient must have only 6 months to live.

Reality: Although in general the prognosis for life expectancy should be in months rather than years, it is often difficult to say for certain how long a patient will live. Unfortunately, this misunderstanding has caused healthcare teams to wait until the last minute before calling in hospice, thereby losing valuable time in which patients and families could be receiving care and counseling that could improve the quality of the remaining time. Also, remember that Medicare allows 210 days (two benefit periods of 90 days and one benefit period of 30 days), which equals 7 months; add to that the indefinite extension. This is fact enough that demise is not "required" in 6 months.

Myth: A 24-hour caregiver is required.

Reality: This one requires careful assessment. We know some patients who had been admitted to hospice who were still independent, although this is rare. Others do well with the 12 to 16 hours of assistance provided. If a patient is terminal, is dependent on others, and does not have a strong support system, then a SNF for terminal care (under Medicare Part A) may be a better choice.

Myth: Nursing home patients cannot receive hospice care.

Reality: Medicare does not pay for the room and board of a SNF under the hospice benefit. However, if the family can fund the room and board or the patient's private insurance policy covers this, as some do, then hospice can be used at the SNF level of care. The bereavement and counseling portion of hospice can then be used; it is an important part of terminal care.

Myth: To be accepted into hospice, all further medical treatment must be forfeited.

Reality: The important distinction here is whether the care is for aggressive, curative purposes or for palliative, comfort means. Radiation therapy has been used for palliation treatment. If someone may have several months to live and cannot tolerate food or tube feedings, total parenteral nutrition has been authorized. The main question to ask is why the care is being given. Hospice patients in distress are readmitted into the hospital; often they are stabilized and sent back home with hospice again. Conditions not related to the hospice condition are treated under Medicare Part A. However, if a patient wants to try chemotherapy with the hope of a cure, he or she will have to leave the hospice benefit period and opt for standard Medicare benefits.

PALLIATIVE CARE

One cannot discuss hospice care without addressing palliative care; it is more frequent today to have a patient consider palliative care long before hospice care. Palliative care can be delivered concurrently with life-prolonging measures and may begin at the time a life-threatening and debilitating illness is diagnosed. Similar to hospice, palliative care is an interdisciplinary approach to care delivery with the main focus of relief of suffering and improvement in the patients' quality of life. Both hospice and palliative care address the physical, intellectual, emotional, social, and spiritual needs of patients and their families.

The five goals of palliative care are:

1. Pain control and management.
2. Sharing of appropriate information with the patient and family, especially that which is essential for informed decision making regarding treatment options.
3. Coordination and facilitation of care activities, especially during transitions from one care setting to another or one provider of care to another.

4. Preparation of the patients and their families for dignified death.
5. Provision of bereavement support to patients and families.

Palliative care is provided in all care settings, including acute care hospitals, rehabilitation facilities, SNFs, outpatient clinics, home, assisted living facilities, and others. Care is provided at two levels: primary and specialized. The primary level refers to the provision of palliative care and services by the same multidisciplinary team responsible for the management of the patient's medical condition. The specialized level refers to palliative care and services provided by a multidisciplinary care team trained, specialized, and credentialed in palliative care.

▶ Home Care Services

Most patients who were living independently before the present episode of illness prefer to return to their own homes. Perhaps they are not completely independent or back to their baseline, but have family support for basic needs. Sometimes home care services provide the vital link to a patient's independence. A thorough social and medical assessment can evaluate the safety of a home health plan. For example, if the patient is a debilitated 94-year-old who lives with her daughter, the daughter also needs to be assessed to see if she can still safely care for her mother (the daughter will likely be in her seventies).

Home health agencies are public or private organizations that specialize in providing both skilled and nonskilled services in a patient's home. This line of service is not new, and several agencies have already celebrated their centennial. Changes in the way that America is delivering healthcare are having a significant effect on the home healthcare industry. There is an increase in patients being sent home, necessitating more nurses. Patients have more medical needs than ever before, requiring clinically and technically astute nurses with developed critical thinking skills and advanced practice degrees (Gookin, 1994). More patients are being sent home on weekends and late in the day, necessitating staff that is available and flexible (Gookin, 1994).

Perhaps the most far-reaching change is occurring because of the Medicare risk contracts or Medicare Advantage Plans. Although this chapter discusses the criteria requirements of the traditional Medicare model, these risk contracts are touching all areas of healthcare, including home health agencies. As more members choose the Medicare HMOs, more hospitals, physician groups, and home health agencies are agreeing to capitation as a means of reimbursement (Gookin, 1994) (see Chapter 3: Reimbursement Concepts for further discussion on capitation). Although this puts home health agencies at some risk, it has some advantages over the traditional Medicare model.

INSURANCE CRITERIA

In the traditional Medicare model, both Part A and Part B cover home health services. Home health visits are authorized only if all of the following five criteria are met:

1. The patient is homebound, which means that he or she is confined to the home or that it would be a great hardship to come to an outpatient facility for treatments.
2. The care required includes intermittent (not necessarily daily, as in the SNF criteria) skilled nursing services and possibly physical, occupational, and speech therapies. These services should be offered on a part-time basis.
3. The care and services must be reasonable and necessary; that is, must be needed based on the patient's health condition and appropriate for provision in the home environment.
4. The patient is under the care of a licensed physician who has set up a home health plan of care and oversees it. The plan is reasonable and necessary and is reviewed at least every 60 days.
5. The home health agency is Medicare certified, which means that the strictest federal standards are met.

INSURANCE COVERAGE

It is doubtful whether this basic criteria set will change. However, the following covered and noncovered services should also be considered. Under the traditional Medicare model, covered home services (if the above criteria are met) include those in the following discussion.

PART-TIME OR INTERMITTENT SKILLED NURSING CARE.   This may include up to 8 hours of reasonable and necessary care per day for up to 21 consecutive days (more, under some circumstances). Few cases are allotted 8 hours per day, and the key phrase is "reasonable and necessary." Most patients who need 8 hours of skilled nursing care are not in the home environment. Occasionally, this does happen. For the most part, stress to your patients that an average home visit from an RN lasts 45 minutes to 1 hour, not 8 hours, and that the services must be skilled.

PHYSICAL OR SPEECH THERAPY. PT and ST may be added if skilled nursing services have been assessed and they are deemed reasonable and necessary. This also opens the gate for OT and home health aide services.

HOME HEALTH AIDE SERVICES. If skilled nursing services have been assessed as necessary and physical or speech therapies have also been deemed necessary, the patient may qualify for intermittent home health aide services. Aide visits occur two to three times per week to help with personal care such as bathing, grooming, and changing linen. Home health aide services are rarely covered under private health insurance plans; check your patient's coverage for the exception.

HOME SOCIAL SERVICES. If skilled nursing services have been assessed, the patient may qualify for home social services. This is at times more effective than a social worker seeing the patient in an acute or subacute facility. The patient is seen and assessed in his or her own environment, and this often elicits a more realistic appraisal of the social situation.

MEDICAL SUPPLIES. Supplies, such as dressings, will be made available if needed by the RN for the patient's care.

NOTE

Skilled Services: Healthcare services that require delivery by a licensed professional such as a registered nurse, a physical therapist, occupational therapist, respiratory therapist, social worker, speech therapist. Examples include wound care, vital signs assessment, health education, psychosocial counseling, catheter care, physical rehabilitation, and intravenous medication administration.

Nonskilled Services: healthcare services that can be provided by a paraprofessional or an unlicensed person such as a home aide. Examples include close observation, bathing, feeding, and transferring from bed to chair.

Custodial Care: Care provided to patients to assist them in meeting the activities of daily living such as bathing and feeding. It also includes the services of a homemaker or housekeeper who can assist a patient in cleaning his or her home, food/meal preparation, or complete grocery shopping.

This is a term sometimes used interchangeably with nonskilled care.

Respite Care: Care provided in an inpatient setting such as a hospital or a SNF for the purpose of offering the patient's usual care giver (family member, friend, or another relative) the opportunity to get some rest. This type of care is common in the case of hospice patients.

DURABLE MEDICAL EQUIPMENT. This equipment must be approved, because not all equipment is covered (Display 5-4). The amount a beneficiary pays for equipment varies based on type of equipment needed. A beneficiary is expected to pay an annual deductible of $131 for Medicare Part B services and supplies before Medicare begins to pay its share. After exhausting the deductible, a beneficiary may still be responsible for 20% coinsurance. For Medicare to cover DME, any needed equipment must be purchased from a Medicare participating supplier. *DME* or *home medical equipment* (HME) are terms that are used for a wide variety of products, services, and equipment. They are often classified into four general groups:

1. Basic mobility aids such as walkers, canes, and crutches.
2. Assistive devices to increase independence for ADLs, such as bathroom equipment (shower chairs, hand rails), kitchen equipment, ostomy supplies, or wound care supplies.
3. Mobility aids such as wheelchairs or electric beds.
4. High-technology equipment such as ventilators, intravenous pumps, parenteral and enteral nutrition, continuous chemotherapy infusion machines, apnea/sleep monitors, and technology that is custom-designed for quadriplegia/paraplegia/rehabilitation patients.

If a patient is in the hospital or other facility and DME is ordered, CMS will allow 2 days before discharge for delivery of the equipment if the purpose of the delivery is to teach the patient how to use the equipment properly; the DME must also be for subsequent use in the patient's home. In the past, early delivery sent up red flags to CMS. Case managers should document why the DME was delivered early and also document the related patient/family teaching sessions. On the billing side, no bills must be rendered for the DME before the date of the patient's discharge from the facility to the home; the date of discharge is deemed to be the date of delivery.

LIST OF DURABLE MEDICAL EQUIPMENT/SUPPLIES COVERED BY MEDICARE

Air-fluidized beds

Blood glucose monitoring devices and related supplies

Canes (except for the blind)

Commodes

Crutches

Dialysis machines

Home oxygen equipment and supplies

Hospital beds

Infusion pumps (and some medicines used in infusion pumps if considered reasonable and necessary)

Nebulizers (and some medicines used in nebulizers if considered reasonable and necessary)

Ostomy supplies

Patient lifts (to lift patients from bed to wheelchair by hydraulic operation)

Suction pumps

Therapeutic shoes

Traction equipment

Walkers

Wheelchairs

Wound care supplies

Some DME, such as oxygen, have strict criteria that must be met. The home oxygen criteria are added here because so many patients, such as those with COPD, diffuse interstitial lung disease, cystic fibrosis, bronchiectasis, or widespread lung cancer, need it for comfort and survival. (If the patient is admitted into hospice, the oxygen guidelines are not as strict.)

To qualify for home oxygen:

1. Arterial blood gases must be drawn on room air (see exception below):
   a. The PO_2 must be 55 or below or with an arterial saturation of 88% or below, or
   b. If the PO_2 is between 56 and 59 mmHg or the arterial saturation is 89% or below, there must also be evidence of one of the following: dependent edema suggesting congestive heart failure; or P pulmonale on electrocardiogram (ECG) (P wave above 3 mm); or erythrocythemia with a hematocrit over 56%.
2. If the PO_2 is between 56 and 59 mmHg or the arterial saturation is 89%, the patient must be retested between the 61st and 90th day of oxygen therapy. A renewal prescription with the qualifying test result will be required in the fourth month for further home oxygen coverage.
3. The physician's documentation must indicate that the patient has severe lung disease and is not getting enough oxygen, and that using oxygen might improve the patient's condition. It also must indicate that using other alternative measures have failed.

Under newer guidelines, the physician must document the applicable diagnosis codes or ICD-9s; physicians previously had a simpler checklist form.

Also, testing of the arterial blood gas or saturation must be performed while the patient is in a "chronic stable state" or within 2 days of discharge. If a patient requires greater than 4 L/min of oxygen, the blood gas must be performed at 4 L/min; if both blood gases and saturation tests are performed, the blood gas results must be used.

Medicare helps pay for the system used to furnish oxygen to the patient, including containers that store oxygen, tubing and related supplies used for the delivery of oxygen, and oxygen contents. A beneficiary is responsible for 20% coinsurance of the Medicare approved amount. Case managers must be aware, however, that Medicare does not cover portable oxygen whether it is used only during sleep or as a back up to a stationary system.

HOME MEDICATIONS. Some intravenous antibiotics, and other select medications, are now offered by Medicare in the home setting (see "Medicare" in Chapter 3 for further discussion).

PSYCHOLOGICAL NURSE ASSISTANCE UNDER SPECIFIC CRITERIA. This service may be needed by mental and behavioral health patients or for social support and counseling for patients immediately post discharge from a hospital stay.

SERVICES NOT COVERED. Services that are not covered under traditional Medicare in the home setting include the following:

▶ General homemaker services such as shopping, cleaning, laundry, and meal preparation.
▶ Standby services such as 24-hour nurse or nurse aide care at home so the patient will not be left alone.

▶ Blood transfusions.
▶ Medications—except when specifically authorized; for example, medications used in a nebulizer and known to be medically necessary.

These strict criteria have been somewhat lifted with the Medicare Advantage Plans. They provide more freedom to choose and use whatever services best meet the patient's healthcare needs and the plan's financial needs. These Medicare plans act more like independent HMOs or even some Medicaid plans; criteria such as a 3-day hospitalization being required before a patient can be placed in a SNF or intravenous antibiotics not being provided for in the home setting no longer makes any fiscal sense.

The previous regulations and limitations on Medicare patients are being lifted with Medicare Advantage Plans. The contracts allow "in lieu of" services. This means, for example, that if a patient could be discharged sooner from the hospital if he or she had, in addition to skilled nursing services, some personal care and provisions for meals, the home health agency has flexibility to do this. The hospital (which may also be capitated on these plans) may choose to reimburse the home health agency for these services in lieu of an extended hospitalization. This allowance of services is carefully monitored. Many studies have been developed to see if Medicare Advantage Plans are providing enough services. These studies have not been conclusive, and although some beneficiaries love the managed plans, others have found them to be inadequate.

Occasionally, the distinction between skilled services and nonskilled services becomes blurred. Essentially a skilled service is one that is performed by a licensed professional such as a registered nurse, physical therapist, respiratory therapist, occupational therapist, or speech therapist. The care given must be for the purpose of patient safety or medical stability. Table 5.2 shows some examples of skilled care and nonskilled care; these may be appropriately applied in any level of care.

Home health agencies are becoming more sophisticated, and many furnish almost any service that can be provided at the acute care level as long as the patient is medically stable. Even if the patient needs blood products (red blood cells [RBCs], fresh frozen plasma [FFP]), many home health agencies can accommodate such treatment/service; often this requires a 24-hour advance notice. However, emergency transfusions must be handled at a higher level of care. It is helpful to know which agencies can provide specified services. Like SNFs, home health agencies differ in their level of acuity. It is important to secure insurance authorization before calling an agency. Many insurance companies use only specific contracted agencies; calling the correct one at the onset can save a hospital day and a dose of aggravation.

When a case manager evaluates a patient for home health, a balance must be considered between what amount of self-care (with or without family help) can be safely attained and what other options are available from the payors. For example, sending a patient home with infusion services requires careful consideration. The patient or family must have cognitive and motor skills to perform the infusion safely, and motivation must be high to minimize poor compliance (especially in long protocols or ones in which there are uncomfortable side effects). Working with the infusion nurses and the patient is a value-added benefit to the case manager. An infusion nurse may also supply much of the patient education and instruction. Psychosocial issues that may only show up "in person" may be revealed. Ongoing on-site supervision is required with many central intravenous lines and also to keep the patient on track; it is also imperative when any type of drug abuse is suspected.

When making a referral to home health, the case manager must be aware of the patient's insurance benefits, limitations, and the amount of benefits already used. Knowing the insurance coverage used and how much remains will assist the coordination of care by preserving enough benefit for the full term (when possible); some very debilitated patients can take their benefits down to the wire by the end of the fiscal year. Although the home health agency must check these benefits (as they are dependent on payment), the case manager must provide the home health agency with some basic information including the patient's name, age, diagnosis, brief medical history, address, telephone number, insurance identification number, Social Security number (which may be different than the insurance identification number), date of birth, and the service(s) requested.

Some rules about referring patients to home health or other agencies and facilities affect case management. One rule, "Nondiscrimination in Post-Hospital Referral to Home Health Agencies and Other Entities," went into effect in 1997. Based on this rule, some issues that apply include:

▶ If any Medicare-certified agency requests to be put on a hospital's referral list, the hospital must comply. However, case managers must know what clinical expertise the patient may require and which facilities have those capabilities.
▶ The hospital cannot specify or recommend any particular agency to a patient. However, it is within the case management/patient advocate

▶ **TABLE 5.2** **Comparison of Skilled and Nonskilled Services**

SERVICE PROVIDED	SKILLED CARE	UNSKILLED CARE
Vital signs	Takes vital signs; may record and report worrisome vital signs to physician; observes cardiopulmonary stability; teaches caregiver how to take and record vital signs and when to call physician	Takes vital signs; may record and report to appropriate person
Medications	Administers medications, injections, sliding scale insulin, suppositories, eyedrops; teaches families about medication, side effects, what to do for side effects, observation of client's ability to comply with medication prescriptions, perhaps teach to give injections; assesses for negative side effects such as toxic levels	May assist in giving medications by reminding client of times to take them or helping open the lid
Skin care	Teaches diabetic skin and foot care; assesses skin for break-down; performs aseptic wound care that may include packing, wet to dry dressings, dry dressing with sterile technique, irrigations; teaches family wound care; takes wound cultures, reports negative assessment to the physician or any negative change in skin condition; provides care for grade 3 or worse decubitus ulcers	Gives baths; applies lotions, ointments, creams, powders; applies nonsterile dressings; may reinforce dressings; provides treatment for chronic, noninfected surgical wounds and minor skin problems
Diet and nutrition	Instructs in special diets such as a low sodium, diabetic, renal, administer TPN, or tube feedings; instructs in administration of TPN or tube feedings; assesses nutritional status, monitors and teaches fluid restriction or fluid status; teaches and assesses fluid intake and output; replaces some indwelling tubes	Helps prepare meals; assists with feeding
Elimination	Inserts straight catheter or Foley; teaches straight catheterizing procedure; observes and teaches signs of urinary tract infection; bowel or ladder training; provides care, observation, and teaching of new ostomy; assesses and reports skin breakdown	Cleans perineal area; empties drainage bags such as colostomies, indwelling Foley; measures urine; tests urine for sugar and acetone; assists client on and off commode; treats incontinence with diapers or rubber sheets; provides general care of colostomies or ileostomies including assisting in appliance changes in stable ostomy
Respiratory	Teaches and administers medical gases in the initial stages; in tracheostomy clients, suctioning and tracheostomy care; instructs client/family in tracheostomy self-care; observes and reports signs of respiratory distress or infection; administers oxygen; respiratory therapists may make ventilator changes per doctor's orders; provides small volume nebulizer and chest physiotherapy treatments and instruction	Administers medical gases after initial stages; provides small volume nebulizer and chest physiotherapy treatments after initial phase; assists in tracheostomy care of stable tracheostomy patient

▶ **TABLE 5.2** **Comparison of Skilled and Nonskilled Services** (*Continued*)

SERVICE PROVIDED	SKILLED CARE	UNSKILLED CARE
Rehabilitation	Assesses and instructs in use of assistive devices, range of motion exercises, gait training, transfers; administers hot packs, ultrasound treatments, TENS units, whirlpools in compliance with doctor's prescriptions; speech therapist assesses and helps with communication problems and swallowing difficulties	Supervises exercises taught to client; performs passive and active range of motion in conjunction with physical therapist; assists in applying and removing prosthesis; assists with use of canes, walkers, wheelchairs, and Hoyer lifts
Miscellaneous	Assesses any complex set of unskilled needs that requires putting together an overall picture of the patient for that Patient's medical safety	

responsibilities to point out which facilities or agencies are in a patient's preferred network; the patients should also be aware that they can choose outside their network, although the costs to them will likely be higher.

▶ If there are any financial interests, the hospital must make that clear on the referral lists.

Compliance with the above rules is necessary for all Medicare-certified facilities. Therefore, documentation of these conversations is important. Some hospitals have entered their referral lists—including home health agencies, DME companies, hospices, SNFs, transportation companies, emergency response centers (Lifeline), hemodialysis centers, and nutrition programs—into laptop computers or hand-held devices; some even include maps, Medicare-specific qualifications, addresses, telephone numbers, and the clinical abilities of each company. Having such tools in place makes it easier for case managers to share such information with the patient and family; the tools allow easy access to such information at the point of care/patient's bedside and enhance consistency in the approach to discharge planning. Documentation should demonstrate which options were discussed, the physician or ordering provider recommendations, which agencies/facilities are financially related to the parent hospital, and the patient/family response to the choices.

▶ Specialty Pharmacy Providers

Case managers are constantly looking for new ways to assist patients in maintaining the quality of their lives. One way to do that is to expedite as much personal independence as possible. In recent years, specialty pharmacy providers have been a case manager's ally in meeting this goal. Pharmacy management is often complex and requires round-the-clock expertise when anxious patients perceive something is wrong or unsure about how/when to administer a medication. A quality specialty pharmacy provider will enhance the case managers' clinical and financial expertise; trained professional pharmacists, nurses, and reimbursement experts add to the case manager's pool of resources when seeking the best alternative to high-cost, specialty biotherapy treatment.

Specialty staff provides teaching about medications as well as ongoing monitoring and evaluating of the patient's pharmacy needs. The additional clinical support enhances other case/disease management goals in patients receiving injectable medications:

▶ Increases patient compliance with recommended therapy.
▶ Increases patient education.
▶ Reduces the potential for patient errors in dosing.
▶ Decreases caregiver and patient anxiety.
▶ Reduces the overall cost of delivery.
▶ May assist the case management organization/department in the collection of medication-related data.

The case manager will find working with these professionals to be of major assistance, but he or she should first make sure that the use of this level of provider is part of the patient's health benefits/insurance plan or can be negotiated. When a case manager makes a referral to a specialty pharmacy provider, the following sequence commences. The physician's office calls or faxes the patient's prescription to the company. The company's intake nurse calls the patient to explain the program and provide education on the medication, self-injection, side effects, and potential drug interactions.

Because this is often provided "long distance," a visit or two from a home health agency may be needed for hands-on teaching about the medication and the self-injection. All deliveries in prefilled syringes are made to the patient's home. Following the initial prescription delivery, the patient is routinely contacted by a patient care coordinator who:

▶ Assesses patient compliance and progress.
▶ Inquires regarding the side effects from the medication.
▶ Arranges the next scheduled delivery.
▶ Verifies the shipping address.
▶ Refers the patient to the clinical staff for any clinical questions.

The company's pharmacists and nurses are available for on-going consultation with the patient, physician, and case manager 24 hours a day. This service has been very successful with long protocols of 12 to 18 months of medications with annoying side effects, and it has appeared to increase compliance. These providers have stringent quality programs. The pharmacies used should be those accredited through TJC.

▶ MEDICARE EXTENDED CARE BENEFIT: THE 3-MIDNIGHT RULE

Within the Medicare list of benefits for beneficiaries is the "extended care benefit" commonly referred to as the 3-Midnight Rule or 3-Day Rule. This benefit means that fee-for-service Medicare beneficiaries are entitled to the extended care benefit only if they have been in an acute inpatient care setting (i.e., hospital) for 3 consecutive calendar days. The days are counted based on the number of times a patient appears on the hospital's midnight census. The 3-Midnight Rule applies only to patients who need posthospital skilled services in a SNF. Such patients tend to require extended care from an acute care stay. The 3-Midnight Rule does not apply to patients whose postacute care stay requires services from a home healthcare agency, or can be transferred to a LTC facility for posthospital rehabilitation (Birmingham, 2008).

The decision of the 3-Midnight Rule was made in the late 1960s based on a national review of care patterns of Medicare patients. This review revealed that patients usually are in an acute care setting for 3 days on average before a discharge plan, including the identification of posthospital services needed, is developed. Although this review is very old, it is currently statutorily mandated and the requirement stands. Case managers must be careful about this rule and ensure

compliance when they develop the discharge plans for their patients (Birmingham, 2008). The 3-Midnight/3-Day Rule is described in 42 CFR, §409.30 of the Social Security Act:

> A claim for extended care benefits generally qualifies for Medicare reimbursement only if the admission to SNF level of care is preceded by an inpatient hospital stay of at least three consecutive calendar days, not counting the date of discharge, and is within 30 calendar days after the date of discharge from a hospital.

In addition to the 3-Midnight Rule to qualify for a SNF admission, a patient must require "daily therapy." This means that the patient must receive skilled nursing services, skilled rehabilitation services, or a combination of both on a 7 days-a-week basis. In the event a patient whose care in a SNF is based solely on the need for skilled rehabilitation rather than skilled nursing services or both, he or she would meet the "daily basis" criteria when he or she receives the skilled rehabilitation services for at least 5 days a week. If the rehabilitation therapy services are provided less than 5 days a week, the "daily" requirement would not be met and the patient would not qualify for the extended care benefit (Birmingham, 2008).

It is important for case managers to track the number of days a patient is in the acute care setting before they finalize a patient's discharge plan to a SNF. For example, if a patient was transferred from another acute care facility where he or she has spent 1 day, this day counts in the new facility toward the 3-Day Rule extended care benefit. In contrast, however, if a patient spends time in the emergency department or at an observation level of care (i.e., "observation status") prior to an admission to a hospital, the time spent in these levels does not count toward the 3-Day Rule even though the patient is in an acute care setting. Another area that is of importance for case managers when deciding whether a patient meets the 3-Day Rule is examining the patient's previous acute care stays; perhaps the most recent discharge from a hospital setting occurred less than 30 days prior to the current admission.

▶ THE INCENTIVES OF CHANGE
▶ Prospective Payment Systems

The Balanced Budget Act (BBA) of 1997 has created new reimbursement rules for postacute services. All postacute services that are reimbursed through Medicare have changed, from the cost-based system to the PPS. These include home healthcare, SNFs, rehabilitation facilities, subacute care facilities and outpatient services/ambulatory care. At this time, there are no plans to limit beneficiaries of the traditional Medicare health plan to panels of contracted providers; however, the Medicare Advantage Plans still use managed care strategies.

Methods of Medicare reimbursement have often been the forerunner of reimbursement changes in other insurance arenas; therefore, it is important for the case manager to see what is changing and formulate strategies to assist patients to secure needed resources. In addition to the changes that occurred in the home health, rehabilitation, ambulatory care, and SNF sectors, case managers must also be well aware of the definition of a hospital discharge for top 10 diagnoses (see "The Discharge/Transfer Rule—The Top 10 DRGs" in this chapter). In domino fashion, this change will affect case management plans through the continuum.

NOTE

Reimbursement in a Box

▶ *Cost-based reimbursement* is based on the actual costs of a patient's care.
▶ *PPS/DRG* is a method of payment to providers at a pre-established rate, regardless of the providers' actual costs.
▶ *Per diem reimbursement* is a fixed daily rate based on the acuity of the patients.

PPS, DRGs, and per diem rates motivate agencies and facilities to practice patient care under various incentives. It is the incentive behind the game plan that must be understood for the case manager to truly advocate for the patient.

Per diem rates tailor the reimbursement to the number of days a patient stays in a facility for care; a set price is paid for each day without regard to actual costs incurred. Traditionally, per diem rates encouraged longer stays, up to the use of all possible days, and there was less incentive to discharge a patient home or transfer to another facility for continued care. However, under the recent federal payment structures, this type of thinking is no longer considered a successful strategy. When a facility is paid on a fixed per diem rate, it must make careful choices of admitting patients who clearly require less expensive and lower levels of medical care. Ventilator-dependent patients in SNFs, for example, may be reimbursed as low as $185 per day in some

geographic locations. With this level of reimbursement, keeping a patient in a facility longer will not equate to more dollars. Per diem reimbursement also supports the incentive to use the least amount of resources per day. Cost-efficient care is critical to survival; however, quality of care must also be maintained.

PPS in a subacute level now tailors the payment to the level of the patient's functional status. This is different from the PPS reimbursement method (i.e., DRGs) applied in the acute care setting, which tailors the payment to the diagnosis. When PPS was instituted in the hospital setting in the 1980s, the hospital incentive was discharge of the patient as early as possible, sometimes bordering on premature discharge. The hospital was essentially paid a set amount (i.e., the DRG case rate) for the episode of care; keeping the patient in the hospital cost the facility more money, but no more funds would be reimbursed. This incentive to move the patient to another level of care as quickly as possible caused the proliferation of subacute centers where care could be rendered to still fairly sick patients.

The result was that the subacute sector of healthcare grew at an alarming rate. In 1996 subacute care in the United States cost about $28 billion; today, the number exceeds $55 billion. At this rate of growth, the Medicare funds simply cannot sustain the costs. Something had to be done. The reimbursement changes we have seen or are now seeing are attempts to stay the tide.

Subacute care has basically been paid on the old fee-for-service model. External case managers who must negotiate costs when moving patients down the continuum of care have, on occasion, come up against a situation in which the subacute costs quoted exceeded the ICU or floor costs in the hospital. These are not isolated cases and explain why the PPS system has moved into the postacute arena. From a subacute perspective, this meant a huge change in reimbursement from more than $1,000 per day to perhaps $300 less per day; this is certainly an incentive to be more efficient in providing care.

CMS and Congress felt that these changes would affect two situations:

1. At least for a set of hospital discharge DRGs, described below, incentives for early discharges would be affected. The incentive would change, as the hospital would not have the incentive to discharge/transfer the patients as quickly. In the future, it will be interesting to note if, for these DRGs, more patients go home rather than to SNFs after the hospital because of the few extra days in acute care.
2. It would control costs at the subacute level.

Changes in the reimbursement structure of the home health industry were also destined to happen; the cost of that care has risen dramatically. For example, in 1990, $3 billion was billed for home health services; in 1997 this escalated to $20 billion. In 1998, at least 3.8 million Medicare beneficiaries received some form of home care. The home health fee-for-service reimbursement structure encouraged providers to use as many services and visits as possible. By changing the reimbursement structure to PPS (and including some cap limits), there is no longer an incentive to prolong services; rather, the intelligent choice would be to structure the care for efficient healing and independence of the beneficiary.

Some of this growth was because patients are using home healthcare as a reasonable and correct level of care; some of the cost has become the target of Medicare's fraud and abuse examinations. It is estimated in some areas of the country that 40% of payments made by Medicare for home health services were improper. Consider that the original intent of Medicare home health benefits was short-term assistance. As many case managers are aware, traditional Medicare patients have received home health for much longer than originally intended. This is not always inappropriate, and those patients may suffer.

Were the reimbursement changes necessary or unfair? Critics of the new reimbursement structure feel that there are many inequities in the home health reimbursement fee schedule. One major complaint is that the reimbursement is based on very old data, a time when patients were not sent home as medically intensive as they are today. Some home health agencies and SNFs (whose per diems are based on old data as well) are feeling the impact to such a degree that they may not survive. However, the changes had to happen; the healthcare funds could no longer sustain the growth. Through governmental agencies, healthcare providers will be observed for fraud and abuse. Underneath it all, CMS is looking for the right incentives: to promote access to care and to provide quality care—the same incentives as case managers. One thing is clear: case management is being mentioned time and again as a critical piece to balance the incentives, control costs, and assure quality and safe patient care.

▶ The Postacute Discharge/Transfer Rule—The Transfer DRGs

CMS became concerned with the lessening of lengths of stay over the years. The DRG-based payment system was originally formulated on reimbursement for a Medicare length of stay that was approximately 40%

higher than was experienced in 1998. The tremendous numbers of transfers to the subacute arena did not go unnoticed. As an outgrowth of the Balanced Budget Act of 1997, and beginning in October 1998, there were 10 DRGs that would no longer be considered a discharge from an acute care setting and an admission to a postacute setting (i.e., rehabilitation facility, SNF, or home healthcare); rather, they were labeled Transfer DRGs. CMS would reimburse hospitals for patients that fell into one of these DRGs under a "post-acute care transfer payment policy."

The original Transfer DRGs were chosen because of their high volume of use in postacute transfers and included strokes, amputations for circulation disorders, skin grafts, hip procedures, and tracheostomies. This ruling also included "swing beds," which was not a popular rule with the American Hospital Association (AHA). The Transfer DRGs at the time accounted for about 30% of the Medicare patients, each representing between 2% and 6% of the total Medicare volume. The number of Transfer DRGs has increased over time; there were 29 Transfer DRGs in Fiscal Year (FY) 2004; 182 by October 1, 2005; and 274 effective October 1, 2007. It is reported that today over 6 million Medicare hospital discharges per year fall into the Transfer DRGs accounting for about 52% of the total Medicare annual discharges.

Patients who fall in one of the Transfer DRGs are considered transfers if:

▶ The patients subsequently receive care in a SNF or a home health agency after discharge from the hospital.
▶ The services are related to the hospitalization.
▶ The services are provided within 3 days of the hospitalization.

From a hospital's fiscal viewpoint, this translates into a situation in which the transfer of any Medicare patient who falls into one of the Transfer DRGs before the "geometric mean day" of the DRG would result in the hospital being penalized. An early transfer patient is one who is discharged more than 1 day sooner than the geometric mean length of stay of patients in that DRG. The hospitals are paid 50% when the patient is admitted; the remaining 50% is divided by the geometric mean length of stay and paid as a per diem. Fiscally sophisticated hospitals analyze the expenditures of the last few days before the geometric mean day to determine if the per diem losses are more—or less—than the actual cost of care. In some cases, it may even be fiscally smarter to transfer sooner (assuming the patient is stable) to a lesser level of care; however, incentives that result in clinically compromising situations would be a poor choice and likely to be noticed. Under PPS, hospitals are given financial incentives to minimize Medicare patients' length of stay; however, these early transfers actually increase Medicare costs because Medicare pays for care in both the acute and postacute settings.

The acute strategies must compliment the needs on the subacute side; with the reimbursement changes at the subacute level, this could pose problems. If lower acuity patients are admitted to SNFs because the hospital kept the patient in acute care until the geometric mean day, their reimbursement level may be less. Networks of acute and subacute providers will be best equipped to work out solutions that are good for everyone. However, it is the case manager, as a patient advocate, who must be aware of any subtle strategies that may not be in the patient's best interests.

Hospital case management can play a huge role in keeping this rule a relatively minor inconvenience. With fraud and abuse monitoring going on at all levels of care, hospitals are being watched for inappropriate transfers to postacute care settings. When a patient is discharged, the hospital may bill under the total DRG rate. When a patient is transferred, the hospital must bill under the per diem rate; if home health or SNF care is ordered, the hospital must bill as a transfer rather than a discharge. This can be a problem because physicians may arrange for SNF placement or home healthcare after a patient is discharged from the hospital. If this happens with these Transfer DRGs, and the hospital bills for the total DRG, it could be considered fraud in the eyes of Medicare. Therefore, hospitals must be aware of orders for postacute services for these patients, even if they are ordered 1 to 3 days after discharge. Case managers are the link between the ordering physician and the proposed care; postacute follow-up care becomes even more essential.

One strategy may be to develop or take a new look at any clinical pathways for these Transfer DRGs. In addition to optimal care, the case manager should also take into consideration the geometric mean day for optimal timing of the transfer to a subacute level of care, such as home health or SNF. An early discharge could lessen the hospital reimbursement. However, an otherwise transferable patient should not be kept in the hospital for fiscal reasons; these are the types of fiscal strategies that CMS is monitoring. If all this sounds like a "between a rock and a hard place" scenario, it may be. Early transfer may be a safe alternative that may fiscally benefit the SNF level of care; it may also penalize the hospital financially. Holding the patient until the geometric mean day will admit a patient to a SNF with less acuity and less SNF reimbursement; it may even

leave the SNF out of the loop if the patient is well enough to go home directly. In those instances, home health agencies may surface as the winners. These are the situations that are destined to twist the already convoluted healthcare system into another curve.

▶ HOME HEALTH CHANGES

Over the past two decades, many changes have taken place in Medicare benefits, especially in the areas of home health and SNF benefits. The cost-based system has been replaced with the PPS, which controls reimbursement to home care agencies; it does not cap the number of visits that a patient can receive or limit the amount of money that can be spent on any one patient. As a result, home health agencies need to look more closely than ever before at what the cost of each patient may be. Admitting practices and policies are likely to change as a result of PPS, and case managers may find that some patients are harder to place in home care than in the past. Case managers need to know how much home health benefit has been used for each patient. For many Medicare beneficiaries, this may entail looking at usage in various states, as many retired people live in different places in the winter and summer (such people are called "snowbirds" in Arizona and Florida). A critical eye on quality of care is more important than ever, as is choice of agency. Just as there are various levels of clinical efficiency within the SNF level of care, home health agencies may start to become more expert in some areas and with certain types of patients than before.

▶ Specific Benefit Changes
VENIPUNCTURE

In the past, any Medicare beneficiary who qualified for home blood draws (venipunctures) was automatically considered eligible for an extensive selection of home services. A new venipuncture plan closes what CMS felt was an expensive loophole. Home blood draws are still a covered item. However, two issues have been addressed: (1) the blood draws are provided by a laboratory technician rather than a home health nurse (unless there are no laboratories in rural areas), and (2) laboratory draws are no longer an automatic trigger that allows all other home care services to be initiated. Any homebound Medicare patient who requires home blood draws will receive them; any homebound Medicare patient who requires blood draws and other home healthcare services will not be denied those benefits. For example, an 82-year-old man was confined to bed after hip surgery. He also suffered from severe rheumatoid arthritis and was status-post stroke. He was eligible for home venipuncture, home PT, and probably some home aide services.

DIABETIC SUPPLIES

Effective July 1998, Medicare coverage for glucose monitors and testing strips expanded. All diabetics now qualify for glucose monitoring devices, strips, lancet devices, lancets, glucose control solutions for checking the accuracy of the test strips, and monitors. This applies, regardless of insulin intake, if a Medicare patient's diabetes would be better controlled through testing blood sugar. However, a 20% coinsurance applies on all diabetes supplies. The patient should ask his or her physician to write a prescription, which should state how often the blood sugar is to be tested; this will indicate how many test strips will be dispensed. Medicare covers the quantity of test strips ordered.

▶ What to Do If You Are an External Case Manager

- ▶ Remember that the physician is the key decision maker. It is ultimately the physician who will assess the patient and determine whether the patient's care is still medically necessary and therefore may still qualify for home healthcare.
- ▶ Be realistic. Some benefits have been generously provided for in the past; with new reimbursement, companies will have to be managing more comprehensively if they are to survive. Personal care services may be one area that will be monitored closely by home health agencies.
- ▶ Keep current about Medicare reimbursement and benefit changes. This knowledge is needed if you are to strategize about how best to meet the needs of your patients.
- ▶ If the patient/family or another case manager calls with home health concerns, reassess the medical condition to evaluate the appropriate level of services. If you feel that the home healthcare that has been ordered remains medically necessary, detail the orders again and document them carefully in the medical record.

▶ What to Do If You Are Employed in a Home Health Agency

- ▶ Educate employees about the new changes in benefits and reimbursement. They must understand reimbursement challenges to help plan for care and services in a way that is beneficial for all parties. Assist employees with

ways to handle beneficiary questions about changes in services. Social workers, trained in role-playing, can be valuable for this function. Emphasize that the patients and families may be traumatized by the impending changes. This may be especially true for fee-for-service beneficiaries who have been receiving ample services; they have a point of comparison and may not like the cutbacks.

- ▶ Use proven strategies to provide quality services in a cost-efficient manner. These may include the use of:
  a. Case management (strongly recognized in the literature as an important strategy).
  b. Clinical pathways/case management plans, especially those that cross levels of care.
  c. Disease management strategies.
  d. Protocols, guidelines, and care plans.
  e. Coordination of care across multiple providers and settings (those involved in the care of a patient or settings being considered for continued care).
- ▶ Monitor provider behavior. It may appear to be an intelligent strategy to only admit low-cost beneficiaries (i.e., "cherry picking") and discharge patients quickly. These strategies present their own challenges, legally and ethically. Overextending services to non-Medicare patients may also lead to negative consequences.
- ▶ Determine new strategies to cope with consolidated billing rules. This may include partnering/contracting with other service providers or using staff strategies such as outsourcing (see "Consolidated Billing" later in this chapter).
- ▶ Use proven case management strategies for quality, cost-efficient patient care. This includes providing the appropriate number of visits, duration of visits, skill level of caregiver, and appropriate use of DME and supplies.
- ▶ Focus on the patient.

▶ SKILLED NURSING FACILITY CHANGES
▶ Reimbursement Changes

Since the 1980s, Medicare has reimbursed the SNF level of care on a cost-based system. Essentially, this meant that SNFs would bill for the costs of care plus a mark-up; this left little incentive to control costs. The old fee-for-service has now been changed, and traditional Medicare is looking more like managed care.

Reimbursement today is based on a PPS method. No one is really sure exactly how it will all play out, except that this level of care (SNFs) will reveal the greatest growth in case management use. There are three reasons for this:

1. SNFs are reimbursed by PPS. CMS will be monitoring for changes in quality of care that potentially accompany the reimbursement changes. Like hospitals that have experienced PPS, SNFs require the skills of case managers to ensure quality of care for the residents while containing costs.
2. The demographics are changing; baby boomers are aging (more demand for SNFs).
3. Life expectancy is increasing (more demand for SNFs). The elderly population today also suffers from increasingly complex health conditions that require higher intensity of healthcare resources.

SNF survival requires some significant changes in the way it does business. Unlike the diagnosis-based DRGs that are used to reimburse acute care (hospitals), resource utilization groups (RUGs) base their SNF payments on the use of resources. The RUGs will adjust the federal rate calculated for SNF reimbursement. The payments will be on a per diem basis and will include routine care, rehabilitation, and other ancillary costs (e.g., laboratory tests, radiographs, medications, etc.). To understand the intensity of the reimbursement issues, consider that in urban areas the most intensive RUGs category will reimburse less than $400 per day; the least intensive RUGs category will reimburse less than $120 per day. The Minimum Data Set (MDS) assessment determines the resource utilization, which in turn determines the per diem reimbursement rate in SNFs.

The MDS 2.0 consists of 109 items; originally the MDS was more of a care plan and clinical assessment than a billing mechanism (CMS, 2009). The assessment established by the MDS 2.0 determines under which of the 44 RUGs a patient will be classified. The RUGs group then sets the prospective per diem rate that each SNF will be paid by Medicare for treating a particular patient. The RUGs III are based on:

▸ A hierarchy of seven major resident types;
▸ The resident's (i.e., the patient's) functionality; and
▸ The intensity of services or additional problems or services.

Resident functionality is measured through ADLs that are calculated based on the assessment in the MDS 2.0; assessment includes functional levels such as bed mobility, transfers, toilet use, and eating (parenteral versus intravenous versus tube feeds). All RUGs III categories are classified using an ADL score; this score can range from 4 to 18, depending on the response to the MDS 2.0 questions. The RUGs III score is not only important on admission to the SNF; the prior activity of the patient may also affect the RUGs rate. The patient may fall under the extensive care category if:

▸ The patient received intravenous or parenteral feeding in the past 7 days, or
▸ The patient received intravenous medication, suctioning, tracheostomy care, or ventilator treatment in the past 14 days.

In effect, the SNF would receive "credit" for prior services rendered to this patient. This is why an on-site preadmission screening by the case manager is so important before admission to the SNF. Although the SNF will have an assessment period, it will still be advantageous to know as much about the patient as possible before admission. This task will certainly require a case manager with the skills of Sherlock Holmes and one who has a reputation with the SNFs of being a trusted professional. Any information used to place a patient in a particular RUGs III category must have adequate back-up documentation both in the SNF and before the SNF admission (7- to 14-day activity). This preadmission screening will be a valuable tool to assess if the patient is deemed skilled by Medicare's standards. Accepting a patient into a SNF with misinformation could cost the facility financially and have painful consequences for the patient and family. The case manager must carefully review all pertinent information and make decisions involving the multidisciplinary care required.

The MDS assessments must be done accurately and on time. Penalties in the form of the lowest default rates are imposed for late assessments; there are no exceptions. When a Medicare beneficiary enters the nursing home for the first time:

▸ A comprehensive, multidisciplinary assessment must be completed by the 5th or 14th day (this day can be chosen by the SNF).
▸ A 5-day assessment must have an assessment reference date of any day between day 1 and 8 (and must be completed by day 14).
▸ A 14-day assessment is required with an assessment reference date that may be as early as day 11 or as late as day 19, because there is a 5-day grace period.
▸ Other assessments are due on days 30, 60, and 90.

▶ PT, OT, ST, AND RESPIRATORY THERAPY CHANGES

In FY 1995, CMS data showed that in SNFs, almost 50% of the charges are for room and board; 30% are for rehabilitation services. In light of these data, many changes have been made under PPS in the rehabilitation services area. PPS reimbursements mandate that the whole rehabilitation service area looks at the way it delivers care. The RUGs III categories include reimbursement for the minutes of therapy delivered directly to the patient. The time required to perform an initial evaluation, develop treatment goals, and create the plan of care for the patient cannot be counted as minutes of therapy received by the patient. Because actual minutes of therapy delivered directly to the patient are so important for the RUGs III level, many therapists have been told to carry stopwatches. Inaccuracy of minutes could result in a lower RUGs III level, which could equate to $30 per day in lost reimbursement for a 1-minute difference. Rounding off the minutes or poor documentation will be a red flag for reviewers. The two highest therapy levels are:

- ▶ Ultra high level: a minimum of 720 minutes of therapy per week.
- ▶ Very high level: a minimum of 500 minutes of therapy per week.

The RUGs III classification pays for minutes of therapy and is not tied to who delivers the therapy. Therefore, as a strategy to optimize reimbursement and reduce labor costs, many SNFs will use "therapy extenders" such as PT assistants or rehabilitation aides. These staff members must be supervised by a licensed or certified individual. Another strategy will be the use of group therapy sessions. This will enhance the ability to deliver many minutes of therapy to patients while only using one staff person. However, Medicare mandates that only four residents per therapist session, and no more than 25% of the patient's total therapy minutes, can be spent in group therapy.

▶ Reimbursement Changes

Beginning in January 1999, Medicare imposed an annual financial cap on outpatient PT, OT, and ST covered under Part B. One potential problem that could arise is if a patient received therapies from unknown sources and the present agency submits a bill in excess of the cap. This is another important reason for case management continuity; a case manager who knows the total expenditures of his or her patient is invaluable. This knowledge is expected for many external case management positions; these case managers must keep track of the amount of benefits the patients have and the amount of benefits that have been exhausted. Can the claims payors help determine how much the patient has used in therapies? Sometimes. However, if the claim has not yet been submitted (and billing may be months behind), then the total expenditures will be incomplete. Sometimes an accurate guesstimate must be made on the total; this may involve going to the individual billing departments of the agencies the patient used for therapies (or other services or DME).

Medicare helps pay for medically necessary outpatient OT, PT, and ST services when the physician or therapist sets up the plan of treatment and the physician periodically reviews the plan to see how a patient is progressing and for how long the therapy will be needed. These services may be obtained from a Medicare participating outpatient provider such as a hospital-based clinic, home health agency, or comprehensive outpatient rehabilitation facility. In private practice settings, Medicare pays for OT and PT services but not for services given by a speech-language pathologist. In these settings and services, the beneficiary remains responsible for 20% coinsurance.

Respiratory therapy is another area that is scrutinized under PPS. Before January 1999, respiratory therapy was a reimbursable service provided to clinically appropriate patients. Medicare would pay a licensed respiratory therapist for the assessment, evaluation, care plan, and respiratory treatments of the patient. In the newer structure, respiratory therapy is included in the per diem rate. The RUGs III grouping takes respiratory therapy into consideration in the three nonrehabilitation groups: extensive services, special care, and clinically complex patients. The MDS 2.0 qualifies respiratory therapy as coughing and deep breathing, "heat nebulizers," aerosol treatments, and mechanical ventilation. These treatments must be provided by a qualified professional; however, it no longer has to be a licensed respiratory therapist. As a result, nurses are being required to perform the respiratory treatments; licensed respiratory therapists will be used more frequently in a part-time, consulting role to set up the respiratory plan of care. Again, documentation to support the RUGs III level is necessary for correct reimbursement.

▶ Suggestions for Managing Therapies

- ▶ Patient and family education must begin as soon as feasible to assist in the therapy process. Self-care has always been a basic case management premise; now it is essential.

▶ In the SNF level of care, 14 of the 18 highest reimbursement categories under the RUGs require rehabilitation services. Patients utilizing these services may become very important to the fiscal health of SNFs. However, this is one area that is being closely monitored.

▶ It must be decided whether hiring therapists or using contracted therapists is in your best fiscal interest. This is a complex and individualized situation that must take many variables into consideration.

▶ PT, OT, and ST have always been covered. However, due to perceived or actual abuses of these services, they will be examined in greater detail. Whether the patient resides in a SNF (thus referenced on the MDS assessment) or is at home, documentation in the medical record should support the following:
a. That the services were ordered by a physician.
b. That a qualified therapist performed an evaluation and plan of care.
c. That the services were provided by or directly supervised by an appropriately licensed individual.
d. That the services were medically necessary.
e. That the services were provided with appropriate frequency and duration.
f. That the plan includes realistic and measurable goals for the patient.

▶ Focus on the patient.

▶ What to Do If You Are Employed in a Skilled Nursing Facility

▶ Become part of an integrated network. This can open up financial options that may be necessary for survival. Strategies to deal with the acute care Transfer DRGs and the transfer to postacute care payment policy (see "The Discharge/Transfer Rule" earlier in this chapter) will benefit from an integrated network. Optimal transfer strategies will require quick and easy access to other levels of care. Several SNFs could unite to share ancillary staff or pharmacy needs, order supplies through group purchasing, or combine staff training efforts.

▶ Educate employees about the new changes in benefits and reimbursement. They must understand reimbursement challenges to help plan care that is both cost-effective and provides safe, quality care for the residents.

▶ Monitor admission requests.
a. Whereas previously the intake coordinator may have spoken to the hospital nurse or case manager and read parts of the medical record, it may be that the admissions nurse should go to the site and actually see the patient; there is often a difference between the "paper patient" and the "actual patient."
b. With the new discharge/transfer rules, the acuity of patients for those particular DRGs may be less on admission to the SNF (because the hospital may keep the patient an extra day or two); the admission of a less acute patient may mean a lower RUG classification and a lower reimbursement level.
c. Under a RUGs-based reimbursement system, one survival strategy may be to control the clinical mix of patients being admitted to the facility. The screening criteria that each SNF sets will be important for survival. However, a little thought here will bring to light many potential legal, ethical, and business dilemmas; only time will tell what the consequences of using this strategy will be.
d. Another RUG strategy may be to place the patient in the highest RUG category while providing the lowest use of resources possible. This "survival" strategy has been cited in the literature as a method to "level the playing field" because the patient's medical condition often changes and can cause higher resource use; however, RUG reimbursement does not change with the patient's condition unless the patient's functional level also changes. Again, this strategy should be used with caution.

▶ Use proven strategies to provide quality services in a cost-efficient manner. These include the use of:
a. Case management (strongly recognized in the literature as an important strategy).
b. Clinical pathways/case management plans, especially those that cross levels of care.
c. Disease management strategies.
d. Protocols, guidelines, and care plans.
e. Coordination of care across multiple providers and settings (those involved in the care of a patient or settings being considered for continued care).

▶ Prove your worth. Learn about outcomes and document cost and quality savings.

▶ Use physician assessment before transfers back to acute care. If a patient is transferred back to the hospital and it is determined that the SNF could have handled the problem, the SNF may be responsible for the bill.

▸ Summarize the MDS accurately and thoroughly. This is the critical tool that will determine revenue entitled to the facility.

   a. Train pertinent staff members to use these documents accurately and thoroughly. A team effort (the nurse case manager, social worker, OT/PT/ST rehabilitation professionals, etc.) may be required to demonstrate fully the range of care provided.

   b. Do not overestimate patient needs; this will be picked up during the fraud and abuse examinations. However, completely document all the care ordered by the physician to maximize reimbursement.

   c. Demonstrate that the care must be provided on a daily basis.

   d. Complete the MDS within the stated time frame. If not done in a timely manner, default per diems will be reimbursed.

▸ Continue appropriate care and services to non-Medicare residents. Overutilization of services to non-Medicare patients will continue to be monitored.

▸ Know your facility's patient mix. Each facility has a unique blend of clinical and cultural situations. Examine where costs are heaviest and look for potential waste. Start a quality improvement (QI) program to set up the most efficient and effective means to achieve quality and financial goals.

▸ Revisit the details of your system. Reevaluate all policies, procedures, clinical pathways, invoicing, billing, forms, and software systems to ensure they are in compliance with consolidated billing requirements and good PPS survival strategies.

▸ Update software systems if necessary; it is mandated for MDS. It will also be essential to adequately document and calculate RUG groupings and electronically transmit the data. With consolidated billing, the software systems will also assist in the tracking of ancillary services and DME/supplies. Lastly, software can assist in outcomes studies, which are more important for survival than ever.

▸ Determine new strategies to cope with consolidated billing rules. This may include partnering/contracting with other service providers or using staff strategies such as outsourcing.

▸ Use proven case management strategies for quality, cost-efficient patient care. As in acute care, perform concurrent review; observe for quality issues; effect and document utilization management strategies; and start post-SNF discharge planning early.

▸ Focus on the patient.

▸ What to Do If You Are a Hospital or External Case Manager

▸ Develop good relationships with referring facilities. SNFs depend on honest assessments of patients for quality of care and financial survival. Report the patient assessment in an objective and thorough manner. The trust between the hospital and SNF case managers is important. Not every patient will "get in," but some frantic Friday afternoon, when there is a last-minute SNF bed desperately required, the SNF case manager will know you are not giving an unrealistic report of a patient just to get that person admitted.

▸ Understand the clinical and reimbursement issues of RUGs and MDS. There is a good chance that it may be more difficult to find placements for high-cost patients. The higher-based per diems translate into less medical costs and more ADL needs. Rehabilitation services may also be in demand. This "cherry picking" could cause ill feelings and frustration all around; work together and understand the constraints the SNFs are under.

▸ Remember that the physician is the key decision maker. It is ultimately the physician who will assess the patient and determine whether the patient's care in a SNF is still medically necessary. However, reimbursement can become a barrier, and advance planning is more important than ever before.

▸ Be realistic. Some benefits have been generously provided for in the past; with new reimbursement, companies will have to be managing more comprehensively if they are to survive. Also, be realistic about the patient's potential for improvement.

▸ Watch for inappropriate denial of SNF admissions. Current literature states that any SNF can produce reasons for refusing patients (e.g., they have no beds, they cannot take that level of acuity, they currently do not have the staff, etc.). The truth is that many SNFs may turn to privately insured patients to offset the PPS reimbursement system as a survival strategy, or facilities may make policy about which patients are/are not to be accepted. The reasons will likely be financial; the underlying fear may be related to survival.

❱ Keep current about Medicare reimbursement and benefit changes. This knowledge is needed if you are to strategize about how best to meet the needs of your patients.

❱ If the patient/family or another case manager calls with SNF care concerns, reassess the medical condition to evaluate appropriate level of services. If you feel that the SNF care remains medically necessary, detail the reasons for this level of care and document them carefully in the medical record.

❱ Remember that the transfer/discharge orders must be very specific. This is good patient care. It is also necessary for full reimbursement for the SNF. An order for a "PT evaluation" is no longer enough.

❱ Try to move patients to SNFs early in the day. The SNFs must heed strict MDS assessment and treatment time limits, and the day of admission is now day 1.

❱ Focus on the patient.

NOTE

Some Internet sites that may be helpful in navigating the Medicare reimbursement changes include the following:

http://www.thomas.loc.gov
  ❱ Will take you to Library of Congress where the rest of the Balanced Budget Act of 1997 can be located
  ❱ Has legislative information of all types
http://www.cms.hhs.gov/NursingHomeQualityI-nits/25_NHQIMDS30.asp
http://www.dhs.state.tx.us/proj/mds.html (this site requires registration)
  ❱ These sites have information on the MDS—the patient acuity measurement tool that SNFs use (with the new PPS reimbursement, accurate assessment using this tool is essential for survival)

❱ OTHER DURABLE MEDICAL EQUIPMENT

Some DME changes have already been discussed, such as glucose monitors and testing strips for diabetics. However, the BBA of 1997 and the Deficit Reduction Act of 2005 have created other new changes that the case manager should be aware of to perform cost-efficient, quality care and be a support to other members of the healthcare team. DME has been deemed "abused," and will be scrutinized carefully. Some changes include:

❱ Physicians must provide ICD-9 codes (which are diagnostic) for DME, orthotics, prosthetics, and supplies billed to the DME arm of the CMS.

❱ Reimbursement has changed from reasonable charges to a fixed payment for such items as parenteral and enteral nutrition as well as home dialysis equipment.

❱ Although glucose monitors and testing strips are covered for diabetics regardless of insulin requirements, a deductible and coinsurance still apply.

❱ Reimbursement for oxygen supplies is also reduced.

❱ Orthotics and prosthetics reimbursement will increase 1% annually.

❱ Mandatory beneficiary ownership of capped rental items of DME after the 13th month of rental.

❱ Mandatory beneficiary ownership of oxygen equipment rental after the 36th month of rental.

❱ Beneficiary paying for service maintenance of DME when such is actually provided.

❱ Beneficiary having a "first month purchase option" for power wheelchairs.

The PPS per diem rate is all-inclusive, and case managers must be aware that most orthotics, prosthetics, and mobility appliances will not be provided in the SNF. The reason for this is simply one of survival: if a prosthetic device costs $10,000, and the highest RUG's reimbursement rate is approximately $400 per day, the SNF would not make a profit and may not even survive. It is imperative that the case manager use all available resources for the benefit of the patient.

Case managers must be more aware than ever of what is going on behind the scenes. DME and HME companies are also realizing deep cuts; in response, they may have to cut some of the value-added services that case managers have taken for granted. For example, oxygen suppliers typically have provided an extra follow-up visit to the patient to ensure that he or she understood the proper use of the equipment and to check for compliance issues. More teaching will have to go on in the inpatient setting. As nurses and respiratory therapists are delivering small volume nebulizer (SVN) or other treatments, they will also need to be teaching the patients at the same time. Case managers will be required to stay on top of these sessions and document them carefully. The same will hold true for all ancillary services; nurses, respiratory therapists, physical therapists, occupational therapists, and speech therapists will need to start home teaching earlier and with more intensity. Although this was always supposed to be done, safe care now depends on it.

Technological advances in home equipment are other changes that are sweeping the world. Case managers must be knowledgeable about the best equipment, the pros and cons of each type of equipment, and the patient's benefits (what will be a covered service). The quality of life and independence of our patients depend on it. This is a challenging part of case management; it can be made easier through working with experts in their fields. Unfortunately, not all contracted companies hire the most knowledgeable employees who will be of assistance in case management decisions; therefore, it is important to find companies who can answer DME—and state-of-the-art—questions when needed.

CMS always monitors the payment/reimbursement systems in all settings, including the SNFs. Some of the issues being watched (and some also apply to home care) include:

- Incentives will be dramatically changed from the past. Do any incentives practiced have the potential to negatively affect quality of care and/or access to services?
- Are there changes in the types of patients who are being admitted to SNFs?
- Are there changes in the average lengths of stay?
- Are appropriate services being provided to patients in SNFs? Are there distinctions between patients who receive rehabilitation therapies versus those who do not? PT/OT/ST reimbursement in SNFs is also going through a change.
- Why are some patients with similar medical conditions and nursing needs discharged from acute care settings to a SNF, whereas others go home with or without home health care? Are there differences in patient criteria or condition? Is there evidence that reflects that the more clinically complex patients go to the more intensive level of care?
- Are there incentives to discharge patients before addressing and treating underlying chronic problems?

- What are the reasons for readmission to acute care? Are they preventable? Is there care needed after hospitalization that is not being addressed?
- Do SNFs have the clinical staffing skill to meet the needs of the complexity of patients they admit?

All these changes may catapult healthcare to where it always needed to be: focusing on the patient. As it becomes more difficult to "win" the reimbursement game, there may be only one thing left to do. Going back to an old nursing medication rule: provide the right care, in the right setting, at the right amount, and for the right reasons.

▶ TRANSFERRING PATIENTS
▶ Transitions of Care

Today, most healthcare needs of patients with chronic and complex medical conditions are being handled in multiple settings and require the involvement of many healthcare providers, often during a single episode of illness/care. Those involved in the care are not limited to the professionals from one single organization where the patient is admitted for care. Others external to the organization are also involved based on the patient's care needs, especially those that are necessary for continued care and postdischarge services such as from an acute care facility. For example, a patient may be admitted to an ICU for a couple of days until his or her condition is stable enough for transfer to a telemetry floor or a regular patient care unit. A few days later, the patient may need a transfer to a SNF or subacute rehabilitation setting for continued care. While in the hospital setting, this patient also may require the care of a specialist depending on the medical condition being addressed (e.g., cardiologist, endocrinologist, diabetologist, neurosurgeon, and so on). As this patient moves across settings and levels of care, or is seen by multiple physicians and other healthcare professionals (e.g., case manager, social worker, physical therapist, and so on), he or she experiences transitions of care.

The term *transitions of care* is defined as a process of moving patients from one level of care to another, usually from most to least complex; however, depending on the patient's health condition and needed treatments/services, the transition may occur in the other direction—from least to most. Some healthcare professionals believe that a change in a patient's plan of care, even if it is as simple as changing the dosage of or discontinuing a medication means a transition of care situation; that is because it changes or interrupts one or more care patterns for the patient.

Tahan (2007) explains that transitions of care cannot take place without an act of "hand off." A hand off, according to Tahan, is an action that facilitates the transfer of responsibility for the care of a patient from one provider to another, from one care setting to another, or from one level of care to another. Although the term *hand off* has been widely used, some healthcare professionals currently are advocating for the use of the term *hand over* instead. Some critics claim that hand off may inadvertently imply the termination of care and accountability while hand over may mean continuity. Regardless of which term one uses, it is essential to relinquish active participation in the care of a patient only after ensuring that the transfer of responsibility and accountability for care has occurred effectively, accurately, safely, at the right time, and to the right person or setting.

A single care transition may constitute multiple hand off/over acts. For example, when a patient is transferred from the hospital setting to a SNF, it requires transitioning the responsibility of care from the hospital team to the SNF team; sharing of information about the plan of care, medications, treatment regimens, allergies, and so on; and communication about the patient's medical history, interests, health insurance status, and numerous other aspects of the care to be provided at the SNF. The following are the five main contexts during which care transitions take place:

1. Transfer of responsibility for care from one healthcare provider to another, such as from a primary care to a specialist physician, from one nurse to another, or from one case manager to another.
2. Change in the environment of care within a healthcare facility, such as moving a patient from the emergency department to the ICU setting.
3. Change in the environment of care from one facility to another, including hospitals, SNFs, outpatient clinic, and others.
4. Change in the plan of care, such as adding a new or discontinuing an existing medication.
5. Change in the payer or health plan, such as changing from a fee-for-service Medicare Plan to Medicare Advantage Plan.

Transitions of care occur during a time when a patient journeys through the healthcare system. This journey may result in vulnerable situations and require an increased need for coordination and continuity of care. During care transitions, patients face significant challenges; they are usually at a higher risk for medical errors, poor quality care, and unsafe experiences. Some of the reasons for these events include system inefficiencies, lack of appropriate follow-up, and poor communication. Transitions of care should be well planned and adequately timed; they must enhance the continuity of care and involve a two-way interaction. Case managers can play an important role in planning and executing transitions of care activities. They are integral to preventing poor outcomes and negative experiences. Safe transitions of care depend on a system approach to care as well as a culture of healthcare professionals working together regardless of place, time, and space boundaries. Case managers are known to be integrators of care and to function in ways that transcend organizational boundaries.

Care coordination, a component of case management, is an effective strategy case managers proactively use in the event of care transition encounters to ensure that care is uninterrupted and patients experience positive outcomes. Additionally, case management is essential for effective care transitions; the case management process (refer to Chapter 6) has been known to facilitate the integration and coordination of healthcare services across consumers of healthcare, providers of care, payors for services, and care settings; that is, across people, space, and time. Contextually speaking, case management facilitates effective collaboration and communication among healthcare team members and across settings, before, during, and after an act of hand off/over or a care transition. These critical interactions ensure patient safety and optimal care outcomes.

Patients at increased risk during transitions of care or hand offs/overs include children with special care needs, the frail elderly, persons with cognitive impairments, persons with complex medical conditions and treatment regimens, persons with disabilities, persons at the end-of-life, the uninsured, those with low income or poor social networks, and those with mental/behavioral health issues. When such patients are transferred to another provider, another level of care, or to another acute hospital, specific information must accompany them. The general transfer packet should include the following:

▶ Physician transfer orders.
▶ Chest radiograph (preferably within 30 days).
▶ Medical history and physical examination results.
▶ Laboratory results.
▶ ECG results.
▶ Urinalysis results.
▶ Preadmission screening (PAS), preadmission screening and annual resident review (PASAAR) forms.
▶ Assessments from nursing, PT, OT, and ST (as needed).
▶ Social service assessments.

▸ Advance directives, do not resuscitate (DNR) forms (if appropriate), living wills, medical power of attorney.
▸ Copies of important information such as results of CT scans, echocardiograms, Dopplers, MRIs, miscellaneous cardiodiagnostic tests, and so on.
▸ A transfer note or summary that provides comprehensive information of the patient's status, the course of treatment received, and the plan for continued care (Display 5-5).

A complete and thorough transfer packet is necessary for continuity of patient care and avoids much trouble and many problems. Patients have been returned to emergency departments for not having a chest radiograph accompany them to the facility. SNFs must ensure that their residents are free from tuberculosis and the necessity of a chest radiograph is usually nonnegotiable. Patients with a positive Mantoux skin test may also need a signed and dated letter from the physician stating that the resident is free from pulmonary tuberculosis or that three consecutive sputum cultures have shown negative results for 3 days in a row.

Another required form in many states is the PAS document. It is also known as a PASAAR form. This program, started by Medicaid in the mid-1980s, was originally designed as a technique to manage LTC costs and utilization of services in nursing homes. It includes an on-site (or hospital) assessment of the patient's needs. In some states, this assessment is extensive and includes an evaluation of physical and mental health, functional status, and formal and informal social supports. Although the PAS program was not deemed successful as a utilization control measure, it was praised for its ability to help assess the level of care and type of facility that is best for the patient. Some PAS programs contain a level I and level II. Level I is essentially used to assess medical necessity for a SNF. Level II indicates whether a psychological referral is needed. This may hold up a transfer to a SNF for a week or more. State laws prohibit SNFs or supervisory homes from accepting patients with active mental illnesses that may cause them to be a danger to themselves or other residents in the SNF. If a patient might need to pass a level II PAS, the paperwork should be started early in the admission.

One last detail: a patient must have an accepting physician at the SNF. If the patient's primary physician cannot follow up at the SNF, the facility often helps to find a physician who can.

▸ Transportation

Safe patient transportation between levels of care is an important consideration for the case manager. Several levels of transportation are available for transferring patients to an outside destination, and the patient's needs must be matched to the appropriate mode of transportation. In many instances, the patient or family is responsible for the cost of transportation. Some rare insurance policies pay for expensive forms of transportation, so if the patient claims to have such a policy rider, check it out. Some family members may request a more intensive level of transportation than the case manager has assessed, and may be willing to pay for it. In one instance, a case manager had assessed that a patient could safely be transported to another hospital using a stretcher van. The family wanted an advanced cardiac life support (ACLS) ambulance plus an RN. Therefore, even when planning the mode of transportation, one must include the patient and family in the decision.

PRIVATE VEHICLES

Private vehicles are the most common mode of transportation. The patient is usually accompanied by family or friends, but occasionally drives him- or herself to the hospital. In such a case, arrangements must be made for the vehicle if the physician feels it is unsafe for the patient to drive. The simplest solution here is for a family member or neighbor to be dropped off at the facility to drive the vehicle and patient home. The facility's personnel can help get the patient into the vehicle. The case manager should assess whether there is enough help at the destination to get the patient inside safely. Assessment is also needed for any equipment needs for the trip. For example, many patients have their portable oxygen tanks at home and must make prior arrangements to retrieve them before they leave the facility. Also, assess the length of the trip and the possible need for more than one oxygen tank. Assess whether the patient can remain sitting for the trip: very ill patients and some orthopedic procedures make this mode of transportation unrealistic. Assess whether the patient has stairs to climb at the other end. If the patient cannot negotiate stairs, a car, taxi, or wheelchair van will not work and a stretcher van should be considered; the stretcher van personnel will take the patient up the stairs and help him or her to get settled.

TAXICAB

Ask some of the same questions as above for taxis, realizing that cab drivers are often less helpful at the other end than family members because of their legal constraints. Also, find out whether the patient can afford a taxi. Many hospitals have funds or cab vouchers to help needy people. From a fiscal perspective, a cab ride is less expensive than a day in the hospital if a

display 5-5

▼ KEY INFORMATION THAT MUST BE COVERED IN THE TRANSFER NOTE

I. Background Information
   a. Patient's name and date of birth
   b. Next of kin or healthcare proxy and contact information
   c. Address and telephone number
   d. Primary language spoken and need for interpretation, health literacy
   e. Health beliefs
   f. Name of primary care provider and contact information
   g. Name of specialist care provider(s) and contact information
   h. Presence of advance directive, healthcare proxy, living will, do not resuscitate
   i. Living situation
   j. Employment status

II. Medical History
   a. Allergies
   b. Chief complaint and summary of healthcare encounter
   c. Medical problems complicating management of current condition
   d. Past medical history including any co-morbidities (chronic illnesses)
   e. Comprehensive list of medications: prescription and over the counter drugs including use of herbal products and vitamins. List should include name of drug, frequency of intake, dosage, and special precautions or instructions
   f. Current or past surgical procedures
   g. Use of durable medical equipment
   h. Other important health information

III. Health Insurance Benefits
   a. Insurance/health plan-related information such as name, policy number, and expiration date
   b. Provider network
   c. Coverage
   d. Any other necessary information

IV. Plan of Care
   a. Goals
   b. Long-term and short-term treatment plans

   c. Areas that require special attention; e.g., health education, use of devices such as a "glucometer"
   d. Psychosocial issues/concerns
   e. Barriers to achieving goals
   f. Wishes regarding end of life care; e.g., life-sustaining measures
   g. Caregiver and ability and willingness to provide ongoing care for the patient
   h. Community level support

V. Educational Plan
   a. Areas patient and/or caregiver knows well
   b. Areas that need further attention or specific follow-up
   c. Plan regarding medications intake
   d. Plan regarding skilled services or treatment regimen

VI. Functional Status
   a. Self-care ability
   b. Ability to make own decisions
   c. Level of dependence or independence
   d. Cognition: impaired, alert/oriented, disoriented
   e. Ability to dress, especially lower extremities
   f. Bathing
   g. Toileting
   h. Ambulation: use of aids such as walker, crutches, prosthesis
   i. Transferring from bed to chair and vice versa
   j. Need for transportation services
   k. Housekeeping assistance

VII. Home Health Services
   a. Name of agency and contact information, if any
   b. Use of home health aide, visiting nurse service, allied health professionals (e.g., physical therapy, social worker)
   c. Frequency and type of visits
   d. Skilled care: wound care, dressing changes, intravenous therapy,

VIII. Durable Medical Equipment
   a. Current needs
   b. Previous use
   c. Name of vendor and phone number
   d. Patient's/caregiver's knowledge and ability of use

patient cannot get someone to take him home until the following day.

WHEELCHAIR VAN

Wheelchair vans are a good choice for several types of patients. If patients who are quadriplegic or who have cerebral palsy use a wheelchair at home, they often have their own wheelchair at the hospital. Notify the van company whether they need to provide a wheelchair or whether the patient has one. If a patient can sit up for a designated length of time but may be slightly confused, he or she may need to be restrained. Careful assessment is imperative when sending a patient needing restraints in a wheelchair van. For example, it would be safer to use a higher level of transportation if the patient is combative or requires maximum restraining. (Consider what the risk management issues would be if the patient is maximally restrained and the van catches fire or goes over the side of a road!) Orthopedic patients can often use wheelchair vans with adaptive equipment such as leg lifts. Specify what equipment is required when ordering the van. Again, assess the whole medical picture before deciding on this level of transportation.

STRETCHER VANS

Stretcher vans allow a patient to lie down for the entire ride. The patient is transferred from the facility bed to the stretcher and taken to the destination, even transported up or down stairs, in the same position. Very ill, debilitated patients who cannot sit for any length of time are candidates for stretcher vans, as are some orthopedic patients or those who must stay on their abdomen or back because of medical considerations such as skin flaps or graft procedures. No form of cardiac monitoring is included in this mode of transportation.

AMBULANCES

There are two types of ambulances: basic life support (BLS) and advanced life support (ALS). BLS ambulances include a BLS paramedic and limited cardiac monitoring. Psychiatric patients or suicidal patients who are being transferred to a mental health unit minimally require this level of care; if the transfer is involuntary and the patient is likely to become combative, extra help should be requested and restraints may be necessary. In general, assess the patient's medical stability and decide whether it would be beneficial to have a BLS paramedic on board.

ALS ambulances include paramedics trained in advanced cardiac life support procedures. Cardiac monitoring and a drug box are available for use. Any patient who has a running intravenous line or who requires medications (including potassium) will minimally require this level of care.

AIR AMBULANCE

Air transport is the most cost-intensive type of transportation available, often costing thousands of dollars for even short flights. When an unstable patient is being transferred to another acute care facility and speed is of the essence, it may be the only safe mode of transfer. As in an ALS ambulance, the air ambulance has cardiac monitoring, a medication box, and ACLS-trained personnel, including a registered nurse.

Almost any patient can be transferred safely, when necessary, with enough support. Some cases require careful consideration and advanced planning. Insurance companies often require their medically stable patients to be transferred to contracted hospitals. One patient had a chest tube and needed an ALS ambulance with a registered nurse on board. Because most ambulance companies retain only a few nurses, it took an extra day to provide the required services. Other patients require detailed coordination of oxygen, stretcher vans, air transport, and accepting facilities. Patients with certain conditions cannot be transferred safely in air transports due to the pressure changes at high altitudes. Transportation needs can be tricky and require early team coordination and planning.

CONSIDERATIONS IN PLANNING TRANSPORTATION

Further important considerations to assess when planning a mode of transportation are as follows.

TUBES AND LINES.   Most tubes can be capped off for shorter rides and require only a physician's order to do so. This may include intravenous lines (peripheral or central), feeding tubes, suction tubes such as nasogastric tubes or percutaneous endoscopic gastrostomy (PEG) tubes, gastrostomy tubes, or jejunostomy tubes. Most modes of transportation—even taxis—allow capped-off tubes, although that is not to say that a taxi is the safest vehicle assessed. If a tube cannot be capped off, an ambulance may be the lowest level of transportation allowed. If, for example, intravenous fluid containing potassium is running, then an ALS ambulance must be used. The transportation company can clear up any questions, because they carry on their business under legal guidelines.

OXYGEN.   Some state laws mandate that oxygen cannot be supplied by the transportation company for wheelchair or stretcher vans. The company can provide oxygen only in a BLS or ALS ambulance. However, if the patient has his or her own portable oxygen tank, a wheelchair van or stretcher van may be provided in conjunction with the patient's personal equipment. The van personnel are not allowed to adjust the oxygen, so that the patient's ability to care for his or her own portable tank must be considered.

PRICES OF TRANSPORTATION.   Because the patient is responsible for the cost of transportation in many instances, the case manager may want to compare the prices of various companies for the best rate. Ambulance prices are essentially set by the government, but taxi, wheelchair van, and stretcher van prices may vary.

TRANSPORTATION REIMBURSEMENT. Insurance companies often reimburse for transportation between two medically necessary levels of care; they usually do not reimburse for transportation to the patient's home. Medicare reimbursement for transportation is very strict and includes only ground ambulance or air ambulance transport.

❭ Ground ambulance may be reimbursed under Medicare Part B for a medically necessary transfer if:
1. The ambulance, equipment, and personnel meet Medicare requirements and approval.
2. Any other mode of transportation could endanger the patient.
3. The destination is to or from a hospital or SNF. This does not include such destinations as hemodialysis facilities, doctor's offices, or ambulatory surgery centers.
4. The transportation is to a local facility (usually). If the facility is outside the local area, Medicare will help pay for the transportation to the nearest appropriate facility.

❭ Air ambulance may be reimbursed by Medicare if:
1. The medical condition seriously endangers the member's life.
2. Immediate medical attention is necessary for the person's survival or necessary to avoid severe health damage.
3. Land ambulance is unavailable or would be so time-consuming that health or life would be further endangered.

STUDY QUESTIONS

1. Discuss the importance of discharge planning regulations and accreditation standards for the role of the case manager.

2. Discuss how discharge planning is affected based on the differences between traditional Medicare and the newer risk Medicare contracts. Do you see these changes positively or negatively?

3. Discuss the Important Message from Medicare and its related appeals review process. How would you handle a family/patient who disagrees with the hospital discharge date or postdischarge services? What steps would you take? What are the financial implications when a patient or hospital does not adhere to the Important Message from Medicare process?

4. Give examples of patients who are appropriate for the custodial level of care, the intermediate level of care, and the skilled and subacute levels of care. Discuss possible pay sources for each level of care.

5. What might constitute a patient being at too high or too low a level for inpatient rehabilitation?

6. Cite an example of a good candidate for a transitional hospital.

7. Cite an example of a good home healthcare patient. Give reasons that may be contrary to home health services.

8. Compare and contrast home health services with hospice care.

9. Cite examples matching patients' needs to safe transportation.

10. Discuss the role of the case manager in safe transitions of care. What can a case manager do to enhance patient safety when a patient is transferred from one provider to another? From one service to another? From one setting/organization to another?

❭ REFERENCES

Anonymous. (1991). CMs find innovative options for patients between the ICU and the acute care bed. *Case Management Advisor, 2*(8), 113–117.

Birmingham, J. (2008). Understanding the Medicare "extended care benefit" a.k.a. the 3-midnight rule. *Professional Case Management, 13*(1), 7–16.

Carr, D.D. (2000). Case management for the subacute patient in a skilled nursing facility. *Lippincott's Case Management, 5*(2), 83–92.

Centers for Medicare & Medicaid Services (CMS). (2007). (accessed 3/13/2008). *CMS manual, Medicare claims processing.* Transmittal Number 1257 (May 25, 2007). [Online]. Available: http://www.cms.hhs.gov/Transmittals/downloads/R1257CP.pdf.

Centers for Medicare and Medicaid Services (CMS). (2009a). (accessed 4/13/2009). Conditions of participation for hospitals, chapter IV: Discharge planning. [Online]. Available: www.cms.hhs.gov/CFCsAndCoPs/06_Hospitals.asp#TopofPage.

Centers for Medicare and Medicaid Services (CMS). (2009b). (accessed 4/13/2009). Minimum data sets 2.0. [Online]. Available: www.cms.hhs.gov/MinimumDataSets20.

Cesta, T., & Tahan, H. (2003). *The case manager's survival guide: winning strategies for clinical practice* (2nd ed.). St. Louis, MO: Mosby.

Gookin, L. (1994). Effects on capitation on home health care. *Geriatric Nursing*, 15(3) 167–168.

Hamilton, M., & Thomsen, T. (1998). Removing the label. *Continuing Care*, 17(9), 26–29, 40.

Kongstvedt, P.R. (2003). *Essentials of managed health care* (4th ed.). Gaithersburg, MD: Aspen Publishers.

National Association of Subacute/Postacute Care (NASPAC). (2009). (accessed 4/13/2009). Frequently asked questions. [Online]. Available: http://www.naspac.net/faq.asp.

Newell, M. (1996). *Using nursing care management to improve health outcomes*. Gaithersburg, MD: Aspen Publishers.

Powell, S. (2007). An important message from Medicare, new rules on July 1, 2007. *Professional Case Management*, 12(2), 1–3.

Tahan, H.A. (2007). One patient, numerous healthcare providers, and multiple care settings. *Professional Case Management*, 12(1), 37–46.

The Joint Commission. (2008). *Comprehensive accreditation manual for hospitals*; Glossary. Oakbrook Terrace, IL: Joint Commission Resources.

Williams. S.J., & Torrens, P.R. (1993). *Introduction to health services*. New York: Delmar.

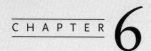

CHAPTER 6

The Case Management Process

"Great opportunities to help others seldom come, but small
ones surround us every day."

SALLY KOCH

LEARNING OBJECTIVES

Upon completion of this chapter, the reader will be able to:

1. Describe each stage of the case management process.
2. List five criteria that qualify a patient for case management services.
3. Determine the essential components of a case management assessment.
4. Develop a case management plan of care, including establishing goals and prioritization of needs.
5. Describe four strategies that ensure effective implementation of the case management plan of care.
6. Recognize the importance of ongoing monitoring and evaluation of the case management plan of care.
7. Identify three strategies for effective closure of case management services.

ESSENTIAL TERMS

Alternative Therapies • Assessment • Care Planning • Case Closure • Case Evaluation • Case Management Assessment • Case Management Outcomes • Case Management Process • Case Plan Goals • Case Screening • Case Selection • Continuous Monitoring • Criteria for Case Management Services • Cultural Diversity • Current Medical Status • External Case Management • Financial Assessment • Functional Assessment • Home Environment Assessment • Implementation • Internal Case Management • Medication Assessment • Nutrition Assessment • Potential Problems • Psychosocial Assessment • Reassessment • Screening • Service Planning • Socioeconomic Indicators

▶ INTRODUCTION TO THE CASE MANAGEMENT PROCESS

This chapter discusses the direction and activities needed to guide a patient through the complex healthcare maze. Nurses will find the process familiar, because it uses some of the same components as the nursing process: assessment, planning, implementation, monitoring, and evaluation. The focus, however, is much broader in case management. In the nursing process, the patient is assessed for changing physical, medical, psychosocial, and safety needs on a shift-by-shift basis. The case manager must also assess the patient's condition before the current illness or event, determine whether his or her environment (physical and social network) will continue

to meet present needs, investigate how the needs will be met financially, and then plan future care. Therefore, the steps may be slightly reordered, new ones added, and the emphasis and purposes altered.

This reordering and altering may also apply when considering different types of case management. Case selection for a hospital case manager may be filtered through the institution's admissions process. An independent case manager may get referrals from a variety of sources such as physicians, insurance companies, and private citizens. Other case managers may select cases according to a predetermined specialty such as spinal cord injuries, asthma, heart failure, AIDS, or cerebral palsy. The monitoring component may be done less frequently for a case manager with patients in private homes or in sheltered care than for a hospital case manager, who may have to monitor patients on a daily (or more frequent) basis.

Follow-up and termination of case management services will depend, in part, on the type of case management work or practice setting. Some hospital case managers are finished with a case at discharge. Others perform posthospital follow-up for a brief time. Hospice case managers may assess their patients in the home or hospital, but they do not actively take on the case until patients are formally "admitted" to hospice care; this may occur when the patient arrives home or to a skilled facility after discharge, or a patient may become a hospice candidate while using home health services. Hospice case managers may follow up the patient until death. Still other case managers follow up their patients in whatever care and service setting the patients' health conditions require.

Responsibilities are also different in various case management positions. Independent case managers and case managers who work outside institutional settings must often obtain signed consents for case management services from the payors or for release of information or medical records. Negotiation and cost-benefit evaluation are daily activities. Reports to consultants and claims managers are very different from the facility-based documentation that internal case managers must provide. Insurance case managers may have varied duties, also depending on where the patient is located. For example, Medicaid case managers rely on hospital personnel and other sources for much of the assessment information, especially for medical and psychosocial aspects. They often work closely with hospital or skilled nursing facility (SNF) discharge planners, case managers, and social workers to fulfill a safe and timely discharge or transfer.

Generally speaking the stages of the case management process are the same regardless of the healthcare provision setting (e.g., outpatient, acute, or rehabilitation), case manager's practice setting (hospital, disease management, health insurance), or type of professional who assumes the case manager's role (e.g., nurse, social worker, rehabilitation counselor).

▶ STAGES OF THE CASE MANAGEMENT PROCESS

Each patient is unique and case management styles are individual; therefore, case management is a very personalized process in every case. Taking this into consideration, the process discussed in this chapter should be used as a guideline: the skills and creativity of each case manager are still the essential ingredients. In general, the case management process involves the following stages:

1. Case selection.
2. Assessment/problem identification.
3. Development and coordination of the case plan.
4. Implementation of the plan.
5. Evaluation and follow-up.
6. Continuous monitoring, reassessing, and reevaluating.
7. Case closure and termination of case management services.

As mentioned earlier, different styles and settings of case management lend themselves to different processes. As a rule of thumb, the stages of Assessment/ Problem Identification, Development and Coordination of the Case Plan, and Continuous Monitoring, Reassessing, and Reevaluating have many universal principles that may apply to several types of case management. However, other stages may vary significantly in different case management settings. Case Selection is different for a medical case manager in an acute care setting than for a disease-specific case manager. A disease-specific case manager may provide services only to a patient population centered around one diagnosis; within that diagnosis, the case manager must prioritize those who need more or less intense case management services. In other words, the amount of case management service is dependent on the risk category the patient falls under, such as low, moderate, or high risk, which mean simple/limited intensity, moderate intensity, or complex/high intensity case management services. Case managers who work in a provider setting may have different functions than those who work in a payor setting. For example, a payer-based case manager may engage in more telephonic triage and utilization management activities while the provider-based case manager may spend more time on activities such as facilitation and coordination of clinical care including treatments, tests, and procedures. This is illustrated in Stage IV: Implementation of the Plan. The stage of evaluation and follow-up is also very specific to the type of case management. The rest of this chapter will attempt to consider case management from many perspectives. However, look to recent journals and magazine articles for information on how other case managers are coping with problems specific to your type of case management.

▶ STAGE I: CASE SELECTION

Case selection is the "first cut" in the process. Basically, this step weeds out patients who probably will not need case management services; thinking differently, it means selecting the patients who would benefit most from case management services. Occasionally, one of the patients placed on the "probably not" list will actually need services. A patient's condition can deteriorate to the point of needing SNF placement or, more simply, a piece of durable medical equipment (DME) may be needed. Sometimes a quirky hitch arises such as a patient losing a lease or being evicted from an apartment by a roommate during the time of hospitalization. On the other hand, not all those who are put on the "probably" list (i.e., needing case management) will need the same degree of case management services; some may need only a bit of education or a walker for safety purposes. All patients need screening for case management services; those patients who are selected need a basic assessment, at the minimum, to determine the type and intensity of the required services.

Universal case management is not necessary. Some cases neither require case management nor benefit from it. Previously healthy people who are admitted for uncomplicated procedures such as hysterectomies, cholecystectomies, transurethral resection of the prostate (TURP), or an occasional exacerbation of asthma or chronic obstructive pulmonary disease (COPD), and who have some social support, usually require little or no posthospital support. However, a simple ailment in combination with a poor social environment may signal the need for further assessment. Diagnosis or chief complaint alone does not determine whether a patient/family would benefit from case management services. However, screening a patient by focusing on the patient/family's total situation (i.e., health condition, financial and insurance status, psychosocial network, availability of community resources, literacy and knowledge, ability for self-care, and so on) is the best strategy for deciding whether to weed a patient out or to place the patient on the probable or definite list. It is necessary for a case manager to complete such screening as early as possible in a patient's encounter with health care services, for example, on admission to the hospital.

In general, if a patient meets intensity of services (degree and amount of resources/services required for safe care) provided and severity of illness (acuity and acuteness of health condition), if no major discharge barriers are identified, if readmission is not a problem, and if there are no financial or psychosocial concerns, case management may not be required. Those patients who may require a case manager include those with moderate-to-complex problems: moderate-to-complex medical conditions and comorbidities, moderate-to-complex discharge needs, or moderate-to-complex social and financial issues. Other criteria may include risk for deterioration, experience of untoward events, or presence of ethical and/or legal issues/concerns. Although

assessment of the patient is considered Stage II, a cursory assessment must be conducted during case selection to make an accurate "cut" about who may require the services of a case manager. Several indicators are commonly used to red flag situations that may require case management services. Some indicators, although useful to trigger a case management investigation, warrant careful use. By their very nature, they are intrinsically flawed and may defeat some of the goals of case management, such as early intervention and cost-containment. Consider the following common indicators:

▶ Length of stay longer than 5 days (or another arbitrary number).
▶ Charges greater than $50,000 (or another dollar amount).

Both indicators exclude the possibility of early case management. Perhaps with early use of case management services, the patient who is now on hospital day 6 could have been discharged by hospital day 4. In addition, if this patient requires intensive needs after discharge, such as a transfer to an extended care facility, it may take an extra day (or more) to plan and implement the discharge or transfer. Such delay could have been prevented if screening was done early on in the hospital stay.

The second indicator (even if the dollar amount is considerably less, such as $10,000) may still pose barriers to the case management process. Again, early case management is precluded. Chances are lost to effect improved utilization of resources, to establish a relationship with the patient and family early in the illness, and to steer any variances back on track. There are situations when a patient does not have health insurance and cannot afford self-pay; in such cases, focusing on cost alone without consideration of reimbursement issues may result in a hospital not getting paid at all for services rendered. Perhaps this patient would meet the criteria for emergency Medicaid. If case management were not involved from the time of admission to the hospital, it is likely that this patient would have been discharged without case management involvement at all; hence, losing the opportunity to apply for Medicaid benefits and ultimately "no reimbursement."

Other commonly used indicators are too general to be used on their own merit and warrant secondary screening for possible case management needs.

▶ The patient lives alone (or with someone with a disability). A psychosocial assessment would be useful in such a case. If the patient lives alone, is there an informal support system strong enough to match the patient's needs? If the patient lives with a disabled or debilitated roommate or family member, can that roommate or family member meet the patient's needs at discharge? Often the patient has been the primary caregiver in the relationship. If so, who is caring for the person left at home?

▶ The patient is older than 65 years. People of all ages may need case management services. (Some facilities use age indicators of 70 or 75 years.) Most case managers have discharged spunky patients in their 90s. On the other hand, as the treatment options for patients with AIDS have advanced, more young men and women are living longer with the disease and need supportive care.

▶ Payor source. Some types of insurance may be clues to possible medical or psychosocial needs such as Medicare disability. Also, patients without any insurance resources may need creative case management and discharge planning.

▶ Readmission within 15 days (or 30 days) for the same problem(s). This may be a quality issue or a sign of an inadequate/early or unsafe discharge plan during the previous admission. It could also signal patient noncompliance, such as a patient with congestive heart failure who loves pretzels and pizza or the diabetic who does not check blood sugar levels, take insulin as directed, or follow a diabetic diet.

▶ Physicians. Some physicians' practices, such as those of trauma surgeons or geriatric specialists, signal a possible need for case management. Other physicians request the services of case management because of its efficacy and patient satisfaction. Another red-flag indicator may be a chart with multiple physicians in consultation or with an extensive multidisciplinary team. Here, the case manager can serve as the conductor, ensuring that all the disciplines are involved in time and playing the same song.

▶ First-time mothers. Giving birth to a first child does not automatically mean a need for case management services. An abundance of family support may limit the degree of case management services needed. Ultimately, a quick assessment of the mother's knowledge, needs, and availability of social support may place the mother and baby on the "weed out" list. In the case of a premature newborn, the story may be much different. Coping with a premature newborn alone may result in the need for case management services.

▶ Diagnosis-related group (DRG). Not all people with a specific diagnosis require case

management services, especially in the early stages of a disease process; educational activities or counseling services may be all that are needed. A chart review and possibly a patient/family interview or assessment will show the level of independence and severity of illness. All complex medical conditions or psychosocial/financial problems will require some degree of case management intervention.

▶ Psychological Indicators

Certain mental health, behavioral, and substance abuse conditions warrant, at the very least, a psychosocial assessment. Often a psychiatric evaluation is also required. The specific case details will guide the case manager to the appropriate referrals. The following are some red-flag indicators.

▶ Overdose (unintentional): unintentional overdoses of prescription medications can result from lack of knowledge about correct dosages or inability to properly self-medicate, as a result of confusion or poor eyesight. Unintentional overdoses can also be of the illegal, polydrug variety.

▶ Overdose (intentional): suicide gestures always need careful assessment and initiation of proper referrals.

▶ Alcohol and drug abuse: may present as a primary or secondary cause of admission.

▶ Eating disorders (e.g., bulimia, anorexia nervosa, "failure to thrive"): psychological causes may warrant psychiatric assessments. Conditions such as anorexia and failure to thrive may also have medical causes. Assessment will determine the extent of case management that may be needed.

▶ Chronic mental illness: may include various psychoses, schizophrenia, neurotic disorders, depression, bipolar disorder, and severe anxiety. Is the mental or emotional condition stable enough for the patient to return to previous living arrangements or is the condition unstable and the patient a danger to self or others?

▶ Alzheimer's/dementia: any form of confusion or disorientation.

▶ Noncompliance: frequent readmissions may be an indicator.

▶ Uncooperative/manipulative/aggressive behaviors: the perpetrator may be the patient, a family member, a friend, or any combination of the above. Often these people create havoc in a case by refusing tests and procedures (delay of diagnosis), "firing" physicians, or making outrageous demands for unnecessary and costly tests (overutilization of resources). Early recognition of potential manipulative behavior and identification of ways to limit these behaviors are necessary.

▶ Miscellaneous conditions such as Münchhausen syndrome or Münchhausen syndrome by proxy: the very definition of Münchhausen syndrome lends itself to overutilization of resources because these people intentionally produce symptoms of illness to assume the sick role. Münchhausen syndrome by proxy is a form of child abuse in which, for example, the parent (usually the mother) produces illness in the child. This, as in all forms of child abuse, is a reportable event. The extent to which one with Münchhausen syndrome will go to receive medical care can be dramatic and often requires investigative work to make the diagnosis of Münchhausen syndrome.

▶ Socioeconomic Indicators

Some socioeconomic factors alert the case manager that further screening for case management is required. High-risk situations, such as reportable events, need immediate and close assessment. The occurrences may include the following:

▶ Suspected child abuse or neglect.
▶ Suspected elder abuse or neglect.
▶ Violent crime.
▶ Domestic violence.

Other socioeconomic red flags include:

▶ Homelessness.
▶ Poor living environment such as inadequate housing, poor sanitary conditions, and lack of water, electricity, or heat.
▶ No known social or familial support systems.
▶ Admission from an extended care facility or other sheltered living arrangement.
▶ Need for transitional care in an extended care facility or sheltered living arrangement.
▶ Out-of-state or out-of-country residence.
▶ Residence in rural community where services are poor or nonexistent, thus limiting posthospital follow-up.
▶ Limited or no financial resources.
▶ No health insurance or inadequate amount of health insurance.
▶ Single parent (assessment of care of minors left at home).
▶ Dependent on others for activities of daily living (ADLs).

▶ Repeated admissions to acute care.
▶ Frequent visits to the emergency department, family physician, or clinic.
▶ Disruptive or obstructive family member or significant other.

Some general clues found in a chart or found on assessment may reveal possible future problems. Appropriate case management, referrals, and support may make a tremendous difference in the patient's quality of life. Be alert for situations such as:

▶ Any condition that will necessitate a major life change or a major quality of life change. Will the patient no longer be able to carry out his or her previous type of employment? Can the patient no longer live in his or her home of 40 years? Life changes may also include behavioral changes such as quitting smoking, refraining from drinking alcoholic beverages, or following a strict diet or exercise regimen.
▶ Any condition that will negatively affect physical or sexual function or self-image.
▶ Unrealistic expectations about the prognosis, treatment, or ability to go back home.

With the exception of reportable events, no single condition or diagnosis is automatically a problem that necessitates full case management services. Certainly, those with obvious home health needs or hospitalizations that include any quality or risk management issues need careful attention. The lists that have been provided here serve as guides, and many patients meeting these guidelines will need some discharge or transition services. The next step is a thorough assessment.

Case management is implemented differently in different organizations. For example, case selection in one organization may be determined based on the case manager screening all patients to determine who would benefit from case management services. In other organizations, case selection is based on a referral from other healthcare providers involved in the care of patients such as nurses and physicians. In some other organizations, screening may not be the practice at all; in such organizations, case managers may be expected to follow all patients regardless of acuity of condition, intensity of resources, or individual patient's needs.

When selection criteria are used, an organization must prospectively determine these criteria and communicate them clearly to all healthcare providers to encourage their use. It is important, however, to avoid the use of generic criteria such as length of stay or cost; criteria must be more specific than that; for example, patients at risk for extended length of stay rather than those of

4 days or greater or patients requiring high intensity of resources rather than those who need a magnetic resonance imaging (MRI) test. Allowing staff to deviate from the use of criteria exclusively for screening and case finding is also important. Sometimes a case manager knows intuitively the importance of providing case management services for certain patients even though those patients do not meet the selection criteria. Personal judgment is necessary in such situations. Follow-up assessment and monitoring may best determine whether to continue the services.

▶ STAGE II: ASSESSMENT/PROBLEM IDENTIFICATION

After the selection process has red flagged a case, Stage II: Assessment follows. Unless it is obvious that at this time the patient needs little or no case management services, a thorough and accurate assessment is done. Assessment determines patient needs and establishes plans that will overcome problems and move the patient forward. Data collecting and analysis focus and direct the case manager to the treatment, resource utilization, care coordination activities, and discharge plans needed for that individual. Potential or actual problems are exposed; goals start taking shape. In this stage, the case manager finds out what gaps need filling, what services are needed, and what quality of life issues need special focus. All anticipated needs are considered for a discharge plan that will allow the optimal quality of life for that patient.

A lengthy discourse on assessment is contained in this section. The reason so much attention is given to it is because assessment is the critical pivot around which the case manager process revolves. If one misses an important enough condition, event, or circumstance, the whole discharge plan becomes unstable. In addition, allocation of resources may be inappropriate, which ultimately affects the utilization management activities. At best, much confusion results and last-minute changes may be needed, sometimes delaying discharge for 1 or 2 days. A case manager once worked hard to set up a complex discharge, complete with high-tech equipment, only to discover at the last minute that the patient's house had no electricity. This was a troublesome situation and was caused by misattention to details. At worst, an inaccurate or poor assessment can lead to an unsafe discharge plan and a possible lawsuit. A complete and concise evaluation of all data is key to holistic and individualized management of the patient. Time spent performing a careful in-depth assessment may be time and money saved

later. Backtracking and changing plans can be confusing and frustrating for the patient and/or family, leaving them perhaps less than confident with the idea of case management.

There are several sources for assessment information. The patient is the primary contributor of data, which include medical, social, functional, financial, historical, and other types of data. If the patient is incapable of an interview, secondary sources can be used, starting with the patient's closest support system: parents and/or foster parents (especially if the patient is a minor), spouse, significant other, adult children, other family members, close friends, and neighbors. When using surrogate sources for information, it is important to ensure that the plan will incorporate what the patient might desire. For example, case managers and other healthcare providers must incorporate in the plan the wishes and interests the patient and/or family has communicated previously to a healthcare proxy or in an advance directive.

Sources for medical information include the family physician and related office records, hospital and ancillary medical staff, and hospital records (both past and present), any supervisory care staff and related medical records, and home health personnel and related records. Dental, hearing, and vision records may also be helpful. Other types of important data can be gathered from physical, occupational, and speech therapists; social workers and discharge planners; and psychiatric nurses.

The patient's home environment is a crucial piece to evaluate for safe discharge planning. Sometimes the insurance company social worker or case manager has visited the patient's home for evaluation purposes and can be asked to share the findings from that review. Other important people who make home visits are therapists, home health nurses, social workers, and psychiatric nurses. They may contribute data needed for a safe discharge plan.

The patient's employer can often be helpful in evaluating the patient's functional capacity before the current illness or event. Care must be taken not to violate confidentialities.

Sometimes in the course of gathering information, conflicting stories are revealed. These contradictions can show up in medical records in which several different physicians are charting medical, social, and functional data. Inconsistencies need further probing. The nature of the incongruity determines the route to clarification. Some contradictions clarify themselves; for example, a patient whose clinical picture is consistent with an alcohol problem may deny such a problem and then experience delirium tremens. In other cases, interviewing the sources of the conflicting data may be necessary. Care must be taken to avoid accusatory or confrontational tones as these make people defensive. The reason for the contradiction may be a seemingly insignificant typographic or dictating error. If resolution of the conflict is vital to the treatment plan (grandma wants full resuscitation measures taken versus only comfort care given), a family or even multidisciplinary team conference may be required to sort out the conflict.

A discussion of several assessment categories follows.

▶ Patient's History and Demographics

▶ Note the patient's name, age, ethnic group, address, marital status, children (with ages), employment, languages spoken, educational level, and religion.

▶ Note all medical history. Most hospital charts contain a "History and Physical" section. This may or may not be comprehensive. A thorough medical history may include all previous diagnoses, diseases, childhood diseases, serious/chronic illness, accidents, injuries, hospitalizations, surgeries, obstetric procedures, and mental health.

▶ Look for complicating factors, chronicity, and comorbidities.

▶ Look at noncompliance issues. They can often be uncovered in the history. Reasons for noncompliance can be explored and hopefully altered. Noncompliance has many causes, some of which can be resolved, such as lack of money for medications and lack of understanding or education about the disease process. Other reasons for noncompliance make behavioral changes more difficult. These reasons can range from burn-out caused by the chronicity of a disease to an "I don't care" attitude (sometimes so severe it appears to be a form of passive suicide).

▶ Note all medications the patient is taking, including over-the-counter drugs, illicit drugs, alcohol, and herbal preparations.

▶ Look at family histories for possible diabetes, cancer, Alzheimer's disease, heart disease, hypertension, epilepsy, sickle cell disease, renal disease, alcoholism, mental illness, and others.

▶ Be aware of allergies: food, drug, and environmental.

▶ Evaluate how your patient uses care facilities. Is he or she inconsistent in the use of medical resources? For example, does your patient rush

to the emergency department when the clinical condition could be taken care of at a lesser level, such as in the physician's office?

▶ Be familiar with the use of nontraditional or holistic modalities. People are increasingly using alternative healing methods, especially patients with incurable diseases or chronic conditions not helped by traditional medicine.

The following are some of the many forms of alternative healing therapies:

Homeopathy	Biomagnetics	Naturopathic
Imagery	Chiropractic	Vitamins/minerals
Acupuncture	Acupressure	Reiki
Shiatsu	Tai chi	Ayurvedic medicine
Reflexology	Prayer	Massage
Herbology	Rolfing	Medicine wheel
Crystal healing	Meditation	Energy healing
Laying on of hands	Bioacoustics	Myotherapy
Sound therapy	Feldenkrais	Biofeedback
Bach flower remedies		

Although many give no credence to alternative healing methods, the National Institutes of Health (NIH) in Washington, DC, has a designated budget for the study of "unconventional" methods of healing. Several medical schools, including Harvard University and the University of Arizona, also offer courses on alternative medicine. Some of the alternative therapies are thousands of years old, and new forms and variations of them are cropping up. It is recommended that case managers have knowledge of some of these modalities, because more patients are using them. Many outcomes studies are taking place to find exactly why millions of patients are willing to spend billions of out-of-pocket dollars on nontraditional healing. Some forms of alternative therapies, although very limited, are being reimbursed by insurance companies, and case managers should be aware of them and their impact on patients' choices of therapy. Examples include chiropractic care and acupuncture.

▶ Current Medical Status

If the patient is at home, interviewing home health professionals can be useful to assess a patient's medical status. Such professionals include physical, occupational, and speech therapists as well as home health nurses, social workers, aides, and homemakers. The family physician may also be able to provide helpful information. If part of your job responsibilities includes a physical appraisal, a head-to-toe assessment can be done.

If the patient is in the hospital or a SNF, all available data can be used: medical charts including laboratory results; special test results; radiographs; MRIs and computed tomography (CT) scans; vital signs; progress notes; nurse notes; physical, occupational, and speech therapist notes; consultations; respiratory therapist notes; surgical reports; allergies; medications, and your personal observations.

The following steps should also be taken.

▶ Assess utilization review modalities. Use of intensity of service/severity of illness criteria, InterQual or Milliman Guidelines, or critical pathways should be reviewed. This alerts the case manager to possible needs for changing the level of care, and it may also be necessary for insurance authorization of resources.

▶ Find out the patient's health goals and major health concerns.

▶ Check assessments of direct care nurses and other care providers.

▶ Evaluate diets. Does the patient follow a special diet for health conditions, religious purposes, or personal preference? Is the diet adequate or is a dietary consultation needed?

▶ Evaluate all skin conditions.

▶ If the patient is in acute care, determine what tubes, catheters, and equipment will continue at discharge. Are urinary catheters, tracheostomies and suction machines and supplies, jejunostomy (J-tube) and gastrostomy tube care, drains, feeding tubes, intravenous (IV) or feeding tube pumps, medication pumps (e.g., insulin), oxygen, and miscellaneous ostomy supplies required? Is any wound care needed?

▶ Review medications. Is the medicine regimen complicated enough to require a visiting nurse to help coordinate and educate about proper intake? Do medications such as anticoagulants and isoniazid require laboratory studies? Assess any over-the-counter drugs for possible problems. Assess patient compliance in the use of medications. Can the patient afford the medications? Is there a problem getting transportation to the pharmacy?

▶ Assess bowel and bladder incontinence.

▶ Analyze patient understanding of conditions and educational needs pertaining to diagnosis/illness.

▶ Assess patient's views and interests pertaining to advance directives. Does the patient have a designated healthcare proxy? Has the patient made his wishes known regarding end-of-life care, do-not-resuscitate status, and withdrawal of life support and nutritional support?

▶ Nutritional Assessment

Proper nutrition is an important factor in a person's health status; it contributes to positive health outcomes and saves healthcare dollars if managed carefully. It is common knowledge that proper nutrition can delay the onset of many health conditions from heart attacks to osteoporosis; early nutritional assessment and intervention is the key to prevention of many complications once a patient is ill. Long-term marginal nutritional status may be the cause of many (or most) of the problems in healthcare today and certainly contributes to functional and cognitive decline.

Nutritional assessments are required by accreditation organizations in most levels of care. The Joint Commission (TJC) requires a nutritional screening within 24 hours of admission to any TJC-accredited facility. This includes nutritional assessment of patients with known nutrition problems (e.g., obesity, anorexia, etc.) or those identified as being at significant risk of a nutritional deficiency (e.g., recent weight loss or gain of 10 pounds or more). Interdisciplinary nutritional care plans are also expected (TJC, 2008). Case managers in other settings (e.g., home care and SNF) are also required to perform nutritional screening.

Research indicates that malnutrition is a serious problem: 30% to 50% of hospitalized patients are malnourished, and 70% of SNF patients are malnourished (Wellman, 1997). Annually, almost 17 million patients are treated for conditions that place them in a high-risk category for malnutrition. Outcome research indicates that personalized nutrition therapy can decrease healthcare costs. Of the 10 leading causes of disease, eight are related to nutrition. Studies document that poorly nourished patients require care for longer periods, have higher complication rates, have higher mortality rates, and require more frequent readmissions and emergency care. In one study by the American Dietetic Association involving approximately 2,400 disease state cases throughout the United States, nutritional therapy saved an average of more than $8,000 per patient (Gibbons, 1998).

Case managers must identify various nutritional needs such as home delivery of meals, assistance with shopping or cooking, or nutritional education; case managers also must be able to assess risk factors for malnutrition. Collaborative work with registered dietitians is worth the effort. Registered dietitians are usually on staff at major hospitals or they also can be accessed by contacting the American Dietetic Association.

NOTE

The American Dietetic Association
Web site: www.eatright.org
Address and Contact Information:

Headquarters
120 South Riverside Plaza, Suite 2000
Chicago, IL 60606-6995
Telephone: (800) 877-1600
Washington, DC Office
1120 Connecticut Avenue NW, Suite 480
Washington, DC 20036
Telephone: (800) 877-087

The following represents some nutritional risk factors. Much of the information can be found in the patient's medical records.

▸ Inadequate or inappropriate food intake: Each diagnosis requires its own variation of foods that can and cannot be tolerated. Compliance with the proper diet is a common problem. Case managers can examine the frequency, amount, and quality of choices for food intake. Is it too little or too much? Is the food of the wrong type (pretzels and fast-food pizza in congestive heart failure patients)? Assess for other issues such as alcohol abuse.

▸ Financial issues: Quality food costs money. Vitamins, minerals, and herbs often touted as helpful are not covered under health insurance plans. Some impoverished people will pay rent and utilities and have little money left for food. Stories are common about elderly people living on cat/dog food or spending the little money they have on food for their pets and leave themselves to starve or eat poorly; unfortunately, these stories are often true.

▸ Social isolation: This can cause a decreased desire to eat; some people hate to eat alone. It can also cause depression, which often results in low appetite levels.

▸ Dental/mouth assessment: If eating is a major source of aggravation or pain due to lack of teeth, poorly fitting dentures, or other mouth

and gum problems, the end result could be decreased nutritional levels.

▸ Ability and disability: Can the patients shop for food? Are they able to prepare food and clean up after the meal?

▸ Weight loss and gain: Has the patient gained or lost 10 pounds recently? A recent change in body weight of 10 pounds is strongly associated with functional and instrumental ADLs; it is also associated with increased healthcare costs (Wellman, 1997). Assess the adequacy of food intake, new prescription or over-the-counter medications, and changed mental or functional status. Certain medications cause nutritional deficiencies and should be assessed carefully. Did the patient have a recent trauma, infection, or surgery that required an additional load of calories? Were the additional needed calories supplied?

▸ Acute and chronic diseases: Assess the patient's history and present health state for clues. Look for major diagnoses, being over- or underweight, mental health issues, and dental and mouth problems.

▶ Medication Assessment

Medication assessment is a part of nearly all other types of assessments in this chapter. Its contribution to health or morbidity cannot be overemphasized. In every level of care, pharmaceuticals must be examined, and this responsibility belongs to many professionals, including physicians, nurses, case managers, pharmacists, and even dietitians. The Institute of Medicine reports that more than 100,000 Americans die in hospitals annually in the United States from adverse medication reactions, both prescription and over-the-counter. In addition, 2.1 million people suffer serious medication-related complications such as gastric bleeding, cardiac irregularities, and allergies.

Case managers should review medications—prescriptive, herbal, and over-the-counter—and carefully assess if the physician or pharmacist should be consulted. Some medication issues to consider include:

▸ Review all allergies.
▸ Review for polypharmacy and consult the physician and/or pharmacist if a problem is possible.
▸ Assess if the patient is taking medications according to physician orders. Assess for general compliance.
▸ Assess lack of transportation as a cause of not obtaining ordered medications.

▶ Assess financial problems as a cause of not obtaining ordered medications. Are generic equivalents a possibility? Would a change to generic make it more feasible for the patient to buy the medication?

▶ Assess insurance for pharmacy benefits.

▶ Assess for adverse interactions and contraindications.

▶ Assess for adverse reactions to common food. Is the patient aware of the potential for an adverse reaction? For example, one common medication was determined to be unsafe when taken with grapefruit juice. Several people became ill before this was discovered.

▶ Because many medications require laboratory monitoring such as anticoagulants, check that scheduled appointments to monitor serum levels or other pertinent blood work are attended.

▶ Assess if the medications are prescribed at the lowest effective dose.

▶ Assess if the supplied medications use the simplest dosing regimen. Sometimes a medication has been taken for many years; meanwhile, advancements have occurred that would allow more simplified dosing.

▶ Assess if the most effective routes have been prescribed for the medications.

▶ Assess whether the medication containers are accessible (e.g., not all arthritic patients can open child-proof containers).

▶ Assess patients with renal or hepatic problems to see if they are taking medications that do not clear through those vital organs.

▶ Carefully assess for educational deficits about medications. Does the patient know:
  1. The name of the medication.
  2. The purpose of the medication.
  3. The dosage of the medication.
  4. The frequency/timing of administration of the medication.
  5. The relationship between taking the medication and meals.
  6. Adverse side effects that require a call to the doctor.
  7. The administration method of the medication: chewed, sublingual, swallowed, swish-and-swallow, crushed, through the feeding tube, etc.

Provide simple explanatory handouts about the medications when necessary. Medication calendars or prepackaging in "Medi-set" containers is often the answer.

▶ Financial Assessment

▶ Does the patient have inadequate insurance coverage or no coverage?

▶ Have you checked for any governmental entitlements (Medicare, Medicaid, Supplemental Security Income [SSI], Social Security Disability [SSD])?

▶ Can the patient/family meet copayments and deductibles?

▶ Can the patient/family pay for necessary supplies, medications, and miscellaneous items not covered by insurance?

▶ If necessary, can the family contribute toward a SNF placement or supplemental home help?

▶ Can the patient meet basic financial obligations (rent, utilities, food) during this illness?

▶ If the patient must be discharged with high-tech equipment, can he or she afford the additional utilities? For example, some air-flow beds may increase electric bills up to $200 per month. Patients on fixed incomes cannot usually afford this monthly increase.

▶ Functional Assessment: Environmental Factors

It is very important to assess for patient safety in discharge planning. Was the patient safe and at an adequate level of care before this event? Many elderly patients fall in the home and are admitted to hospitals. If hospitalization has been caused by an unsafe home environment, can it be modified for safety or is a more supervised setting needed?

It is also vital to look at the patient's level of independence. How well did the patient perform functional tasks before this event? Was he or she independent in all ADL and ambulatory, or was there a prior psychomotor deficit?

THE HOME ENVIRONMENT ASSESSMENT

The home environment assessment is a key activity for safe discharge planning. The following should be checked:

▶ Stairs: Can the patient get into and out of the house or apartment safely? Are there stairs inside that the patient needs to negotiate?

▶ Telephone: Telephone communication is especially important to consider if the patient lives alone or is alone for several hours at a time. Can the patient see and hear adequately to use the telephone? If not, can adaptations be readily made?

▸ Toilet, tub, and shower: Check for conditions and safe access. Does the patient require the use of an elevated toilet seat or bars in the shower and tub for assistance in mobilization? Is the floor condition unsafe? Does it place the patient at risk for slipping, falling, or tripping?

▸ Utilities: Check electricity, heat, fans, and air conditioning to ensure that they are in working order. Many older people are admitted to hospitals with dehydration or heat stroke in the summer and with pneumonia in winter, both caused by poor environmental conditions. Gas heaters and heat from gas stoves are often major fire hazards. Is the electrical wiring safe for the DME use?

▸ Sanitation: Are running water, working toilets, and clean conditions available? Are rodents or roaches a problem? We have seen more than one patient readmitted with maggots invading postsurgical wounds, caused by poor sanitary conditions.

▸ Equipment needs: Does the patient have a bed? Does he or she require a special hospital bed, other DME, a Hoyer lift, or portable ramps?

ADL ASSESSMENT

Both prior and present self-care deficits and present learning capabilities are to be noted. If the patient is currently less independent in daily activities than at a prior time, discharge compensations may be needed. The discharge disposition must match and compensate for the patient's deficits. The following questions about the patient's capability for self-care must be addressed:

▸ Can the patient dress and undress?
▸ Can the patient put on vision and hearing aids and stump prosthesis?
▸ Does the patient have the ability to perform the following hygiene tasks:

▸ Bathing.
▸ Shaving.
▸ Brushing teeth or dentures.
▸ Testing temperature of bath or shower water.
▸ Entering and exiting the tub/shower safely.
▸ Lowering and raising self from toilet.
▸ Cleaning self after elimination?

▸ Can the patient handle nutritional needs: shopping for and preparing food, using utensils, chewing, and swallowing? Is extra help needed, such as for shopping and food preparation or perhaps Meals on Wheels?
▸ Is the patient able to do housekeeping and yard work?

▸ Can the patient take prescription medications as ordered or is the task too complicated, requiring home health nurse supervision? Are wrong doses or expired medications still in the patient's possession?

▸ Can the patient handle transportation needs to get to the store, pharmacy, or place of worship?

▸ Does the patient have balance and coordination problems? Does he or she tend to fall or have difficulty with motor skills?

▸ What is the patient's ability to see, hear, speak, read, and write? Is his or her native tongue English? Are translators or bilingual nurses needed?

▸ If patient uses a wheelchair, is this a new development? Is the previous dwelling accessible to the wheelchair? If not, can modifications be made or does the patient need to change living arrangements? Is the wheelchair the correct size and type, with properly fitting cushions and trays?

▸ Does the patient know how to telephone for emergency services? This is especially important in areas without 911 capabilities. Does the patient have telephone numbers for utility companies and medical equipment supply companies in case of equipment malfunction or a need for medical supplies?

▸ The big question—is safe home care a possibility for this patient? (The psychosocial assessment is the other major factor that affects the patient's ability to be discharged home safely).

▸ Psychosocial Assessment

In the psychosocial part of the assessment process, the case manager treats the whole family unit as the patient. The family, significant other, and close friends are an extension of the patient, and all needs and desires should be heard. The family's effect on the patient is too important to overlook. In some social cultures, the extended family is a primary social unit; the parents are the decision makers and not the patient.

A relationship does not necessarily exist between the severity of the illness and psychological functioning; therefore, the patient's response to the illness or event must be assessed, along with the family's adjustment to it. This is most important in the case of a chronic illness that is life-altering in nature, especially when it is a new diagnosis.

▸ What other stresses are taking a toll in the patient's family life at the time of the illness? These possibilities include divorce, moving, a death in the family, job change/loss, or a new baby. What family dynamics are revealed? How do the patient and family usually cope with stress? These methods can include religious activities, meditation, sports, talking with friends or a professional counselor, anger, physical violence, and the use of alcohol and drugs. Even if the family dynamics were functional and safe before this event, will they continue to be so now?

▶ Who is at home? If the patient is a single mother, are the children safe? If the patient is a casualty of the "sandwich generation" and is responsible for caring for an ill parent, who is caring for that parent now? If the patient is elderly, is there a spouse (or other relative) at home who is unable to care for his or her own needs without the patient's assistance? Are there pets at home that need attention?

▶ Assess the family for exhaustion and burn-out. Can respite care be provided to help ease the burden?

▶ Ask about hobbies and recreational activities. One case manager once shared with us that she had a chronically ill patient who loved to sew as a diversion, but she lost an arm. With her primary form of entertainment made so much more difficult, the case manager needed to find another way for her to relax. For this type of situation, it is necessary to explore other relaxation outlets.

▶ Assess the formal support system. Is it adequate, inadequate, lacking, or dysfunctional?

▶ Assess the patient's informal resources such as neighbors, church or synagogue groups, friends, and relatives. Can these be expanded if more help at home is needed?

▶ School or employment records may be assessed as appropriate or if job placement is part of your particular case management responsibilities. Patient or family-signed release forms may be required. School records may be necessary if dealing with a pediatric patient.

▶ Assess the patient's level of care before current illness. Can the patient return to the same environment, or is short- or long-term SNF or subacute rehabilitation care needed? Do the people associated with the previous living arrangement agree to have the patient discharged back into their care? Some even family members have reached their limit, but the decision to send the patient to a SNF is a challenging one, especially when the patient is

fairly lucid and wants to go home. Early intervention with family or team conferences should begin.

▶ Secondary gains to illness often serve conscious or unconscious needs. Some patients do not want to get well. They like the special attention from family and medical staff. Some feel it is a way to gain power over others. For others, dependency needs are met while ill. For still others, a hospital stay represents a warm or cool place to sleep and eat. Occasionally, the hospital is a refuge—a safe place—where a parent or spouse cannot abuse them. Patients such as these are often the "frequent fliers," who are admitted regularly for exacerbations of their basic problem (often rotating from hospital to hospital). A psychiatric consultation with possible referrals to outpatient support groups may assist such persons. Depending on the problem, an Adult Protective/Child Protective Services referral may be needed. If the patient is homeless, referrals to shelters may help or, preferably, a social service plan can provide a more permanent solution.

▶ Cognitive or mental status assessment may be needed. Not infrequently, a patient at home or in a hospital desires an unsafe or detrimental disposition (in the medical team's professional judgment). If that person is otherwise alert and oriented, ancillary assistance may be all you can provide. If the person's mental capacity is in question, the next step would be a psychiatric referral to evaluate the patient's judgment, competence, and orientation. If the psychologist or psychiatrist feels this person is incompetent, court action may be necessary, especially in the case of a patient without a healthcare proxy, or one who has no family members or other relatives. Mental incompetence sometimes must be verified in a court of law.

▶ The brick wall syndrome. Occasionally, a psychosocial situation occurs in which a very ill patient requires intensive care, 24 hours a day. Family members insist that they can handle the patient at home. Your instincts as the case manager are that it will not work, that the family will not be able to get enough rest, or that the patient may not be cared for adequately. Families have the right to try to care for their loved one, and all necessary equipment and available help can be provided. Many times, after this plan has been implemented, reality sets in. The family members "hit the brick wall" and realize that they are unable to handle the care of the patient alone, and therefore, request SNF placement. If there is a considerable chance that the home placement will not succeed, making necessary copies of the medical record for a SNF placement before the chart goes to the hospital records department may ease and speed a transfer request by the family. Suggestions for supervisory homes may also be given to the family just in case.

▶ Cultural and Religious Diversity

To provide appropriate case management services, the case manager must be aware of cultural and religious differences; this is both confusing and gratifying. Evaluate patients according to their beliefs, value systems, and traditions.

- ▶ Gestures: Nonverbal body language is an important communication method. However, this is not always clear when caring for individuals from various cultures. The same gesture may mean "good-bye" in one culture and "come here" in another. A smile and a nod "yes" may not indicate agreement, but rather the wish to be polite and respectful.

- ▶ Language barriers: This reaches beyond simply not speaking the same language. Misunderstood basic language concepts can hinder the case manager relationship. Ruth Beebe Hill (1979) writes in her introduction to *Hanta Yo:*

  > Admit, assume, because, believe, could, doubt, end, effect, faith, forget, forgive, guilt, how, it, mercy, pest, promise, should, sorry, storm, them, us, waste, we, weed—neither these words nor the conceptions for which they stand appear in this book; they are the Whiteman's import to the New World, the newcomer's contribution to the vocabulary of the man he called Indian. Truly, the parent Indian families possessed neither these terms nor their equivalents.
  >
  > The word "maybe" is another concept not readily understood by some Native American tribes, and use of this word may instill lack of trust in a relationship.

- ▶ Cultural traditions, differences, and taboos: Some people do not approve of eye contact, either feeling that it is impolite or believing that it robs them of their spirit. Others do not like casual touching. Silence is essential in some cultures and uncomfortable in others.

Some ethnic groups are uncomfortable discussing topics that medical professionals and case managers may consider necessary. In some cultures, healthcare decisions are the responsibility of the elder family members (parents/grandparents) rather than of the patient. Expressions of pain, from stoic to expressive, vary among different cultures. Knowledge that the patient may be acting stoically can help you to determine how to offer optimum comfort.

- ▶ Religious and spiritual beliefs: For some, the spiritual belief system is a major source of strength. Assess the feasibility of pastoral/rabbinical visits or tapes and reading material for spiritual nourishment. If daily prayer or meditation was previously an important part of the patient's life, an effort to include time alone without interruption could be arranged for this purpose.

  Some religious practices may affect healthcare subtly, such as dietary practices or beliefs that illness is a punishment from God. Overt practices, such as the Jehovah's Witness's rejection of blood transfusions, can affect the treatment plan and have far-reaching consequences. Consideration should be given to all spiritual and cultural differences because they can affect the patient–case manager relationship.

- ▶ Cultural and religious conflicts within the individual. Humanity is in the global information age. Cultures are merging, and information on anything is at one's "beck and call." This can create conflicts within people. An example of such a conflict is below.

  > A large Navajo tribe lives in Arizona. A Navajo newspaper reporter once wrote about this conflict when her father died.
  >
  > Like most Navajos, she follows the Earth-based traditional faith of Hozho—a concept about beauty, stability, and order—yet traditional Christianity also plays a strong role in her life and the lives of many of her extended Navajo family. It took her 4 years to write about the conflict. During her father's illness and struggle with Parkinson's disease, she prayed to and cursed two gods—the Christian God and the Holy People, who show themselves as lightning, dawn, rain, wind, snow, water, and fog.
  >
  > She asked much of her Christian God during the difficult college years; *maybe she asked too much and used up her quota of assistance. Maybe she was being punished for holding on to her Navajo beliefs.* Among taboos of the Navajos are avoid contact with dead bodies, do not stare straight into a person's eye, never

drive away from a coyote that crosses your path without sprinkling corn pollen in his tracks, and never say harsh words because they have the power to kill. *Maybe the Holy People were punishing her for not covering her eyes quickly enough during a bloody scene she had to witness for her newspaper job. Maybe the power of words (which she uses to craft her work) has caused harm to Navajos or others.*

During the burial process, many other conflicts arose. Her father was a traditional Navajo who never saw the inside of a Christian church; he followed the way of the Holy People. Traditional ceremonies for the dead do not mesh well with hermetically sealed coffins that preserve dead bodies for many years. The Christian and traditional factions of the family had differing needs.

At times, providing culturally relevant care may be better left outside the realm of case management. The above conflict was solved among a large family in their own unique way. However, case managers must be aware of these conflicts, be prepared to not fully understand, and yet be nonjudgmental and supportive when these issues arise. If, by chance, you have personal cultural knowledge to assist more fully, then your patients are indeed fortunate.

NOTE

Some resources about cultural competencies include:

MINORITY HEALTH RESOURCES

Office of Minority Health Resource Center
Families USA
The Voice for Health Care Consumers
1201 New York Avenue NW, Suite 1100
Washington, DC 20005
Telephone: 202-628-3030
E-mail: info@familiesusa.org
Web sites: http://www.familiesusa.org
http://www.familiesusa.org/issues/minority-health/resource-center/

CULTURE, HEALTH, AND LITERACY

Office of Minority Health Resource Center (OMHRC)
P.O. Box 37337
Washington, DC 20013-7337
Telephone: 800-444-6472
E-mail: info@omhrc.gov
Web site: http://www.omhrc.gov/

▶ Care Planning Activities

Some types of case management require care plans. A care plan is a written agreement that spells out actual and potential case problems (patient's and family's), goals, timing, and funding according to the assessment of the case's strengths and weaknesses. Because of the unique needs of each patient, care planning must be customized for each situation. The care plan is based on the comprehensive assessment performed by the case manager and on the patient's/family's preferences. Care planning is a collaborative activity that must include the case manager, the patient/family unit, the physician(s), and other pertinent members of the multi-disciplinary team, including the social worker, the physical therapist, occupational therapist, home care nurse and so on. The care plan should include:

- ▶ Actual and potential problems.
- ▶ Patient/family/physician preferences.
- ▶ Problem-oriented goals and outcomes.
- ▶ Potential services required to achieve the goals; this may be from paid services and/or unpaid family or other sources of support.
- ▶ A timetable to reach the goals, including a section on the persons responsible for each goal: the case manager, patient, physician, family, friends, church group, home health agency, etc.
- ▶ The interventions and treatments necessary (indicated by the patient's health condition and situation) to achieve the goals and outcomes.
- ▶ Estimated costs and who is responsible for these costs.

After the care plan has been written, the next step is implementation of the case management actions. This includes such activities as referrals, negotiations, monitoring, utilization management, communication and coordination with all necessary professionals/family/patient, educating the patient and family for self-care and to maximize independence, and anticipating changes in health status. The care plan is also a living document that can change as the patient's health status and situation improve or deteriorate.

▶ Screening and Assessment Tools

Assessment and screening are related tasks, but there are some distinctions. Assessment is the process of gathering information about a patient to determine needs—clinical, physiological, financial, social, psychological, educational, discharge (or postdischarge), and others. From the assessment, the case manager determines which case management interventions will likely assist the patient to the greatest degree. Experts have formulated several assessment tools that cover many of the categories for a thorough assessment. Some organizations either modify standard assessment tools or write their own for customized needs. The tools can be a good "reminder system" so that basic assessment areas do not get missed during the interview. Assessment tools can bring to light patient problems; they assess the patient's present situation and future needs.

Screening tools identify beneficiaries/individuals who are at risk for potential health problems. They can "predict" future problems. Health risk assessments (HRAs) are essentially screening tools and are also used in a predictive way. HRAs identify lifestyle behaviors, such as smoking or not wearing seatbelts, which could put the person at high risk for illness or injury. They also identify genetic predispositions, such as height versus weight ratios and short/bald/male. HRAs can assist the case manager in pinpointing high-risk populations.

The SF (short form) 36 or 12 is an example of a screening tool. The use of the Health Status Survey (SF-12 or SF-36) has gained credibility in the healthcare arena. The Health Status Survey is a patient's self-assessment of perceived quality-of-life issues and has been proven to be a predictive tool that may indicate a potential for a hospital admission in the next 6 to 12 months. Physicians have often ignored patients' perceptions of their health when determining medical care; patients' perceptions were considered "soft" data, compared with the "hard" (or objective and quantifiable) data of laboratory results and CAT scans. The SF-36/12 tool has changed that. The importance of considering perspectives has been documented by John E. Ware, Jr., PhD, and the Health Outcomes Trust. The Health Status Survey is used to determine the patients' health status perspective on eight dimensions of functioning that are considered critical to quality of life. Data taken from many years of using this tool have determined that there is a definite correlation between people's perception of their health and the potential for hospital admission within 6 to 12 months. By early utilization of this tool and early identification of possible problems, a disease management plan can be implemented to attempt to avoid or delay progression of disease and increased use of emergency department visits or hospitalization. This tool can be administered early in the case management process; it can then be readministered at 6-month intervals to assess the patient's perception of his or her health curve.

There are various health status tools. The SF tools are perhaps the most commonly used in healthcare. The numbers, 12 or 36, describe the number of survey questions for the patient to answer; an SF-8 has also been tested and found valid and reliable. The SF-12 takes about 2 minutes to complete. According to experts, the SF-12 and 8, although shorter, are as predictive as the SF-36 in determining use of future healthcare resources. Scoring of the results is most easily done by a proprietary computer program, but can be done manually for smaller groups.

The eight domains of health assessed in the health status survey follow.

1. Physical functioning assesses a range of physical activities such as self-care, walking, climbing stairs, and performing vigorous activities.
2. Role physical assesses the effects of physical health on the patient's life roles and regular daily activities.
3. Bodily pain assesses the severity of bodily pain and its interference with work inside or outside the home.
4. General health assesses perception of general health, health outlook, and resistance to illness.
5. Vitality assesses the frequency of feeling tired versus energetic.
6. Social functioning assesses the extent and frequency of limitations in social activities due to health problems.
7. Role emotional assesses the effects of emotional problems on the patient's life roles and regular daily activities.
8. Mental health assesses anxiety, depression, and loss of behavioral/emotional control versus psychological well-being.

One caution about the health status tools is that data were collected on large groups of people. Therefore, they are more predictive on a group or population scale; they are not as accurate on an individual scale. Another general caution is that even the best of the screening instruments are not 100% accurate all the time. The case manager must use all the knowledge and judgment at his or her disposal to form a total picture to determine the best course of action.

▶ STAGE III: DEVELOPMENT AND COORDINATION OF THE CASE PLAN

If assessment aids the case manager in deciding where to go with a particular case, then Stage III helps the case manager to choose the best way to get there. In this stage, the needs and services are matched into a seamless plan based on the assessment data and the desires of the patient and family/caregiver. Creativity is the keynote at this point; often there is more than one "best" way to do something. Maintaining a patient/family-centered approach to care coordination is essential for choosing what is best for the case. Flexibility is another important factor; the patient and family may desire changes, or the patient's condition may change. Amending the plan based on these changes is necessary for meeting the goals designed for the case. It also is essential for maintaining a case plan that is relevant to current condition of the patient. Here is where the role of patient advocate becomes most evident. Creatively finding ways to meet the basic needs of your patient is reflected in quality treatment and discharge plans. The "gift" a patient advocate gives to the patient is a case plan that promotes the patient's optimal level of self-care and control over his or her life.

The case manager has just spent many hours amassing a thorough clinical and psychosocial assessment. The patient's individual strengths, weaknesses, resources, and lack of resources have been identified. Now the multidisciplinary team, which can include several professionals such as the case manager, social worker, physical or occupational therapist, pharmacist, patient, family/caregiver, physician, payor, and others in the patient's case, must decide the following:

▶ What needs to be done.
▶ How best to do it.
▶ Who will provide necessary services.
▶ When each need will be met.
▶ Where and when the next level of care will be provided.
▶ How the patient/family can best manage after discharge (post this episode of care).

For this planning stage to be successful, the patient and family must actively participate in all decisions, including any changes in the case plan. If the patient or family is not in agreement with the plan, it most likely will not be successful. The family can add to a successful plan by identifying any informal resources that may be needed to fill in the gaps. These informal resources may be friends, neighbors, or volunteers from religious organizations or community agencies.

▶ Establishing Goals

The first step in this stage of coordinating and developing treatment and discharge plans is establishing goals. What must be accomplished by when? For example, the family must agree on a SNF for grandmother, and all transfer details must be approved and completed within 72 hours, assuming that the patient is stable for transfer.

Most goals are composed of many smaller goals or tasks that must be met for successful completion of the main goal. Missed details can delay or hinder the smooth sequence and progression of the case plan. Objectives such as home safety at discharge or the promotion of an optimal level of independence for the patient may require two, three, a dozen, or more modifications in the home setting to make the goal of home safety a reality. Grandmother's transfer to the SNF may consist of several tasks, such as finding an appropriate SNF, finding a physician who will follow-up at the SNF, setting up appropriate transportation and DME, copying all the necessary medical records, notifying the family of transfer time, obtaining physician's orders for her care at the SNF, coordinating transportation to the SNF, and obtaining reports from the multidisciplinary team. The ultimate goal of case management is quality of care and efficient use of resources. This entire book is dedicated to the smaller tasks needed to ensure that these two major goals will be met.

Establishing long-term and short-term goals may also be required. Consider short-term goals for a previously independent, elderly gentleman who recently had total hip replacement surgery. These goals may include the removal of all tubes and drains, stable blood tests, transfer from bed to a chair with assistance, and walking a few steps with assistance. This man's long-term goals—possibly in a SNF—may be walking 300 feet or more with a walker or cane and independence in ADLs, which would allow the patient to return home safely.

▶ Prioritizing Needs and Goals

The second step in the planning stage is to prioritize the needs and goals that were assessed. Again, the patient's and family's input is insightful here. What is their idea of the most pressing problem? Each person views life and adversity from his or her own perspective and value system. A "can't live without" for one person might be a minor irritation to someone else.

There may be times when the patient's or family's idea of a priority problem does not match the professional staff member's idea of a priority. One case manager had a case that involved an elderly lady who was in the terminal stage of cancer. While the case manager, physicians, and social worker repeatedly tried to speak to the daughter about hospice care, the daughter focused on her mother's dental cavity. The prospect of hospice was too much for this daughter, so she narrowed down the problem into something she could handle. Sometimes hard reality is just too overwhelming. Starting to work with the patient and family at their stage of acceptance of a health condition, diagnosis of a terminal illness, or prognosis is necessary to get to the most important discussions or decisions regarding the case plan. Neglecting this makes it too much of a challenge to address the important issues. This strategy allows the patient and family to be more involved in the care and the related decisions.

At other times, families or patients may adamantly disagree with the assessed priority needs. An alert and oriented elderly lady may insist on going home alone, when a short-term SNF placement is the obvious safe choice. Perhaps a patient is readmitted to the acute care level within 1 week of discharge. During the first admission, the family and patient refused services that the case manager deemed a priority and in need of immediate attention. Through education and negotiation, a revised plan may be successful the second time.

Some limiting factors often narrow the choices, which may make prioritization of treatments and activities easier but treatment and discharge plans less than optimal. Consider financial and insurance resource allocation and limitations. The limitation may be as simple as the fact that the health insurance company will not pay for both a front-wheeled walker and a wheelchair, which both the patient and case manager feel are needed. On the other hand, the limitation may be as critical as a need for bone marrow transplantation with no payor source. Therefore, concentrating on conditions that can be improved is one way to prioritize. Because not all circumstances can be "fixed," the focus should be on attaining the best quality of life possible.

▶ Service Planning and Resource Allocation

After priority goals have been ascertained, the case manager compensates for assessed deficits, fills in healthcare gaps, and reduces duplication through coordination of services. This third step, service planning and resource allocation, requires knowledge of public and private organizations that may be helpful. Medical insurance companies are often the first place to try for funding needed services, and they usually consent to medically necessary requests. If your idea of medical necessity does not coincide with the insurance company's idea of medical necessity, you have the options of negotiating, speaking to the company's medical director for clarification, or finding other resources such as charitable agencies.

Resource allocation for a patient with no or inadequate health insurance is a challenge and requires creative case management. The second place to look is "informal" resources such as the patient's family,

friends, neighbors, community-based agencies and religious groups. Matching the patient with government entitlements such as Medicare, SSD, or Medicaid may be helpful, but may sometimes require long waiting periods. Geographically convenient resource books are a funnel of information for local social services. Make use of social service personnel, who sometimes can provide invaluable help.

The unique features of each case will determine the service planning and coordination details. If a patient can be independent with intensive education and a few follow-up home health visits for education and review of the skills taught, then education and home health are provided. If long-term placement is needed, a facility is matched with the patient's skill needs and available resources. If the family and multidisciplinary team agree that hospice and a duplication of the hospital room at home are required, the case manager will coordinate these services. Discharge plans can be simple or multifaceted and complex, but they are always personalized to meet the needs and interests of the patient and family.

Even with the best intentions and the most careful planning, changes, stops, and detours are common. During busy winter seasons, many SNFs and shelters may be full, with waiting lists of several days to several weeks. If one SNF gives you a "definite maybe" for 2 days hence, it may be good insurance to place the patient on a second waiting list that also meets with the family's approval. An unexpected deterioration (or improvement) in the patient's medical status may necessitate an entirely new service plan. A change of heart/mind of the family members may overthrow the plan. Sometimes families, overcome by guilt, refuse SNF placement at the last minute or, overcome by exhaustion, feel incapable of taking the patient home again. Family and team conferences should be convened as soon as possible to prevent additional unnecessary/avoidable hospital days. New goals and new plans may have to be evaluated.

With some patients who undergo planned, elective surgeries, discharge planning may be done before surgery. If complications occur and are serious enough, those plans may need reassessing. Anything can happen, so a "plan B" or an alternate plan is always a good idea. A "plan B" strategy keeps the case manager ahead of the game.

Coordinating treatments and services during a hospitalization is another important function of the case manager. Efficiency not only saves valuable resources but can also save entire hospital days. This may be accomplished in several ways. Clinical pathways are a chosen tool for decreasing lengths of stay. Observation for correct sequencing of tests can also prevent unnecessary additional hospital days. Most case managers have witnessed patients who have required barium clean-outs (sometimes requiring 2 days), when the barium tests could have been scheduled last on a list of diagnostic tests.

Several consultants treating one patient often make their own individual plans. The case manager can bring those plans into alignment to cause the least trauma to the patient. For example, if a patient needs major debridement for osteomyelitis and requires 6 weeks of intravenous (IV) antibiotics, the case manager can coordinate a long-term venous access placement to be done concurrently with the debridement. Perhaps a patient requires a TURP (genitourinary surgeon) and a hernia repair (general surgeon). If the patient and physicians are in agreement, a single coordinated surgery saves the patient from two general anesthesias, saves operating room time, saves postoperative hospital time, and cuts down on the use of miscellaneous resources. However, good clinical judgment is necessary when suggesting a "better way"; poor or unsafe suggestions at the very least diminish the case manager's credibility.

The team has assessed the problems, ascertained what needs to be done, orchestrated a time frame (pending medical stability of the patient), and determined the contributions and limitations of the health insurance company. Informal supports are verified and available. Referrals are in for SNFs, rehabilitation facilities, mental health facilities, home health agencies, community-based resources such as Meals on Wheels, and whatever else the patient needs. Transportation needs are assessed. DME is approved. Educational factors—what needs to be taught to whom—have been evaluated. This stage culminates when assessed needs are linked with chosen interventions and desired outcomes.

▶ STAGE IV: IMPLEMENTATION OF THE CASE PLAN

Implementation is the process of putting the plan into action. In the implementation of the plan, the patient's assessed needs have been linked with private and community services. The gaps are filled, there is no duplication of services, and the patient and support systems are in agreement with the case plan. The goal of this stage is to maximize the safety and well-being of the patient, using the most independent and necessary level of care. A cost-effective setting must match the patient's health condition, needs, capabilities, desires, and financial abilities. This is where the case manager shows a talent for coordination and facilitation. The

patient is now discharged home, transferred to a supervised setting, or remains in the same setting but with a more appropriate service and treatment plan because of case management.

By this stage in the case management process, the case manager has accurately assessed the patient's and family's needs. Weaknesses have been delineated and problems solved. The treatment plan may have made a few detours off the expected clinical path, but variances were expediently identified and promptly brought back in line. The total case has been assessed, reassessed, negotiated, and coordinated. The treatment and discharge plans are realistic and workable and have been approved by the multidisciplinary team, patient, family, and third-party payor.

The case manager has the companies and facilities chosen and the patient/family, team, and payor have approved the choices. All informal supports are in place. The case manager is comfortable that this plan will work, but still is flexible and has a pretty good idea what "plan B" might entail if needed. The team and family are depending on the case manager to take care of all the details and to get it right.

There are as many types of implementation of a case management plan as there are types of case management programs. For simplification purposes, this section will separate essential issues by the division of internal and external case managers.

▶ Internal case managers are those within a facility or agency, such as a hospital, acute rehabilitation facility, SNF, home health agency, or hospice; some refer to this as "within-the-walls" case management. Internal case managers are employed by the providers of care. They are on-site case managers.

▶ External case managers are those who work outside facilities, such as insurance/third-party payor case managers, health maintenance organization (HMO)/preferred provider organization (PPO) case managers, or those private/independent or contracted with self-insured plans or union groups. External case managers essentially work for payors of care. They often work telephonically and may also function on site according to contracts.

There are no distinct lines that can be drawn in the separations of duties below; all case managers may be responsible for any of these tasks. Knowing what is expected of you by your employer, the clients who refer the patients, and by state and federal laws, is essential for effective case management services.

Those case managers who work in settings in which they are the primary case manager through the continuum, such as some disease-specific case managers, may perform another set of tasks. These may be related to tracking and trending of various outcomes through the use of quality indicators; other tools include disease-specific forms, clinical pathways, HRAs, or SF-36/12/7 surveys. Examining case management interventions and resulting outcomes is a growing trend in case management.

It may be useful for your organization to assess the issues below. Make a permanent check sheet for your charts with these points (see sample checklists); also brainstorm other pertinent job responsibilities necessary for your organization. The check sheet can help to ensure that no important information or steps will be missed. When there are perhaps hundreds of details to take care of in each case—and each case manager has "too many cases"—even the most basic of responsibilities may be overlooked (i.e., checking the PPO status or benefit status of a provider or service).

▶ Case Managers Within Facilities (Internal)

Case managers working within acute and postacute facilities can benefit from the support of external case managers. The external case managers are knowledgeable about patients' benefits and about which agencies and facilities are contracted with the patient's health insurance plan. This information is valuable and can save time when seeking follow-up care.

BEFORE DISCHARGE

☐ Medical stability and discharge screens are monitored (see "InterQual" in Chapter 4).

☐ Education continues and return demonstrations identify any misinformation or incomplete learning processes. Teaching is stepped up for patient's discharge the following day. If home health is required, home health professional staff is notified of learning weaknesses.

☐ Evaluate pain control and attempt to change to oral pain management, if possible.

☐ Anticipated tests (hemoglobin and hematocrit, room air, arterial blood gases for supplemental oxygen, prothrombin time/partial thromboplastin time, and so on) are ordered. Results are reported to attending physicians.

☐ Transportation needs are evaluated. If the patient is from out-of-state or county (or even out of country), transportation plans need clarification as early as possible. If the patient requires a ground or air ambulance or stretcher van, calls should be made 24 hours in advance; cancellation may sometimes be necessary but is preferable to holding up a discharge because an appropriate transport vehicle is not available. Wheelchair vans may also require 24-hour notice. Families can confirm approximate pick-up times on this day if they can transport the patient home.

☐ Find out when the attending physician and consultants need to see the patient after discharge and, if necessary, help the patient make follow-up appointments.

☐ Confirm outpatient physical therapy, occupational therapy, and speech therapy appointments and give the patient the times, days, and a contact telephone number.

☐ Any needed outpatient IV therapy (such as antibiotics, chemotherapy), wound care, and scheduled tests and procedures need orders and appointments. This is often needed for patients who are not homebound and therefore do not qualify for home health services.

☐ Coordinate the DME. Delivery of all large equipment that must be brought to the home or apartment needs to be timed appropriately so that someone is there to accept it at the door. Smaller DME (e.g., small volume nebulizer [SVN] machines, portable oxygen tanks) can be sent to the hospital. Often a patient cannot go home without continuous oxygen; a smaller oxygen tank must go to the hospital before discharge and the larger unit needs to be coordinated at the house. When assessing equipment needs, ask about room sizes and space availability. This should be done as soon as DME need is assessed. Many patients require a hospital bed but must move home furniture around to make it fit into the room. Even three-in-one toilets do not always fit if the patient lives in a small trailer. Shower equipment also needs to fit in the type of bathroom facilities the patient has (full-size bathtub, smaller trailer-size tubs, or shower stall).

☐ Get all supplies ready for wound care, tracheostomy, ostomy, or other procedures. Some home health agencies want the patient to go home with a few days' worth of supplies for continuity of care purposes. This is especially important on weekends.

☐ Confirm hemodialysis days and times with the accepting facility. Confirm transportation needs.

☐ Call the home health agency and/or IV infusion therapy company to confirm impending discharge, and update the company(s) on the social and medical status of the patient. Discuss any change of instructions.

☐ For transfers to a SNF, call for validation that the patient's bed is still available. Update the SNF on the social and medical status of the patient. Ask whether the SNF supplies transportation from the hospital to the facility or set it up. Confirm that there is a physician to follow up; if not, find one. If possible, get transfer orders written, get reports from the multidisciplinary staff, and copy pertinent parts of the medical record.

☐ Get confirmation from the patient, family, and attending physician that they still agree with the discharge plans (whether home or SNF transfer).

☐ Make a list of all pertinent agencies, companies, and community referrals and their telephone numbers. Give this to the patient and family.

☐ Call the insurance company with up-to-date medical and discharge data; obtain authorization for the final hospital day (many insurance companies pay for the day of admission but not the day of discharge) and obtain authorization for any discharge disposition services.

☐ Gather any other details specific to a particular case.

THE DAY OF DISCHARGE

☐ Monitor medical stability and discharge screens.

☐ Give written discharge instructions. Work on fine-tuning any assessed educational insufficiencies.

☐ All test results have been reported to the physician. Those that are not normalizing have been discussed, and documentation verifies the physician's notification and permission to continue with discharge as planned.

☐ Transportation to home or another facility is set up and confirmed. The patient/family and physician is notified of final times for pickup.

☐ The patient and family are given written instructions for follow-up with physician(s).

☐ The patient and family are given written dates, times, and addresses for any outpatient needs (physical therapy, occupational therapy, speech therapy, IV therapy, tests, hemodialysis, and so on).

☐ DME is delivered to the home or hospital.

☐ Supplies are delivered to the home or hospital.

☐ Home health agencies are called for medical updates and for confirmation of time and day when a first visit will commence. Often a home health agency will not begin servicing a patient until the day after discharge if the care can be completed in the hospital on the day of discharge. If a patient needs a twice daily treatment or IV antibiotics, the home healthcare worker will come on the day of discharge. Communicate these arrangements to the patient and family.

☐ For SNF transfers, calls are placed with medical updates and to confirm transfer on that day. Final validation is obtained that physicians/ family/patient all agree with the transfer; transportation is set up, a physician will follow up, the chart is copied, orders are complete and correct, and all reports are included.

☐ Gather any other details specific to a particular case.

▶ Case Managers Outside Facilities (External)

The above internal case management responsibilities may also be required of external case managers. Because of the different healthcare relationships in these two types of case management, additional responsibilities often are incurred with external case management. Many of the tasks are more in alignment with business, rather than clinical job descriptions. External case managers are frequently required to document and report differently than those in hospitals or SNFs. Proof of negotiation and pricing agreements must be in writing, confidentiality and release of information forms may be required, and often even agreement and consent for case management services may need to be obtained. Reports to consultants and claims to payors demonstrating the improvement in quality of life and cost-benefit savings because of case management services are required on a regular basis. Return-to-work plans and life-care planning documentation is required for some external case managers. In addition, careful chart documentation is required on a day-to-day basis for both external and internal case management.

Some external case management responsibilities are included in the following checklists.

INITIAL CHECKS (FOR EXTERNAL CASE MANAGERS)

Date:
___ 1. ☐ Fill out facesheet.
___ 2. ☐ Verify insurance coverage:
- When does patient coverage end? (Date) _____.
- Do benefits require working status for continued coverage:
  ☐ Yes ☐ No
  #hours/week _____
- If there is more than one type of benefit package for employees (e.g., retired versus active benefits, HMO versus PPO)? Use the proper benefit book for the patient.
___ 3. ☐ Check benefit coverage:
- Is the service/procedure/equipment a covered benefit?
  ☐ Yes ☐ No
- Check limitations of benefits.
- Check exclusions of benefits.
- Check for "carve-outs" for certain conditions (e.g., bone marrow or other transplants).
___ 4. ☐ Check PPO status:
- Provider in PPO network?
  ☐ Yes ☐ No
- If "no"—options:
  1. May negotiate rates with non-PPO provider, **or**
  2. Change to PPO provider.
___ 5. ☐ If medical event is the result of an accident/trauma:
- Is it covered under auto insurance?
  ☐ Yes ☐ No
- Is it covered under workers' compensation?
  ☐ Yes ☐ No
- Is it covered under another third-party insurance plan?
  ☐ Yes ☐ No
  If "yes"—call client: does the client want case management services?
  ☐ Yes ☐ No
___ 6. ☐ Check for patient's extended benefits options or disability insurance options (for long-term or catastrophically ill patients).
___ 7. ☐ Check for multiple insurance coverage necessitating coordination of benefits.
___ 8. ☐ Initial call to patient or family.
___ 9. ☐ Initial call to physician/nurse.

INTERMEDIATE CHECKS (FOR EXTERNAL CASE MANAGERS)

Date:
___ 1. ☐ Revision of case plan or case management goals, if needed.
___ 2. ☐ Reports written in time frame per contract. Reports include:
- Negotiations signed.
- Physician advisor bills.
- Other.
___ 3. ☐ Reports to finance for billing.
___ 4. ☐ Reports to secretary for mailing.
___ 5. ☐ Ongoing communication with precertification/utilization management division about admissions to acute hospital and services authorized (if a precertification is required).
___ 6. ☐ Intermittent checks: physician advisor required?
___ 7. ☐ Intermittent checks: quality issue?

Case Closed
___ 8. ☐ Final report written with date closed.
___ 9. ☐ Customer/patient satisfaction survey (in long cases, every 6 months).
___ 10. ☐ Client satisfaction survey.
___ 11. ☐ Final report to finance.
___ 12. ☐ Report to secretary for mailing.
___ 13. ☐ File case folder in main locked cabinet.
___ 14. ☐ Notify precertification/utilization management division of case closure or death.

SIGNED LETTERS OF AGREEMENT/RECORDS

(Choose those applicable during initial assessment of case)
Date:
___ 1. Agreement with client: goals of case management.
2. Release of information/confidentiality statement:
___ ☐ Sent out.
___ ☐ Signed and returned.
3. Consent for case management:
For clients: include expected goals of case management:
___ ☐ Sent out.
___ ☐ Signed and returned.
For patients: simple consent to cooperate with case management:
___ ☐ Sent out.
___ ☐ Signed and returned.
4. Physician orders/medical records:
___ ☐ Requested.
___ ☐ Received.

(continued)

(Continued)

5. Physician documentation of medical necessity:
   ___ ☐ Requested.
   ___ ☐ Received.
6. Provider service agreement (used for negotiated rates, benefit plan exceptions, DME [evaluate rent versus purchase], and other major decisions):
   ___ ☐ Sent out.
   ___ ☐ Signed and returned.
   ___ ☐ Included in case management report.

▶ STAGE V: EVALUATION AND FOLLOW-UP

The stage of evaluation and follow-up is an important one; it ensures case continuity and sends the patient and family a caring message. The job responsibilities of your particular type of case management determine what you do in Stage V and how you do it. Episodic case management is done for a specified encounter of care in a patient's life. Some hospital case managers follow a patient in the hospital during an illness but do little follow-up after discharge. Other case managers start their responsibilities after the patient is discharged. Home health case managers follow up on the patient/family in the home setting; extended care facility case managers follow up patients while they reside in that facility; hospice case managers follow up their patients from admission into hospice until death (unless the patient or family opts otherwise); other case managers manage their patients throughout all levels of care until independence, formal release of the case, or death.

Postdischarge follow-up from a setting such as a hospital, rehabilitation center, or SNF may be done by telephone or in person. The follow-up may be as minimal as one or two telephone calls or visits or as significant as an extensive rehabilitation transitional period. This follow-up is usually appreciated, and often needed, by the patient and family. Many times after discharge unexpected events occur, questions surface, and ordered services fall through the cracks or do not meet expectations. Equipment does not arrive or is different from the type that the family was taught how to use in the facility. Perhaps the patient/family expected more hours of help or had a different idea of needed help from that of the home health agency or that approved by the health insurance plan. Caring for the patient may present more challenges than the family had anticipated; perhaps proper encouragement and a couple of added services would be all that are needed to turn the situation from one of panic to one of

success. In addition, a family may be having a difficult time securing a medication. The family may not know which pharmacy is contracted with their health plan, or the medication is not covered and they cannot afford the expense. A patient may feel that a physician is not responsive to telephone calls; on the other hand, some patients and families would rather ask questions of a case manager than "bother" their physician. Any number of unanticipated situations may surface.

This follow-up contact can be a vehicle to answer questions, discuss possible solutions, reassure the patient/family and often prevent complications or even readmissions and trips to the emergency department. One or several telephone calls may be needed. Telephone calls to the physician, the home health agency, the DME company, social service agencies, or any other part of the case plan within question may be required.

▶ Familial Needs

Several research studies have been conducted to find what families with chronically ill family members need to help them cope with illness and hospitalization. The original landmark study was conducted by Molter in the late-1970s. The universal need identified as extremely important was the need for hope (Molter, 1979). Another study distilled the responses of 17 previous studies and revealed that 14 of the top 21 needs were concerned with obtaining information about the family member (Hickey, 1990; Kleinpell, 1990). Case managers are often the disseminators of the information that the family needs to cope. Families are a total system in which a change in one member (e.g., the ill patient) directly affects all other members (the family), often disrupting the equilibrium of the whole system (Kupferschmid, 1987). By the case manager sharing accurate information, the family becomes empowered to make informed decisions; in this way, the case manager helps the family to gain understanding and a feeling of control over a difficult situation (Bouley, Von Hofe, & Blatt, 1994).

Fifteen of the most important family needs are discussed in this chapter. The needs may have been ranked differently, depending on the study performed, and the year that a study was performed has influenced its findings. Earlier studies show comfortable furniture in the waiting room as well as waiting room and bathroom locations ranking higher in importance than do later studies. A reason for this may be that many hospitals have addressed these issues, and they no longer loom today as major concerns.

It is interesting how often a case manager can make an impact on the 15 most important needs. When appraising the final evaluation of a case, assess the success and impact that case management services have had in meeting these needs.

1. To feel there is hope. Hope helps people to cope with a current life crisis by helping them to believe that the future holds promise; it is the universal need expressed. There is a delicate balance that case managers must achieve between giving too much hope or too little. We must often talk about the gravity or difficulty of a situation. It is not always easy to do this without destroying hope. Assess how well this was done in some of your most challenging cases.

2. To have questions answered honestly. People respond to sincere honesty and expect it. In 10 studies, 100% of the respondents rated this need as extremely important (Hickey, 1990). Even grave news has the benefit of preparing family members for the worst. Less than honest answers—or providing false hope—can leave a family member in shock and disbelief if they were not told of the possibility of a poor outcome before its occurrence. This is especially difficult if the physician or family member wants information kept away from the patient or another family member. Assess how well this was done in a difficult situation.

3. To be assured that the hospital personnel care about the patient and that the best possible care is being given to the patient. Families want to be assured that their ill relative and loved one is important to the staff and is treated kindly, respectfully, and with total honesty. They also need to know that the care is appropriate for the illness. Clinical pathways, when shared with patients and families, have been noted to ease the worries of this point. If the patient is moving along the pathway fairly steadily, the family can see that the care is standard protocol and the family member is responding as expected. Using patient- and family-focused clinical pathways enhances patient and family control over the situation, alleviates their anxiety concerning the type of care/treatments to be provided, and allows them to anticipate their role in the treatments to be provided and understand their responsibilities.

4. To know the prognosis. Often after the family is told the prognosis by the attending physician, they have many questions that do not surface immediately. The case manager can act as a safety net, being there to allow the family to vent, grieve, or ask questions as they come up and perhaps to make one of the most difficult decisions—whether to sign a do-not-resuscitate (DNR) order.

5. To know specific facts about the patient's progress on a daily basis. This knowledge was also an extremely important need to 100% of the respondents in 10 studies (Hickey, 1990). Some of the angriest family and patient complaints have resulted from their feeling that they were not updated regularly about the patient's progress and could not get the information they needed. Frequent visits by case managers to answer questions and clarify any misconceptions can prevent unnecessary anger and anxiety. Assess the patient's/family's satisfaction on this point.

6. To have explanations given in understandable terms. There is an art to explaining complicated concepts in easy-to-understand language. Some physicians are excellent at this; other times it may be necessary for the case manager to assess for gaps and misunderstandings in the patient or family. When a patient is in pain or a family is in crisis from the acute, severe nature of the illness or injury, even clear and simple explanations may be more than a person can process. The explanations then must be simple, concrete, and clear, with only the most immediately necessary facts conveyed. Speaking slowly and calmly and making eye contact aid this process. Assess whether the family/patient received this kind of attention.

7. To see the patient frequently. This is more difficult in some areas of case management than in others, such as when the patient is in an intensive care unit. The inability of a family to see, touch, and assess how their loved one is doing is a constant reminder of the threat of permanent loss of that person (Mathis, 1984). This is especially true in sudden, acute situations such as traumas. One case manager remembers when, as a fairly new bride in the late-1970s, she was called at work with information that her husband had been involved in a motorcycle accident. She arrived at the scene and stayed with him for 45 minutes until the ambulance came. During that time, he was in and out of consciousness, his pupils were dilated, and it was obvious that several bones were broken, including his clavicle, which was protruding through the

skin. In the 7 hours that followed—during which he was in the emergency department—the only information volunteered to her was the name of the ward to which he was being transferred. The only time she saw him was when she sneaked into his room in the emergency department and was then promptly ushered out. The anxiety she felt was intense; it could have been eased greatly by regular updates and closer physical proximity.

Perhaps because of that experience, that case manager now uses more cots on her unit—and has been known to run out of them—than are used on other units. Both patients and families usually respond with decreased anxiety when they can be near each other. Case managers who work in ICUs or emergency departments can plan times that are acceptable to the area and the family for visitation. Keeping the patients and families informed of what is going on is essential to reducing their anxiety and ultimately increasing their cooperation and involvement in care and decisionmaking. Assess family satisfaction on this point as part of the final evaluation.

8. To know exactly what is being done for the patient and why it is being done. This is important in helping patients and families to make informed decisions. The case manager aids the family by sharing accurate and consistent information. This is a shared responsibility with the physician and has legal ramifications when this information is used for the purpose of signing an informed consent. As in all informational needs, assess how well this was covered in the case plan.

9. To talk to the physician every day. Usually a patient, if alert and oriented, speaks daily to the physician. Issues occur when family members and significant others are unable to make contact with busy physicians. After a couple of days pass with no word from the patient's doctors, family members are likely to become upset, displaying attitudes that lead the staff to label them as "difficult," "manipulative," or "interfering." Again, anxiety is often the cause of this behavior and it can be diminished by a physician telephoning the family, sometimes supplemented with information offered by the case manager.

One communication disaster paired a physician with a less-than-empathetic bedside manner with an angry man whose grandfather—his only living relative—was in the hospital. As the patient's hospitalization stretched longer and longer, the worried grandson threatened lawsuit after lawsuit, fired multiple physicians, and became tangential in his conversations. The physician withdrew, doing his best to avoid communication. The situation was reaching a dangerous point, because staff nurses were becoming frightened of the grandson. When the case was transferred to another unit, the case manager there made a deal with the physician that if he would speak daily—at least briefly—to the grandson, she would fill in the gaps. The grandson agreed to this arrangement, after she assured him that she was available for further informational needs. Working on the tangential nature of his personality was a little more challenging, however. She limited the number of main points for each conversation (frequent reorientations back to those main points were necessary), and the main points were written down for the grandson to hold onto. At first, the grandson asked the same questions over and over without seeming to hear the answers. Within 3 days, he was much less hostile and the frequency of repeated questions was dramatically reduced. Finally, the patient was transferred to an extended care facility with the same physician following up, and the grandson was in agreement with the plan.

In the final evaluation, assess whether the family and patient were comfortable with the one-on-one attention from the attending physician and other staff involved in care.

10. To be called at home when the patient's condition changes. Because case managers are not present 24 hours a day, the responsibility of calling to update families may fall on the staff nurses or physicians. Many nurses are very conscientious about this. If the family is upset over poor communication, staff teaching and support may be needed.

11. To have a specific person to call if the family cannot make it to the facility. The three-shift structure of facilities that give 24-hour care translates into many caregivers for each patient. Families often feel more peace of mind if they have a single contact person who they can ask for by name. The case manager is a reasonable choice that benefits everyone. The family has a

knowledgeable contact, and the case manager often picks up important information about discharge planning from these conversations. Information appears to be a vital need for families, and the case manager can be a primary link between that information and the family. If too many people are calling from one family unit, it helps to have the family appoint a spokesperson to call the case manager. The other family members can then call this designated person. In the final case evaluation, assess your role in this pivotal communication position.

12. To be told about transfer plans. When a patient is being transferred to another unit in the hospital, let the family know. It frightens family members when they visit and find an empty bed, especially if the patient is critically ill. When the transfer is to another facility, the plans should be agreed to by the family and coordinated with them. One uncomfortable type of situation occurs when a family approves of the hospital where the patient is, but the health insurance company wants the patient transferred to one of their contracted hospitals. The present hospital could suffer financially if the transfer is not made, and few families can afford to pay for a hospitalization. In the final evaluation, assess transfer coordination with the family.

13. To feel accepted by the hospital staff. Family members often feel like "strangers in a strange land" and need to feel supported if they are to be a support for the ill family member. A case manager remembers one very difficult case involving a husband and wife. The wife was a large woman who was essentially a quadriplegic as a result of multiple sclerosis. She had many chronic conditions, including infections that frequently necessitated IV antibiotics. Although she required 24-hour care, the husband adamantly refused nursing home placement. He was a difficult person, and many home health agencies could no longer deal with his demands. Therefore, this case manager's challenge became finding a home health agency that would accept the wife each time she was discharged. The staff always groaned when this patient was admitted; although she was extremely pleasant, the husband could not be satisfied. One afternoon, while making rounds with the nurse manager of the unit, the husband went into his usual tirade of complaints and demands. The nurse manager approached him in a way no one else had. She touched his arm and gently asked how long he had been caring for his wife in this condition. He looked surprised but answered, "Seventeen years." "And who," she asked, "takes care of you?" Breaking into tears the man said quietly, "No one." Suddenly someone had accepted him. This nurse manager's compassion opened a door and the man responded with a remarkable mellowing.

Some patients and family members are also afraid that if the staff disapproves of them, they will not receive good care. This fear is not uncommon. If the case manager or the staff cannot connect with the family, perhaps a minister, rabbi, or psychologist may be able to do so. In the final evaluation, assess whether the case manager was instrumental in helping the family to feel accepted and welcome.

14. To have directions about what to do at the bedside. Families are often afraid to touch the ill family member, especially if there are many tubes and machines in use. Neonatal intensive care nurses routinely show parents how to handle the "preemies" and sick newborns. Parents of older pediatric patients are also routinely given directions for safe handling of the child. Many family members, especially spouses, would like to do more for the patient but are not sure what is allowed. The staff nurse and case manager can explain any invasive lines, assess the extent to which the family member would like to help with basic care, and help dispel any fears. Assess family satisfaction in this area.

15. To talk about the possibility of the patient's death. Some people have a great need to talk about their loved one's possible death; it is almost as if, by rehearsing it, they might be better prepared when it happens. Others will not verbalize the possibility as if, by talking about it, they might bring it on. Sensitivity to the family's needs on this point is critical, and some families prefer to speak to a member of the clergy. In the final evaluation (if this is applicable), assess whether the family's needs were met.

▶ Case Evaluation

In general, families want reassurance that their loved one is well cared for, that they have access to the patient, and that they have all the information they can handle.

If these points are addressed, the family is usually satisfied. Overall, how well did the patient/family unit respond to the case plan? The following are some general questions to ask in case evaluation and follow-up.

1. Were the goals and objectives met? Essentially, there are only three possibilities: the goals were met, partially met, or not met at all. Any shade of gray must be addressed. Determine why the goals were partially (or not) met:
   ▶ Were the goals realistic?
   ▶ Were appropriate treatment, procedures, or case management interventions selected? Were all the essential needs of the patient and family identified and addressed? Did other issues come to light after the initial interventions that demonstrated a new strategy might be more successful or necessary?
   ▶ Was the patient or family motivated?
2. Were all services delivered as planned?
3. Were there any problems with the agencies or companies that were set up?
4. Are new needs surfacing that are serious enough to destabilize the whole case plan?

Some cases do not go smoothly and the case manager is not surprised. Perhaps the patient wanted more than the health insurance agency would pay for and refused other options. Perhaps the patient's needs and the available resources were a poor match. What if the case management interventions appeared to go fairly routinely, yet later the patient or family expressed disappointment or resentment? The following are some possible questions to ask.

▶ Did the patient and family truly agree to the plan, were they pressured or coerced, or did they simply lack understanding?
▶ Was the family or patient unrealistic or in denial about the options?
▶ Did the patient's medical status change after discharge or transfer, necessitating revisions?
▶ Was poor or inadequate planning responsible for the disappointment?
▶ Was the suboptimal intervention due to the fact that the patient had virtually no resources (socially or financially/insurance) and refused other available assistance (shelters, community assistance)?
▶ Was the follow-up agency/facility less than adequate, or was poor "chemistry" with the staff to blame? Case managers are responsible for using credible resources; however, sometimes even reliable agencies and facilities have intermittent problems.

There are as many reasons for case management interventions and plans to falter (in whole or in part) as there are details to a particular case. If improperly evaluated and executed, any detail can destabilize the whole plan.

▶ Case Management Outcomes

Outcomes evaluation is not precisely a step in the case management process, but it is essential for case management to continue to grow and be recognized as a value-added part of the healthcare system. In discussing the Standards of Practice for Case Management, the Case Management Society of America (CMSA) focuses on the following standards of care:

1. Assessment/case identification and selection.
2. Problem identification.
3. Planning.
4. Monitoring.
5. Evaluating.
6. Outcomes.

The final standard of care, outcomes, is important because case management is a goal-directed process. Case managers collaboratively determine goals with the patient/family unit, the physician, and the multidisciplinary team. Next, case management interventions are set in motion that will have the greatest likelihood of achieving those goals. Then, we identify what the outcomes, or results, of those case management interventions will be. For a new stroke patient with left hemiplegia, for example, the goal may be ambulating 50 feet with a walker. The time frame may be in weeks or months, depending on the severity of the paralysis, and the general health condition of the patient, and the involvement of the family in care. Both the goal in feet and the goal in a specified time frame are measurable. That is the key—any outcome must be the result of a measurable goal.

On a more global level, case management outcomes may not necessarily be patient-related in a quality-of-life or clinical sense. Rather, outcomes in case management can also be measured in terms of cost-effectiveness because of a given case management intervention. Does case management presurgical teaching shorten lengthes of stay? Does diabetic education reduce the frequency of hospitalizations due to diabetic ketoacidosis or uncontrolled diabetes? Does close monitoring of pharmaceuticals in a congestive heart failure patient lessen the number of readmissions to the hospital or emergency department visits?

Proof of good case management outcomes, for both cost and quality, is expected in today's healthcare environment. The key purpose of measuring case management outcomes is to quantify and qualify the impact of case management services. In fact, the role of an outcomes manager is becoming one of the hybrid case management roles in many settings today. Hands-on case managers are being asked, at the very least, to collect the information used for outcomes analysis. Administrative case managers may be required to develop quality improvement projects.

Outcomes management is, at times, a frustrating and complex activity requiring knowledge about topics such as how to develop and improve outcomes; how to identify and develop quality indicators that are measurable, reliable, and valid; and how to interpret the data. It is not, however, an activity that will disappear anytime soon. Accreditation projects standards are written with outcomes in mind, and accreditation status depends on them. The healthcare industry is demanding evidence of quality care, customer/patient satisfaction, and efficiency of care delivery.

▶ STAGE VI: CONTINUOUS MONITORING, REASSESSING, AND REEVALUATING

Case management monitoring, reassessing, and reevaluating continue until the case is officially closed. Therefore, it is not really a stage, but rather a review process. Ongoing activities include monitoring, reassessing, and reevaluating the patient's status, treatment, case plan, and discharge plans. Rarely does the case management process proceed directly from Stage I to Stage VI, in which the patient is miraculously being fully and perfectly cared for! More often, this continuous reassessment and monitoring reveals changes in the patient's medical condition or hidden social circumstances hitherto unknown, necessitating changes in the case plan. Through the activities of this step, the service plan is revised, refined, and fine-tuned. This back-and-forth flow may occur several times before implementation of the final plan becomes reality.

The stability and type of the case determine the frequency of the monitoring and reevaluating. Some hospital cases need more than daily attention, whereas a stable patient residing in a long-term facility may need only weekly visits (although the patient would be monitored daily at the facility). Disease-state case management monitoring depends on the issues of the particular disease. Other types of case management require care plans and have policies about exactly

when the care plans must be reviewed. Reassessment may also be required at specific intervals by state laws in long-term care programs. Each case management model has its own challenges and unique clientele, requiring customized monitoring and reevaluating.

For some types of case management (mostly external case managers), the payor of case management services must also be monitored. There are times when details of a case change so that the payor may not want to continue providing case management services. Some patients may eventually qualify for Medicare or another insurance as a primary payor; most payors do not want to continue to pay for case management services because they are not financially liable, but some (a few) continue because case management can benefit the patient. The details of the patient's condition may change so that the payor of case management services may decide on a new goal for case management. Perhaps initially case management was called on to find a perfect placement for a hard-to-place patient, complete with reasonable per diem negotiations. That was all the case manager was hired to do. However, once in the facility, problems may develop with the family and care; case management may be asked to stay on for a longer period of time.

The process of case selection eliminates patients who are essentially stable. The remaining cases, by their very nature of severity and instability, require continuous monitoring. Like a domino effect, a change in the patient's medical status could affect the entire continuum from the treatment plan to the final disposition. As the case manager monitors the medical and psychosocial stability of the patient, a moderate-to-severe change could necessitate the reassessment of the total balance of services planned for in previous stages. The change may be minor, such as a new need for home oxygen, which would be added to any other home health needs that were previously evaluated. Perhaps a major reevaluation of the whole service, treatment, care plan, or transfer plan may be needed. Most case managers have at some time needed to upgrade a discharge disposition from home-based services to admission at a SNF because of medical deterioration; the reverse may also take place. Following is an example of the importance of continuous case management.

> Mrs. Bolton was 97 years old and lived with her 79-year-old daughter. Mrs. Bolton had a medical history that included hypertension, osteoarthritis, congestive heart failure, and colon cancer necessitating J-tube feedings for nutrition. She was admitted to the hospital in a cachectic condition with hypotension, dehydration, acute renal failure (creatinine, 4.3 mg/dL), and pneumonia.

Within 48 hours of admission, Mrs. Bolton was unresponsive, with a temperature of 34°C. A DNR order was signed, and comfort care and gentle IV hydration were provided. It was also decided that IV antibiotics would be continued for the pneumonia. The next day her stools became grossly heme-positive and her hemoglobin and hematocrit levels dropped significantly. The daughter and physicians decided to transfuse 1 unit of red blood cells and monitor her hematocrit and hemoglobin daily. The family did not wish the patient to undergo a colonoscopy. By the week's end, the doctors assessed the prognosis as "grim."

The following Monday morning, the case manager noted that Mrs. Bolton's name was still on the census board. She checked with the unit secretary and was told that she was indeed still on the unit. Imagine the case manager's surprise when, in the morning report, the night charge nurse mentioned that Mrs. Bolton was ambulating with assistance through the hallways! While the family and medical team were making "final disposition" plans, Mrs. Bolton had other ideas. She remained in the hospital for an additional 7 somewhat rocky days, during which time her pneumonia and gastrointestinal bleeding both cleared. Her creatinine decreased to a reasonable level, and physical therapy helped with strengthening. Once her J-tube feedings were tolerated at the prescribed rate, she was discharged home with her daughter.

It is said that the only constant thing is change; this is certainly true in case management. Constant change is the prime reason why this stage of continuous monitoring and reevaluating is so essential. Each case has unique features and important aspects that need monitoring. The following represent some basics that need to be monitored.

▶ Changes in Medical Status (Improvement or Deterioration)

Change in medical status (improvement) is the desired outcome when a patient enters the hospital. When a patient comes in sick, it is hoped that the illness can be changed to a more homeostatic condition. If the lungs are wheezy, physicians try for clear lungs and to achieve acceptable arterial blood gases. If bowels are obstructed, the medical team attempts to clear the obstruction with conservative or surgical methods. A multisystem failure patient or a level I trauma victim may deteriorate further or may stabilize at a level of health that is less than the previous baseline. All body systems, laboratory results, and vital signs must be monitored. Patient changes may signal the need for change in the treatment plan. Anything that varies from the patient's baseline may indicate a need for compensations in the discharge plan.

Medical status changes often must be monitored for utilization and insurance authorization purposes. Clinical pathways, intensity of service, severity of illness, and other utilization modalities may demonstrate a need for a change in the level of care and the case plan. A patient who is not in an appropriate level of care may be at risk medically if a more acute level of care is needed; he or she may be overutilizing resources if a less acute level of care is available to treat the medical condition.

▶ Changes in the Social Stability of the Patient

Life changes that occur while a patient is in the hospital or in the convalescent phase of an illness can sometimes be more trying than the illness itself. A lost lease or apartment may leave a patient homeless and worried about his or her possessions. If pets or family members also live there, the emotional trauma is multiplied. During hospitalizations and convalescent periods, patients can lose roommates, significant others may depart, parents may die, spouses may also need to be hospitalized, pets may be left uncared for, bills pile up, utilities are turned off, and employment is terminated—all these may have a significant effect on the total psychosocial picture and often cause stress-related exacerbations of illnesses. Prompt attention from social services and modifications of the discharge plan may be needed.

▶ Quality of Care

Acceptable standards of care and careful, ethical treatment of patients and their medical conditions are the minimal expected norms. Unfortunately, accidents and oversights take place. A clinically astute case manager can often prevent or impede an adverse outcome. Ideally, a maloccurrence can be averted. If that is not possible, quick action may minimize the negative consequences. If an undesirable outcome takes place, it may be wise to call the risk management department and follow the facility's protocol (see Chapter 7, Quality Management and Outcomes).

▶ Changes in Functional Capability and Mobility

Functional changes are especially important for older adults who may have been independent prior to the current ailment. Some conditions preclude early mobilization; recent surgery (especially in those patients with orthopedic conditions), profound weakness, deep vein thromboses, and hemiparesis are examples. An aggressive approach to early mobilization is essential to prevent further weakness and decline. Patients often feel that illness and bed rest are a natural marriage, whereas nurses know that bed rest may lead to a host of possible comorbidities. Sometimes the physician's order for restorative nursing, physical therapy, or ambulation is missing and therefore not considered until late in the admission. Patients who may be restrained for safety purposes often are capable of walking with assistance. Case managers should guard against extra lengths of stay due to minimal mobilization until late in the hospitalization. It jeopardizes the independence of some patients and may cause insurance denials at the acute care level.

▶ Evolving Educational Needs

As the patient or family is ready, knowledge deficits about the disease process, its course, and treatment should be identified and educational sessions can be added. Opportunities for teaching seem endless. Education by staff nurses or other healthcare professionals concerning the disease process, dressings, medical equipment, nutrition, rehabilitation activities, tube care, medication usage, medication interactions and side effects, suctioning, and many other techniques and informational aspects of care are essential. As case managers, the teaching aspect expands into areas such as explanations about the individual's health insurance coverage, deductibles, copay plans, DRGs, prescription costs, and location of contracted pharmacies and hospitals. Patients are often uncertain who their primary care physicians are or how to access the medical system. Overuse of emergency departments is often a clue to the latter knowledge deficit. Community resources and how to access these may be important to many individuals.

Patients retain only approximately 10% of the information given to them in teaching sessions (Ferrell & Rhiner, 1994). Visual demonstrations, books, and audiovisual handouts are helpful. As the patient's and the family's readiness and receptivity increases, they can review the education materials as needed. Studies have shown that informational materials are best understood when written at the sixth grade reading level or lower, in large print, and including several illustrations (Ferrell & Rhiner, 1994). Tapes should be interesting but concise, because people who are ill often have short attention spans. If headphones are available, they can be used to block out distractions.

Education of patients and their families is not merely an option but a mandate by TJC. According to TJC, the goal of educating the patient and family is to improve the patient's health outcomes by prompting recovery, speeding return to function, promoting healthy behavior, and appropriately involving patients in their care and care decisions. Patient and family education should:

▶ Facilitate patient/family understanding of the patient's health status, healthcare options, and consequences of options selected.
▶ Encourage participation in decision making about healthcare options.
▶ Increase patient/family potential to follow the therapeutic healthcare plan.
▶ Maximize care skills.
▶ Increase the patient's/family's ability to cope with the patient's health status/prognosis/outcome.
▶ Enhance patient/family role in continuing care.
▶ Promote a healthy lifestyle (TJC, 2008).

Physical and psychosocial influences must be taken into consideration when assessing a patient's readiness to learn. Pain, weakness, nausea, and drowsiness from medications weigh heavily on a person's ability to learn. A person who is still in shock over a new diagnosis may be too depressed or in the denial stage, and therefore, unreceptive to learning. Body image is another powerful force. Occasionally, a previously independent patient who lives alone may need to go to an extended care facility after a colostomy or tracheostomy because of refusal to accept—and subsequently care for—the tracheostomy or colostomy. Some people simply need more time. Learning cannot be forced; the information must be accepted and absorbed in cooperation with the free will of the patient.

▶ Pain Management

Pain management is one aspect of care that often brings out the "judge" in the medical staff. Perhaps it is because pain is a subjective experience that often does not correlate with objective criteria. This is further complicated by an individual's tolerance to pain and psychological, sociologic, and cultural elements.

Studies have shown that although pain is cited as the most common reason why people seek medical attention, the management of pain often is inadequate (Henkelman, 1994).

CAUSES OF INADEQUATE PAIN RELIEF

The reasons for the inadequate relief of pain are many and include factors and misconceptions by the patient/family unit and by medical personnel. Patients and families may be concerned about addiction and therefore ask for too little pain relief (McCaffery & Ferrell, 1994). They may also fear a tolerance ceiling of the pain medication and therefore may anticipate a time when further pain relief will not be possible (McCaffery & Ferrell, 1994). Medical staff may suspect ulterior motives when some patients with "drug-seeking behavior" ask for increased dosages. This is likely to happen in the case of patients with chronic illnesses and chronic pain conditions. Medical staff also may be concerned about addiction or about harm caused by higher doses, such as respiratory depression. Communication differences also may cause less than adequate pain relief. Persons in some cultures are stoic in their responses to pain and will not ask for relief. Others may not look as if they are in pain while they are asking for pain medication, causing doubt among the medical personnel about the level of discomfort. Some patients may smile and use laughter as coping mechanisms while being in excruciating pain (Acute Pain Management Guideline Panel, 1992).

Case managers may find that much teaching is necessary for patients, families, and the medical staff. Misconceptions are common on this subject. However, relief of pain is essential. Pain-relieving strategies vary with different causes of pain. Postoperative pain medications are scheduled differently from those for a patient with terminal cancer who is readying to go home with hospice care. The postoperative patient will most likely be weaned off IV and intramuscular injections and be discharged with oral pain medication. The cancer patient may be admitted for intractable pain and may reach a comfort level only with a morphine patient-controlled analgesia (PCA) pump (see Figures 6.1 and 6.2 for surgical pain flow charts).

The bottom line is that early and adequate pain management is part of our obligation to relieve suffering as much as possible. It also produces earlier mobilization of patients, shortened hospital stays, and reduced costs (Anonymous, 1994). Because home health agencies rarely send nurses out on an as-needed (PRN) basis for a pain shot, a stable patient may stay in the hospital or transfer to an extended care facility for final management of pain when all systems are ready for discharge except for the pain management piece. Sometimes this is unavoidable; at other times, medical attention has been focused on other parts of the treatment plan and has caused a delay in assessing this important aspect of care. Just like early mobility, early attention to pain management is essential when a discharge plan is being assessed. Constant monitoring and reevaluating of pain medications and the patient's response are essential.

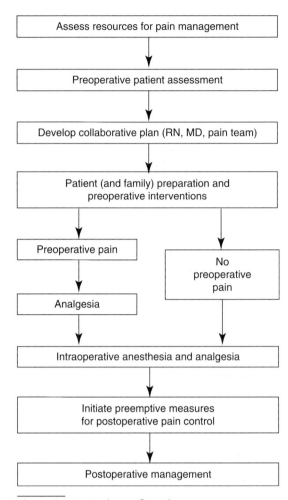

Figure 6.1 Surgical pain flow chart.

APPROACHES TO PAIN MANAGEMENT

Patients should be made aware that a goal of total absence of pain may be unrealistic, although pain control is considered an important part of the treatment plan. Nonpharmacologic methods may be used successfully as an adjunct to pharmacologic methods and often are especially helpful for chronic pain conditions (see Tables 6.1 through 6.3 for both pharmacologic and nonpharmacologic pain-relieving techniques). These techniques include the use of heat, cold, massage, vibration, counterirritants, distraction, relaxation, acupuncture, imagery, music, biofeedback, patient education, and transcutaneous electrical nerve stimulation (TENS) units.

Many excellent books and articles have been written about pain management. There always are new treatments for pain, new medications, and new methods of pain-relieving delivery being discovered and produced. The National Institutes of Health (NIH) has demonstrated that acupuncture is a major reliever for

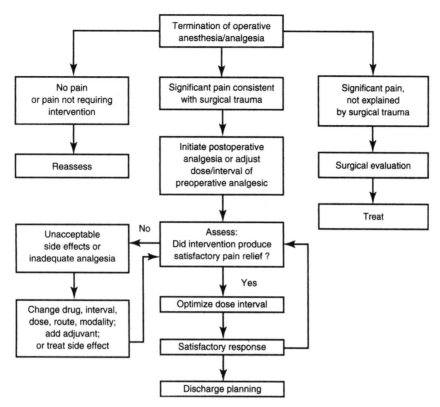

Figure 6.2 Pain treatment flow chart: postoperative phase. From Acute Pain Management Guideline Panel. (1992). *Acute pain management: Operative or medical procedures and trauma.* (AHCPR Publication No. 92-0032). Rockville, MD: Agency for Health Care Policy and Research, Public Health Service, U.S. Department of Health and Human Services.

back pain. New, smaller patient-controlled anesthesia (PCA) pumps allow home use of this self-controlled pain-relief method. New medications and new forms of old medications are frequently in the news and in magazine articles.

The psychosocial aspect of pain control is important for the case manager to consider, and some comprehensive pain management clinics include psychosocial care and alternative methods in their programs. Pain management programs at numerous institutions such as the Beth Israel Deaconess Medical Center in Boston teach relaxation, stress reduction, and meditation as a pain reduction plan. The goal of the 10-week program is to address four components of pain:

1. Somatic.
2. Affective.
3. Behavioral.
4. Cognitive.

The first week introduces patients to the pathophysiology of pain. They are given a pain diary and requested to record notes about their pain medication use and side effects. The second session teaches relaxation and breathing exercises, and patients are given a relaxation audiotape to listen to; they are encouraged to continue the pain diary. In the third session, patients are taught how to pace themselves and how to describe pain in specific, qualitative terms; they are encouraged to continue the pain diary and the relaxation work. The fourth session teaches nutritional guidance related to pain management and simple yoga exercises; the diaries and relaxation techniques are still encouraged. The fifth through tenth sessions of the program focus on cognitive restructuring. Patients are assessed for problem-solving skills, communication skills, and coping strategies. The success of such programs was noted to reduce the rate of clinic visits up to 36%.

The perception of pain is perhaps the most important component in pain control. Humans have a unique way of experiencing pain, one that is mixed with fear; when the fear component is missing, the experience is very different from what is typically witnessed in adults after a stay in the hospital. The Beth Israel Deaconess pain clinic found that if patients could modify the way they perceived pain, the pain often lessened.

▸ **TABLE 6.1 PHARMACOLOGIC INTERVENTIONS**

INTERVENTION	COMMENTS
NSAIDS	
Oral (alone)	Effective for mild to moderate pain; begin preoperatively; relatively contra-indicated in patients with renal disease and risk of or actual coagulopathy; may mask fever
Oral (adjunct to opioid)	Potentiating effect resulting in opioid sparing; begin preoperatively; use cautions as above
Parenteral (ketorolac)	Effective for moderate to severe pain; useful when opioids are contraindicated, especially to avoid respiratory depression and sedation; expensive
Opioids	
Oral	As effective as parenteral route in appropriate doses; use as soon as oral medication tolerated; route of choice
Intramuscular	Standard parenteral route, but injections painful and absorption unreliable; avoid this route when possible
Subcutaneous	Preferable to intramuscular when a low-volume continuous infusion is needed and intravenous access is difficult to maintain; injections painful and absorption unreliable; avoid this route for long-term repetitive dosing
Intravenous	Parenteral route of choice after major surgery; suitable for titrated bolus or continuous administration (including PCA) but requires monitoring; significant risk of respiratory depression with inappropriate dosing

NSAIDS, nonsteroidal antiinflammatory drugs; PCA, patient-controlled analgesics.

Adapted from Acute Pain Management Guideline Panel. (1992). *Acute pain management: operative or medical procedures and trauma.* (AHCPR Publication No.92-0032). Rockville, MD: Agency for Health Care Policy and Research, Public Health Service, US Department of Health and Human Services.

IMPORTANT PAIN MANAGEMENT CONSIDERATIONS

▸ Establish a positive relationship with the patient and family as early as possible and get them involved. Find out the pain management preferences of the patient. Some people prefer to avoid pain as much as possible, whereas others may opt for less obtundation while tolerating some level of discomfort.

▸ **TABLE 6.2 PHARMACOLOGIC INTERVENTIONS**

INTERVENTION	COMMENTS
Opioids	
PCA (Systemic)	Intravenous or subcutaneous routes recommended; good steady level of analgesia; popular with patients but requires special infusion pumps and staff education; see cautions about opioids in Table 5.1
Epidural and intrathecal	When suitable, provides good analgesia; significant risk of respiratory depression, sometimes delayed in onset; requires careful monitoring; use of infusion pump requires additional equipment and staff education; expensive if infusion pumps are used
Local anesthetics	
Epidural and intrathecal	Limited indicators; effective regional analgesia; opioid sparing; addition of opioid to local anesthetic may improve analgesia; risks of hypotension, weakness, numbness; requires careful monitoring; use of infusion pumps requires additional equipment and staff education
Peripheral nerve block	Limited indications and duration of action; effective regional analgesia; opioid sparing

PCA, patient-controlled analgesics.

Adapted from Acute Pain Management Guideline Panel. (1992). *Acute pain management: operative or medical procedures and trauma.* (AHCPR Publication No.92-0032). Rockville, MD: Agency for Health Care Policy and Research, Public Health Service, US Department of Health and Human Services.

▸ Whenever possible, discuss pain management options and elicit preferences preoperatively. Develop a plan for pain assessment and management. As in the doctrine of informed consent, the patient has a right to know what options are available to make informed choices about these options.

▸ Fear and anxiety play a major role in the perception of pain. Preoperative guidance often helps dispel much anxiety, but only elective surgeries allow for this luxury. Many conditions other than surgery create pain. The case manager can help by being there to answer questions, dispel fears, and give appropriate information. Some patients respond well to active participation in their pain management. For those who would feel less anxious by

▶ **TABLE 6.3 NONPHARMACOLOGIC INTERVENTIONS**

INTERVENTION	COMMENTS
Simple relaxation (begin preoperatively)	
Jaw relaxation Progressive muscle relaxation Simple imagery	Effective in reducing mild to moderate pain and as an adjunct to analgesic drugs for severe pain; use when patients express an interest in relaxation; requires 3-5 minutes of staff time for instructions
Music	Both patient-preferred and "easy listening" music effective in reducing mild to moderate pain
Complete relaxation (begin preoperatively)	
Biofeedback	Effective in reducing mild to moderate pain and operative site muscle tension; requires skilled personnel and special equipment
Imagery	Effective for reduction of mild to moderate pain; requires skilled personnel
Education/instruction (begin preoperatively)	
	Effective for reduction of pain; should include sensory and procedural information and instruction aimed at reducing activity-related pain; requires 5 to 15 minutes of staff time
TENS	Effective in reducing pain and improving physical function; requires skilled personnel and special equipment; may be useful as a adjunct to drug therapy

TENS, transcutaneous electrical nerve stimulator

Adapted from Acute Pain Management Guideline Panel. (1992). *Acute pain management: operative or medical procedures and trauma.* (AHCPR Publication No.92-0032). Rockville, MD: Agency for Health Care Policy and Research, Public Health Service, US Department of Health and Human Services.

taking the medication at regular intervals, a blood level is maintained that relieves pain continuously (Ferrell & Rhiner, 1994).

▶ Discuss the side effects of analgesics and the comfort measures to decrease them. These side effects may include dry mouth, constipation, drowsiness, and nausea. Teach that nausea often goes away in 3 to 5 days (Ferrell & Rhiner, 1994).

▶ If pain is poorly controlled, assess more frequently. Revise the pain management plan as necessary. Teach the patient that factual reporting of pain is necessary to gain good control and to avoid either stoicism or exaggeration of symptoms.

▶ Pain assessment tools are often helpful. Visual tools such as those in Figures 6.3 and 6.4 are good guides, or simply ask the patient to describe the pain on a scale of zero to 10, with zero expressing no pain and 10 being the worst possible pain. Make sure the pain assessment tools are developmentally appropriate. Children 4 to 12 years old often respond well to face scales, which show faces in different levels of distress. Vital signs and behavior as a sign of pain intensity should be used only if self-report (the most reliable indicator) by the patient is not possible (Anonymous, 1994).

▶ On discharge from the hospital, SNF, or ambulatory setting, patients should be provided with a written pain management plan. Pertinent discharge instructions related to pain management include specific drugs to be taken, frequency of drug administration, potential side effects of the medication, potential

actively participating in their pain management, a PCA device is often successful. Studies have shown that in the short-term, postoperative patients who are able to self-medicate report less pain, are more satisfied with their pain relief, and tend to be discharged earlier than those who are given PRN drugs by the nurse (Acute Pain Management Guideline Panel, 1992).

▶ Teach the principle that "pain is easier to control when it is prevented than when it gets out of control and must be brought back in line." This means that analgesics may be administered regularly instead of PRN. By

NOTE

For information about clinical guidelines, including the *Pain Management Guideline Manual,* call:

AHRQ Clearinghouse
Telephone: 800-358-9295 or 301-495-3453

Or write:

Center for Research Dissemination and Liaison
AHRQ Clearinghouse
P.O. Box 8547
Silver Spring, MD 20907

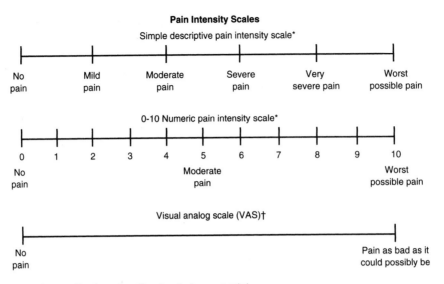

Figure 6.3 Examples of pain intensity and pain distress scales. Adapted from Acute Pain Management Guideline Panel. (1992). *Acute pain management: Operative or medical procedures and trauma.* (AHCPR Publication No. 92-0032). Rockville, MD: Agency for Health Care Policy and Research, Public Health Service, U.S. Department of Health and Human Services.

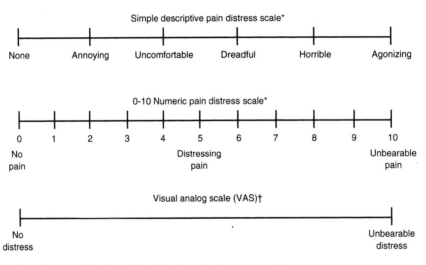

Figure 6.4 Pain distress scales. Adapted from Acute Pain Management Guideline Panel. (1992). *Acute pain management: Operative or medical procedures and trauma.* (AHCPR Publication No. 92-0032). Rockville, MD: Agency for Health Care Policy and Research, Public Health Service, U.S. Department of Health and Human Services.

food and drug interactions, specific precautions to follow when taking the medication (e.g., physical activity limitations, dietary restrictions), and name of person to notify about pain problems and other medical conditions.

▶ Document all discussions and teaching in the patient's chart.

These guidelines are in the public domain (i.e., may be copied for clinical use) and contain charts and flowsheets that may be beneficial in clinical practice.

▶ Changes in Patient or Family Satisfaction

The patient or family may exhibit changes in level of satisfaction with the treatment or discharge plans.

Ensure that the service plan continues to match the needs of the patient/family. Attitudes change and vacillate for a variety of different reasons. Sometimes the patient or family feels as if the attending physician is unresponsive to their questions or telephone calls. Perhaps it is information that the case manager can provide, or a call to the doctor may be appropriate. Occasionally, families are so demanding that the physician (and/or other healthcare professionals) backs away and would appreciate help from the case manager. Attitudes may shift because the patient/family gets frightened or feels guilty about the service plan. Should we have signed Dad's DNR order? Should we put him in a nursing home? A family conference may be needed to explore feelings and refocus back on the patient and on what is needed to ensure the best quality of care and of life. If revisions in the plan are needed, the case manager should keep the patient, family, physician, and other pertinent members of the multidisciplinary team informed and in full participation of the changes.

▶ Goals

It is important to assess and reassess if all the goals determined to be essential to a case continue to be realistic and appropriate as the case evolves and unfolds. Priorities change as patients either improve or become more accepting of their current situations. Life care plans must be modified when patient/family goals are changed or the patient's condition changes. Perhaps the major goal was to keep the patient at home; after major mental deterioration, the burden may become so large that a residential placement is in order. The case manager's role may shift to assisting the family to find a place where they feel the care will be good for their loved one; grief counseling for the family may also be needed, as this is a major life shift.

▶ STAGE VII: CASE CLOSURE AND TERMINATION OF CASE MANAGEMENT SERVICES

Sometimes, one of the most challenging tasks a case manager must complete is saying "good-bye." Case managers who follow patients throughout the continuum of healthcare services have been invited to birthday parties, retirement parties, and even funerals. Obviously a patient's death terminates case management services, but there are other reasons for termination, including:

▶ The patient, provider, or payor requests termination.

▶ The patient is no longer eligible for the insurance that is paying for case management services.

▶ Changes in the medical condition warrant closure: a well baby is born, the medical condition is stabilized, or disease-specific education and monitoring have been maximized.

▶ The patient/case management goals have been achieved.

▶ The patient and/or family opt for a change in the case manager or the private case management company.

▶ The patient died.

▶ The case manager is no longer available; for example, relocation, change in job, change in organization/employer.

▶ The case management company closed or relocated.

▶ The case management program was discontinued.

Case closure or termination of case management services requires special skills and talents. Terminating services is as challenging as building a trusting relationship between the case manager and the patient/family. Case managers should exercise caution in how they go about closing a case or terminating a relationship with a patient and/or family. They are advised to:

▶ Educate the patient and family about the need for case closure.

▶ Share the expectation of case closure with the patient and family at case selection and intake time.

▶ If case closure is done due to relocation or change in insurance company or provider, the case manager involved should transition the case to the next case manager or provider to maintain continuity of care.

▶ Answer patient and family questions.

▶ Alleviate patient and family anxiety.

▶ Reintroduce the need for case closure a few days prior to the last date of involvement in the case.

The case management process is not an easy one, but a skilled and experienced case manager can usually overcome obstacles, regardless of what they are or when they occur. Most patients and families are very appreciative of the case management process and the guidance and support extended to them. The final question, the answer to which will test the efficacy of the whole case management process, is: did case management efforts improve or at least optimize the quality of life for this person and this family unit? Within this question lies the heart of case management.

STUDY QUESTIONS

1. How does the case management process differ from the traditional nursing process? How is it similar?

2. Cite an example of a case that was not selected for case management but should have been. How did this case fall through the cracks? What did you do to prevent such mistakes from happening in the future?

3. Discuss the importance of a thorough assessment. What are some barriers to a thorough assessment?

4. Discuss the steps needed to coordinate and develop a treatment or discharge plan. What are some barriers to this stage of the case management process?

5. How would you go about developing a list of community resources and agencies in your area?

6. Discuss changes that must be monitored in the case management stage of continuous assessment and monitoring. Evaluate how one change can affect the structure of the whole case plan.

7. Cite a case example in which a discharge was held up because all services were not evaluated and set up by the day that the patient was ready for discharge. What could have been set up the day before discharge? Would this have allowed the discharge to go on as scheduled?

8. Discuss the important issues cited by families. How can a case manager help meet those needs?

9. Consider a case that you managed. Were all the steps and stages included? What would you do differently?

10. Discuss a case where closure was challenging. What were the issues? What strategies were effective? What activities were ineffective?

▶ REFERENCES

Acute Pain Management Guideline Panel. (1992). *Acute pain management: operative or medical procedures and trauma.* (AHCPR Publication No.92-0032). Rockville, MD: Agency for Health Care Policy and Research, Public Health Service, US Department of Health and Human Services.

Anonymous. (1994). Acute pain management in adults: operative procedures—quick reference guide for clinicians. *MEDSURG Nursing, 3*(2), 99–107.

Bouley, G., Von Hofe, K., & Blatt, L. (1994). Holistic are of the critically ill: meeting both patient and family needs. *Dimensions of Critical Care Nursing, 13*(4), 218–223).

Ferrell, B., & Rhiner, M. (1994). Managing cancer pain: a three-step approach. *Nursing 94, 24*(7), 57–59.

Gibbons, R. (1998). Cost-effectiveness of nutrition services. *Home HealthCare Consultant, 5*(3), 19–22.

Henkelman, W. (1994). Inadequate pain management: ethical considerations. *Nursing Management (Critical Care Edition), 25*(1), 48A, 48B, 48D.

Hickey, M. (1990). What are the needs of families of critically ill patients? A review of the literature since 1979. *Heart & Lung, 19*(4), 401–415.

Kleinpell, R.M. (1990). Needs of families of critically ill patients: a literature review. *Critical Care Nurse, 11*(8), 34–40.

Kupferschmid, B. (1987). Families of critically ill patients. *Critical Care Nursing Currents, 5*(2), 7–12.

Mathis, M. (1984). Personal needs of family members of critically ill patients with and without acute brain injury. *Journal of Neurosurgical Nursing, 16*(1), 36–44.

McCaffery, M., & Ferrell, B. (1994). How to use the new AHCPR cancer pain guidelines. American Journal of Nursing, 94(7), 42–46.

Molter, N. (1979). Needs of relatives of critically ill patients: a descriptive study. *Heart & Lung, 8*(2), 332–339.

The Joint Commission. (2008). *Comprehensive accreditation manual for hospitals.* Oakbrook Terrace, IL: Joint Commission Resources.

Wellman, N. (1997). A case manager's guide to nutrition screening and intervention. *The Journal of Care Management, 3*(2), 12–24.

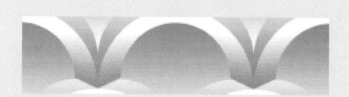

Key Concepts in Case Management

"Quality is never an accident; it is always the
result of high intention, sincere effort, intelligent
direction and skillful execution; it represents the
wise choice of many alternatives."

WILLA A. FOSTER

CHAPTER 7

Quality Management and Outcomes

LEARNING OBJECTIVES

Upon completion of this chapter, the reader will be able to:

1. Define performance management, outcomes management, risk management, and core measures.
2. Describe the relationship between case management and quality management.
3. Describe the process of quality reviews.
4. Explain the role of the case manager in quality and outcomes management.
5. List five strategies in case management practice that enhance patient safety.
6. Describe the role of the case manager in the reporting of outcomes (core measures).

ESSENTIAL TERMS

Adverse Patient Outcome (APO) • Core Measures • Important Aspects of Care • Incident • Incident Report • Indicators • Occurrence Report • Outcomes • Outcomes Management • Patient Safety • Performance Improvement (PI) • Performance Management (PM) • Potentially Compensable Event • Quality Assurance (QA) • Quality Improvement (QI) • Quality Management (QM) • Quality of Care • Risk Management (RM) • Total Quality Management (TQM) • Variances

The present healthcare climate contains several factors that leave it open to accusations of compromised patient safety and quality of care. Among these factors are utilization review and management criteria that are becoming stricter each year and that demand prompt transitioning of patients to lower levels of care. Additional factors are the increased scrutiny of the use and allocation of healthcare resources; capitation and risk contracts that place hospitals and other types of healthcare organizations at increased fiscal risk; and in an effort to be cost-effective organizations, cost-cutting activities that ultimately change the professional staff-to-patient ratios.

Quality improvement (QI)—also referred to as quality management (QM) and traditionally referred to as quality assurance—has long been a function mandated by regulatory or accreditation agencies such as The Joint Commission (TJC), previously known as the Joint Commission on Accreditation of Healthcare Organizations (JCAHO). Some TJC requirements that improve various aspects of quality care include the creation of hospital

policies and procedures; job descriptions; personnel performance evaluations; credentialing of professional staff; the provision of educational programs to ensure that knowledge, competencies, and clinical skills are up-to-date; and continual monitoring activities. TJC mandates the demonstration of multidisciplinary performance improvement (PI) efforts using specific indicators and processes. Rather than merely emphasizing quality assurance, which is often episodic in its assessments, today the emphasis is on the concept of quality improvement (QI) and performance management (PM) (TJC, 2008a). Gleaned from the industrial sector that is typical of the Japanese automotive management philosophies since World War II, QI attempts to meet or exceed the customer's needs. The customer is no longer the patient only but everyone associated with the healthcare industry, those who work for your organization and for other organizations (Fanucci et al. 1993).

The continuous QI (CQI) concept, sometimes referred to as total quality management (TQM), has gained strength in the healthcare industry and is closely related to QI processes and risk management (RM) activities. The intent of all improvement processes, whether labeled QI, QM, PI, or another acronym, is to provide excellent care in the first place, evident through patient safety and quality of care, thus lessening chances of adverse events that will need RM attention. QI and PM emphasize a proactive rather than a reactive approach; they provide the compass that leads the way to quality services. The result, excellent quality of care, is the measuring rod.

Another frequently used term for similar activities is *performance improvement* (PI), which uses the processes of design, improvement, measurement, and control. The design step is responsible for designing new (or modifying existing) functions, processes, and services based on the mission and vision of the organization, the concerns identified, the expectations and needs of the customers, and the most up-to-date information regarding the focus of improvement. The improvement step focuses on implementation of the strategic and well-thought-out changes prompted by the identified concerns or problems and the desired outcomes. The measurement step evaluates the effectiveness of the redesigned process(es); thus identifying opportunities for further improvement/modification as necessary. The focus of measurement includes areas of care that are high-volume, high-risk, high-cost, and problem-prone. Integral to the measurement step is an assessment that provides a systematic approach to determine whether the goals and priorities for the redesigned process have been met and how further improvement can be made. The control step includes implementation of specific activities or strategies to maintain and sustain the improvement and the redesigned process. This is important for ensuring that the improvements achieved become part of the regular process.

The following quote from Kongstvedt still holds true today. It emphasizes the movement from a punitive quality assurance model (find the bad apple) to the QI model of quality performance.

> Effective quality management is both a continuous and a systematic endeavor. Instead of centering on crisis, wrongdoing by individuals, and conformity to correct processes established by experts, quality management should engage everyone in the organization in continuous efforts to raise the organization's level of performance (Kongstvedt, 1993, p. 167).

This ideal of a high level of performance is the goal of QI and RM programs. Unfortunately, because mistakes do take place, we must also continue to focus on crises when they occur and to monitor potential or actual problems. This troubleshooting is done through

safety checks, infection control surveillance, incident reports, RM activities, care evaluations, outcomes management, and case management assessments and use of tools such as clinical pathways. Quality assurance cannot "assure" that risks and maloccurrences will not happen, but through the previously mentioned activities and prompt identification of problems, the risk (and quality) manager can initiate the appropriate intervention to minimize crescendoing consequences.

RM and QI are closely related programs with similar goals. This chapter clarifies the similarities and differences of traditional QI-RM programs, illustrates the importance of the case manager's role to QI-RM activities, and describes circumstances, claims categories, and indicators that warrant close attention. Through the course of a case manager's responsibilities, chart reviews and discussions with others on the healthcare team often expose potential problems in care or services.

▶ QI AND RM RESPONSIBILITIES

Traditional QI is a process that determines whether the care provided meets medical and nationally recognized and accepted standards (Sederer, 1987). QI activities are designed to monitor, prevent, and correct quality deficiencies. In that sense, QI is a proactive model. It is a continuous effort to raise the organization's quality level and performance. This is accomplished through quality assessment, which is the process by which quality of care is examined and evaluated. It also is achieved through the implementation of tools, methods, or strategies so that quality of care and patient safety are assured at all times. In this regard, quality assurance activities are performed on an ongoing basis, with the goal of QI. However, this traditional effort of quality assurance has changed, routinely incorporating more QI, QM, PI, and RM techniques, which is having the effect of making quality assurance even more proactive. The first step is no longer monitoring, but rather doing it right the first time and all the time.

Traditional RM is the "art and science of how not to be successfully sued" (Sederer, 1987, p. 214). Ideally, the major emphasis is on identifying potential risk areas and on interventions that will enhance patient safety and prevent losses, including untoward events, before they occur. In reality, in many organizations the RM department is called in after the undesirable event has occurred. Its function then is to control and minimize losses through legal methods and public relations efforts. Because of this, risk management sometimes has been characterized as the "damage control" entity: "an attempt to remedy the effects of internal failures before they can become external embarrassments" (Kongstvedt, 1993, p. 166).

In this sense, RM is a reactive model, but risk cannot always be prevented. Some adverse events do not become apparent until after the fact. Consider a case in which a patient received standard treatment for a disease and in which patient care was of high quality during the treatment phase: good quality management. Unfortunately, the disease was misdiagnosed: poor RM potential. This case is not likely to be reported through routine QI channels at the time of misdiagnosis.

To avoid the reactive nature of risk management activities, healthcare organizations have implemented risk mitigation programs that allow them to identify proactively potential risks or failures and to implement specific interventions (checks and balances) to prevent these potential problems from occurring. The following are examples of risk mitigation activities:

▶ Pressure ulcer prevention programs.
▶ Falls risk assessment and injury reduction programs.
▶ Infection control surveillance: MRSA screening, central line-associated blood stream infections (CLABSI), incision/surgical site infection, hand hygiene, and water safety testing.
▶ Prevention of complications: anticoagulation therapy, deep vein thrombosis prophylaxis, ventilator-associated pneumonia prophylaxis.
▶ Failure mode analysis: examining processes of care to identify potential risk for failure and instituting an intervention to prevent such risk; for example, requiring two-person check for chemotherapeutic agent use/administration or requiring two-person check for blood and blood product administration; use of a magnetic resonance imaging (MRI) safety checklist.
▶ Daily review of throughput and patient flow activities: among other indicators, this involves bed capacity evaluation, bed management, an examination of emergency department patient volume, hours of diversion, and percentage of "waiting to be admitted" patients; an examination of postanesthesia care unit patient volume and length of stay; and turnaround time for admitting patients to an inpatient bed.

▶ HOW QI AND RM CONTRAST AND COMPARE

Like case management, the direction in QI emphasizes looking at the big picture and efficiently coordinating the whole system. Classic QI, with its inherent limitations and flaws, is still necessary and required by regulatory agencies such as TJC. Therefore, an understanding of how QI and RM differ, and how they work together, is important.

QI and RM differ in the following ways (Northrop & Kelly 1987):

▶ Their focuses are different. RM is concerned with acceptable care from a legal and financial perspective and attempts to minimize the costs of liability insurance and the liability of claims. QI emphasizes patient care issues and related outcomes rather than financial concerns.
▶ RM looks at all hospital exposures: environmental, patient safety, visitor safety, and so on. QI emphasizes patient-care–focused issues, which includes all services involved in patient care: optimal quality of care, adherence to professional standards, and reasonable and prudent delivery of care.
▶ RM focuses on loss prevention activities. QI facilitates the improvement of the processes of care and ultimately their associated outcomes.
▶ Overall, RM aims to decrease the probability of adverse patient outcomes (APOs). QI, on the other hand, aims to increase the probability of quality patient outcomes.

The following are areas of common concern in RM and QI (Northrop & Kelly 1987):

▶ Both are concerned with anything that may cause risk of injury to the patient. Both attempt to identify and avoid APOs.
▶ Both involve the monitoring of trends to identify risk patterns or problems in patient care.
▶ Both require and emphasize the need for complete and clear documentation.
▶ Both require cooperation and information from the multidisciplinary team to assess trends and resolve problematic issues. This is of particular importance to case managers, who play an integral role in RM, especially identifying potential risk while engaged in medical record review as well as communication with members of the multidisciplinary team. Being on the front lines, case managers often are privy to discovering impending or completed adverse occurrences.
▶ Many of the tools used are effective for both QI and RM purposes.
▶ Both attempt to correct identified problems by educational methods, changes in policies and procedures, or disciplinary action.

▶ QI AND RM TERMINOLOGY

Some terms frequently used during QI and RM activities are self-explanatory: *mishap*, *patient safety problem*, *maloccurrence*. Others require further definition.

▶ Outcomes

Outcomes describe the results and consequences from the care received; outcomes also result from care that was not received. Outcome studies look for trend patterns and potentially adverse events. Poor outcomes revealed through outcome studies often lead to policy and procedural changes and additional training and education of personnel in an effort to improve the problem. Sometimes they may result in a change of job descriptions.

▶ Outcomes Management

Outcomes management is a process that applies outcomes research to practice, allowing the delivery of evidence-based care and treatments. It involves assessment and measurement of performance (based on specific indicators) at one point in time; monitoring and evaluation of performance using the same outcomes over time and at specific intervals (longitudinal approach); analysis and interpretation of the results to identify issues or concerns; and taking specific or strategic actions to improve quality and performance.

Combining outcomes and case management enables us to improve our patient care practices and performance by highlighting opportunities for:

- ▶ Enhancing patient care quality and safety.
- ▶ Implementation of evidence-based standards, protocols, and treatment options.
- ▶ Conducting systematic evaluation of performance, including the effectiveness of programs such as case management.

Case managers are frequently involved in the evaluation of the effectiveness of the case management programs of which they are a part. Such activities cannot be done without a focus on identifying key and strategic case management-related outcome indicators: assessment, measurement, and monitoring of these indicators; analyzing and interpreting the data; and finally improving the effectiveness of case management where the opportunity for improvement exists. These activities are nothing but outcomes management in itself. As a result of these activities, case managers are only then able to improve quality of the care patients receive and ensure that it also is safe.

Examples of outcome indicators/measures case managers evaluate include those listed in Table 7.1.

Healthcare organizations report their performance on these outcomes on a regular basis (e.g., monthly or quarterly) using a report card, dashboard, or scorecard format. They usually trend their performance over time (longitudinal approach) and compare it against predetermined targets, using either internal or external benchmarks, or both. Executives of case management programs also use these reports to communicate the contribution of case management to patient care quality, safety, and outcomes, including return on investment. Such reports are perceived as powerful tools to demonstrate the effectiveness of case management and its impact on patient care and healthcare services.

▶ Adverse Patient Outcome

An *adverse patient outcome* (APO) is defined as any adverse patient occurrence that, under optimal conditions, is not a natural consequence of the patient's disease process or the end-result of a procedure (Northrop & Kelly 1987). Many organizations detail a severity coding system for APOs. In general, severity ratings separate acceptable and unacceptable ranges of outcomes. For example:

Level I. There is a confirmed quality problem with minimal potential for significant adverse effect(s) on the patient. The problem may be a discharge with mild bacteriuria and pyuria and without follow-up plans for further evaluation. Events that are predictable within an expected standard of care also may be included in level I; these are events such as urinary retention after a total abdominal hysterectomy.

Level II. There is a confirmed quality problem with the potential for significant adverse effect(s) on the patient. Perhaps the wrong intravenous fluid or medication was administered but was quickly discovered and corrected before harm occurred.

Level III. There is a confirmed quality problem with significant deviation from expected levels of care, resulting in an unexpected injury to patients. These events represent gross departures from expected standards and may result in serious impairment such as loss of a limb or function of a body part, psychological injury, or death. An example would be operating on the wrong side, such as the left instead of the right hip, or removing the wrong kidney.

Healthcare organizations have a process in place for identifying, reporting, investigating, and correcting such events. An example is a root cause analysis

▶ **TABLE 7.1** **Examples of Outcome Measures Relevant to Case Management Programs**

CATEGORY	EXAMPLES OF OUTCOME MEASURES
Cost	▶ Length of stay ▶ Cost per case ▶ Cost per day ▶ Cost per diagnosis-related group ▶ Cost per service or product line
Utilization	▶ Average number of laboratory tests (e.g., complete blood count, chemistry, pathology) per case ▶ Average number of radiologic tests (e.g., chest x-ray, computerized tomography scan, magnetic resonance imaging) per case ▶ Denials rate ▶ Appeals conversion rate (by case manager) ▶ Appeals conversion rate (by physician advisor) ▶ Number of avoided days ▶ Conversion of observation status to inpatient status ▶ Volume of one day admissions ▶ Turnaround time on tests ▶ Turnaround time on procedures ▶ Surgical delays ▶ Surgical cancellation
Transitional planning and throughput	▶ Delays in discharge ▶ Re-admissions within 72 hours of discharge ▶ Re-admissions within 1 week of discharge ▶ Re-admissions within 30 days of discharge ▶ Volume of discharges to home without services ▶ Volume of discharges to home with home care ▶ Volume of discharges to another facility (e.g., skilled nursing facility, acute or subacute rehabilitation facility) ▶ Return to operating room ▶ Returns to intensive care unit ▶ Turnaround time on admission from emergency department ▶ Turnaround time on admissions from postanesthesia care unit ▶ Appropriateness of the level of care ▶ Effective hand offs/hand overs: completion of transfer of key information (verbal and written) from one provider or setting to another
Clinical	▶ Achievement of intermediate outcomes (e.g., switching from intravenous to oral medications) as expected in the clinical pathway ▶ Achievement of discharge outcomes (e.g., no fever for 24 hours prior to discharge) as expected in the clinical pathway ▶ Morbidity/complication rates (e.g., nosocomial infections) ▶ Mortality rates ▶ Relief of signs and symptoms of a disease condition ▶ Compliance rates with core measures (refer to table 7.2 for additional information) ▶ Medical errors or significant events ▶ Pain management
Satisfaction	▶ Patient experience ▶ Satisfaction scores ▶ Patient and family education ▶ Comfort ▶ Physical ability and level of independence ▶ State of well-being
Variance/ Delay in care	▶ Patient- and family-related variances ▶ System-related variances ▶ Community-related variances ▶ Practitioner-related variances

(RCA) process, which involves a multidisciplinary team that includes representation from risk management and quality and patient safety departments. Some of these events may require reporting to your state's Department of Health and/or to accreditation agencies such as TJC. Usually your organization will have an administrative procedure in place describing these events, the RCA process, and the reporting process.

The RCA process may include the following:

❭ Study of the involved environment, systems, and processes to identify the critical steps and decision points.
❭ Identification of the personnel, actions, and equipment necessary for the proper functioning of the system or process, and critical to its outcomes.
❭ Finding links between variables involved in performance.
❭ Ranking of the frequency of causes.

Investigating APOs by applying the RCA review process almost always results in recommendations for improving a patient care flow process, enforcement of a process, adding a new process, or eliminating an existing process. In addition, it may result in additional training and education of certain personnel, especially those intimately involved in the process. After a change has been implemented, monitoring of outcomes is usually necessary.

❭ Potentially Compensable Event

A potentially compensable event is one in which the end-result could be litigation (Northrop & Kelly 1987). For more information, refer to Chapter 8.

❭ Incident

An incident is an accident, error, or the discovery of a hazardous condition that is inconsistent with standards of care or standards of practice (Northrop & Kelly 1987).

❭ Incident Report (Also Known As Occurrence Report)

An incident report is a communication tool to record adverse events or unusual occurrences. Incident reports assess potential liabilities, are used for discovering existing problems, and assess the need for revising current policies or procedures. State law determines whether they are confidential or discoverable in court. It is not advisable to document in the medical record that an incident report has been filled out, although the events of the incident may be recorded in the patient's chart if

they are important to future care and treatment. Be objective, factual, clear, and complete. Refrain from speculation, subjectivity, or drawing judgment. This is important because incident reports may be discoverable in court.

❭ Variances

Variances are deviations from expected care. Four types of variances exist: practitioner, system/institutional, community, and patient/family (see "Lag Days and Variances" in Chapter 4 for a more complete discussion).

❭ Important Aspects of Care

These aspects of care occur frequently, affect large numbers of patients, or place patients at risk for serious consequences if not provided for optimally. These aspects of care are often the target of performance improvement activities and therefore must be measurable.

❭ Core Measures and Other CMS-Related Measures

Core measures are a national, standardized performance measurement system that was implemented to improve the quality of health care. First begun by TJC in 1997 as a voluntary effort for the management of the quality and performance of healthcare organizations, they were known as the ORYX measures and later renamed core measures. More recently, the Centers for Medicare & Medicaid Services (CMS) implemented a core measures system that is in alignment with TJC. The CMS system is also known as National Quality Measures and endeavors to help hospitals improve the quality of patient care by focusing on the actual results (outcomes, consequences) of care. The measures are medical information retrieved from patients' records and converted into a rate or percentage that shows how well hospitals care for their patients. The core measures include the following (see Table 7.2):

❭ Eight measures related to heart attack care.
❭ Four measures related to heart failure care.
❭ Seven measures related to pneumonia care.
❭ Five measures related to surgical infection prevention.
❭ Three measures related to asthma care for children only.

Today, participation in the public reporting of data on these core measures is an expectation by CMS. Although public reporting of data on core measures is not mandatory, if a hospital (for example) does not publicly report its data, its reimbursement by CMS will

▶ **TABLE 7.2   Core Measures/National Quality Measures**

DISEASE CATEGORY	CORE MEASURES
Pneumonia	▶ Oxygenation assessment ▶ Pneumococcal vaccination ▶ Blood cultures performed within 24 hours prior to or 24 hours after hospital arrival for patients who were transferred or admitted to the intensive care unit (ICU) within 24 hours of hospital arrival ▶ Blood cultures performed in the emergency department prior to antibiotic administration in the hospital ▶ Adult smoking cessation advice/counseling ▶ Initial antibiotic received within 4 hours of hospital arrival ▶ Initial antibiotic received within 6 hours of hospital arrival ▶ Initial antibiotic selection for community-acquired pneumonia in immunocompetent patient ▶ Influenza vaccination
Surgical care improvement/ surgical infection prevention	▶ Prophylactic antibiotic received within 1 hour prior to surgical incision (or 2 hours if receiving Vancomycin or Fluoroquinolone) ▶ Prophylactic antibiotic selection for surgical patient ▶ Prophylactic antibiotic discontinued within 24 hours after surgery end time ▶ Cardiac surgery patients with controlled 6 AM postoperative blood glucose ▶ Surgery patients with appropriate hair removal ▶ Colorectal surgery patients with immediate postoperative normothermia ▶ Surgery patients on beta-blockers therapy prior to admission who received a beta-blocker during the perioperative period ▶ Surgery patients who received appropriate venous thromboembolism prophylaxis ordered
Heart failure	▶ Discharge instructions (including diet, activity, follow-up, medications, symptoms worsening, and weight monitoring) ▶ Evaluation of left ventricular systolic function ▶ Angiotensin-converting enzyme (ACE) inhibitor or angiotensin receptor blocker (ARB) for left ventricular systolic dysfunction ▶ Adult smoking cessation advice/counseling
Acute myocardial infarction/heart attack	▶ Aspirin at arrival ▶ Aspirin prescribed at discharge ▶ ACE Inhibitor or ARB for left ventricular systolic dysfunction ▶ Adult smoking cessation advice/counseling ▶ Beta-blocker prescribed at discharge ▶ Beta-blocker at arrival ▶ Median time to fibrinolysis ▶ Fibrinolytic therapy received within 30 minutes of hospital arrival ▶ Median time to primary percutaneous coronary intervention ▶ Primary percutaneous coronary intervention received within 90 minutes of hospital arrival ▶ LDL cholesterol assessment ▶ Lipid-lowering therapy for discharge
Pediatric asthma	▶ Relievers for inpatient asthma (age 2–17 years) overall ▶ Relievers for inpatient asthma (age 2–4 years) ▶ Relievers for inpatient asthma (age 5–12 years) ▶ Relievers for inpatient asthma (age 13–17 years) ▶ Systemic corticosteroids for inpatient asthma (age 2–17 years) overall ▶ Systemic corticosteroids for inpatient asthma (age 2–4 years) ▶ Systemic corticosteroids for inpatient asthma (age 5–12 years) ▶ Systemic corticosteroids for inpatient asthma (age 13–17 years) ▶ Home management plan of care/document given to patient/caregiver

Source: U.S. Department of Health and Human Services. http://www.hospitalcompare.hhs.gov/Hospital/Static/About-HospQuality.asp?-dest=NAV%7CHome%7CAbout%7CQualityMeasures. Accessed August 26, 2008:

be affected. Therefore, hospitals tend to report their data to maintain acceptable reimbursement rates. The core measures are derived largely from a set of quality indicators defined by CMS. They have been shown to reduce the risk of complications, prevent recurrences, and otherwise treat the majority of patients who come to a hospital for treatment of a condition or illness. Under each category, key actions are listed that represent the most widely accepted, research-based care process for appropriate care in that category.

Other CMS-related measures are the Hospital Outcome of Care Measures, which include 30-day risk-adjusted death (mortality) rates and are produced from Medicare claims and enrollment data using a complex statistical model. The model predicts patient deaths for any cause within 30 days of hospital admission for heart attack, or heart failure, or pneumonia, whether the patients die while still in the hospital or after discharge. Thirty-day mortality is used because this is the time when deaths are most likely to be related to the care patients received in the hospital. Deaths that occur outside the hospital within 30 days are included along with deaths that occur in the hospital, because some hospitals discharge patients sooner than others. By *risk-adjusted* we mean that the model calculates a death (mortality) rate that adjusts for the kinds of patients who go to that hospital, so that hospitals that take care of sicker patients won't have a worse rate just because their patients were sicker before they arrived at the hospital.

As part of the ongoing effort to improve the quality of care, CMS also developed the first readmission outcome measure for hospitals in 2008: a 30-day risk-standardized readmission measure for heart failure (HF) patients. This measure responds to the recent call by the Medicare Payment Advisory Commission (MedPAC) to develop readmission measures, with HF as a priority condition. The measure includes fee-for-service (FFS) Medicare beneficiaries of at least 65 years of age with a principal discharge diagnosis of HF. In September 2008, CMS conducted a national "dry run" of the implementation of the 30-day HF readmission measure. The dry run was designed to educate hospitals about the HF readmission measure and to test the public reporting of outcomes on this measure. Similar to the 30-day-risk-adjusted-death rates, the readmission measure will also affect hospital reimbursement.

The 30-day-risk-adjusted-death rates and the HF readmission measure, in addition to the rest of the core measures, are important for case managers. The role case managers play in transitional and discharge planning relates directly to these outcomes. For example, if a patient were discharged prematurely from the hospital or patient's care needs after discharge were not appropriately coordinated, resulting in an unsafe discharge, the patient would have a much higher chance of experiencing serious deterioration in health condition and therefore an increased risk for death after discharge.

In addition, CMS requires hospitals to evaluate patient and family satisfaction with care received, using the Hospital Consumer Assessment of Healthcare Providers and Systems (HCAHPS) measure. This is a national, standardized survey of hospital patients. HCAHPS was created to publicly report the patient's perspective on hospital care. The survey asks a random sample of recently discharged patients about important aspects of their hospital experience. Included in this assessment of patients' experiences are questions about how prepared they were for discharge and how informed they were about new medications—two important case management responsibilities. Similar to data on the core measures, the HCAHPS results are also publicly reported and posted on the Hospital Compare Web site to allow consumers of healthcare to make fair and objective comparisons among hospitals, and of individual hospitals to state and national benchmarks. For more on HCAHPS information, visit the official HCAHPS Web site (www.hcahpsonline.org).

▶ HOW CASE MANAGEMENT, QUALITY MANAGEMENT, AND RM WORK TOGETHER

Case managers constantly oversee all aspects of patient care: assessing, reassessing, evaluating, monitoring, and reevaluating. For this reason, case managers are critical team members in the QI-RM process. Consider the following six high-risk areas for healthcare professionals, including nurses; after reviews of occurrences and actual claims against nurses, these deficits have been deemed areas of practice that can become major sources of liability (Northrop & Kelly 1987). Many of these "failures" can be spotted through astute chart reviews; hopefully, this can prevent an APO (Northrop & Kelly 1987).

1. Failure to take or properly assess a patient's history. *Example:* a missed medication allergy.
2. Failure to perform a nursing procedure according to nursing standards. *Example:* failure to properly administer medications.
3. Failure to follow a doctor's order promptly; failure to follow a doctor's order correctly. *Example:* failure to follow the organization's chain of command if the nurse or case manager thinks something is wrong or lacking in the orders. It may also be that the correct

procedure was followed; however, it may not have been fully documented.

4. Failure to report deviations from accepted practice. *Example:* again, this may also be a lack of complete documentation of what really transpired.

5. Failure to properly supervise the patient. *Example:* patient falls, intravenous line failures or infiltrates, patient extubation. These may be from inadequate monitoring; they may also be due to staff covering more patients than is humanly possible.

6. Failure to summon the medical attending physician appropriately. *Example:* a related but frequent allegation is failure to communicate appropriate and complete information to the physician.

Keeping these high-risk areas of concern in mind, consider how important a case manager's skills and responsibilities are from a QI-RM perspective. As patient advocates who are involved in all areas of patient care, case managers are always alert for hindrances to optimal outcomes. Case management is a highly prized RM tool in many ways.

▶ Case Managers Identify and Anticipate Potential Problems

▶ Case managers are adept at identifying circumstances that make the patient vulnerable to high-risk incidents, optimally before they happen but certainly before they have done maximum damage. Related to this is the identification of potential safety issues in confused and/or frail patients. For example, quality chart reviews reveal that a patient had a high potassium level, yet no one discontinued potassium from the intravenous solutions. Review also shows that a medication that was listed under allergies was ordered for a patient.

▶ Case managers identify traits in patients that could make them vulnerable to high-risk incidents and adjust the case plan for maximum safety.

▶ Case managers act as patient advocates; they function in a capacity in which they hear many patient and family complaints. Sometimes the case manager can appropriately intervene; sometimes it is important to call the RM department. The wise choice is always to practice good communication and documentation skills.

▶ Case managers act as liaisons among the patient, the facilities where they work, other providers of care, and the insurance company. In this capacity, case managers assist in developing treatment and discharge plans. The case manager ascertains the best plan to meet the individual needs of the patient—all within the constraints of the payor (insurance company). This often takes thought, creativity, and negotiation skills in today's resource-conscious atmosphere. At times, it is necessary to do some bargaining to meet the basic needs of the patient. Perhaps without the case manager's assessment of the need for these services—and negotiation skills—this patient would be a future risk liability; many insurance companies realize this concept and are willing to cooperate by authorizing plans that have been negotiated by the case manager to enhance the patient's safety. The authorization may include more discharge supports than are normally covered, such as a noncovered service or piece of equipment.

▶ Quality Reviews

Quality reviews refer to screening the clinical content of the patient's medical record and treatment to determine if professionally and nationally recognized standards of care were met. Many times a careful review of the medical record will reveal issues or situations that warrant a closer inspection of the care provided. Any condition that may indicate poor or incomplete patient care, occurring either inside a facility or as an outpatient service, requires QI or RM notification. In general, the sequence for handling quality reviews goes as follows:

1. Identification of a quality concern. This concern may be revealed in a chart review or in a discussion with a member of the multidisciplinary team or patient/family member.

2. Determination if a quality problem indeed exists. If a significant breach of the standards of care is suspected, it must then be validated by appropriate professionals. The case manager must decide how to proceed, and that may depend on the type of organization. For a hospital case manager, the first line is usually a call to the RM department; in a health maintenance organization or other organization, a medical director or administrator may need to be notified. The case manager should make details of the concern and appropriate documentation available to the medical director or other specialist to determine if there is, in

fact, a problem. Organizations usually have policies and procedures that mandate the sequence of events that must take place when a quality of care issue is suspect. Depending on the issue or concern at hand, an RCA may be completed.

3. Confirmation of the existence of a quality problem. The organizational policy and procedure usually detail how, in what time frame, and to whom the information is communicated.

When reviewing charts, a quality review may identify poor or incomplete patient care (see Appendix 7.A), clues to possible delayed diagnoses, and admission concerns.

DELAYED DIAGNOSES

Be aware that reasons other than missed early clues—such as patient noncompliance—can cause some of these delayed diagnoses:

▶ First admission for advanced disease processes including, for example, advanced metastatic cancer, perforated ulcer, advanced tuberculosis.

▶ Diagnosis such as a perforated appendix when a chart review reveals an emergency department visit 3 days before admission to the hospital for abdominal pain.

▶ Severe diabetic ketoacidosis (watch for noncompliance or "brittle" diabetes).

▶ Shock (various types) or septicemia.

▶ Possible poor monitoring of a patient's condition. Examples include pregnancy-induced hypertension (preeclampsia, eclampsia, and toxemia) and diabetic ketoacidosis.

ADMISSIONS CONCERNS

▶ Admissions for diseases for which immunizations are available. Did the pediatrician or primary care physician offer the immunizations? Did the parent (or patient, if an adult) refuse them or not take the child to the primary care physician for them?

▶ Admissions from complications following an outpatient or emergency department procedure. Examples include poorly set fractures, neurologic defects, and wound infections.

▶ Admissions for side effects of outpatient drug therapy. Did the patient take more, or less, than was ordered? Did the physician or nurse improperly or incompletely educate the patient about the medication? Were the patient's blood levels adequately monitored

for the medication? Examples include gastrointestinal bleeding resulting from the patient taking aspirin while also taking Coumadin or hypokalemia while the patient is taking a potassium-depleting diuretic.

▶ Readmission for the same condition within 2 weeks or 30 days of discharge for same problem/chief complaint. This can happen with any condition or diagnosis. The causes may range from patient noncompliance (a woman with heart failure who goes home and eats pretzels) to poor outpatient monitoring or premature discharge.

OTHER EXAMPLES OF QUALITY REVIEWS

Sometimes critical thinking and investigative work must precede the discovery of poor management of the care of a patient or the occurrence of adverse events. For example:

▶ During a gastrectomy, the spleen is removed. Because this is not standard protocol for a gastrectomy, the curious case manager would investigate. No explanation is found in the progress notes or the operative procedure report. The pathology report states that the splenic artery had been injured, necessitating the removal of the spleen.

▶ Perhaps a hysterectomy patient returns postoperatively with bloody urine. A further review shows the ureter was inadvertently transected and repaired.

▶ A 6-week-old infant is admitted for seizures. A review of his birth chart reveals that labor was prolonged and difficult; it necessitated midforceps delivery.

▶ An infant with congenital heart disease develops severe bradycardia and arrhythmia and dies. An autopsy report shows his digoxin level was 10 times above the normal range.

▶ An infant with an Apgar score of 3 requires resuscitation. A review of the maternal predelivery record shows that the mother had been given excessive doses of narcotics.

▶ RM Recommendations and Prevention Skills

CONSULT A RISK MANAGER

When in doubt about anything that may preclude an RM event, call a risk manager in your organization for clarification and evaluation.

WARN THE RM DEPARTMENT

A goal of RM is never to be served with a lawsuit of which the facility agency was previously unaware. Through warnings by the case manager, the RM department would have time to flag the chart, review the medical records, and possibly review court records.

DO NOT AVOID ANGRY CLIENTS

When a patient or family has complaints, listen and be responsive. Many families and patients are angry because they feel no one is listening to them. Listening may not avert all lawsuits, but it is true that people get angrier if they feel ignored.

NOTIFY A RISK MANAGER OF POTENTIAL SUITS

If a patient or family member mentions a lawsuit or attorney, a call to the risk manager may be appropriate. Although unreasonable expectations may be the cause of the threat, it is still better to notify the RM department for its assessment.

BE INCLUSIVE

Include the patient/family unit in the decision-making process about various aspects of care. Those inside the boat are less likely to rock it.

CAREFULLY CONSIDER READMISSIONS

Readmissions soon after a discharge from the hospital need careful consideration. This is especially true if the previous admission had the possibility of suboptimal treatment or an inappropriate discharge (either a premature discharge or the result of poor discharge planning).

PAY SPECIAL ATTENTION TO HIGH-RISK NEONATES

Adverse outcomes in neonates need attention. All parents reasonably expect a positive outcome—a healthy newborn; events that deviate from this expectation could benefit from an RM evaluation.

PRACTICE QUALITY DOCUMENTATION

Documentation is a vital aspect of RM. This theme surfaces often throughout this book. Its importance cannot be overstated and is especially critical in the courtroom when proving whether negligence or malpractice has occurred. The old adage, "if it's not documented, it did not occur" is important; what is documented versus what is not documented can determine the outcome of a case. Documentation in a medical record may be the only evidence available to indicate whether a standard of care was met. Because years usually have gone by between the care and the court date, important details may be lost without thorough documentation.

The RM department also depends on quality documentation for determining how to handle a particular case. What the old adage does not do is give specific guidelines that may be helpful if a case does go to litigation. The following are some further recommendations regarding documentation:

▶ Ask yourself whether you would mind if your charting was read aloud in court. If the answer is "yes" on any case, assess why you feel discomfort. For example, did subjectivity, judgment, or frustration show up in your notes? Were your notes incomplete? Use this assessment for personal growth and improvement.

▶ Document all communications between yourself, the patient/family, other healthcare professionals, and physicians. Include dates and times calls were initiated, response time, doctor's response to the reason for the call, and your intervention. Number 6 in the previous list of high-risk areas for nurses was a failure to summon medical attention. Perhaps in some cases the physician was summoned but, without documented proof, the nurse had to assume the responsibility for a poor outcome. If a physician is paged and does not answer within a reasonable amount of time and after a reasonable number of attempts, go through the chain of command until a physician who will address the problem can be reached. Document all efforts and their outcomes.

▶ Falls are a major cause of litigation, especially when due to failure to properly supervise a patient. Document close observation, falls assessment, implementation of fall prevention activities, use of side rails, and visits to a patient's room for treatment and monitoring purposes. This is especially important for case managers who are also direct care nurses.

▶ Follow some basic record-keeping rules. To begin, remember to include the date and time on all entries. This is especially true in emergency situations. Furthermore, state all information clearly, factually, objectively, and completely. This should ensure that standards of care are met. Any measures used to prevent complications should be noted, because they may show good faith in the future. Avoid ambiguity. "Feels warm," "high blood pressure," and "lower temperature," are too nonspecific. Chart the facts—the actual values.

Use words that are not susceptible to multiple meanings.

▶ In a court of law, the appearance of the chart is often as important as the content. Use TJC-approved abbreviations and recommendations. Using a whiting-out agent to delete errors is not permissible in court and leaves room for suspicion of falsifying information. The chart for one case involving whiting-out agent had to be x-rayed to determine what was underneath. Use a single line to cross out an error. Write "error" over the single line and initial it. Sign all completed entries. Also, make sure all blanks and boxes are filled in or checked. Always write legibly and with permanent black ink.

▶ If electronic documentation is used, be aware that the time of documentation may not necessarily be the actual time of observation, treatment, or evaluation. Remember to include the time of such activities in your documentation to avoid the problem of wrong time and the need to explain that in a court of law; those who review the chart may assume the electronic and automated time stamp is the actual time if the time has not been amended in your notes.

▶ Good follow-through should be evident from the chart. If a critical laboratory value or patient condition is noted, as stated above, keep track of the person to whom you reported it and what the response was. Note all patient responses to any treatments or medications given (again, this is especially important for case managers with direct patient care responsibilities). If a physician's order is not carried out, explain the reason(s).

▶ When documenting complications or mishaps, be factual, thorough, and objective. Do not assign blame or fault.

▶ Threats and complaints can be documented, but it is best to quote, if possible. Document follow-up actions to the threat or complaint.

▶ Patient or family concerns or worries can also be documented. Identify who expressed concern, what was said (quote if possible), your verbal responses, and any interventions that were done in response to the concern.

▶ Patient noncompliance needs to be documented, including what the patient is or is not doing. A diabetic eating candy or a patient allowed nothing by mouth found munching on crackers is not an uncommon occurrence. Nevertheless, such situations can delay surgical procedures and extend length of stay. In many cases, noncompliance can harm a patient and interfere with optimal patient care.

▶ Document informed consent about medical procedures (more on this subject is discussed in "Informed Consent" in Chapter 8).

▶ Document information about transferring patients to other facilities. Record on the chart who was spoken to and what was agreed on. This may include conversations or telephone calls to the patient's family, the skilled nursing facility, and the attending physician. Note who made the decision to transfer, when the transfer took place, and who approved the transfer. If there is a suboptimal outcome during or after a transfer, and there is no documentation that the family supported the transfer decision, repercussions can occur.

▶ QUALITY INDICATORS

Quality indicators are measurable, specific, and clear guides for monitoring and evaluating important aspects of patient care. Indicators may be written for any area that enhances patient care, from ambulatory services and social services to nuclear medicine and case management. Each service has its own specific indicators to monitor potential problems or opportunities to improve patient care. Ongoing monitoring should reveal trends and opportunities for improvement. Several years ago, one study revealed a high rate of pneumothorax after central line insertions. Astute detective work disclosed a problem with a discrepancy between the insertion site and the use of an appropriate length of catheter. As a result, standards/protocols to address the prevention of such problems are followed.

Appendix 7.A includes several sample indicators from various service lines. A visit to the facility's QI and patient safety (QIPS) department is likely to reveal several books on quality screens and monitors. A review is recommended, especially in your specific service line or case management practice setting. Such reviews often raise red flags about certain situations, and the case manager can then alert the QIPS or RM departments. Appendix 7.B displays sample clinical indicators of generic quality screens advocated for by accreditation agencies and CMS. A review of the CMS generic screens demonstrates some circumstances that may signal inadequate quality of care. Appendix 7.C includes a compilation of 10 types of claims categories gleaned from the National Practitioner's Data Bank. These categories are used by RM departments as a possible indication of suboptimal quality of care. A review of the indicators, the CMS generic screens, and the claims categories should arm the case manager with enough cues so that an "off" case will signal further investigation and monitoring and possibly a call to the RM or quality management departments.

Quality indicators also include those described earlier in this chapter: case management outcome indicators/measures (Table 7.1) and core measures (Table 7.2). When examining quality in your organization, look for all the indicators your organization reports on, whether they are directly or indirectly related to the case management program of which you are a part. Often you will find that going beyond the case management program leads you to a better understanding of the total picture of quality and patient safety in your organization. Such understanding will also provide you with more appreciation of your role in, and contribution to, quality and the reputation of your organization. As you identify opportunities for improvement, you are better able to package a PI project beyond the immediate boundaries of your case management program, and therefore you are able to sell your improvement project idea to the executives in your organization so that they can invest in making it happen. Communicating the value and benefits of your proposed improvement from the patient's perspective and experience as well as its potential impact on organizational performance are usually effective strategies for obtaining buy-in.

▶ PATIENT SAFETY AND CASE MANAGEMENT

Across the healthcare continuum and settings, patients are routinely transferred from one care provider, service, or setting to another. During these transitions, the risk of providing suboptimal care may exist. If case managers are careful during these transitions, exercise their patient/family advocacy role, and assume responsibility and accountability for ensuring patient safety, quality of care, and satisfaction with the experience, safe, optimal and effective care is guaranteed. This "guarantee" is strengthened when case managers ensure the transfer of key and necessary information (both in verbal and written forms) between providers and settings. As a result, medical errors are prevented, safety is enhanced, continuity of care is maintained, and ultimately, quality is ensured.

Case managers integrate patient safety activities into every phase of the case management process: for example, advocacy, medication reconciliation, timeliness of care activities or treatments, timely completion of necessary tests, communication among providers of care, and communication with payers. From assessment and planning, to monitoring and evaluation of outcomes, the case management process provides an excellent opportunity for implementing a proactive approach to patient safety by ensuring access to quality, safe, effective, timely, patient-centric/family-centric, and efficacious care and outcomes.

NOTE

Key Organizations That Focus on Patient Safety

The Joint Commission: http://www.jointcommission.org

National Patient Safety Foundation: http://www.npsf.org

World Health Organization/World Alliance for Patient Safety: http://www.who.int/patientsafety/en/

Agency for Healthcare Research and Quality/Patient Safety Network: http://www.psnet.ahrq.gov/

Institute for Healthcare Improvement: http://www.ihi.org/IHI/Topics/PatientSafety/

United States Department of Veterans Affairs/National Center for Patient Safety: http://www.va.gov/ncps/

Consumers Advancing Patient Safety: http://www.patientsafety.org/

United States Food and Drug Administration/Patient Safety News: http://www.accessdata.fda.gov/psn/index.cfm

---

One of the original and most popular organizations to promote patient safety is TJC. It approved its first set of National Patient Safety Goals (NPSGs) in July 2002. These goals included specific requirements for improving quality and patient care safety in healthcare organizations. Today, almost 50% of TJC's standards are directly related to safety. Assessment of safety during an accreditation survey is "front and center" to the survey. The standards address specific issues that affect patient safety during an episode of care and illness (TJC, 2008b). Case managers can play an important and integral role in assisting an organization to adhere to the standards and the NPSGs. For example, case managers can prevent accidental harm by ensuring that the medication reconciliation process is completed for every individual patient and that the hand off/hand over communication includes the transfer of key information (e.g., medical regimen, medications, allergies, plan of care, and so on) from one provider or setting to another is timely and complete.

▶ **TABLE 7.3   2009 National Patient Safety Goals (NPSGs)**

GOAL	REQUIREMENTS	DESCRIPTION
1: Patient identification	NPSG 01.01.01	Use at least two patient identifiers when providing care, treatment, and services.
	NPSG 01.02.01	Prior to start of any surgical or invasive procedure, individuals involved in the procedure conduct a final verification process, such as time-out, to confirm the correct patient, procedure, and site using active, not passive, communication techniques.
	NPSG 01.03.01	Eliminate transfusion errors related to patient identification.
2: Communication	NPSG 02.01.01	For verbal or telephone orders or telephone reporting of critical test results, the individual giving the order verifies the complete order or test result by having the person receiving the information record and "read-back" the complete order or test result.
	NPSG 02.02.01	There is a standardized list of abbreviations, acronyms, symbols, and dose designations that are not to be used throughout the organization.
	NPSG 02.03.01	The organization measures, assesses and, if needed, takes action to improve timeliness of reporting, and the timeliness of receipt of critical tests, and critical results and values by the responsible licensed caregiver.
	NPSG 02.05.01	The organization implements a standardized approach to hand-off communications including an opportunity to ask and respond to questions.
3: Medications	NPSG 03.03.01	The organization identifies and, at a minimum, annually reviews a list of look-alike/sound-alike medications used by the organization and takes action to prevent errors involving the interchange of these medications.
	NPSG 03.04.01	Label all medications, medication containers (for example, syringes, medicine cups, basins), or other solutions on and off the sterile field.
	NPSG 03.05.01	Reduce the likelihood of patient harm associated with the use of anticoagulation therapy.
7: Healthcare-associated infections	NPSG 07.01.01	Comply with current World Health Organization or Centers for Disease Control and Prevention hand hygiene guidelines.
	NPSG 07.02.01	Implement evidence-based practices to prevent healthcare associated infections due to multiple drug ressistant organisms in acute care hospitals.
	NPSG 07.03.01	Manage as sentinel events all identified cases of unanticipated death or major permanent loss of function related to a healthcare-associated infection.
	NPSG 07.04.01	Implement best practices or evidence-based guidelines to prevent central line-associated bloodstream infections.
	NPSG 07.05.01	Implement best practices for preventing surgical site infections.
8: Medications reconciliation	NPSG 08.01.01	A process exists for comparing the patient's current medications with those ordered for the patient while under the care of the organization.
	NPSG 08.02.01	When a patient is referred or transferred from one organization to another, the complete and reconciled list of medications is communicated to the next provider of service and communication is documented. Alternatively, when a patient leaves the organization's care directly to his/her home, the complete and reconciled list of medications is provided to the patient's known primary care provider, or the original referring provider, or a known next provider of service.
	NPSG 08.03.01	When a patient leaves the organization's care, a complete and reconciled list of the patient's medications is provided directly to the patient, and the patient's family, as needed, and the list is explained to the patient and/or family.
	NPSG 08.04.01	In settings where medications are used minimally or prescribed for a short duration, modified medications reconciliation processes are performed.

(continued)

▶ **TABLE 7.3   2009 National Patient Safety Goals (NPSGs)** *(Continued)*

GOAL	REQUIREMENTS	DESCRIPTION
9: Falls	NPSG 09.02.01	The organization implements a falls reduction program that includes an evaluation of the effectiveness of the program.
10: Influenza and pneumococcal disease risk	NPSG 10.01.01	The organization develops and implements protocols for administration of the flu vaccine.
	NPSG 10.02.01	The organization develops and implements protocols for administration of the pneumococcal vaccine.
	NPSG 10.03.01	The organization develops and implements protocols to identify new cases of influenza and to manage outbreaks.
11: Surgical fire risk	NPSG 11.01.01	The organization educates staff, including licensed independent practitioners who are involved with surgical procedures and anesthesia providers, on how to control heat sources, how to manage fuels while maintaining enough time for patient preparation, and establish guidelines to minimize oxygen concentration under drapes.
13: Patient's active involvement in own safety	NPSG 13.01.01	Identify the ways in which the patient and his or her family report concerns about safety and encourage them to do so.
14: Pressure ulcers	NPSG 14.01.01	Assess and periodically reassess each resident's risk for developing a pressure ulcer (decubitus ulcer) and take action to address any identified risk.
15: Safety risks	NPSG 15.01.01	The organization identifies patient's risk for suicide.
	NPSG 15.02.01	The organization identifies risks associated with home oxygen therapy such as home fires.
16: Recognition of changes in patient's condition,	NPSG 16.01.01	The organization selects a suitable method that enables healthcare staff members to directly request additional assistance from a specialty trained individual(s) when the patient's condition appears to be worsening.
Universal protocol (UP)	UP 01.01.01	Conduct a pre-procedure verification process.
	UP 01.02.01	Mark the procedure site.
	UP 01.03.01	A time-out is performed immediately prior to starting procedures.

Source: National Patient Safety Goals according to The Joint Commission. Available online at http://www.jointcommission.org Accessed August 27, 2008.

The 2009 NPSGs are listed in Table 7.3. Table 7.4 shares the applicability of each of the goals to the various types of healthcare organizations. It also identifies the goals where case management programs and the role of the case manager can affect the organization's ability to adhere to the NPSGs. The goals where case management is most valuable include those in the following areas:

▶ Communication among members of the healthcare team, especially in reporting of test results and hand offs or hand overs.
▶ Use of evidence-based practice standards/protocols such as anticoagulation therapy.
▶ Prevention of healthcare-associated infections, especially through the use of evidence-based practice standards/protocols (e.g., prevention of surgical site infection through use of antibiotic prophylaxis; prevention of central-line associated blood stream infections).
▶ Medications reconciliation.
▶ Patient involvement in own safety through patient and family education of healthcare safety activities (e.g., hand hygiene).
▶ Safety risks at home, especially if the patient is on oxygen therapy (e.g., oxygen therapy safety and prevention of fires) or of dependent physical functioning (e.g., barrier-free environment and use of mobility-assist devices). This is best accomplished through the case manager's role in transitional/discharge planning and patient/family education.

▶ TABLE 7.4 Application of the 2009 NPSGs to Various Healthcare Organizations and CM Impact

GOAL	REQUIREMENTS	AHC	BHC	CAH	DSC	HOSP	HHC	LAB	LTC	LT-CMS	OBS	CM IMPACT*
1: Patient identification	NPSG 01.01.01	X	X	X	X	X	X	X	X	X	X	
	NPSG 01.02.01						X	X	X	X		
	NPSG 01.03.01	X		X		X					X	
2: Communication	NPSG 02.01.01	X	X	X	X	X	X	X	X	X	X	
	NPSG 02.02.01	X	X	X	X	X	X	X	X	X	X	
	NPSG 02.03.01	X	X	X	X	X	X	X	X	X	X	X
	NPSG 02.05.01		X	X	X	X	X	X	X	X	X	X
3: Medications	NPSG 03.03.01	X	X	X		X	X		X	X	X	
	NPSG 03.04.01	X		X		X					X	
	NPSG 03.05.01	X		X		X	X		X	X		X
7: Healthcare-associated infections	NPSG 07.01.01	X	X	X	X	X	X	X	X	X	X	
	NPSG 07.02.01	X	X	X	X	X	X	X	X	X	X	X
	NPSG 07.03.01			X		X						X
	NPSG 07.04.01	X		X		X	X			X		X
	NPSG 07.05.01	X		X		X					X	X
8: Medications reconciliation	NPSG 08.01.01	X	X	X	X	X	X		X	X	X	X
	NPSG 08.02.01	X	X	X	X	X	X		X	X	X	X
	NPSG 08.03.01	X	X	X	X	X	X		X	X	X	X
	NPSG 08.04.01	X	X	X	X	X	X		X	X	X	X
9: Falls	NPSG 09.02.01			X	X	X	X		X	X		
10: Influenza and pneumococcal disease risk	NPSG 10.01.01					X			X	X		
	NPSG 10.02.01					X			X	X		
	NPSG 10.03.01					X			X	X		
11: Surgical fire risk	NPSG 11.01.01	X									X	
13: Patient's active involvement in own safety	NPSG 13.01.01	X	X	X	X	X	X	X	X	X	X	X
14: Pressure ulcers	NPSG 14.01.01								X	X		
15: Safety risks	NPSG 15.01.01		X			X						X
	NPSG 15.02.01						X					X
16: Recognition of changes in patient's condition	NPSG 16.01.01			X		X						X
Universal protocol (UP)	UP 01.01.01	X		X	X	X					X	
	UP 01.02.01	X		X	X	X					X	
	UP 01.03.01	X		X	X	X					X	

*NPSGs where Case Management and the Role of the Case Manager can impact on

X indicates that the goal applies in this care setting

NPSGs, National Patient Saftey Goals; AHC, Ambulatory Health Care; BHC, Behavioral Health Care; CAh, Critical Access Hospital; HHC, Home Health Care; DSC, Disease-Specific Care; LAB, Laboratory; LTC,Long-Term Care; LT-CMC, Long-Term Care-Medicare and Medicaid Certified Programs; OBS, Office Based Surgery; Case Management

Source: National Patient Safety Goals according to The Joint Commission. Available online at http://www.jointcommission.org Accessed August 27, 2008.

▶ Recognition of changes in patient's condition, which is achieved by engaging the right healthcare provider at the right time to address deterioration in patient health status, preventing delays in treatment, and enhancing patient's access to care.

STUDY QUESTIONS

1. Describe a significant event or adverse patient outcome you identified in your practice that resulted in a root cause analysis. How did you go about identifying the event? What was your role in the review process? What was the value of having case management represented on the root cause analysis team?

2. What outcomes does your organization monitor and report on that relate to the case management program? How does your role as a case manager enhance your organization's performance in these outcomes?

3. How does your organization incorporate the national patient safety goals into the role of the case manager? If it does not, how do you suggest it should? Why?

4. Describe how the role of the case manager in transitional and discharge planning impacts quality, outcomes, and core measures.

5. Describe how the role of the case manager in utilization review and management impacts quality, outcomes, and core measures.

▶ REFERENCES

Fanucci, D., Hammil, M., Johannson, P., Leggett, J., & Smith, M.J. (1993). Quantum leap into continuous quality improvement. *Nursing Management*, 24(6), 28–30.

Kongstvedt, P.R. (1993). *The managed health care handbook*. Gaithersburg, MD: Aspen Publishers.

Northrop, C.E., & Kelly, M.E. (1987). *Legal issues in nursing*. St. Louis: Mosby.

Sederer, L.I. (1987). Utilization review and quality assurance: Staying in the black and working with the blues. *General Hospital Psychiatry*, 9, 210–219.

The Joint Commission. (2008a). *Comprehensive accreditation manual for hospitals*. Oakbrook Terrace, IL: Joint Commission Resources.

The Joint Commission. (2008b). (accessed 8/27/2008). 2009 *National patient safety goals*. [Online]. Available: http://www.jointcommission.org.

- Some of these indicators are "undeveloped" and lacking specific criteria; your institution's indicators will likely contain objective criteria to match the needs of the organization.
- Many of these indicators are for inpatient and outpatient settings; indicators can be written for any organization.
- These indicators do not represent a complete list of potential complications; the case manager can use these as guideposts.

CARDIOLOGY AND CARDIOVASCULAR INDICATORS

- Readmission within 30 days of discharge
- Congestive heart failure—not present on admission
- Pericarditis—not present on admission
- Pulmonary embolus—not present on admission
- Cardiac/respiratory arrest following cardiovascular (or other) procedure
- Postoperative neurologic deficits
- Complication of thrombolytic therapy
  Gingival bleeding
  Hematemesis
  Hematomas at puncture sites
- Unplanned transfer to special care unit
- Injury to organ/structure during cardiovascular procedure

- Return to operating room for postoperative thoracic bleeding
- Return for percutaneous transluminal coronary angioplasty (PTCA) of some lesion within 72 hours
- Post-PTCA complications such as hematoma at insertion site requiring evacuation or vascular intervention
- Patients undergoing nonemergent PTCA with subsequent occurrence of either an acute myocardial infarction (MI) or coronary artery bypass graft (CABG) surgery needed within the same hospitalization
- Patient undergoing attempted or completed PTCA during which any lesion attempted is not dilated

PEDIATRIC CARDIOVASCULAR INDICATORS

- Return to surgery for exploration of bleeding or other complication
- Infection of device or graft
- Sepsis with positive blood cultures
- Postoperative neurologic deficits
- Wound infection or dehiscence
- Pulmonary emboli not present on admission

- Cardiac or respiratory arrest
- Complication of device or graft such as occlusion or malfunction
- New-onset renal failure requiring dialysis
- Readmission for complication of surgical procedure within 30 days of discharge
- All deaths related to surgical procedures

PEDIATRIC INDICATORS

- Apgar scores less than 6 at 1 minute and less than 8 at 5 minutes
- Newborn injuries
- Transfer to neonatal intensive care unit after 24 hours of age
- Readmission to hospital within 72 hours of discharge
- Physical or sexual abuse

- Fever of unknown origin
- Errors in diagnosis and management
- Inpatient mortality including perioperative mortality
- Unscheduled admissions following ambulatory procedure
- Unscheduled return to ICU within 48 hours of transfer

NEUROLOGY AND NEUROSURGICAL INDICATORS

- Unplanned readmission within 15 days of discharge
- Unplanned transfer to a special care unit
- Injury to an organ or structure during a procedure or treatment
- Pulmonary emboli or deep vein thrombosis (DVT) not present on admission
- More than five consultations
- Complication of neurodiagnostic procedures
- Neurologic deficits not present on admission
- Organ failure not present on admission
- Cardiac or respiratory arrest

- Discharges against medical advice (AMA) or patient/family dissatisfaction
- Deaths
- Unplanned return to operating room
- Unplanned removal, injury, or repair to an organ or structure during an operative procedure
- Acute MI during or within 48 hours of an operative procedure
- Wound infection or dehiscence
- Pulmonary edema not present on admission
- Unplanned transfusion of greater than 2 units of blood
- Acute hemorrhage or wound hematoma postoperatively

(continued)

APPENDIX 7-A—*CONTINUED*

INTERNAL MEDICINE INDICATORS

- Complications from invasive, diagnostic, or monitoring procedures
- Management errors including errors of omission or commission
- Death (see death indicators below)
- Delays or inadequacies in diagnosis increasing length of stay
- Adverse reactions to medications
- Unplanned admission to special care unit
- Pneumothorax following central line insertion
- Unplanned readmission for same reason within 30 days of discharge
- Unplanned transfer to special care unit
- Cardiac-respiratory arrest
- Patient/family dissatisfaction or AMA discharge
- Pulmonary emboli or deep vein thrombosis (DVT) not present on admission
- Complications of anticoagulation therapy
- Organ failure not present on admission
- Urinary tract infection (nosocomial)

UTILIZATION INDICATORS

- Hospital admission not meeting acute criteria
- Readmission within 30 days for incomplete management of problems of previous hospitalization
- Peer review organization/quality improvement organization issue needs attention
- Readmission within 15 days for same diagnosis
- Receipt of Medicare denial
- Inappropriate observation status
- Delays in diagnosis increasing length of stay

ANESTHESIA INDICATORS

- Malintubation or reintubation
- Morbidity or mortality for complications such as hose disconnection, incorrect gas flow, or too much or too little medication
- Patient's developing postural headache within 4 postprocedure days following use of spinal or epidural anesthesia administration
- Dental injury following procedure involving anesthesia care
- Ocular injury during procedures involving anesthesia care
- Unplanned admission within 2 postprocedure days following outpatient procedures involving anesthesia
- Vocal cord paralysis after intubation that was not present before intubation

SOCIAL WORK INDICATORS

- Recognition of psychosocial needs such as crisis intervention
- Timeliness of interventions
- Quality of counseling/interventions
- Interdisciplinary collaboration
- Abuse (child and elder)
- Appropriateness of discharge or referrals
- Lack of health insurance

AMBULATORY INDICATORS

- Unscheduled returns to the emergency department within 72 hours
- Cancellation of ambulatory procedure on day of procedure
- Unplanned admission to acute care related to surgery or complication
- Patient not accompanied home by a designated person post ambulatory procedure
- Morbidity: vascular, neurologic, pulmonary, cardiac, drug reactions, or infections
- Local anesthesia supplemented with general anesthesia
- Adequate patient education for safe self-care
- Lack of patient/family education

EMERGENCY SERVICES INDICATORS

- Registered patients in emergency department more than 6 hours or delayed evaluations or treatment
- Registered patients who leave emergency department before completion of treatment or AMA emergency department discharges
- Transfers to another acute care facility
- Return visit for similar or same complaint
- Misadministration or adverse drug reaction
- Death after arrival and within 48 hours of admission
- Consultant responds within reasonable time
- Complications related to caseload

(continued)

APPENDIX 7-A—*CONTINUED*

DIETARY SERVICES INDICATORS

- Appropriateness of diet order versus diagnosis
- Adequacy of dietary counseling/teaching
- Adequacy of parenteral nutrition

- Duration of nothing by mouth (NPO) status without nutritional support
- Adequacy of nutritional values of diets
- Diet orders/errors or ambiguous or improper dietary order

PATHOLOGY INDICATORS

- Monitoring unnecessary tests
- Evaluating appropriate sequencing and frequency of tests

- Evaluating of inadequate or improper specimens
- Lost or inappropriately labeled specimen

NUCLEAR MEDICINE INDICATORS

- Turnaround time for studies
- Comparison between nuclear medicine and pathologic diagnosis for inconsistencies

- Appropriateness of study requested for the diagnosis
- Misadministration of, or adverse reaction to, radionuclide agents

---

RADIOLOGY INDICATORS

- Turnaround time for studies
- Number of "repeat" films
- Compare radiologic and pathologic diagnosis for any inconsistency
- Consistent reading by radiologist and nonradiologist (attending physician or others)

- Appropriateness of radiologic study to symptom/disease
- CT scan when headache is an isolated symptom
- Upper GI series in asymptomatic duodenal ulcer patient
- Routine chest radiographs
- Studies meet utilization review criteria or guidelines

OBSTETRIC CLINICAL INDICATORS

- Any maternal death
- Fetal mortality in pregnancy over 20 weeks (stillborns)
- Delivery-related hemorrhage requiring transfusion
- Any Apgar score of less than 6 at 1 minute and less than 8 at 5 minutes
- Third- or fourth-degree birth canal laceration
- Malposition accidents and/or extractions
- Anesthesia-related problems

- Intrahospital neonatal deaths of infants with birth weights 750 to 1,000 g who were born in a hospital with an neonatal intensive care unit (NICU) stay
- Readmissions of the mother within 2 weeks of delivery
- Infants weighing less than 1,800 g delivered in a hospital without an NICU
- Unattended delivery
- Unplanned return to obstetric or surgery unit
- Newborn injuries

INTENSIVE CARE UNIT INDICATORS

- Mortality
- Medication errors
- Appropriate admission and discharge criteria
- Patient returned to ICU/premature transfer
- Incidence of DVT
- Ventilator-associated pneumonia

- ICU psychosis
- Physician response time to calls
- Response time to "code blue" alerts (cardiopulmonary arrests)
- Complications of immobility
- Incidence of urinary tract infection
- Incidence of MRSA

RESPIRATORY CARE INDICATORS

- Hypoxemia is documented for oxygen therapy (exception: MI)
- Arterial blood gases (ABGs) criteria Patient's clinical condition changes (exception: continuous ventilation therapy) For home oxygen authorization (room air ABGs)

- No PRN oxygen
- Mechanical ventilation is based on established criteria
- Premature extubation
- Self-extubation

(continued)

APPENDIX 7-A—*CONTINUED*

REHABILITATION INDICATORS

- Timeliness of referral into rehabilitation unit
- Appropriateness and adequacy of treatment plan and goals
- Quality of treatment techniques
- Number and types of readmissions
- Adequacy of interdisciplinary collaboration
- Patient's understanding of instructions
- Availability of inpatient and outpatient services
- Therapy sessions missed versus reasons

PHARMACEUTICAL INDICATORS

- Time response to medications orders
- Accuracy of medication, dosage; dispensing errors
- Appropriateness of medication ordered
- Identification of interaction, compatibilities, allergies
- Preparation of all mixtures
- Food or drug interactions or compatibilities
- PRN medications administered without documentation of effects
- Medication errors

DEATH INDICATORS—CRITERIA GUIDELINES

Note: If a patient meets three of the four expected death criteria (below), the death may not be a quality issue.

EXPECTED DEATH CRITERIA

(Must have three of the four criteria [any combination])

Unexpected Death Criteria

1. Death within 24 hours of hospitalization
2. Death within 24 hours of a do not resuscitate (DNR) order
3. Death that occurs after a steady downhill course with multiple interventions
4. Death within 24 hours of surgery or other procedures

1. Clearly documented prognosis that death is expected
2. Patient/family/next of kin are aware of, and in agreement with, medical plan
3. Interventions are for comfort care only (hospice care)
4. DNR status is documented in orders and progress notes

ADEQUACY OF DISCHARGE PLANNING

- No documented plan for appropriate follow-up care or discharge planning as necessary, with consideration of physical, emotional, and mental status needs at the time of discharge

---

MEDICAL STABILITY OF THE PATIENT AT DISCHARGE

- Blood pressure on day before or day of discharge: systolic, <85 mm Hg or >180 mm Hg; diastolic, <50 mm Hg or >110 mm Hg
- Oral temperature on day before or day of discharge >101° F or rectal, >102° F (38.3° C oral/38.9° C rectal)
- Pulse <50 beat/min (or <45 beat/min if patient is taking a beta blocker) or >120 beat/min within 24 hours of discharge

- Abnormal results of diagnostic tests not addressed or explained in the medical record (e.g., pneumonia on chest X-ray, abnormal results of blood tests)
- Intravenous fluids or drugs on the day of discharge (excludes the ones that keep veins open [KVOs], antibiotics, chemotherapy, or total parenteral nutrition)
- Purulent or bloody drainage of postoperative wound within 24 hours before discharge

---

DEATHS

- During or after surgery
- After return to intensive care unit, coronary care, or special care unit within 24 hours of being transferred

- Other unexpected death

NOSOCOMIAL INFECTIONS

- Temperature increase of more than 2° F more than 72 hours from admission

- Indication of infection after an invasive procedure (e.g., suctioning, catheter insertion, tube feedings, surgery)

PATIENT FLOW

- Delay in admission to the hospital
- Admission to wrong level of care or patient care unit
- Lack of inpatient bed availability
- Diversion status in the ED

- Premature transfer out of an ICU
- Premature discharge or transfer to another facility such as skilled nursing facility (SNF) or subacute rehab
- Care is not provided at the right level such as staying in emergency department (ED) when requiring an ICU level of care
- ED overcrowding

UNSCHEDULED RETURN TO SURGERY WITHIN SAME ADMISSION FOR SAME CONDITION AS PREVIOUS SURGERY OR TO CORRECT OPERATIVE PROBLEM (EXCLUDES STAGED PROCEDURES)

Trauma suffered in the hospital

- Unplanned removal or repair of a normal organ (i.e., removal or repair not addressed in operative consent)
- Fall with injury or untoward effect (including but not limited to fracture, dislocation, concussion, laceration)
- Life-threatening complications of anesthesia
- Life-threatening transfusion error or reaction
- Hospital-acquired decubitus/pressure ulcer
- Care resulting in serious or life-threatening complications not related to admitting signs and symptoms, including but not limited to neurologic, endocrine, cardiovascular, renal, or

- Major adverse drug reactions or medication errors with serious potential for harm or resulting in special measures to correct (e.g., intubation, cardiopulmonary resuscitation, gastric lavage), including but not limited to the following:
    1. Incorrect antibiotic ordered by physician (e.g., inconsistent with diagnostic studies or patient's history of drug allergy)
    2. No diagnostic studies to confirm which drug is correct to administer (e.g., culture and sensitivity)
    3. Serum drug levels not measured as needed

(continued)

APPENDIX 7-B—*CONTINUED*

UNSCHEDULED RETURN TO SURGERY WITHIN SAME ADMISSION FOR SAME CONDITION AS PREVIOUS SURGERY OR TO CORRECT OPERATIVE PROBLEM (EXCLUDES STAGED PROCEDURES)

respiratory body systems (e.g., resulting in dialysis, unplanned transfer to special care unit, lengthened hospital stay)
- Hospital-acquired urinary tract infection
- Hospital-acquired deep vein thrombosis (especially post surgery or procedure)
- Hospital-acquired ventilator associated pneumonia
- Hospital-acquired MRSA or other types of infections

4. Diagnostic studies or other measures for side effects not performed as needed (e.g., blood urea nitrogen, creatinine, intake and output)

DIAGNOSIS-RELATED

- Failure to diagnose (i.e., concluding that patient has no disease or condition worthy of further follow-up or observation)
- Wrong diagnosis (misdiagnosis, i.e., original diagnosis is incorrect)
- Improper performance of test
- Unnecessary diagnostic test
- Delay in diagnosis
- Failure to obtain consent or lack of informed consent

ANESTHESIA-RELATED

- Failure to complete patient assessment
- Failure to monitor
- Failure to test equipment
- Improper choice of anesthesia agent or equipment
- Improper technique or induction
- Improper monitoring of conscious sedation
- Improper equipment use
- Improper intubation
- Improper positioning
- Failure to obtain consent or lack of informed consent
- Premature discharge postambulatory procedure

SURGERY-RELATED

- Failure to perform surgery
- Improper positioning
- Retained foreign body
- Wrong body part/surgery on the wrong site or side
- Improper performance of surgery
- Unnecessary surgery
- Delay in surgery
- Improper management of surgical patient
- Failure to obtain consent for surgery or lack of informed consent

MEDICATION-RELATED

- Failure to order appropriate medication
- Wrong medication ordered
- Wrong dosage ordered of correct medication
- Failure to instruct on medication
- Improper management of medication regimen
- Failure to obtain consent for medication or lack of informed consent
- Failure to medicate
- Strong dosage administered
- Wrong patient
- Wrong route
- Improper technique
- Medication administration-related (NOC)

INTRAVENOUS- AND BLOOD PRODUCTS-RELATED

- Failure to monitor patient
- Wrong solution
- Improper performance
- IV-related (NOC)
- Failure to ensure contamination-free
- Wrong type
- Improper administration
- Failure to obtain consent or lack of informed consent

OBSTETRICS-RELATED

- Failure to manage pregnancy
- Improper choice of delivery method
- Improperly performed vaginal delivery
- Improperly performed cesarean section
- Delay in delivery (induction or surgery)
- Failure to obtain consent or lack of informed consent
- Improperly managed labor
- Failure to identify or meet fetal distress
- Delay in treatment of fetal distress (i.e., identified but treated in untimely manner)
- Retained foreign body—vaginal or uterine
- Abandonment
- Wrongful life or birth

(continued)

APPENDIX 7-C—*CONTINUED*

TREATMENT-RELATED

- Failure to treat
- Wrong treatment or procedure performed (also improper choice)
- Failure to instruct patient on self-care
- Improper performance of a treatment or procedure
- Improper management of course of treatment
- Unnecessary treatment

- Delay in treatment
- Premature end of treatment (also abandonment)
- Failure to supervise treatment or procedure
- Failure to obtain consent for treatment or lack of informed consent
- Failure to refer or seek consultation

MONITORING

- Failure to monitor
- Failure to respond to patient

- Failure to report on patient condition

BIOMEDICAL EQUIPMENT/PRODUCT-RELATED

- Failure to inspect/monitor
- Improper preventive maintenance
- Improper use
- Failure to respond to warning
- Lack of equipment

- Failure to instruct patient on use of equipment/product
- Malfunction or failure
- Wrong equipment used

MISCELLANEOUS

- Inappropriate behavior of clinician (i.e., sexual misconduct allegation, assault)
- Failure to protect third parties (i.e., failure to warn or protect from violent patient behavior)
- Breach of confidentiality or privacy

- Failure to maintain appropriate infection control practices
- Failure to follow institutional policy or procedure
- Other (provide detailed written description)
- Failure to review provider performance

NOC, not otherwise classified.

CHAPTER 8

Legal Issues in Case Management

Lynn S. Muller, RN, BA, CCM, JD

"Keep away from people who try to belittle your ambition. Small people always do that, but the really great people make you feel that you too can become great."

LEARNING OBJECTIVES

Upon completion of this chapter, the reader will be able to:

1. Distinguish negligence from malpractice.
2. Recognize the importance of documentation in avoiding risk for litigation.
3. List four strategies to ensure appropriate patient's discharge or case closure.
4. Describe the informed consent process.
5. Explain the role of advance directives in the planning and case management of patient's care.
6. Identify five strategies case managers may use to reduce legal risk.

ESSENTIAL TERMS

Administrative Law • Advance Directives for Healthcare • Affidavit of Merit • Competency • Confidentiality • Continuity of Care • Contract • Deposition • Discoverable/Discovery • Documentation • Do Not Resuscitate (DNR) • Elder abuse • Employee Retirement Income Security Act of 1974 (ERISA) • Expert Witness • Health Insurance Portability and Accountability Act of 1996 (HIPAA) • Implied consent • Incompetence • Informed consent • Interrogatory • Interstate Case Management • Living Will • Malpractice • Negligence • Negligent Referral • Negligent Utilization Review • Mandatory Reporting • Patient Abandonment • Patients' Bill of Rights • Patient Self-Determination Act of 1990 • Pre-trial • Power of Attorney (POA) • Professional Negligence • Reportable Events • Statute of Limitations • Surrogate

The complex relationship between medicine and the law requires healthcare providers to be careful about the way they deliver healthcare services to those who need them. Case managers are uniquely suited to work in a cooperative manner throughout the care continuum, having knowledge of both medical information and an educated appreciation for the law and its rules and regulations. Healthcare and case management have moved out of the shelter of hospitals into the community and every setting of care. However, the concept of community is more global than ever before. The advent of advanced technology in both medicine and communication has opened opportunities for case management around the globe. With increased opportunity comes greater responsibility, as well as greater

legal risks to all players in the healthcare theater; as professionals, case managers are exposed to legal risk more than ever before. Each of the legal issues discussed in this chapter repeatedly surfaces in the course of the case managers' responsibilities.

This chapter starts with a description of general legal concepts that apply to case management and ends with a set of techniques case managers may employ to minimize liability exposure. Depending on the practice setting, not all types of legal exposure may apply to case management. For example, a hospital-based case manager who may or may not perform direct patient care has different potential risks than a telephonic case manager with a strong utilization management role.

Laws change and vary from state to state. Even federal law can have different applications in the various states. Therefore, it is critical that case managers learn the legal statutes for the state or states where they practice, especially because they are charged with the responsibility of knowing the law and acting in accordance with it whether they know it or not. With the advent of the Internet, it is easier to find state and federal laws, particularly those legal issues that relate to nursing, social work, case management practice, pharmaceuticals, research, and other areas. Some healthcare-related law books are broken down into clinical areas (e.g., medicine, surgery, mental health, obstetrics, perinatal care, and cardiac care). They contain reviews of actual court cases in these areas, many of which are enlightening and can help the case manager to avoid mistakes. However, it is important to remember that the law is not stagnant; it is an ever-changing and developing body of knowledge. It also is important to remain current on your institution's policies and procedures and updated on changes in the law. If you have any doubt about a proper course of action, call your risk management department for assistance or guidance. Many institutions retain lawyers/legal counsels who can answer questions and offer potential solutions. You may contact an attorney familiar with medical-legal issues to obtain information on protecting your license while providing high quality case management services. Additionally, you may consult with your professional organization or licensing agency for an opinion on a situation you may be facing. Seeking expert advice is helpful when unsure of the best course of action.

▶ NEGLIGENCE

The very word, *negligence*, sends chills down a healthcare worker's spine. Most people enter the healthcare field with a genuine sense of caring for others and a sincere commitment to doing the best job they can. Mistakes or oversights are far too common and occur even with the best of intentions or under the best circumstances. In your day-to-day life, such as in the case of driving your car, you are held to a simple or regular negligence standard. Negligence is the failure to act as a reasonable person would in a given situation. The plaintiff, the individual who believes he or she was harmed by another (the defendant) and initiates a lawsuit by filing a complaint, must meet four very specific requirements to show that negligence has occurred. If one of these four elements is missing, the plaintiff will likely lose the case (Ovando & Thies, 1997); the court may consider the complaint unfounded.

The four elements of negligence are:

1. *Duty.* A legal obligation based on relationship or statute, such as parents' obligation to rescue their child; an obligation that a stranger does not share.
2. *Breach.* A failure to act in accordance with a recognized duty.
3. *Causation.* The required nexus or direct link between the breach of duty and the resulting harm; proof that the breach of duty actually caused the injury.
4. *Harm.* Injury experienced as a result of the breach.

Negligence is a tort, a civil wrong. It is distinguished from a crime in that it is one individual harming another, where money (known as dollar damages) can provide a remedy. Crime deals with victims who have been harmed by someone who has violated a state or federal statute. Victims leave the criminal courtroom empty-handed (Keaton, Dobbs, Keaton, & Owen, 1984). Many states provide for Victims' Funds, but these funds rarely give a victim more than a meager amount of money. Regular or simple negligence is a minimum standard and is based on a "reasonable person" standard. For example, when you are driving down the street you are expected to act in a reasonable and prudent manner, similar to the way other reasonable drivers would. A failure to do so, resulting in the injury of another, can subject you to liability; that is why we have automobile insurance.

▶ PROFESSIONAL NEGLIGENCE

Professional negligence, commonly referred to as *malpractice*, is a higher standard of obligation, a greater duty than simple or regular negligence. It is based on the idea that someone with specialized knowledge and skill, by virtue of education and experience, should know how to act in his or her specialized field. That special or superior knowledge is referred to as the Standard of Practice or Standard of Care (Keaton et al., 1984, § 32). The first level of scrutiny for case manager's liability is the underlying profession of that individual case manager (e.g., nursing, physical therapy, medicine, social work). If the case manager is a nurse, the Nurse Practice Act in the state of licensure is controlling; a doctor would be viewed consistent with state law in his or her state of licensure. In addition, the so-called "geography rule," applies a standard to similarly situated professionals in the relevant geography/locale. For example, a practitioner in a remote and isolated village or Native

American reservation with limited services would not be held to the same standard as a practitioner in a large metropolitan medical center with state-of-the-art equipment. However, with the advent of high-tech wireless and satellite communications, this distinction is not as great as it once was. Within minutes, an ill or injured person can be transported from one location to another, even from the most remote area; therefore, the need for the geography rule appears to be diminishing. For links to all state boards of nursing and their Nurse Practice Acts, go to https://www.ncsbn.org/index.htm. For social work, refer to the National Association of Social Workers (NASW) (http://www.socialworkers.org). For certified case managers, refer to the Commission for Case Manager Certification (CCMC) (http://www.ccmcertification. org). Generally speaking, you may refer to the licensing services of your state education department for further information on your practice act as a licensed professional in your area of specialization.

▶ Affidavit of Merit

In most states, before a professional malpractice case can be filed in court (or shortly after filing), an Affidavit of Merit must also be filed; otherwise, the lawsuit will be dismissed. In the Affidavit of Merit, a like-kind professional (nurse for a nurse, case manager for a case manager, etc.) must state under oath that there is reasonable probability that the case will succeed.

The following is an example of a law requiring an Affidavit of Merit.

> The plaintiff in a professional negligence case must prove the four elements of negligence: duty, breach, causation, and harm. The plaintiff also must prove that the health-care professional deviated from a recognized and accepted standard of practice. In any action for damages for personal injuries, wrongful death, or property damage resulting from an alleged act of malpractice or negligence by a licensed person in his profession or occupation, the plaintiff shall, within 60 days following the date of filing of the answer to the complaint by the defendant, provide each defendant with an affidavit of an appropriate licensed person that there exists a reasonable probability that the care, skill, or knowledge exercised or exhibited in the treatment, practice, or work that is the subject of the complaint, fell outside acceptable or recognized professional or occupational standards or treatment practices. The court may grant no more than one additional period, not to exceed 60 days, to file the affidavit pursuant to this section, upon a finding of good cause (NJ ST. §2A:53A-27 Affidavit of Merit, June 29, 1995).

There is no requirement that the professional who submits the Affidavit of Merit be the same individual who testifies at trial as an expert witness.

▶ Expert Witness

No medical or other professional negligence case can be litigated without an expert witness. The only way for the plaintiff to prove the case is to rely on the testimony of one or more expert witnesses. The Federal Rules of Evidence (adopted in whole or in part by most states) set forth the requirement that a like-kind expert testifies to the deviation from expected standards of practice and/or that no reasonable and similarly situated professional would have acted in the way that the defendant did, given similar circumstances (Fed. R. Evid. Article VIII, Rule 703 [2009]).

Some states have developed special panels or tribunals that examine the facts in the case along with the Affidavit of Merit to determine whether the lawsuit can be filed at all (Gen. Laws Massachusetts, Part III, Title II, Ch. 231, §60B). In those states, a preliminary hearing is conducted based on the plaintiff's allegations contained in the complaint and documented by an expert witness. If the plaintiff fails at the panel stage, the lawsuit is dismissed before it starts.

▶ Case Manager Liability

The law is an ever-changing and growing body of knowledge. Nowhere is this truer than in case management practice. Case management is required by law in certain circumstances and states, such as Georgia, and under federal law for certain beneficiaries of Tricare, the medical benefits system for United States military and their dependents. Failure to provide statutory case management services can be a violation of law in itself. For information about Tricare benefits refer to http://www.tricare.mil/.

In most situations, case management services are provided through a contractual relationship. A client may have case management services through employment as either a direct benefit or through the state's workers' compensation system. Some businesses are using the services of absentee management companies that offer case management services as a component of a variety of health and wellness services for their employees. More and more today, case management may occur within the traditional hospital setting, in the form of transitional/discharge planning and continuity of care services, or may be available through home health services. Judges and juries decide cases based on statute, case law, or both. With ever-changing practice settings and case management applications, the law lags behind. Until a case comes through the courts identifying a new and different aspect of liability, the old rules still apply. Many cases are brought and settled out of court and the facts of those cases, even if known, do not change the body of case law.

Some examples of potential case management negligence are as follows:

▶ Premature discharge from a hospital, home care, or skilled nursing facility (SNF).
▶ Negligent referral to alternative care centers.
▶ Negligent hiring and retention of employees.
▶ Inadequate communication with physicians or other healthcare professionals involved in patient care.
▶ Inadequate communication (e.g., withholding information) with a patient or family.
▶ Failure to comply with physician orders.
▶ Patient abandonment.
▶ Improper telephone triage.
▶ Failure to maintain medical record confidentiality.
▶ Adverse payment decisions, particularly those based on price alone, without an assessment of quality.

In addition to these concerns, case managers may also be placed in a precarious position due to competing pressures of the gamut of stakeholders. Healthcare has become an aggressively competitive market. There continue to be frequent mergers and acquisitions as well as bold and aggressive marketing ploys by companies; some even go so far as to market directly to consumers on television, in print media, and on the Internet. This may place case managers in a position where unrealistic expectations cannot be met or may be limited by contract. Marketing strategies can actually create a situation in which there is breach of contract, fraud, or misrepresentation.

The standards of professional practice are one of the gold standards that lawyers use to prove that the case manager did or did not breach the standard of care. However, keep in mind that case management remains a dependent credential—a supplement to one's primary profession.

▶ If You Are Named in a Lawsuit

If you are served with a summons and complaint, which are documents that initiate a lawsuit, you should behave in the following manner:

1. Don't refuse or avoid receiving these documents.
2. Don't argue with the process server.
3. Report receipt of the summons and complaint immediately to your attorney and your employer, as well as your employer at the time in question if different.
4. Obtain and review the record. Review it completely to refresh your recollection of the case. Lawsuits are typically filed up to 2 years after the incident, although this varies from state to state.
5. Follow your attorney's advice. If that individual is not fully familiar with your area of practice, explain your practice fully to that person, so he or she can best assist you.
6. Be sure to tell the attorney about standards of case management practice, policies and procedures, protocols, and other information that were in effect at the time of the occurrence and may be helpful in court.
7. ONLY discuss the matter with your attorney and not with co-workers.
8. Be honest with your attorney. He or she cannot help you without accurate information. Don't tell what you wish happened; rather tell exactly what happened.
9. Don't panic. An allegation is just that, a claim unless and until it is proven. Often, several defendants are eliminated from a lawsuit before the matter ever goes to court.

PRE-TRIAL

The time between the filing of a complaint (the document that starts a lawsuit by a plaintiff) and the trial itself is the pre-trial phase of the case. Discovery is the fact-finding process that occurs in this pre-trial phase and permits the attorneys on both sides to prepare their case. Discovery includes investigation, review of documents, and pre-trial testimony. There are two methods in which sworn testimony is obtained before trial: interrogatories and depositions.

INTERROGATORIES *Interrogatories* are a formal request for additional information in a case; a series of questions that a party to a case, or witness in a case, must answer. After answering the questions, the individual signs a document that contains answers to the questions, certifying to the truth and accuracy of the information provided. Later at deposition or at trial the answers that the same individual gives can be compared to the interrogatory answers included in the signed document. Inconsistencies must be explained and may affect the credibility of the witness. These tools are used to obtain background information and clarify facts surrounding the case.

DEPOSITION A *deposition* is a question-and-answer session conducted in a lawyer's office under oath. The witness, known as the deponent, is sworn in just as if in court. The proceeding is recorded by a court reporter and transcribed into a booklet referred to as the *transcript*. The deposition transcript may be used for further pre-trial investigation, or to impeach or challenge a witness's testimony at trial. In certain circumstances a video deposition also may be used. It is an essential method: if during the trial the witness cannot be present in court, the video deposition can then be shared.

STATUTE OF LIMITATIONS

In most states, the statute of limitations for adults in personal injury cases is 2 years. That is the time that a person has to file a lawsuit. However, Kentucky is an example of a state that only permits a 1-year statute of limitations (Ken. St. Title 36, Chapter 413, Sec. 413.140). Some states measure the time for filing a lawsuit strictly from the date of injury. Other states extend the time to include a period when the patient knew or should have known of the discovery that a certain event caused a newly discovered consequence (illness or injury).

In the case of children, the date for filing may be extended past the first 2 years (or other statutory limit) and up to 2 or more years after the child reaches the age of maturity. This is one area where there is greater variation from state to state. Each state has its own definition of adulthood; there is no national standard. However, even in those states that would extend the filing date for an injured child, the statute of limitations may remain only 2 years for any out-of-pocket costs or damages claimed by the parents related to their child's claim. For a complete list of state statutes of limitations and access to each state's legislative Web site, refer to http://law.freeadvice.com/resources/personal_injury_statute_of_limitations.htm.

One reason for a statute of limitations is that few people remember intimate and complex details from years past. Another is to limit the time a reasonable practitioner must retain records and be expected to remember complex details from any particular case.

DOCUMENTATION

Courts in general and juries often believe that what is written and properly documented in the normal course of business is more credible than live testimony. Therefore, your documentation as a case manager is critical to your professional practice, no matter what the setting is, and in particular if you find yourself the defendant in a professional liability/malpractice lawsuit.

Following are four general criteria for documentation, no matter what documentation tools (electronic or manual) are used:

1. Chart the facts. Be objective. Subjective complaints are acceptable if a patient states them (i.e., "Mr. Jones stated, 'My left abdomen pain is much worse.'"). On the contrary, subjective statements or those that are judgmental or opinionated in nature when made by a case manager should be considered carefully, as they will take on an entirely different meaning out of context. For example, unless the occurrence was actually witnessed, the case manager should write, "patient found on floor" (with details), not "patient fell out of bed." Documentation should be complete and correct. If true, you might even go as far as stating, "when I returned from the Code Blue two rooms away, I found Mr. J on the floor. Immediately I performed an assessment of his condition and especially checked for signs of bleeding, bruising, etc.; I stayed with Mr. J and called for help." Two or more years later, there would be no confusion or alternate interpretation of what happened and why you were not there. Throughout my lengthy nursing history, there have been many schools of thought on charting; too much, too little; signing clearly, scribbling your name so it cannot be identified, etc. At the end of it all, documentation is the case manager's best friend and protector.

2. Use The Joint Commission, URAC, or other approved abbreviations (e.g., those adopted and enforced by your healthcare organization). This discourages ambiguity and prevents potentially harmful misunderstandings. Refer to your organizational policies for an approved list of abbreviations. These policies are developed based on nationally recognized standards and usually describe where your organization stands in relation to abbreviations. They also explain what is allowed and what is forbidden. If unsure, it is best to spell things out; this prevents confusion, misinterpretation, and miscommunication.

3. Use legible penmanship. It would be embarrassing to have your own documentation shown on a giant screen in court and you yourself are unable to decipher it. It may affect your credibility. More and more, healthcare organizations (hospitals and other agencies) are changing to computer-based documentation, both complicating and simplifying this issue.

4. Record your information as promptly as possible so that details are not lost or forgotten. Use actual times accurately and chart in chronological order. If you must chart information at a later time, due to an emergent

situation or simply that you forgot, DO NOT squeeze it in or backdate the information. Make your note the next entry and state clearly and accurately why you are charting out of order. For example, "1/1/08, 2:10 PM I was called away to a code and failed to chart Mr. Jones' blood sugars this morning; however, they were taken on time and insulin coverage given to the patient immediately." It is only this entry that was delayed. Attorneys later use these times to reconstruct the case, as in a play. For example, if you called a physician at 5-minute intervals or gave sublingual nitroglycerine according to protocol, providing the times will be to your advantage. Honesty remains the best policy.

▶ NEGLIGENT REFERRALS

Negligent referrals is an area that has been growing as a danger point for case manager liability and is closely related to the discharge-planning role. From the lawyer's standpoint, the problem with these cases is proving measurable damages, but this does not limit the potential for liability for case managers. If the plaintiff can prove that, because of the case manager's choice or recommendation, he or she chose a particular product or service that resulted in injury, delayed recovery, or worse, the case manager will be defending how and why a particular vendor, facility, or product was selected. The case manager may find himself or herself as a party to a lawsuit containing, among other causes of action, a negligent referral claim.

Many health maintenance organizations (HMOs) and preferred provider organizations (PPOs) have large networks of providers (hospitals, healthcare professionals such as physicians, home care agencies, SNFs, and other institutions) who have contracted with the HMO/PPO or other entities to provide products (e.g., durable medical equipment such as wheelchairs, canes, bedside commodes) and services at a reduced rate. In addition, large medical centers across the country have developed extensive integrated healthcare networks, including subacute, long- and short-term rehabilitation centers, stepdown facilities, and even durable medical supply and medical transport companies. Case managers who work in these environments are often faced with a difficult ethical dilemma. Their employers instruct them (either openly or covertly) to refer patients only "within network" and they have learned through experience that one or more of the network businesses or providers are of lesser quality. One of the goals of medical centers is to keep costs down for themselves and/or the insurance

companies in which they participate. Liability exposure for case managers in such cases occurs when there is a poor or harmful outcome from one of the contracted network providers where it can be shown that the case manager knew, or should have known, but ignored the fact that a high-quality, cost-effective (albeit out-of-network) option was geographically and financially viable.

If the case manager participated in the referral process and did not critically and objectively assess the provider, or even perform a cost-benefit analysis comparing providers, courts in California, New York, Alabama, and elsewhere have recognized the responsibility of case managers to adhere to the standard of practice. Case managers can minimize these risks by considering the following:

▶ Credentialing in any organization is a key safety net and is now required by recognized credentialing bodies, such as the CCMC, URAC, or The Joint Commission. A periodic review of the credentials, complaint logs, and certifications of providers of all types is an important task to decrease this liability.

▶ Compare costs and ask questions to determine the quality of products and services offered by a provider. Negotiate price for equivalent products even in network or more importantly, when you identify a higher quality choice and successfully negotiate a competitive out-of-network rate.

▶ Physicians are becoming more and more resistant to making direct referrals due to their fear of liability exposure. Patients or families may ask the case manager for recommendations. When making recommendations and referrals, always give the patient and family several options to choose from and let them make the ultimate decision. If the patient's plan has a provider network, have the patient choose from among those listed in the reference book once you have assessed their quality. However, make the patient aware that paying privately for a product or service that is out-of-network is an alternative, especially if the individual is unhappy with the choices within the plan. This possibility may not be financially viable in every case, but it is the client/patient who should make the choice. Your duty as a case manager is to provide fair and honest information.

Cost-benefit analyses are part of the case manager's patient advocacy responsibility. The concept of client-centered case management services implies a responsibility to always act in the best interest of the patient/client. Document that a reasonable process was applied; show the steps taken; demonstrate that you (the case manager) were, in fact, acting in the best interests of the patient and/or family.

A thorough, accurate, and ongoing credentialing process is the **best prevention** for negligent referral claims.

▶ HEALTH INSURANCE PORTABILITY AND ACCOUNTABILITY ACT OF 1996 (HIPAA)

The Health Insurance Portability and Accountability Act (HIPAA), Public Law 104-191, was enacted on August 21, 1996, and is a significant piece of civil rights legislation.

Since the 1960s there have been two significant pieces of health-related civil rights legislation. The first is the Americans with Disabilities Act (ADA), which many confuse with labor law; the second is the Health Insurance Portability and Accountability Act (HIPAA) of 1996. HIPAA affects more people than ADA, as it affects every person in the United States, rather than a unique and protected group. HIPAA is intended to improve the portability and continuity of health insurance by protecting individuals against laws regarding preexisting conditions and other restrictions. A preexisting condition is a medical condition diagnosed or treated before an individual changes to a new health plan. In the past, healthcare for a preexisting condition was not covered in a new health insurance plan until after a waiting period. The new law changes the rules. It is called the portability act because it protects a person's ability to maintain insurance coverage when changing jobs or insurance plans; in effect, even with preexisting conditions or chronic illnesses insurance is portable.

Health insurers must offer insurance to individuals who lose coverage for reasons such as a change in employment, a job not offering health insurance, or job termination. To qualify, the individual must first exhaust a full 18 months of Consolidated Omnibus Reconciliation Act of 1985 (COBRA) coverage and be ineligible for other programs such as Medicaid and Medicare.

The Privacy Rule was published on December 28, 2000 (67 C.F.R § 82462), with the goal of providing consumers with greater rights for protection of individually identifiable health information. Modifica-tions of the Privacy Rule were published in final form on August 14, 2002 (65 C.F.R. §53182). In the spring of 2003 there were further modifications to the Final Privacy Rule. HIPAA is here to stay; the key to HIPAA is demonstrating compliance. Case managers must understand these laws and adhere to them at all times to reduce the risk for, or completely avoid, negligence or malpractice actions.

The best resource for HIPAA Compliance is the federal Office of Civil Rights (OCR) (http://www.hhs.gov/ocr/hipaa). There are Guidance Documents on the OCR Web site on such topics as government access, business associates, protected health information, incidental uses and disclosures, public health, workers compensation, and others. Other resources include the HIPAA confidentiality and privacy policies and procedures of the healthcare organization to which you belong.

▶ EMPLOYEE RETIREMENT INCOME SECURITY ACT OF 1974

The Employee Retirement Income Security Act (ERISA) is primarily concerned with the regulation of pension plans. ERISA was originally enacted so that employers who hire employees in multistate areas would not be encumbered by multiple state laws. For example, coordination-of-benefit state laws do not apply to ERISA employers. This means that if a patient has more than one insurance plan, state rules about who is the primary source of insurance and who is the secondary source of insurance do not apply; however, ERISA employer plans must comply with federal laws.

From a case management perspective, those who work with employer plans or self-funded plans must consider the other aspects of this act: the benefit plan becomes the controlling document and establishes coverage, coordination of benefits provisions, claims processes, appeals procedures, and essentially all rules and regulations governing the rights of beneficiaries and plan participants, including the liabilities of the plan administrator (Gammage & Burham, 1997). Case managers must be aware of the specific guarantees and exemptions written into the benefit plans. MCOs have successfully used ERISA as a shield against malpractice lawsuits. Many case managers have heard stories of tremendous loss where no punitive damages were awarded because ERISA protected the plan administration. Recovery of damages under ERISA cannot exceed the cost of the benefit that should have been provided; therefore, if a bone marrow transplant was in question, and the patient died, approximately $91,000 would be allowed in damages. In other words, only the denial of benefits can be the focus of an ERISA lawsuit (Robbins, 1998).

In the past several years a number of lawsuits have been filed that address ERISA issues. One bottom-line ERISA issue is whether or not the claim "relates to" the ERISA benefit plan. Essentially, if the court determines that a claim relates to ERISA, then the patient is not likely to receive any recovery of damages. That is essentially what happened in the case of *Corcoran v. United Healthcare, Inc.* (Mellette & Kurtz, 1993). For safety reasons, Mrs. Corcoran's physician wanted 24-hour fetal monitoring for her last trimester of pregnancy. She was already admitted to the hospital when she was told her health plan would not cover the admission but would cover 10 hours of home nursing services per day. She returned home and, during one of the gaps without monitoring, the fetus went into distress and died. No wrongful death damages were rendered to the mother because ERISA rules preempted other laws. On the other hand, if the court determines that the claim does not relate to ERISA, damages can be won.

ERISA issues are a complex problem best left to legal experts. This is further complicated by state statutes that challenge ERISA, and even specific aspects of HIPAA. Case managers who work with patients under ERISA may require expert counsel in some predicaments. This situation is a moving target; in fact, due to new laws being considered and being enacted (both federally and statewide), no one is quite sure how several case management/managed care legal situations will play out. Still, the following are a few preventive actions case managers can take:

▶ Know the plan documents, including the coverage and payment decisions.
▶ Call the plan's consultant for anything that is unsure, whether it is the fine points of a covered service or a nebulous definition such as medical necessity. Be persistent. If consultants are unsure, they often go to their supervisor or legal counsel for the answers.
▶ Make sure the utilization management criteria are consistent with the plan's standards and benefits.
▶ Do not forget to tell the patient of the right to appeal when a service is not included in the benefits or is deemed not medically necessary by a physician advisor.
▶ Keep abreast of changing legislation.
▶ Consult with legal experts at your own organization.

Certain health care plans are controlled by federal law under the Employee Retirement Income Security Act of 1974. [ERISA]. (29 U. S. C. §§ 1001-1461 (2000).

Since ERISA is federal law, in most cases where there is a conflict, federal law preempts or supersedes state law. This is true in cases where the administration of the ERISA plan is at issue; however, in 2003 in the case of *Villizon v. PruCare* (843 So.2d 842 [2003]), the Florida Supreme Court held that "Upon an appropriate finding, the trial court may dismiss the estate's direct negligence, corporate liability and implied contract claims for a lack of subject matter jurisdiction [due to federal preemption]. However, in no event may the vicarious liability count be dismissed, as the same does not 'relate to' an employee benefit plan" (*Citing Estate of Frappier, 678 So. 2d at 88, 888, Fla. 4th DCA 1996*). Therefore, the vicarious liability suit was heard in Florida State Court. In this case there was delay in diagnosis due to the "hoops" that claimants and their HMO physicians had to go through before a specialist could make timely referral to diagnostic testing and evaluation. The primary care physician was found to be liable for delayed diagnosis and PruCare was vicariously liable when a cancer was not appropriately and timely diagnosed.

▶ NEGLIGENT UTILIZATION MANAGEMENT/REVIEW

One of the first cases to address potential managed care organization (MCO) liability for negligent utilization management and review was *Wickline v. State of California* (29 Cal.Rptr at 818.2). In this landmark decision, the physician was deemed responsible for treatment decisions; however, the court also indicated that in some situations, third-party payors "can be legally accountable when medically inappropriate decisions result from defects in the design or implementation of cost-containment mechanisms as, for example, when appeals made on a patient's behalf for medical or hospital care are arbitrarily ignored or unreasonably disregarded or overridden" (Sturgeon, 1997, p. 68). Ultimately, the California Appellate Court held that the HMO was not liable and that the *Wickline* decision was limited to its unique facts.

Subsequently in *Wilson v. Blue Cross of Southern California*, the court determined that even though a treatment decision and a payment decision are two distinct subjects, if the payment decision is made negligently and is a factor in subsequent harm to the patient, the MCO (and its agents) can be liable. However, other courts do not agree that physicians will be improperly influenced by utilization review systems (Sturgeon, 1997).

When appeals made on a patient's behalf are arbitrarily ignored or unreasonably disregarded or overridden, they are considered negligent utilization review. This type of negligent utilization review will be less common as mandatory appeals protocols go into effect (see "Denials and the Appeals" later in this chapter).

> When performing utilization management activities, apply utilization review criteria **consistently** to avoid negligent utilization review practices. The utilization review criteria applied must be those that are recommended and used by the health insurance or benefit plan such as InterQual or Milliman Guidelines.

In 1995, the New Jersey Supreme Court held in *Dunn v. Praiss* (606 A.2d 862) that an HMO was liable for the contribution toward the malpractice of a physician they hired as an independent contractor. Logically it would follow that a case manager performing telephonic or field case management services for an HMO who deviates from the "accepted standards of practice" could be held liable for his or her actions. In addition, the HMO could share in that liability. This is known as joint liability.

More recently in *Basil v. Wolf* (193 N.J. 38, 67 [2007]) the same New Jersey Supreme Court would not extend liability to a workers' compensation insurance company for the malpractice of a physician who performed an independent medical examination (IME) on its behalf and failed to diagnosis cancer metastasis over a period of 2 years. These cases are important to case management as the selection of a physician, including IME physicians, is often left to the case manager. One should make a reasonable inquiry into the physician's qualifications and past practices. At a minimum, one should check the state medical board's Web site to determine if the physician is in good standing or if any board action is pending. Similar inquiries should be made for pharmacies, pharmacists, home care companies, and other practitioners to whom referrals are considered.

In an Alabama case, *Reid v. Aetna Casualty & Surety Co.* (1997), the allegation by a plaintiff/employee, "that the nurse [case manager] was more concerned with saving money than with the employee's recovery," was found to be insufficient to support a claim. In this case, the client was offered a variety of choices for the treatment of pain management and the provider chosen was also the least expensive. In addition, there was an allegation of fraud on the part of the defendant or insurance carrier, in that they had suppressed the following material information (among other things): "that the nurse [case manager] was not acting as a registered

nurse with the normal professional obligations toward the worker [client]" (*Reid v. Aetna Casualty & Surety Co.*, 1997). The court held that even if that were true (and made no finding that it was true), there was no evidence that the actions of the case manager caused any harm to the patient. "It is undisputed that Aetna hired [a case management company] to perform medical case management, that the [case manager] was employed as a registered nurse … and that she worked on the client's case." Although the patient claimed that the case manager "prevented her from undergoing beneficial treatments," she failed to offer proof of such alternative beneficial treatments, and the case was dismissed (*Reid v. Aetna Casualty & Surety Co.*, 1997).

▶ DENIALS AND APPEALS

The courts have mandated that MCOs have a duty to inform patients of their right to appeal insurance denials. In the case of *Sarchett v. Blue Shield of California*, (43 Cal.3d 1, 10 [1987]) Blue Shield denied a patient's hospitalization on the grounds that it was not medically necessary and the insurance company did not mention to the patient the right to appeal. The California Supreme Court held that the insurance company breached its covenant of good faith and fair dealing by failing to inform the insured of the right to appeal. Rather, the insurance company's conduct appeared designed to mislead the insured into giving up the right to impartial review (Sturgeon, 1997). Case managers must be familiar with denials, appeals (both expedited and standard appeals), grievances, reconsiderations, and patient rights, because here is another role for the case manager: that of mediator.

▶ Grievances, Expedited and Standard Appeals

An *appeal* is a request to reexamine a healthcare decision, usually one in which the patient and physician believed that the procedure or service was medically necessary, but the authorizing agent denied the procedure or service. Depending on the state laws and the insurance procedures, the process may vary. However, the appeals process is one with which a case manager must be familiar for several important reasons.

First, the case manager may be asked by the patient or physician to help obtain services for the patient. If the insurance benefits are vague or the services are not authorized, the appeals procedure may be the first line of defense. It may also be that the case manager agrees that this is not only a necessary service, but also one that is inappropriately denied and is a covered benefit. The appeals process exists precisely for such a scenario.

As a patient advocate, see that every opportunity is provided to the patient to receive services that the physician deems important for the patient's health and well-being. This is not just a nice thing to do, but legally wise. When cases go to court, the case manager who has walked through the appeals procedure with the patient, family, and physician will be viewed as an advocate, not an adversary. This can have important ramifications for the case manager on the witness stand.

Common reasons for denial of claims of which case managers must be careful include, but are not limited to, the following:

▶ Errors in the information shared with the funding source or payor.
▶ Additional supporting documentation was needed. This may include manufacturer pricing and a description of the item (if equipment is being requested, for example).
▶ The physician failed to supply clear, supporting information or documentation.
▶ Consumer expectations exceed the limitations of their insurance coverage.

Often, the first part of the appeals process involves a simple reconsideration, which is a request by telephone or fax for additional review of a utilization review determination not to certify. This is performed by the peer reviewer who reviewed the original decision, based on submission of additional information; sometimes, it is a peer-to-peer discussion. In other words, when a service or procedure is denied, the physician who is providing care to the patient speaks with the physician at the payor/insurer organization who reviewed (and denied) the service and discusses the case. More patient information may be all that is needed. If the service is then approved, the appeals process does not need to go any further. If this does not settle the matter, it will become a formal appeals consideration.

An appeals consideration is a clinical review conducted by appropriate clinical peers, who were not involved in the clinical review, when a decision not to certify a requested admission, procedure, or service has been appealed. There are two types of appeals: expedited and standard.

▶ An *expedited appeal* is a request by telephone or fax for additional review of a determination not to certify imminent or ongoing services, requiring a review conducted by a clinical peer who was not involved in the original decision not to certify.
▶ A *standard appeal* is a request to review a determination not to certify an admission, extension of stay, or other healthcare services,

conducted by a peer reviewer who was not involved in any previous noncertification pertaining to the same episode of care.

Various credentialing organizations and state and federal laws mandate specific time frames and conditions in which to perform an appeal procedure. The expedited appeal is for "imminent or ongoing services" that must be attended to quickly (usually within 1 business day) for patient safety. The physician (clinical peer) who is allowed to perform the expedited appeal must not be the same physician who made the initial determination to deny the service. A standard appeal is usually for retrospective services that do not require immediate attention (usually within 30 days of receiving the documentation). A physician who was not involved in any other part of the appeals process can perform this level of appeal. Standard appeals are initiated in writing and include examining parts of the medical record. Other requirements may also be expected in appeals (e.g., board certification of a physician who is knowledgeable about the type of case being reviewed).

A *grievance* is a "formal written request by a member for a hearing by the (provider) regarding: (1) a complaint about care or services received from the network or from a network provider, or (2) an appeal of a decision made by the network with regard to the provision of a requested service." This is a complaint that is usually made when no urgency of medical care is needed. It may precede a standard appeal or it may stem from a complaint about an expedited or standard appeal decision (often called a determination).

As more Americans opt for Medicare benefits under the HMO plans (i.e., Medicare Advantage Plans) rather than the traditional fee-for-service design, case managers are increasingly expected to perform utilization review and precertification for services rendered or to be rendered to Medicare Advantage Plans beneficiaries. As a result, there is an increased chance that some services and procedures will be denied and appeal procedures will be indicated. The Medicare appeals process may vary from private insurance appeals processes (which could also vary from state to state). (For more information, refer to Chapter 4, Utilization Management.)

Medicare expedited appeal reasons are similar to those of commercial insurance providers; they imply that expedited appeals are used for "imminent or ongoing services." The expedited appeal is used when:

▶ The health plan refuses to provide services that the beneficiary believes should be furnished or arranged for by the health plan.
▶ The beneficiary has not received the services outside the health plan and it is believed the

beneficiary requires those services or an adverse health condition may result.

▶ The health plan discontinues services when the beneficiary believes there is a continuing need for the service.

▶ Exhaustion of benefits occurs and a medical need is still present; depending on the circumstances, this may become an expedited or a standard appeal process.

The standard appeal is used when less emergent services are denied such as:

▶ Precertification denial when the physician or beneficiary thinks the service is necessary and a covered benefit.

▶ Nonpayment of claims for which the physician or beneficiary believed the care was necessary and a covered benefit; this nonpayment could be for the total bill or a part of the bill.

▶ Emergency or urgent services were billed and the health plan does not feel they were urgent.

▶ Discontinuation of services while the physician or beneficiary feels those services are still needed.

▶ Exhaustion of benefits occurs and a medical need is still present; depending on the circumstances, this may become an expedited or a standard appeal process.

▶ Who May Request an Appeal

1. A Medicare beneficiary can request an appeal. A beneficiary may request, either orally or in writing, an expedited appeal if he or she believes that health, life, or ability to regain maximum function may be jeopardized by the standard appeal process, which sometimes may take up to 60 days. It is not necessary for the beneficiary to enlist the support of the physician for an expedited appeal (although it may be a wise choice); the health plan cannot require this. It is the health plan's responsibility to decide whether the request for an expedited appeal meets the criteria. If the beneficiary desires a standard appeal, and no expedited appeal has been filed, the standard appeal request is made in writing.

2. A Medicare beneficiary can request a representative to file an expedited or standard appeal. The beneficiary must provide his or her name, Medicare number, and a statement that appoints the individual as the representative. The beneficiary must also sign and date the

form and have the representative sign and date the form.

3. A physician can request an appeal on behalf of the beneficiary. A physician may provide oral or written support for a beneficiary's request, or a physician may act in the beneficiary's interest by requesting an expedited appeal as the beneficiary's representative. The same paperwork as stated in number 2 must be provided. The expedited appeal can be initiated verbally or in writing by fax. The physician should be very clear that he or she believes the situation is time sensitive and/or the review should be conducted within 72 hours or less as medically necessary or appropriate.

4. A court-appointed guardian or an agent under a healthcare proxy can request an appeal. This must be in accordance with what is provided by state laws.

5. If the beneficiary is an inpatient in the hospital and disagrees with the decision to be discharged, the case manager should steer the patient to the use of the hospital-issued notice of noncoverage (HINN) procedure, rather than an expedited appeal process. This can be done by calling the state's peer review organization/quality improvement organization (PRO/QIO).

▶ What to Do to Reduce the Need for Appeal Procedures

▶ Check to ensure the bill/claim was accurately coded. Incorrect coding may lead to denials, and coding may differ between companies; a claim will be denied if it is not found in *the insurance company's* list of covered items or services.

▶ Communicate the patient's condition and the medical necessity of the service or equipment. It is not uncommon for a request or claim to be denied due to lack of some important information. Payors want medical justification for spending medical dollars. Sometimes a claim is denied for not-so-obvious reasons.

▶ Make sure that the insurance company/payor receives the claims and the utilization review information or case management reports. The reports should include the information needed to adjudicate the claims.

▶ Document carefully and fully. Keep the benefits in mind while you are documenting and match the patient's condition with the requested service or equipment. Validate that the service or equipment is medically needed and is the most appropriate for the situation, as well as where it fits into the benefit design. If convenience or preference is conveyed, it will be more difficult to obtain authorization. In most cases this information must be written by a physician. The case manager can assist by understanding and suggesting what must be communicated, including pictures or consumer letters if appropriate.

▶ Speak plainly at the appeals board. Use pictures if it would help. Many people in the appeals process do not have medical backgrounds.

▶ Explain the benefit limitations and the appeals process to the patient and family. Often it is the case manager's role to explain coverage limitations to patients. Assess if consumer expectation is a contributing factor to the problem. However, it is also the case manager's role to be a patient advocate when medical needs truly exceed benefits.

▶ Use a cost-benefit analysis approach. Occasionally, benefits will be altered if the case manager can prove that the suggested treatment, service, or piece of equipment is the best and most cost-efficient for the patient and the payor. Using this approach before a denial notice may avoid a need for an appeal in the first place. However, an informed analysis requires complete and accurate data. Information that may be needed for the analysis will need input from the patient's multidisciplinary team and will include some or all of the following:
  ▶ Complete history and physical assessment.
  ▶ Proposed treatment plan.
  ▶ Timing for implementing treatment plan (with estimated length of treatment or equipment need).
  ▶ When and what changes may be made to the treatment plan.
  ▶ How the treatment plan will be evaluated and monitored; expected outcomes.
  ▶ How often the patient is seen.
  ▶ How long the patient was evaluated before developing the treatment plan.

▶ Explore product support programs as an option. Many case managers are aware of community support programs for various diseases, and pharmaceutical help for required medications when a patient cannot pay. Less well known is that pharmacies and high-tech medical device companies have case managers that act as representatives for the products. These case managers are highly trained in insurance and reimbursement issues and claims processing; they assist in verifying benefits and answering questions about denials. They conduct a comprehensive funding search, identify trends in reimbursement, and approach the payor to resolve problems.

▶ In some states, very specific language can be found that will help in the appeal process. As a case manager you should be familiar with the language and the laws in your state.

▶ INTERSTATE CASE MANAGEMENT PRACTICE

In the United States today, a professional may practice only in the state or states in which he or she is licensed and in good standing. A nurse, for example, must be licensed in the state where the patient/client is located. Otherwise, the nurse would not be able to provide care to the patient. This appears to be complicated by the move to a global economy where health care organizations are securing multistate and offshore sites.

Each nurse's practice is controlled by the law in the states(s) where he or she is licensed, typically, by the Nurse Practice Act of that state. The advent of the Nurse Licensure Compact places nurses on notice that interstate practice is only recognized in those states that have passed legislation, rules, and regulations adopting the compact (24 Del. Laws c. 19A, §1901A). The Compact permits nurses whose home state participates in the Compact to practice in any other state participating in the Compact. In the absence of such law being adopted by one's home state, a nurse must be licensed in each and every state in which he or she practices, even if the practice is limited to services such as telephonic triage. With less than half the states included in the Compact, the majority of nurses are left having to be licensed in each and every state in which they practice nursing.

In December 2005, the Case Management Society of America (CMSA) took an official position on this issue and incorporated its position in the *CMSA's Standards of Practice for Case Management* which clearly states that: "The case manager practices in accordance with applicable local, state, and federal laws. The case manager has knowledge of applicable accreditation and regulatory statutes governing sponsoring agencies that specifically pertain to delivery of case management services."

▶ CMSA encourages case managers and case manager employers to work aggressively with state Boards of Nursing to encourage compliance and entry into the National Council of State Boards of Nursing (NCSBN) as the Compact states so that appropriate multistate nursing licensure might continue appropriately and cost effectively.

▶ Alternatively, CMSA encourages the enactment of federal legislation mandating the recognition of nurse licensure in all states.

▶ CMSA has added its name to the growing list of those organizations supporting and endorsing the Nurse Compact. A copy of the CMSA Position Paper can be obtained through its Web site, www.cmsa.org (Powell & Tahan, 2008, pp. 591–593).

A telephone conversation may quickly transform from informational to nursing practice when it stops being about an appointment or delivery of a product and the simple question is asked, "How are you doing?" If the nurse case manager uses that information to assess the client's condition, then he or she is practicing nursing. Clients offer symptoms over the phone and in person and nurses are trained to make nursing assessment, based on such symptoms. That is nursing practice and it requires a license to practice in the state where the patient is located.

The question often arises: "But what if the patient is a pilot or sales representative and is traveling?" Although there are no cases to date, the controlling law states two (sometimes conflicting) rules. If the case is a workers' compensation case, the law that applies is the law where the individual was hired. For example, pilots employed by certain airlines are presumed to work where the airline's corporate office is located, even if they receive treatment around the globe. In general health or more traditional employment scenarios, the state of the patient's residency applies. Obtaining an additional license by waiver (entry into another state without examination) is the way in which a professional learns and is kept up-to-date on changes in the law and the legal requirements, such as specific continuing education training. It is reasonable for a case manager to request contribution by the employer for the cost of the additional license while employed in a multistate field for telephonic case management setting. This is something that can be discussed at the time of interview or after the case manager is hired and learns that the assignment will require case management across state lines.

▶ USE OF COMMUNITY STANDARDS IN THE UTILIZATION MANAGEMENT ROLE

A patient with multiple sclerosis was receiving a standard treatment protocol for the condition but was having side effects that led to at least two hospitalizations. The physician wanted to try a commonly used treatment protocol for multiple sclerosis in Arizona. However, the patient's primary insurance company was in Massachusetts and denied the treatment because it was not a standard treatment on the east coast. The request to change protocols was reasonable (and medically necessary). The argument was one of the "right to use treatment protocols" according to the standards of the medical community in which the patient resides.

Lawsuits against MCOs can be based on the theory that the MCO did not make a utilization decision in accordance with the standard of medical necessity of the local community. In the case of *Hughes v. Blue Cross of Northern California* (215 Cal.App.3d 832 [1989]), the issue was whether a third-party payor acted in bad faith by using a standard of medical necessity significantly at variance with that of the medical community when making insurance coverage decisions. In a mental health case, the hospital's utilization review department determined that the hospitalizations for the illness were medically necessary; the insurance company denied most of the claims, saying they were not medically necessary. The court held that Blue Cross used a standard of medical necessity different from the standard of the community, and that Blue Cross also denied benefits based on a cursory review of incomplete records (Sturgeon, 1997). "Thus, good faith mandates that the reviewer apply a standard of medical necessity consistent with community medical standards" (Sturgeon, 1997, p. 68).

In response to *Hughes* and other similar cases, effective January 1, 2001, the California State Legislature passed new laws, including California Civil Code § 3428, to protect HMO members. The law establishes liability for insurance carriers and by extension their employees (including case managers)

for any and all harm legally caused by its failure to exercise ordinary care when both of the following apply:

(1) The failure to exercise ordinary care resulted in the denial, delay, or modification of the health care service recommended for, or furnished to, a subscriber or enrollee and (2) The subscriber or enrollee suffered substantial harm

(See Display 8-1, California Civil Code, Section 3428.) The significance of this law, besides the recognition

CALIFORNIA CIVIL CODE SECTION 3428 [Liability of Health Care Service Plans]

a. For services rendered on or after January 1, 2001, a health care service plan or managed care entity, as described in subdivision (f) of Section 1345 of the Health and Safety Code, shall have a **duty of ordinary care** to arrange for the provision of medically necessary health care service to its subscribers and enrollees, where the health care service is a benefit provided under the plan, and shall be **liable for any and all harm legally caused by its failure to exercise that ordinary care** when both of the following apply:

   ▶ (1) The failure to exercise ordinary care resulted in the denial, delay, or modification of the health care service recommended for, or furnished to, a subscriber or enrollee.

   ▶ (2) The subscriber or enrollee suffered substantial harm.

b. For purposes of this section:

   ▶ (1) substantial harm means loss of life, loss or significant impairment of limb or bodily function, significant disfigurement, severe and chronic physical pain, or significant financial loss;

   ▶ (2) health care services need not be recommended or furnished by an in-plan provider, but may be recommended or furnished by any health care provider practicing within the scope of his or her practice; and

   ▶ (3) health care services shall be recommended or furnished at any time prior to the inception of the action, and the recommendation need not be made prior to the occurrence of substantial harm.

c. Health care service plans and **managed care entities are not health care providers** under any provision of law, including, but not limited to, Section 6146 of the Business and Professions Code, Sections 3333.1 or 3333.2 of this code, or Sections 340.5, 364, 425.13, 667.7, or 1295 of the Code of Civil Procedure.

d. A health care service plan or managed care entity **shall not seek indemnity**, whether contractual or equitable, from a provider for liability imposed under subdivision (a). Any provision to the contrary in a contract with providers is void and unenforceable.

e. This section shall not create any liability on the part of an employer or an employer group purchasing organization that purchases coverage or assumes risk on behalf of its employees or on behalf of self-funded employee benefit plans.

f. **Any waiver** by a subscriber or enrollee of the provisions of this section is contrary to public policy and shall be **unenforceable and void**.

g. This section does not create any new or additional liability on the part of a health care service plan or managed care entity for harm caused that is attributable to the medical negligence of a treating physician or other treating health care provider.

h. This section does not abrogate or limit any other theory of liability otherwise available at law.

i. This section shall not apply in instances where subscribers or enrollees receive treatment by prayer, consistent with the provisions of subdivision (a) of Section 1270 of the Health and Safety Code, in lieu of medical treatment.

j. Damages recoverable for a violation of this section include, but are not limited to, those set forth in Section 3333.

k. [Exhaustion of IMR]

   ▶ A person may not maintain a cause of action pursuant to this section against any entity required to comply with any independent medical review system or independent review system required by law unless the person or his or her representative has exhausted the procedures provided by the applicable independent review system.

   ▶ Compliance with paragraph (1) is not required in a case where either of the following applies:

      ▶ Substantial harm, as defined in subdivision (b), has occurred prior to the completion of the applicable review.

      ▶ Substantial harm, as defined, in subdivision (b), will imminently occur prior to the completion of the applicable review.

   ▶ This subdivision shall become operative only if Senate Bill 189 and Assembly Bill 55 of the 1999–2000 Regular Session are also enacted and enforceable.

l. If any provision of this section or the application thereof to any person or circumstance is held to be unconstitutional or otherwise invalid or unenforceable, the remainder of the section and the application of those provisions to other persons or circumstances shall not be affected thereby.

of liability on the part of the insurance provider, is that it lowers the standard from one of professional liability and its prerequisites (discussed earlier in this chapter) to the lesser standard of "ordinary care." Ordinary or simple negligence is far easier to prove and therefore provides greater protection to the public.

Proving a community standard for professional liability was not all that difficult in the multiple sclerosis case, it was just time consuming. The neurologist who was a local expert in treating multiple sclerosis had written a letter, as did an Arizona pharmacist. There were also two articles from case management magazines stating that this particular protocol was used. Finally, the article cited in the above paragraph was submitted. Standards are being tested in so many facets of healthcare, including the use of alternative treatments, that case managers may require the perspective of "consistent community standards" in some of their cases. Conversely, case managers who perform interstate utilization management for MCOs should be aware of community standards in other regions. However, as more disease-specific guidelines and protocols become accepted, community-based standards may become a thing of the past.

Two themes repeat throughout any discussion of interactions between case managers and their clients: documentation and communication. The fact that our society has become more litigious is no secret. However, one should remember that good, culturally sensitive, and effective communication, which includes thoughtful efforts that demonstrate caring when someone is ill or injured, goes a long way to avoiding litigation. Clear, factual, objective, nonjudgmental, and complete documentation and communication make litigation less likely or more importantly, should a lawsuit occur, make case managers less likely to be the target. Remember the following:

▶ When making observations either visually or through telephonic communications, the words that you choose can make all the difference.
▶ Describe objectively, rather than characterizing observations; for example:

> **Do** say/write "The client expressed his upset with delays, when he said, 'I've called three times and I simply can't get an MRI appointment.'"
>
> **Don't** say/write "The client was raving and carrying on about the MRI appointment."
>
> **Do** say/write "The condition of Ms. X's home made mobility difficult. We discussed a plan to eliminate unnecessary obstacles.
>
> **Don't** say/write "Ms. X is a slob, her house is a mess; she's going to fall."

A study of lawsuits reveals that the underlying cause of litigation is often lack of information, lack of patient understanding, discourtesy, and other communication failures. Patients with chronic illnesses, for which the medical profession can only temporarily abate the symptoms and distress, are especially prone to frustration. In the 1980s, a study performed nationally with U.S. Postal Service employees revealed that a simple follow-up after an employee went home ill or injured reduced workers' compensation litigation and days lost from work by a great percentage. People need to know that someone cares; that's where communication comes in.

The case manager can be acutely successful by simply calling an injured or ill employee on the day of injury or a few days into the illness to inquire if needed services are in motion. Have you been able to get an appointment with the physician? Have you been able to get your prescriptions filled? How can we (employer) help you? Sometimes, just asking the question is enough, other times facilitating and coordinating medical services is exactly what case managers do.

In my own experience, I supervised a team of case managers for the sheriff's department in a suburban area. We would receive an accident report via facsimile within 24 hours following a work injury. A courtesy call was made within 24 hours of receiving the report and most times little or nothing but a few well-invested moments of time were needed and the officer returned to work appropriately. By reviewing accident reports from the same facility over and over again, a pattern of time, location, and type of injury appeared. It turned out that there was a slow-dripping water leak in the ceiling, above a concrete stairwell. Officers on rounds on the night shift were falling and sustaining a variety of sprains, strains, and fractures. I made a site visit, met with the administration, who called building maintenance. The problem was identified and fixed, and the injuries stopped. When you take into consideration that these employees received unlimited full-pay sick time due to their particular employment, even if the injury was a simple slip and fall, the cost savings were enormous and turnover was greatly reduced. Case management, when effectively implemented, can save time, improve safety, reduce litigation, and save thousands of dollars.

▶ DOCUMENTATION

In any case related to medical treatment, whether within a facility or in the community, the first place an investigation begins is with the record. The record can be an office or hospital chart or merely case management notes or reports. It is not uncommon for medical records to be incorrect and incomplete. For example, one individual went to the emergency department with severe nausea, vomiting, watery diarrhea, and abdominal pain. During the emergency department admission he was administered a medication that caused his blood pressure to drop; intravenous (IV) fluids were infused, and he was placed in a Trendelenburg position. The emergency department medical record stated that he came in with complaints of chest pain; no mention was made of the reaction to the medication or the subsequent treatment. Many nurses and case managers have had similar experiences. This particular case didn't become a legal issue, but if the same set of facts occurred today, it very well could have. It is critically important that case managers incorporate assessment and document the results of that assessment. Whether you are face to face or on the telephone, you are expected to meet the obligations of your professional practice/license.

You might receive a referral of a person with an orthopedic problem, perhaps a fracture. During your initial telephonic assessment of the individual he mentions that his toes are cold and the small toe used to hurt, but it stopped and he can't feel it anymore. These acute symptoms of impaired circulation could easily be overlooked and go undocumented. Three days later when that small toe is amputated due to a gangrenous state, the lack of documentation could very well be linked causally to the loss of the toe. Would the same standard of liability exist if the case manager was a social worker by education, license, and experience? Probably not! A social worker doesn't receive the same training as it relates to disease processes, nursing assessment, and nursing diagnosis. A nurse must be able to identify deviations in body systems as cause for emergent medical intervention. Each person does the best they can with his or her unique education and training.

It is also very confusing to case managers when we read contradictory statements; one or the other must be wrong. What about missing documentation of drug reactions that is needed for a thorough assessment? Case managers must procure the correct facts (as must all medical professionals) and must document them accurately.

For a long time, The Joint Commission, formerly known as the Joint Commission on Accreditation of Healthcare Organizations (JCAHO), *Accreditation Manual for Hospitals* (1985) gave an excellent overview of the main points to document. Although it was originally written for staff nurses, much of the following quote is important for the case manager.

> Documentation of nursing care shall be pertinent and concise and shall reflect the patient's status. Nursing documentation should address the patient's needs, problems, capabilities and limitations. Nursing intervention and patient response must be noted. When a patient is transferred within or discharged from the hospital, a nurse shall note the patient's status in the medical record. As appropriate, patients who are discharged from the hospital requiring nursing care should receive instructions and individualized counseling prior to discharge, and evidence of the instructions and the patient's or family's understanding of these instructions should be noted in the medical record. Such instructions and counseling must be consistent with the responsible medical practitioner's instructions (Joint Commission, 1985, pp. 98–99).

The question that we need to examine in the modern case management setting is, "Has technology changed anything?" The case manager's initial answer is probably "Yes. It's great; we just click on the buttons in the case management program (software application) and no more awful narrative reports." Any abbreviated method of charting is a double-edged sword, however. The time-saving aspects are wonderful and those programs that can provide outcomes, statistical information, and cost-savings can further assist the case manager in many expected functions, but there is a down side.

The law is slow to catch up with technology in medicine as well as in other industries. Legal requirements of complete and accurate charting have not changed. If you review the Nurse Practice Act in the state in which you practice, you will find a documentation obligation. In October 2007, the state of Illinois updated its Nurse Practice Law. Title 68 §1300 states, in the relevant part, that a nurse must take a complete history and do a complete physical assessment, including all body systems, to develop a nursing care plan.

Case management shares the requirement as Illinois' Nurse Practice Act; however, for those case managers who are not also direct caregivers, it translates simply into an obligation for a case manager to perform a complete assessment, including all body systems, in the development of the case management plan. That requisite assessment can be performed at arm's length or telephonically over great distances. The only way to demonstrate compliance with this very common and basic requirement is to document the assessment and resulting interventions and recommendations contained in a Case Management Care Plan. In over 20 years of case management practice, the tools have changed, but the essential elements of practice have not. Documentation remains a case management obligation and an ally in demonstrating compliance with laws, rules, and regulations, as well as quality case management practice standards.

Documentation in medical records is discoverable, meaning it can be requested for use in court. More documentation recommendations are discussed under specific issues.

The key to successful case management documentation is to present a clear and objective picture and to demonstrate that the chronological progression of events was within the standards of care of the documenter's professional scope of practice, based on the underlying professional license and case management standards of practice.

▶ PRIVACY RULES

The *Standards for Privacy of Individually Identifiable Health Information* (Privacy Rule) establishes, for the first time, a set of national standards for the protection of certain health information. The U.S. Department of Health and Human Services (HHS) issued the Privacy Rule to implement the requirement of HIPAA (Pub. L. 104-191, 1996). The entire rule is available online, along with numerous valuable resources (http://www.hhs.gov/ocr/hipaa).

The final regulation, the Privacy Rule, was published on December 28, 2000 (67 C.F.R § 82462), with the goal of providing consumers with greater rights for protection of individually identifiable health information. Modifications to the Privacy Rule were enacted on August 14, 2002 (65 C.F.R. §53182). In the spring of 2003 there were further modifications to the Final Privacy Rule. Now HIPAA is here and it is here to stay. The key is to have an organized system of demonstrating HIPAA compliance. HIPAA is a *minimum* mandatory national standard. If you, your state, or your individual practice is stricter than the declared HIPAA requirements, there is no need to change.

Medical records can legally be used for billing, auditing, utilization review, quality assurance studies, and research. When they are used for this purpose or when a patient makes his or her medical condition the basis for a lawsuit, HIPAA privacy protections are waived by the patient in a limited fashion to allow permitted uses of the information contained in the record. The key to HIPAA compliance is informing the patient of his or her rights, documenting that you have informed the patient, and taking necessary steps to assure that the patient's expressed wishes are carried out.

▶ THE MEDICAL RECORD

The medical record is created through documentation. Whether it is a hospital chart, a field case management record or a telephonic log, the goals are the same. The quality and completeness of the documentation determine the effectiveness of the record.

Today more than ever, hospital case management is becoming the norm rather than the exception. The contents of the medical record must be complete and accurate and contain the necessary documents that the hospital or other healthcare facility requires. In many states, state law (often found in the state's administrative code) specifically mandates the type of medical record used and its contents. Services provided and then submitted for either private insurance payment or a government program such as Medicare or Medicaid must be "clean" if payment is to be forthcoming. It is the role of the case manager to ensure that his or her contribution to the record does not interfere with these requirements. A complete medical record enhances continuity and coordination of patient care by providing interdisciplinary guidance to the entire treatment team. The medical record is more than a medical history and plan of care; it is a legal record and, for the reasons described, the medical record will supply evidence that a standard of care was (or was not) met.

In the case of third-party reimbursement, insurance companies and other payment sources scrutinize patients' charts for several reasons:

▶ To determine whether services billed for were actually provided. All orders, tests and their results, medication administration, supplies, and other procedures will be perused. Insurance companies may not reimburse if the evidence for the billed items is not in the chart.

▶ To determine whether this hospitalization or procedure was medically necessary. Nursing and physician documentation should support admitting diagnosis completely and factually, with symptoms, vital signs, and treatments listed. Specific communications with the patient, family, or others, documented accurately, can explain long after discharge the events that might otherwise be vague or confusing with simple entries. Even with computerized charting, narrative notes are still the most valuable tools for professionals to protect themselves and explain events they might otherwise have forgotten.

▶ To establish length of hospital stay. Any changes in the patient's condition may lend support to an increased length of stay; therefore, it is important for nurses to help identify and document complications and additional problems. Case managers should collaborate with staff nurses and other professionals in emphasizing the importance of accurate charting in this area. The case manager's role may include requesting and justifying additional hospital days; the charting is necessary to aid the case manager when advocating for needed extra days. There is a trend for insurance companies and governmental benefit plans to refuse to pay for those parts of hospitalizations they determine are due to complications caused by something that the institution could have prevented (hospital-acquired conditions [HACs] or Never Events). Therefore, complete and accurate documentation is not only a professional duty, but also a legal obligation. The Joint Commission also places great emphasis on evaluating the completeness of patient records when determining whether the agency will attain accreditation status.

Similarly, URAC scrutinizes medical records, policies, and procedures to determine whether core case management standards are being properly utilized. URAC standards cover several critical operational categories for any quality case management program including:

- Staff structure and organization.
- Staff management and development.
- Information management.
- Quality improvement.
- Oversight of delegated functions.
- Organizational ethics.
- Complaints.

(For more information, see the URAC Web site, http://www.urac.org/programs/prog_accred_CM_po.aspx.)

Who owns the medical record? The actual physical document belongs to the institution that created it; the institution is the custodian of the hard copy. The hospital owns the hospital medical record; a physician owns his or her office records. The information, however, belongs to the patient. The patient is entitled not only to this information but to other items, such as actual radiographs, computed tomography (CT) scans, pathology slides, gallstones, and others. In most cases, failure to provide a patient with requested records is grounds for a civil suit. With the advent of HIPAA, much of this confusion is eliminated, however, the burden remains on patients to request their records, follow through to overcome improper denials of access, and to report HIPAA violations. (The HIPAA Complaint Form with instructions is available online at http://www.cms.hhs.gov/enforcement/downloads/complaintinwriting.pdf.)

The patient can also authorize the release of medical records to others. Because the institution is responsible for the confidentiality and security of these records, a signed Authorization of the Release of Records Form is required. Under HIPAA, even family members are not entitled to the records unless the patient has died. Here are some special situations:

- The parent or legal guardian of a minor may or may not have access to records. A noncustodial parent, following a divorce, may or may not have rights to the medical record. Such access is specifically addressed in Judgments of Divorce and associated agreements. These have the effect of a court order. Consult your institution's attorney or risk management department before participating in release of records or patient information based on a claim of right under such a document.
- Since the advent of HIPAA, a subpoena alone is not sufficient to obtain medical records. The subpoena must be accompanied by an Authorization for Release of Medical Records signed by the patient or other authorized person. If served with a subpoena, immediately contact the facility's attorney or risk management department, as policy requires. A court order may be required to release information.
- Some records are protected by law. Drug and alcohol records from a drug/alcohol detoxification program and mental health records may need a court order before information is released. It is suggested that case managers be familiar with their own state laws in these instances.
- In many states, HIV/AIDS medical records are protected far beyond HIPAA's minimum standards.

To avoid a trip to the courthouse, in most states custodians of medical records are permitted to certify medical records as being complete, true, and accurate. This is accomplished with an affidavit or certification being attached to the records and signed by the custodian. The HIPAA Compliance Officer in a facility must oversee this function, along with other compliance issues. They are very aware that computerized charting, although wonderfully efficient, exposes the risk for potential privacy abuses.

▶ DISCHARGE PLANNING AND PREMATURE DISCHARGE

Discharge planning and continuity of care are two of the most important responsibilities of the case manager.

A case manager can complement, and be an extremely valuable asset to, a healthcare team; the accuracy of the financial and psychosocial assessment can make or break the discharge plan. The best discharge planning starts on admission. That is true whether we are talking about an acute hospital stay or a referral for an injured employee. The case management assessment should take into consideration all stakeholders, including but not limited to, the client, family, employer, payor(s), and ancillary services that may be needed for short- and long-term outcomes. The important thing to remember is that the assessment is a living document that can be changed and updated as new information is learned or the client's condition changes. The need for client and/or family teaching or support should be considered throughout.

There is a crisis in America today and time-honored systems for safe and efficient continuity of care are being challenged in the name of healthcare cost-containment. More than ever, case managers are needed to promote an atmosphere of safe and efficient planning. Cost-efficiency and safe, thoughtful continuity of care need not be mutually exclusive.

Because of this, the likelihood of allegations such as abandonment or premature discharge is increased. Premature discharge is often associated with adverse payment decisions by third-party payors and delayed decisions by payors. "Both nurse managers/supervisors and nurses in direct patient care positions are accountable for providing safe nursing care to their patients" (N.J. Board of Nursing Patient Abandonment—Position Statement, 2007).

> *An important documentation consideration:* the physician is the discharging agent. In your case management documentation, *never* make it look like the case manager discharged the patient.

▶ Adequacy of Discharge Planning

The adequacy of discharge planning describes the discharge plan, with the case manager as the link between the patient and community resources. A complete discharge summary report is necessary for the prevention or avoidance of legal and risk management issues. Many outcomes management projects and accreditation mandates include discharge planning issues (e.g., medications on discharge, education before discharge). The questions to be addressed when engaged in discharge planning activities are as follows: Is the plan appropriate and adequate for this individual? Does the plan consider physical, emotional, social, mental health, and safety needs? Is follow-up care addressed? Are educational needs addressed?

The following are guidelines to help the case manager with discharge planning:

1. Before you make any referrals, obtain consent from patient, family/significant other, and physician, consistent with HIPAA and state regulations.
2. Document all communications with patient and family, including agreement or rejection of recommended services. Record the patient's and/or family's direct quotes, if possible.
3. Document the patient's limitations and refusals in an objective manner.

    Consider the following example:

> Mr. Grant, an 82-year-old unmarried male, refuses a SNF. Your assessment demonstrates that he needs continued care that can be provided in a SNF. Patient states he lives alone with intermittent visits from one neighbor. You have an obligation to explore available options, even if they are not your first choice. Physical therapy charts, "Patient can walk 10 feet with front-wheeled walker and maximum assist of two." Now your discharge work begins. This may show that the patient is unsafe for discharge home alone, but have you asked enough questions to assess the home environment? Maybe Mr. Grant lives in a senior community that is barrier-free, with assistive devices already installed in the bathroom, kitchen, and hallways. The options in that environment are far different if Mr. Grant lives in an older building with a two-flight walk-up. Many times patients later agree to a short stay in a SNF for the purpose of improving strength and endurance while home modification can be accomplished.
>
> Your goal is complete, unbiased assessment and reasonable recommendations in a cost-effective manner. Before discharge, an appropriate discharge agreement must be reached and documented, with steps shown to facilitate the plan. Your documentation might be as simple as, "Visiting nurse will do complete home assessment on morning of discharge and order necessary assistive devices, along with home care, including physical therapy." Documentation can protect you from a lawsuit later on should Mr. Grant fall at home in a manner that could not have been foreseen.

4. If the discharge plan changes, as is often the case, document the change, including who requested the change, the reasons for the change, and your activities now to make possible necessary changes. Mr. Grant may agree to home healthcare with aides and private duty nursing. Before the actual discharge, he may decide that a SNF is the best alternative temporarily. Sometimes deterioration of the patient's condition or an unexpected improvement deems the plan change appropriate. Document the medical status of the patient to substantiate the necessary change, including the physician's contribution to the discharge plan, such as orders for homecare, including physical therapy, home infusion, etc., or prescriptions for medications.

5. Document all interventions and the patient's responses to them as well as interactions with the treatment team.

6. On the day that a patient is transferred to another facility or discharged home, document communication with the family; this is a must. This is especially important when the patient is going home with many discharge needs. You want to document who the primary caregiver will be and that you've communicated with that person.

7. Document contacts with other agencies and institutions, as well as times, dates, with whom you spoke, and what was said and agreed on. Fax or e-mail a confirmation to such agencies to demonstrate your compliance with the plan and that you've properly notified and perhaps transferred responsibility for the patient to another professional.

8. Documenting patient/family education and teaching is extremely important. If anything goes wrong after discharge, documentation can be evidence of proper and adequate teaching. If documentation is inadequate and the patient is readmitted, insurance companies may attempt to deny reimbursement, based on a supposition that the member was inadequately taught or prepared for discharge. Chart:
   ▶ How much time was spent teaching.
   ▶ What was taught.
   ▶ To whom the information was given (e.g., caregiver, patient).
   ▶ How well the "student" comprehended the information.

   ▶ The outcomes of the teaching.
   If follow-up teaching is necessary, include plans for such teaching and, when completed, add notations. If someone other than you did the teaching, identify the person in your notes.

9. Whenever possible, provide written as well as verbal instructions and provide demonstrations. Document the teaching tools used.

10. It is critical to chart confirmation of the patient's caregiver's understanding of what is being told such as special diets, treatments, potential complications, follow-up doctor visits, wound care, medications and side effects, and activity level.

11. It is not enough to explain and document potential side effects and complications of medicines and treatments. Today, there are programs available in hospitals and online that provide standardized patient teaching and discharge information. Although these tools are useful, they merely provide a baseline of information. It is important to modify these "cookie cutter" documents, as needed, to properly and completely inform the individual of their specific needs.

12. The patient or caregiver must also know what to do if complications arise; that is, to seek medical attention. Some people, hearing from a physician about a possible side effect, may wrongly interpret that side effect as being normal and expected and may continue with whatever caused the problem. Document that the patient and caregiver were told what to do if anything unusual occurs.

13. Many patients go home with durable medical equipment (DME), such as oxygen, suction machines, bipap ventilators, feeding pumps, and IV delivery systems, including pumps. Without sufficient instruction, this equipment can become more of a hazard than a help. Document what equipment is being used, the teaching that was done (and any follow-up required), and who was taught, along with their comprehension. Documentation of coordination—that the equipment will be available when the patient arrives home—is also important.

14. Educational needs should be addressed as soon as possible; last minute teaching is typically quick and often inadequate.

15. Document the patient's clinical condition at discharge. If psychosocial stresses or mental

health conditions are present, document the patient's status at discharge.

16. Medications and discharge planning are often chosen as quality indicators (core measures) to measure. Documentation of these two aspects of care is essential to provide evidence that these expectations were met.

17. Medical stability of patients within 24 hours of discharge from a hospital: Documentation of medical stability may include vital signs (blood pressure, pulse and respiratory rates, and temperature); laboratory and radiology tests, including results, especially if abnormal findings were noted; IV fluid therapy or medications intake (especially last dosage administered); and condition of wounds, incisions, or drainage tubes/catheters. Documentation should also include any abnormalities, notification of physicians of abnormalities, interventions instituted, and patient's response. In addition, documentation should reflect the physician's agreement with the discharge despite the presence of an abnormality.

▶ INFORMED CONSENT

The first thing that any healthcare practitioner needs to understand is that informed consent is a legal requirement that rests with the physician. It is not simply "nice" if the physician gets it signed; it is the physician's legal and ethical responsibility to provide his or her patient with sufficient information to permit the patient to make a knowing and intelligent informed consent or refusal. Further, *Case Management Standards of Practice* say that the client must consent to case management services (Case Management Society of America, 2002).

Informed consents are used specifically for treatments and procedures that are invasive or that have potentially dangerous side effects or complications. Depending on the institution's policies and procedures, state laws, and the emergent need of the procedure, a signed informed consent form is required. Implied consent may be appropriate in an emergency situation in which lack of action may cause greater harm than the potential risks of the treatment. The classic example of implied consent to medical intervention is the unconscious patient. In many states there is a legal presumption that an unconscious patient gives consent for life-saving treatment simply based on the presentation of symptoms and an inability to communicate due to those conditions.

Before a patient is informed of anything, that patient must be capable of comprehending what is being said. It is important to document the patient's ability or inability to understand, particularly in those cases when the information is being given in a language that is not the patient's or family's native language. Capacity versus incapacity is based on a patient's ability to understand the information, to make choices, and to communicate verbally or nonverbally. A patient under chemical sedation may be only temporarily incapacitated, but nevertheless unable to give consent for a period of time. Advance Directives for Healthcare can avoid this problem even in the case of sedation. Only a court of law and a judge's order can find a person legally incompetent. Legally incompetent persons, no matter their age or level of consciousness, cannot sign on their own behalf.

There are two basic steps to the informed consent process: the disclosure of information and the signature.

▶ The Disclosure of Information

The following, at the minimum, needs to be discussed with the patient (or surrogate) (Feutz-Harter, 1991):

▶ The patient's condition or problem.
▶ The nature and purpose of the proposed test, therapy, or procedure.
▶ Any hazards, risks, or potential complications of the proposed test, therapy, or procedure.
▶ Any feasible alternatives to the proposed test, therapy, or procedure.
▶ The expected outcome of the proposed test, therapy, or procedure.
▶ The risks and prognosis if the proposed test therapy or procedure is not done.

Most litigation surrounding disclosure issues addresses the healthcare professional's or physician's failure to reveal "material" risks or dangers. When a complication arises and the patient was unaware of its possibility, liability may attach. Yet there is a delicate balance between disclosing too little and too much. Patients can become so overwhelmed with frightening, potential dangers and risks that they are no longer capable of sifting out the important information and making appropriate choices. The case manager can be very helpful to the patent/client and physician by being able to restate complex issues in simplified terms. Except in those states that acknowledge that Physician's Assistants or Advanced Practice Nurses have a specifically identified statutory duty or ability to obtain informed consent, the responsibility never shifts from the physician to provide the requisite information and obtain the signature.

Complete documentation is essential to demonstrate compliance with the state's requirements for informed consent. Often a patient will claim he or she was not fully informed, even in those cases where there was complete, truthful, and accurate information provided in a manner that the individual could or should have been able to comprehend. The case manager's notes describing the event can be affirmative proof that all legal requirements were satisfied.

Notations describing obtaining informed consent may include:

▶ Who informed the patient.

▶ The information discussed—including the above list of topics.

▶ Who the explanation was given to and who else was present.

▶ How long the discussion took.

▶ Teaching materials used, such as videos, flip charts, booklets, or drawings.

▶ Offering the patient the opportunity to ask questions and have them answered.

▶ Indication of comprehension, and whether more thought, time, and discussion are needed before the decision can be made.

Incomplete or inaccurate information could deem the dispenser of the information liable. Take time to chart comprehensively, objectively, and accurately.

▶ Signing of the Informed Consent

Many times the case manager is told to present the informed consent form to the patient sometime after the disclosure of information. Often the case manager did not even witness the disclosure. Therefore, the case manager must be skilled in assessing the adequacy of the information and patient comprehension. As a patient advocate, the case manager has a legal and ethical responsibility to protect patients from misinformation, omissions, and errors. If lack of understanding is assessed about the treatment, hazards, alternatives, risks, expected outcomes, or prognosis if therapy is not performed, the case manager can fill in omissions and clarify misunderstandings if he or she feels qualified to do so. Your role as a case manager is really that of a witness to the signature and nothing more. One legal source has this to say about nurses answering questions regarding procedures and informed consents:

> If the patient doesn't understand the information or wants more information, you can answer any questions that are within the scope of your knowledge. You aren't obligated, however, to answer any of the patient's questions. As a witness, you are not legally responsible for disclosing all relevant information to the patient. The doctor retains this responsibility, and he cannot delegate it to you. If you see that a patient is

confused, and you can't provide the information he needs, document your observation in the patient's chart and make sure the patient gets the information from his doctor or another appropriate source (Andrews, Goldberg, & Kaplan, 1996, pp. 73–74).

Notification of the physician regarding problem areas is advised, along with complete documentation of the lack of understanding and of the time and date that you have notified the physician. If you believe that the patient requires more explanation from the physician, communicate that to the physician and document your concerns in the medical record. In today's world of electronic charting, there is always some additional screen for notes or comments, even in those cases where narrative charting is limited.

Where informed consent for minors is concerned, parents and legal guardians must sign consent forms. One rare exception is an emancipated minor, who would be able to show documentation of that fact in the form of a court order. There is great variation from state to state but, as in all things, documentation is your protection. Ask questions; document your questions, and document the answers you relied on.

> **Court Orders and Legal Documents**: As a general rule you must see and should keep a copy of the order or other documents in the chart. Never accept a person's word that such documents exist.

Once fully informed of the risks and benefits of a procedure, a competent adult may elect to refuse a treatment or other intervention. Some facilities have a Refusal of Treatment Release Form. It is the patient's right to do so, and that right must be honored. A patient's refusal of care can only be overridden when:

1. The patient is not mentally or legally competent.

2. There are compelling reasons to overrule the patient's wishes. These may include such issues as the refusal may endanger the life of another (if a pregnant woman's refusal threatens the life of her unborn child), it threatens a child's life (for parental refusal), the patient is refusing treatment but also stating that he or she wants to live (i.e., noncongruence), and when the public interest outweighs the patient's right. In large medical centers and in state or county government there are Offices of Patient Advocacy and Ombudsmen; Protective Services

for Adults, Seniors, and Children, all of whom can be contacted for guidance and assistance.(In New York State [http://pubadvocate.nyc.gov], in New Jersey [http://www.state.nj.us/ publicadvocate/public/issues/ civilombudsmaninto.html], or the United States Ombudsman Organization [http:// www.usombudsman.org/index.cfm]).

▶ CONFIDENTIALITY

Both federal and state law control confidentiality. HIPAA is the national minimum mandatory standard; however, some states have exceeded the federal standard and provided citizens with even greater protection. Statutory mandate gives legal clout to professional relationships. Privilege is the statutory protection of the physician–patient (and in some states nurse–patient) relationship. New York was one of the first states to recognize the nurse–patient relationship as a separate and distinct confidential relationship. Unless state law specifically recognizes the relationship, privilege does not apply.

It is incumbent on the prudent practitioner to see the document authorizing the sharing of information, such as an "Information Release Form." In case management, it may feel awkward asking for documents, but remember you are acting not only as an advocate for your client by protecting his or her rights under HIPAA, but also ensuring that his or her wishes are given paramount consideration as you develop the case management plan (CMSA, 2002).

Maintaining patient confidentiality is not an easy task. Consider some of the members of the multidisciplinary medical team who may access the patient's medical records: attending physicians, residents, interns, medical students, nurses, nursing students, physical therapists, occupational therapists, speech therapists, social workers, case managers, utilization review personnel, insurance company case managers, hospital utilization reviewers, auditors, coders, billers, quality improvement organization (QIO) review teams, The Joint Commission accreditation teams, hospital quality assurance, researchers, and many others. As a case manager, you will be speaking to many people on each case. Care must be taken in each conversation to reveal only what is necessary. Give only the portion of information that the other party requires. Social services needs are different from an insurance company's utilization review requirements. It is important to remember that although persons or entities (such as insurance companies) may be entitled to information contained in the medical record for a specific purpose, such as paying a claim, they are not necessarily entitled to the entire medical record. If a patient is being treated today for a simple fracture of a forearm, the patient's 20-year gynecologic history is irrelevant and may not be released. HIPAA mandates that only necessary information be released.

Two basic questions to ask yourself are:

1. What patient information needs to be given?
2. What patient information cannot, need not, or should not be given?

If a patient/client makes a written request to access, review, or copy his or her own medical record, do you know how to respond? Patients have the right to access their medical records (45 C.F.R.§164.528). In other words, a person who is the subject matter of the medical record has a legal right to see its contents. However, it is incumbent on the covered entity to record who, when, what, and why any disclosure is made. Telephonic requests for confidential information should be rejected; however, you may simply ask the caller to fax a signed written request on a letterhead, along with necessary releases. It is far safer for the case manager to follow an established procedure to protect a patient's rights to confidentiality than to give instant gratification to an unknown caller. Well-intended calls from family members and friends to find out how a patient is doing can be a confidentiality nightmare if the case manager is not careful. Know your facility's policy and adhere to it; for most hospitals, the policy is to give a general statement of condition, by a nonmedical staff member, rather than exposing the professional staff to potential risk.

Those case managers who work with self-insured employer groups have even more reasons to be concerned. These case managers often are required by the groups to provide reports on the patients receiving case management services. HIPAA specifically safeguards employees in such circumstances, requiring "firewalls" to protect employee health information. Health records must be kept separate from employment records and persons with the authority to hire, fire, promote, or demote staff generally have no access to this information, in case they might let a medical diagnosis affect their authority and the decisions they make. Failure to keep protected health information (PHI) private can lead to accusations of invasion of privacy, defamation of character, and intentional infliction of emotional distress, and of course, a HIPAA violation.

Case managers, particularly those in the occupational health/workers' compensation arena must take certain actions to protect employee information. For example,

▶ Abide by federal (HIPAA) and state laws.
▶ Abide by federal laws such as the ADA and the Family Medical Leave Act.

▶ Establish and abide by a well-defined policy on the use of "firewalls" to protect employee PHI and limit access to unauthorized persons.

There are some situations where public safety may outweigh confidentiality; but in each of these cases an agency may not be entitled to the patient's entire medical record. In the case of communicable diseases, for example, public interest outweighs patient privacy and states have reporting requirements for such things as tuberculosis, measles, and other diseases that can spread through the population. In some states, failure to report certain situations may result in criminal culpability. The only exception to the authorization requirement besides those identified in the privacy rule itself (45 C.F.R. § 164.512), such as public health and communicable disease reporting, is a court order signed by a judge. If the request is merely for access to medical records and review of information, HIPAA requires that access be provided within 30 days (45 C.F.R. §164.524). An example of a state where compliance differs is California, which requires the same access to be provided within 10 days.

Confidentiality has become an even bigger issue because disease management programs and outcomes management projects are moving so much information to computerized databases. Electronic data are easy to access and patient consents are not always obtained for use in these managed care modalities. It is critical that any case manager involved in such projects or studies either obtain patient-signed consents or ensure that the organization is not using patient identifiers. This could save endless legal trouble in the confidentiality arena.

Fax machines pose another legal concern. Nearly every case manager has depended on the convenience of fax machines for both sending and receiving patient-specific information, especially for utilization management and review purposes and between the provider of care and the insurance company/health plan. Nearly every case manager has wondered if, at some point, confidential patient information may end up at the wrong place. Some fax precautions you may apply to avoid risk include:

▶ Double-check the number you are to send the fax to before you hit the "start" button; program commonly used numbers into the fax machine to lessen chances of inadvertently misdialing.
▶ Call the other party advising him or her that you are about to send the fax, then confirm that it has been properly received.
▶ Use a cover sheet that includes a confidentiality statement based on your organization's policy.
▶ Be sure that nothing is faxed that the recipient does not have a right or a need to know.

▶ Make sure that appropriate patient releases have been obtained before faxing anything.

Other actions for better management of information and for ensuring privacy include the following:

▶ Locate fax machines in secure areas with limited access to others.
▶ Assign a staff member to monitor faxes sent to each machine. The staff member's responsibilities should include:
  a. Collecting each document as soon as it arrives.
  b. Checking each document to be sure that it has arrived in its entirety and is legible.
  c. Sealing each document in an envelope and routing it to the addressee.
▶ Institute a system that ensures that incoming documents are routed to the appropriate people.
▶ Furnish contingency procedures to follow in the event that a document is misrouted. This information can be included as part of the confidentiality statement on the fax cover sheet.
▶ Physician orders should be signed. Orders that are not signed should not be followed until verified with the physician.
▶ State laws differ; make sure that you are not restricted from faxing patient information about HIV/AIDS or mental health issues. Know what your state requires and adhere to it.

▶ E-MAIL

The use of e-mail is becoming the norm rather than the exception. You must assume that it is simply not secure. Know your facility's policy regarding e-mail and what information may or may not be transmitted in this manner. E-mail policies should cover a broad variety of topics, including but not limited to:

▶ Permitted and prohibited use of e-mail.
▶ E-mails containing libelous, defamatory, offensive or other objectionable material that can expose the employer to liability.
▶ Forwarding and/or use of confidential and/or PHI.
▶ Copying messages and other materials without permission.

The same rules that would apply to a written letter, message, or other communication also apply to e-mail. One positive aspect of e-mail is that documentation takes care of itself. Storing e-mails either electronically or as printed hard copies provides documentation of the content, time, date, and parties to a communication. Personal use of company computers should be discouraged, especially on a system containing PHI. Informal personal use of e-mail in an environment containing PHI is an increased security risk, as unintentional disclosures of PHI could occur. Although HIPAA accepts and tolerates incidental disclosures (i.e., hearing your neighbor's name called out on the pharmacy waiting line), there should be great concern if there are no safeguards in place to protect against PHI getting into personal e-mail. The "minimum necessary" rule (45 C.F.R. §§ 164.502[a][1][iii]) applies, no matter what the method of communication is.

▶ ADVANCE DIRECTIVES FOR HEALTHCARE

The right of an individual to direct his or her own destiny is a constitutional right. As a patient advocate, there may not be a more important task than the discussion of advance directives, that is, getting a patient's wishes for care and treatment in writing—and fulfilled. Prolonging life for the sake of prolonging life is passé. Transitioning with as much comfort as possible is more often the goal.

In compliance with the Patient Self-Determination Act of 1990, hospitals, subacute care facilities, home health agencies, and hospices are federally mandated to counsel patients about their right to accept or refuse treatment and their right to the use of advance directives (Bosek & Fitzpatrick, 1992). Advance directives are legally executed documents, drawn up while the individual is still competent. They can be used only if the individual becomes incapacitated or incompetent. In this situation, patients are directing their own care in advance of the need (before incapacity). Individual autonomy is the end result, because the person is able, without coercion, to make some extremely important decisions about him- or herself.

The two most recognized advance directives are the living will and the medical power of attorney (POA), also called the durable POA for healthcare. A third advance directive is a pre-hospital medical care directive. This directive focuses on several aspects of a resuscitation event, such as defibrillation, chest compressions, assisted ventilation, intubation, and advanced life support medications (Perin, 1992). The individual can choose all, none, or any number of the above treatments. Case managers today are working with greater numbers of very ill young and older adults. Many may know little about documents such as medical POA, but most have thought a lot about dying and feel very little control over it. Although no one controls the death process, people can sometimes maintain authority over the events surrounding death and can make sure their last wishes are carried out.

Case managers and social workers are often asked to initiate discussions about advance directives; most institutions keep the forms to sign on hand. It is recommended that case managers understand advance directives and feel comfortable discussing the subject with patients and their families. Workshops about advance directives and those addressing death and dying are helpful; another way to learn about advance directives is to choose a medical POA for yourself or become a medical POA for a close family member or friend. The process is enlightening. Due to changing laws and various state mandates, it is an extra protection to attach a state-specific advance directive to the original. These are offered free by hospitals, state or city health departments, and the American Bar Association.

Another innovative move in advance directives is one recently launched in several states by a Florida-based nonprofit organization, Aging With Dignity. This do-it-yourself, fill-in-the-blank living will speaks plainly to people about a subject that is not clear to many; the added burden of trying to understand lawyer-speak or doctor-speak is gone. People finally understand the difference between "cure" and "palliative care." The goal of the advance directives document is to prompt discussion about a topic few of us like to discuss. This document addresses five areas, called *five wishes*, and goes beyond feeding tubes and ventilators. Five Wishes is now valid in 40 states and addresses all of a person's needs—medical, personal, emotional, and spiritual—at a time when unable to speak for oneself and suffering a serious and terminal illness.

NOTE

Aging With Dignity
Five Wishes
Mail to: P O Box 1661
Tallahassee FL 32302-1661
Office: 820 E. Park Avenue, Suite D 100
Tallahassee, FL 32301-2600
Telephone: (888) 5 WISHES/ (888) 594-7437
E-mail: fivewishes@agingwithdignity.org
Web site: www.agingwithdignity.org

The five wishes, or decisions, in the new living will are:

1. The person I want to make care decisions for me when I cannot is _____. This provides the name of the medical POA.
2. The kind of medical treatment I want/I do not want. Here, a checklist of medical treatments is provided. The checklist may include defibrillation, chest compressions, assisted ventilation, intubation, nutritional support, and advanced life support medications.
3. How comfortable I want to be.
4. How I want people to treat me.
5. What I want my loved ones to know.

The document is eight pages long. Questions 1 and 2 are generally legal/medical issues. The last three sections provide more than just clinically based functions. They address such personal issues as does the person wants someone by the bedside praying for him or her; does the person want poetry or music around; does the person wish his or her hand held; does the person want to be alone at the time of death; what are the person's thoughts on pain management; the last question provides memories, if the person so chooses, that can be used for a memorial. Simple, humane, and comforting information is included. Some attorneys feel that this is too simple, that the law is not clear or black and white: time will tell. Courts often honor advance directives if there is evidence that the patient has discussed end-of-life decisions with the family and physician. Although the document uses the word "wishes," the information gathered really reflects the patient's final "expectations." No one relishes this discussion, but even young, healthy baby boomers like myself have to agree that if Mick Jagger needs a hip

NOTE

Information on Living Wills and Advance Directives
Compassion and Choices/Choices in Dying
Address: P O Box 101810
Denver, CO 80250-1810
Telephone: (800) 247-7421
Web site: www.compassionandchoices.org

replacement and Jerry Garcia is mortal, perhaps this is a subject everyone must address.

▶ PROTECTING YOUR LICENSE

Most health professionals fear malpractice lawsuits over anything else. What they fail to understand is that civil liability exposure is only one aspect of risk. Malpractice insurance is designed to protect you financially from a damaging lawsuit. Professional practice is an area where several bodies of law control both the federal and state levels; civil, criminal, and administrative laws all regulate certain aspects of this practice.

In 2006, the notorious nurse serial killer, Charles Cullen, was sentenced to 11 consecutive life sentences in New Jersey and 18 in Pennsylvania after pleading guilty to murdering at least 35 people between 1998 and 2003. Cullen, a registered nurse, was labeled the "Angel of Death" when he admitted to administering overdoses of medications to terminal patients or those with fatal diagnoses to "spare them from being coded." New laws have followed this horrific series of deaths at the hands of one individual and placed all nurses and other health care providers under a new level of scrutiny.

During the investigation of these deaths and Cullen's behavior, it was revealed that he moved from hospital to hospital without notice, due to lax or absent reporting requirements. In response to this case, the New Jersey State Legislature enacted strict laws requiring background checks, including mandatory fingerprinting of healthcare professionals (Display 8-2). "The Health Care Professional Responsibility and Reporting Enhancement Act (N.J. Stat. § 45:1-33 [2007]) requires that a criminal history background check be conducted for all healthcare professionals licensed or certified by the Division of Consumer Affairs by 2009." Further information is available at http://www.state.nj.us/lps/ca/chbc/chbcinfo.htm (accessed on 3/18/2008). In addition, nurses who choose to leave one facility to improve their career opportunities or simply because they wish to work closer to home, find themselves answering probing questions by investigators of the Board of Nursing. In those cases where a nurse is terminated by a facility, the investigation can be lengthy and quite worrisome. Good and caring health professionals are now viewed with a cynical eye by their licensing authority because of the criminal acts of one individual.

BACKGROUND CHECKS

display 8-2

N.J. ST§ 10:48A-2.1 General standards

a. N.J.S.A. 30:6D-63 to 72 requires that the Department shall not contract with any community agency for the provision of services unless it has first been determined that no criminal history record information exists on file in the Federal Bureau of Investigation Identification Division, or in the State Bureau of Identification in the Division of State Police, which would disqualify the community agency head or the community agency employee from such employment.

b. **Fingerprints** shall be taken electronically through a "live scan" process. The agency staff shall be responsible to call a toll free number to schedule an appointment to have **fingerprints** taken. The State Bureau of Identification will **check** its own records and forward an inquiry to the Federal Bureau of Investigation.

c. It shall be the responsibility of the community agency head to assure compliance with this chapter.

d. If the criminal history record indicates a conviction for certain criminal or disorderly persons offenses, the employee shall be terminated from employment unless he or she affirmatively demonstrates to the community agency head or the community agency board, if the individual is the community agency head, clear and convincing evidence of his or her rehabilitation.

e. If a prospective employee refuses to consent to or cooperate in securing a **background check,** the person shall not be considered for employment.

f. If a current employee refuses to consent to or cooperate in securing **fingerprints** for the purpose of a **background check,** the person shall be immediately removed from his or her position and the person's employment shall be terminated.

g. A **background check** shall be conducted at least once every two years.

h. The community agency head and all employees who may come in contact with persons served by the agency, shall submit their **fingerprints** upon employment to the Department of Human Services office as directed by the Division.

i. If the **background check** of the community agency head reveals a criminal record as identified below, the community agency board shall determine within 15 working days, if the community agency head has been rehabilitated in accordance with N.J.A.C. 10:48-3.4.

j. The community agency head shall ensure that each employee who may come in contact with persons served by the agency shall be fingerprinted in accordance with the procedures contained in this chapter.

k. All employees shall sign a written consent to the criminal **background check** (refer to chapter Appendix A, incorporated herein by reference) prior to the time the **fingerprints** are taken. This consent shall remain on file in the agency.

l. Individuals shall be disqualified for employment for any of the following crimes or disorderly persons offenses in New Jersey:

1. Any crime or disorderly person offense (See Note Below) involving danger to the person as set forth in N.J.S.A. 2C:11-1 et seq. through 2C:15-1 et seq., including the following:
    i. Murder;
    ii. Manslaughter;
    iii. Death by auto;
    iv. Simple assault;
    v. Aggravated assault;
    vi. Recklessly endangering another person;
    vii. Terroristic threats;
    viii. Kidnapping;
    ix. Interference with custody of children;
    x. Sexual assault;
    xi. Criminal sexual contact;
    xii. Lewdness; or
    xiii. Robbery.

2. Any crime against children or incompetents as set forth in N.J.S.A. 2C:24-1 et seq., including the following:
    i. Endangering the welfare of a child; or
    ii. Endangering the welfare of an incompetent person;

3. A crime or offense involving the manufacture, transportation, sale, possession or habitual use of a controlled dangerous substance as defined in N.J.S.A. 24:21-1 et seq.; or

4. In any other state or jurisdiction, conduct which, if committed in New Jersey, would constitute any of the crimes or disorderly persons offenses described in (l)1 through 3 above.

NOTE: New Jersey does not use the term misdemeanor; a "disorderly persons offense" is one that is punishable with a potential sentence of up to 180 days in jail and $1000 in fines or both. A crime is a felony offense punishable with more than one (1) year in jail.

▶ MANDATORY REPORTING

All states have laws that require mandatory reporting by healthcare professionals of acts of abuse, injury, or violence that they observe. Refer to Display 8-3 for an example of mandatory reporting (New Jersey State Board of Nursing mandatory reporting guidelines). In recent years the scope of this requirement has broadened from reporting suspected child abuse to include protection of the elderly and disabled. Criminal penalties can be imposed if those events are not reported to the proper authorities, because the law recognizes the need to protect the public. When such a report is made based on a reasonable cause and in good faith, most states provide civil immunity to the reporter for possible repercussion. It is critically important that you document objective information and personal, objective observations, especially in abuse cases. Most states require that health and education professionals complete a course in identifying abuse and the specifics of the reporting requirements.

Some states require professionals to report co-workers who appeared to be under the influence of drugs or alcohol. Teachers are under a similar mandate. Mandatory reporting is required of case managers specifically. The CCMC Code of Professional Conduct (the Code) requires that certified case managers (CCM) possessing knowledge that another CCM has committed a violation of the Code must promptly report that knowledge to CCMC (CCMC Code of Professional Conduct for Case Manager, G-26) and are required to assist with the enforcement of the Code (CCMC Code, G-27) (CCMC, 2005).

▶ Domestic Violence

Violence in America is not limited to street crime. All too often domestic violence affects the workplace, the classroom, and the sanctity of the home. Case managers, as health professionals, must be ever vigilant and sensitive to their patient's/client's symptoms and injuries, and listen to what they are saying, recognizing that it is difficult for victims of domestic violence to speak out and ask for help. Domestic violence as a topic has been incorporated in many nursing curricula. In the past decade, domestic abuse has been identified as a health problem of epidemic proportion by such organizations as the Institute of Medicine, American Medical Association, American Nurses Association, and the American Association of Colleges of Nursing (AACN). The AACN position statement calls on nurses to "be aware of assessment methods and nursing interventions that will interrupt and prevent the cycle of violence (AACN, 1999). Case managers should be encouraged to participate in continuing education programs that focus on domestic violence identification and prevention.

Case managers may find themselves dealing with a completely unrelated illness, injury, or topic with their client when the trust that is established between clients and case managers invites a victim to reach out. Learn and maintain a list of area resources so that appropriate referrals can be made in a timely basis. If the present opportunity is lost for a victim to reach out for help, it may be months or years before he or she feels safe enough to tell the story to someone else or to call the police. More information on how one can help victims of domestic violence is available on the National Coalition on Domestic Violence Web site, accessible at http://www.ncadv.org. A list of sources for information regarding domestic violence is available in Display 8-4.

▶ Child Abuse

Child abuse is an issue that can produce rage in the most nonjudgmental case manager. Child abuse has many variations and is not limited to any ethnic or socioeconomic group. Not only is reporting of suspected child abuse mandatory, but if a classic case is not reported and the child suffers further danger or even death, healthcare professionals involved in caring for the child can be charged criminally, as well as being found to be negligent. It is clear that case managers, nurses, social workers, teachers, and others charged with a duty of care must report acts of child abuse that they either witness or identify the symptoms thereof. In observing the behavior of children, there are signs that must be learned to help in identifying these problems. One classic sign is a child who wears clothing that is not seasonally appropriate. For example, why would a child wear a winter jacket or long-sleeve sweatshirt on a hot summer day?

Definitions of child abuse speak of nonaccidental injuries from mistreatment, sexual abuse, or exploitation such as child prostitution and deprivation of necessities. The perpetrator can be a parent, legal guardian, uncle or aunt, grandfather or grandmother, baby-sitter, boyfriend, or stranger. Many books and articles have been written on how to recognize child abuse. Some classic signs are certain types of bodily harm (especially with radiologic evidence of older, healing fractures); failure to attend to medical, physical, or hygiene problems; sexually transmitted diseases; apprehensiveness or secretiveness; bruising or bleeding near genitalia; overly compliant behavior; suicidal attempts or gestures; and failure to thrive (which can

NEW JERSEY BOARD OF NURSING MANDATORY REPORTING GUIDELINES

What should be reported?

LEVEL I—Always requires reporting to the Board of Nursing

▶ Conduct that clearly violates expected standards of care and may result in various degrees of harm

▶ Conduct that demonstrates a pattern of poor judgment or skill

Examples: suspected drug diversion, misappropriation, theft, physical/verbal abuse, sexual abuse or exploitation, falsification of documents, cover-ups, a single serious medication error, repeated medication errors or charting errors, signing out without a physician's order or failing to account for wastage of controlled medication, serious medication errors, arrests, indictments and convictions, intoxication on duty and patient neglect (such as failing to properly assess, treat, monitor, notify or intervene).

LEVEL II—Depending on an analysis of the facts, may require reporting to the Board of Nursing.

▶ There is no list of what should or should not be reported under this category. It is a matter of judgment for the person(s) making the report, based upon a review of all the relevant factors.

▶ Conduct that may be indicative of a more serious problem should be reported.

LEVEL III—Does not require reporting to the Board of Nursing.

▶ Low-level infractions that do not involve patient care, professional judgment or wrongdoing.

Examples: co-worker disputes, personality conflicts, absenteeism, tardiness, labor-management or employer-employee disputes, fee or wage disputes, unanticipated adverse outcomes independent of anyone's fault (such as equipment failures or allergic reactions) and minor policy infractions.

Who should report?

▶ All licensed nurses have an affirmative obligation to report suspected violations of the Nurse Practice Act and the Uniform Enforcement Act to the Board of Nursing.

▶ Generally, in the work setting (e.g., licensed health care facility or agency) the highest nursing officer should take responsibility for reporting to the Board (e.g., Director of Nursing/Vice President of Patient Care) However, it is also appropriate for the Director of Security, the Director of Human Resources or Risk Manager to file a complaint. If the facility or agency's administrators refuse or delay a report, it is appropriate for a staff nurse or nurse manager to take responsibility for reporting to the Board.

▶ The Board also receives complaints from consumers/patients, families of consumers/patients, the Ombudsman for the Institutionalized Elderly, the Department of Health and Senior Services and the Criminal Authorities.

How should a report be made?
INITIAL REPORTS TO THE BOARD OF NURSING SHOULD:

▶ Be in writing (except for emergent matters involving suspected drug diversion/misappropriation or sexual abuse complaints).

▶ Contain basic information about the "who, what, where, why and how" of the incident.

▶ Contain the name of a contact person and a telephone number and address where he/she can be reached during business hours.

ALL PERSONS MAKING A REPORT TO THE BOARD OF NURSING SHOULD BE PREPARED TO:

▶ Provide legible copies of all relevant records, materials and information as requested by the Board's representative.

▶ Speak with the Board's representative by telephone, in writing or in person, as requested.

▶ Assist the Board's representative in gaining access to all relevant information, witnesses or other persons, as requested.

▶ Follow through and agree to appear before the Board, if necessary.

For purposes of these guidelines, the Board's representative may include any one of the following individuals: The Board's executive director, paralegal, deputy attorneys general or Enforcement Bureau investigators.

Where should a report be made? All letters of complaint should be made

Board of Nursing

P.O. Box 45010

124 Halsey Street, Sixth Floor

Newark, New Jersey 07101

Tel. Number: (973) 504-6457

Emergent complaints of drug diversion or sexual abuse may be made by telephone to the Board of Nursing at (973) 504-6457, or to the Deputy Attorney General at (973) 648-7093 or the Enforcement Bureau of the Division of Consumer Affairs at (973) 504-6300.

FOR LINKS TO ALL BOARDS OF NURSING IN THE UNITED STATES GO TO:

http://www.medscape.com/viewarticle/482270

display 8-4

DOMESTIC VIOLENCE RESOURCE LIST

If you, or someone you know, are a victim of domestic violence, please call:

National Domestic Violence Hotline

1-800-799-SAFE (7233)

1-800-787-3224 (TTY)

If you, or someone you know, are a victim of sexual assault, please call:

▶ Rape, Abuse, and Incest National Network (RAINN) 1-800-656-HOPE (4673)
▶ National Sexual Violence Resource Center (NSVRC) 1-877-739-3895

▶ American Bar Association Commission of Domestic Violence http://www.abanet.org/domviol/home.html
▶ For a complete list of State Domestic Violence Coalitions http://www.ovw.usdoj.gov/statedomestic.htm
▶ Shelter Our Sisters (New Jersey) http://www.shelteroursisters.org/
▶ Pennsylvania Domestic Violence Resources http://www.dvresources.org/
▶ The National Criminal Justice Reference Service http://www.ncjrs.gov/

also be caused by medical problems; however, a medical cause must first be ruled out).

Verbal reports are acceptable initially to a law enforcement officer and state agency (these agencies go by various names, from state to state; for example, Child Protective Services). You should know your state's reporting requirements and keep the hotline number readily available. When you make a report, it is very important that you do not guess or give personal opinions. Report only the facts that you have seen or heard. Providing basic facts will give the agency investigator the necessary information to determine whether there has been an act of child abuse or merely an unfortunate accident or justifiable series of events. Kids get hurt, but it is not for us to assume or guess and make excuses for what we suspect. Our duty is to factually and properly report accurate information to the state mandated investigatory agency. When in doubt, let the police be your first point of contact. They, too, can make appropriate referrals.

▶ Adult/Elder Abuse

Elder abuse has many of the same characteristics as child abuse. It is also an event that brings with it mandatory reporting requirements. As with reporting child abuse, if done in good faith and with reasonable cause, the person reporting has state immunity against libel or slander claims in most states. Adult abuse can also take many forms, including physical abuse, neglect, exploitation of property or pets, unreasonable confinement, sexual assault, medical neglect, psychological abuse, or failure to thrive not caused by medical conditions. Most definitions include the stipulation that the adult is incapacitated or vulnerable and helpless to defend him or herself (Perin, 1992). Just as was discussed for child abuse, the case manager should contact the appropriate state agency to report the situation

and document completely what was discussed and to whom he or she spoke. Also include in your notes what steps were discussed; in other words, what will happen next.

Some states have an Adult and/or Senior Protective Services for reporting and investigation. These cases are investigated on a priority basis, taking emergency cases first. These agencies also have an arsenal of resources available to them and make referrals to public health and other services. The case manager can make such referrals; using public services can increase your client's ability to access resources, particularly when finances are at or near the poverty level.

Elder abuse in long-term care or subacute care has gotten much press. It can cost the facility its Medicare and Medicaid license; more importantly, it simply should not be part of the fabric of medical and case management practice. Many families, including those of case managers themselves, find their time and resources divided between multiple generations. With a large aging population and life expectancies greater than they have ever been in history, states have found it necessary to enact laws, rules, and regulations to protect seniors both in medical facilities and in their own homes. The federal Administration on Aging, under HHS, was created in response to these needs. Congress passed the Older Americans Act of 2006 (Display 8-5) with the intent to ensure equal opportunity for all Americans to have access to healthcare, community services, employment opportunity, etc. The term *caregiver* is broadly defined in subparagraph 18(A) of the Act as an "individual who has the responsibility for the care of an older individual, either voluntarily, by contract, by receipt of payment for care, or as a result of the operation of law and means a family member or other individual who provides (on behalf of such individual or of a public or private agency, organization, or institution)

display 8-5

▼ **OLDER AMERICANS ACT OF 2006**

Title I—Declaration of Objectives; Definitions

Declaration of Objectives for Older Americans

Section. 101.

The Congress hereby finds and declares that, in keeping with the traditional American concept of the inherent dignity of the individual in our democratic society, the older people of our Nation are entitled to, and it is the joint and several duty and responsibility of the governments of the United States, of the several States and their political subdivisions, and of Indian tribes to assist our older people to secure equal opportunity to the full and free enjoyment of the following objectives

1. An adequate income in retirement in accordance with the American standard of living.

2. The best possible physical and mental health which science can make available and without regard to economic status.

3. Obtaining and maintaining suitable housing, independently selected, designed and located with reference to special needs and available at costs which older citizens can afford.

4. Full restorative services for those who require institutional care, and a comprehensive array of community-based, long-term care services adequate to appropriately sustain older people in their communities and in their homes, including support to family members and other persons providing voluntary care to older individuals needing long-term care services.

5. Opportunity for employment with no discriminatory personnel practices because of age.

6. Retirement in health, honor, dignity—after years of contribution to the economy.

7. Participating in and contributing to meaningful activity within the widest range of civic, cultural, educational and training and recreational opportunities.

8. Efficient community services, including access to low cost transportation, which provide a choice in supported living arrangements and social assistance in a coordinated manner and which are readily available when needed, with emphasis on maintaining a continuum of care for vulnerable older individuals.

9. Immediate benefit from proven research knowledge, which can sustain and improve health and happiness.

10. Freedom, independence, and the free exercise of individual initiative in planning and managing their own lives, full participation in the planning and operation of community based services and programs provided for their benefit, and protection against abuse, neglect, and exploitation.

(42 U.S.C. 3001)

---

compensated or uncompensated care to an older individual"(Sec. 102[18][B]). It is incumbent on the case manager to be familiar with the Act, which can be found in its entirety at http://www.aoa.gov/oaa2006/Main_Site/index.aspx. In fact, the term *fiduciary*, discussed previously in this chapter, is specifically defined by the Act:

A. means a person or entity with the legal responsibility –
   i. to make decisions on behalf of and for the benefit of another person; and
   ii. to act in good faith and with fairness; and
B. includes a trustee, a guardian, a conservator, an executor, an agent under a financial power of attorney or health care power of attorney, or a representative payee.

Therefore, when dealing with this population, this definition is the minimum mandatory national standard and state laws cannot limit these duties. State laws can, however, provide additional protections to older Americans and often do.

With the advent of HIPAA, many of the protections found in the Omnibus Budget Reconciliation Act (OBRA) of 1987, such as the right to privacy, to receive notice before a room or roommate change, to voice grievances, to meet with other residents, and to participate in the planning of care or treatment, as well as freedom from physical or mental abuse, involuntary seclusion, or the use of physical or chemical restraints for the purposes of (staff) convenience or punishment, are not encompassed in these two very extensive pieces of legislation. Like child abuse, elder abuse cannot be tolerated in any level of care. All medical professionals have an affirmative duty to report elder abuse. Failure to report elder abuse can lead to the same criminal consequences as if the negligent reporter was the actor.

▶ DO NOT RESUSCITATE—NO "CODE BLUE"

In most states a physician's written order is required in addition to an Advanced Directive for Healthcare or

Living Will for a Do Not Resuscitate Order. In 1998, Ohio adopted a Do Not Resuscitate (DNR) law. Ohio's DNR law gives individuals the opportunity to exercise their right to limit care received in emergency situations in special circumstances. "Special circumstances" include care received from emergency personnel when 911 is dialed. The law authorizes a physician to write an order letting health care personnel know that a patient does not wish to be resuscitated in the event of a cardiac arrest (no palpable pulse) or respiratory arrest (no spontaneous respirations or the presence of labored breathing at end of life). (For more information, refer to Probate Court, Franklin County, Ohio, 1998.)

The intent of such laws is to provide assurances that patient rights will be respected, even when a 911 call is made. If a patient is competent, the right to choose or refuse resuscitation measures belongs solely to that person. Incapacitated patients need a prior signed advance directive or a Surrogate Decision Maker. DNR orders must be written prior to their need. In other words, in the event of an emergency situation or "code" where there is the cessation of breathing, heartbeat, or both, a physician cannot telephonically give a No Code or DNR order. The order must predate the need, even if it is within a matter of seconds. Without the existence of a DNR order, a full code must commence and continue until successful or a physician determines that death is irreversible.

Historically, "slow codes" and "partial codes" have loomed as legal and ethical quagmires. These codes are illegal in some states and carry liability because of their vagueness. Hospital policy consistent with state law clears up the uncertainty. Rather than fear a conversation regarding end-of-life issues, a case manager can provide an individual and family members with a well-trained and sympathetic ear. A well-drawn Health Care Directive will reference DNR and express the individual's wishes, providing the healthcare representative/proxy and the physician with guidance for end-of-life choices. Caution should be used with menu-like directives, as individuals don't have the medical training and knowledge to distinguish between life-saving cardiopulmonary resuscitation (CPR) and life-sustaining interventions, such as intubation and use of a respirator.

Families often are confused about what DNR means, feeling that their loved one will not get necessary treatment. It must be clearly explained that DNR is not the same as do not treat, that the patient will not be abandoned, and that everything will be done for the patient up to the point where life saving is no longer possible.

If that is not complex enough, living wills stating no extraordinary measures are contested in some states. In Georgia, for example, the physician must obtain the patient's permission or other authority to write a DNR order; in the absence of that, the physician must get another physician's concurrence or use the hospital ethics committee as a second vote. Patient's wishes in a living will are not enough. In Georgia, the living will statute only applies to three clinical conditions: if the patient is terminally ill, in a vegetative state, or in an irreversible coma. Alternatively, other states allow unilateral decisions by physicians that do not require any other consent for a DNR order (Banja, 1998). In 2000, New Jersey established additional administrative rules (with full force and effect of law) to protect persons with dementia, including Alzheimer disease, who live in rooming and boarding houses. Even if there is a DNR order, the law requires, "Even if a resident has a 'Do Not Resuscitate' (DNR) order, staff must call 911 for appropriate assistance in the event of an emergency, so that appropriate medical staff can assist the resident and act, if appropriate" (N.J. Stat.§ 5:27-13.1[f]). In addition, home health agencies or subacute care facilities must include in their medical record of any individual, particularly when there is a transfer in or out of one subacute facility to another, "a notice of the existence of an advance directive and/or Do Not Resuscitate (DNR) order" (N.J. Admin. Code § 8:42-11.2[d][7]). The bottom line is that the case manager must know the patient's wishes, communicate those wishes to the next provider of care or setting, and follow state law and facility policies.

▶ DEATH, ANATOMICAL GIFTS, AUTOPSY

Most states define death as an irreversible cessation of cardiopulmonary functions or an irreversible cessation of brain function. This is essentially an irreversible loss of consciousness and function (Feutz-Harter, 1991). An example of this would be the persistent vegetative state, in which there is seemingly no awareness of anyone or anything. These patients live at a primitive reflex level and often have eye-blink reflexes and react to noxious smells, sound, pain, or light. Although their prognosis is poor, diagnosis as a form of death strains the definition.

In most institutions, the physician must "pronounce" the patient and fill out the paperwork. As stated in the section on coroner's cases, under certain conditions such as home hospice care, nurses may pronounce the patient and fill out paperwork. Often the case manager is tending to family or attempting to contact family. If the family is en route to the hospital after their loved one has died, every effort should be made to meet them before they reach the room.

A thorough review and documentation is warranted in situations when deaths (1) occur during or after elective surgery, (2) occur after returning to an intensive care unit (ICU) or within 24 hours of being transferred out of an ICU, or (3) occur unexpectedly. Documentation should include, but not be limited to, complete patient assessments, prompt responses to any changes in patient's condition (laboratory test results, vital signs, cardiac rhythms, breathing patterns, pain, bleeding, and drug reactions), timely physician notification, equipment malfunctions, and interventions. If the staff believes that an equipment malfunction played a significant role in the demise of the patient, the case manager may want to strongly suggest that the hospital hold on to the piece of equipment, whether it is a ventilator or a pacemaker. The hospital would like to prove that it was equipment failure and not user failure; the manufacturer would like to prove that it was not equipment failure.

▶ Organ and Tissue Donation

Anatomical gifts can be voluntarily donated by anyone 18 years or older. Driver's licenses and durable medical POA for healthcare documents are two ways to check a person's wishes about organ donation. If there are no indications that the person had any objections, the following can approve donations, in order of legal priority: (1) spouse (or parent if younger than 18 years), (2) adult child, (3) either legal parent, (4) adult siblings, (5) legal guardian, and (6) the person responsible for burial (Perin, 1992).

With the modernization of technology and medicine, organ and tissue donation and transplantation can mean amazing life-saving or life-improving results. Organ procurement organizations (OPO) are the state designated and authorized agencies for donation. Some OPOs cover vast regions and others are limited to the boundaries of a single state. In 2009 the number of people waiting for transplants will reach and perhaps exceed 100,000 (UNOS, 2009). When the case manager is given an opportunity to answer questions, or if it is part of your job to initiate the discussion, it is important to have up-to-date information on organ procurement and transplantation from a reliable source. Myths and misconceptions contribute to the length of the waiting list (see Display 8-6). This is obviously a very sensitive job, and case managers may, at one time or another, be left with the task, amid enormous grief.

Transplant Speakers International, Inc., a nonprofit charitable organization, is dedicated entirely to the advancement of education regarding organ and tissue donation. Through its free user-friendly interactive e-learning program (http://www.transplant-speakers.org),

you can learn about organ and tissue donation, dos and don'ts for speaking with families, how to address potential religious and ethnic objections, and much more, in a nonthreatening environment from the privacy of your desk at home or at work. Transplant Speakers is unique in its blended learning approach. It provides live teams, composed of both organ recipients and donor family members, at little or no cost.

▶ Autopsies

Autopsies (postmortem examinations) are usually required in coroner's cases. In other cases, they may not be mandatory. Similar to organ donation, the following can give authorization for autopsy: (1) spouse (or parent if the patient is a minor), (2) adult child, (3) legal guardian, and (4) next of kin. If none of these is found, the person responsible for the burial can give consent (Perin, 1992).

Coroner's cases must be autopsied. Other reasons for autopsies may be for informational purposes or because the results of the autopsy may be required in the future (i.e., for lawsuits). Autopsies should be considered in the following situations:

▶ When deaths resulted from high-risk infections or contagious diseases.
▶ When the cause of death was not absolutely known, and an autopsy could help to explain the circumstances and ease concerns of the family or the public.
▶ Unexpected or unexplained deaths; may have occurred spontaneously or during/after a diagnostic procedure or therapy.
▶ Obstetrical, neonatal, or pediatric deaths.
▶ When the autopsy could reveal a suspected illness that might affect survivors.
▶ If organ donation is a possibility.
▶ When the death was suspected of being the result of environmental or occupational hazards.
▶ When the deceased participated in experimental or approved clinical trials.
▶ When the patient is dead on arrival at the emergency department, the death occurred within 24 hours of admission, or if the patient sustained an injury during the hospitalization.

A case manager may be asked about who pays for autopsies. Many hospitals perform autopsies as a courtesy to the medical staff. Hospitals often perform autopsies at no charge even when the patient had left the hospital previously and subsequently died. There

display 8-6

DONATE LIFE AMERICA

There is a severe organ shortage in this country. Despite continuing efforts at public education, misconceptions and inaccuracies about donation persist. It's a tragedy if even one person decides against donation because they don't know the truth. Following is a list of the most common myths along with the actual facts:

Myth: If emergency room doctors know you're an organ donor, they won't work as hard to save you.

Fact: If you are sick or injured and admitted to the hospital, the number one priority is to save your life. Organ donation can only be considered after brain death has been declared by a physician. Many states have adopted legislation allowing individuals to legally designate their wish to be a donor should brain death occur, although in many states Organ Procurement Organizations also require consent from the donor's family.

Myth: When you're waiting for a transplant, your financial or celebrity status is as important as your medical status.

Fact: When you are on the transplant waiting list for a donor organ, what really counts is the severity of your illness, time spent waiting, blood type, and other important medical information.

Myth: Having "organ donor" noted on your driver's license or carrying a donor card is all you have to do to become a donor.

Fact: While a signed donor card and a driver's license with an "organ donor" designation are legal documents, organ and tissue donation is usually discussed with family members prior to the donation. To ensure that your family understands your wishes, it is important that you tell your family about your decision to donate LIFE.

Myth: Only hearts, livers, and kidneys can be transplanted.

Fact: Needed organs include the heart, kidneys, pancreas, lungs, liver, and intestines. Tissue that can be donated include the eyes, skin, bone, heart valves and tendons.

Myth: Your history of medical illness means your organs or tissues are unfit for donation.

Fact: At the time of death, the appropriate medical professionals will review your medical and social histories to determine whether or not you can be a donor. With recent advances in transplantation, many more people than ever before can be donors. It's best to tell your family your wishes and sign up to be an organ and tissue donor on your driver's license or an official donor document.

Myth: You are too old to be a donor.

Fact: People of all ages and medical histories should consider themselves potential donors. Your medical condition at the time of death will determine what organs and tissue can be donated.

Myth: If you agree to donate your organs, your family will be charged for the costs.

Fact: There is no cost to the donor's family or estate for organ and tissue donation. Funeral costs remain the responsibility of the family.

Myth: Organ donation disfigures the body and changes the way it looks in a casket.

Fact: Donated organs are removed surgically, in a routine operation similar to gallbladder or appendix removal. Donation does not change the appearance of the body for the funeral service.

Myth: Your religion prohibits organ donation.

Fact: All major organized religions approve of organ and tissue donation and consider it an act of charity.

Myth: There is real danger of being heavily drugged, then waking to find you have had one kidney (or both) removed for a black market transplant.

Fact: This tale has been widely circulated over the Internet. There is absolutely no evidence of such activity ever occurring in the U.S. While the tale may sound credible, it has no basis in the reality of organ transplantation. Many people who hear the myth probably dismiss it, but it is possible that some believe it and decide against organ donation out of needless fear.

Information obtained from http://www.unos.org/news/myths.asp (accessed 4/27/2008)

is usually a time limit in this case; 6 months is an average.

Most facilities have an authorization for autopsies form that must be signed. However, this was not always the case, and the issue of autopsies is very personal to some people. I will never forget the grief one woman suffered when she discovered that her husband was mistakenly autopsied against his wishes. If this is within your realm of job responsibilities, make sure to document to whom you spoke and the decision made concerning postmortem examination.

▶ TECHNIQUES TO MINIMIZE LIABILITY

There is no guaranteed method of totally eliminating legal risk in today's litigious environment. Anyone can file a lawsuit; the question of proof is entirely different. There are some fundamental, common sense case management tenets that will certainly minimize the chances. Remember, trial lawyers will analyze each word of your job description to determine whether you performed all required and expected aspects of your job or if you overextended your role by stepping into the realm of another professional, such as the physician. In addition, participate in the creation, maintenance, and updates of the policies and procedures in your unique work environment. Failure to follow one's own protocols may be worse than having no protocols and policies at all.

▶ COMMONSENSE SAFEGUARDS

1. Learn where to find state and federal laws; www.findlaw.com and http://www.law.cornell.edu/states/listing.html both provide a good launch point for all states.

2. Know and incorporate the standards of case management practice into your activities, as well as the standards of the certifying agency of the credential you possess (e.g., CCMC for the CCM- www.ccmcertification.org), or the credentialing/accreditation agencies of your program such as URAC (http://www.urac.org) or The Joint Commission (http://www.jointcommission.org), where applicable.

3. Look at the Protected Health Information Authorization form. Don't assume you know what it says. Once you've confirmed whether the patient has limited disclosure, which is his or her right, keep your patient and family informed consistent with their wishes.

4. Do not make decisions for others that they should make for themselves.

5. Offer all known options, whether in or out of network. Private pay is always an option.

6. Remember the three "C's." Communicate, Communicate, Communicate. Communicate your role clearly to the patient/client and family. Advise them truthfully, from your first contact, what will happen to information they share with you.

7. Remember the three "D's." Document, Document, Document! Documentation demonstrates compliance with the standard of care and offers evidence.

8. Do not practice medicine. Do not give the impression that the case manager is the medical authority. Refer medical decisions to physicians or those authorized to prescribe and work in a cooperative manner with physicians to facilitate case management goals. REMEMBER, the obligation to obtain informed consent remains with the physician and cannot be delegated in most states.

9. Understand how risk managers and legal consultants can assist you and use this resource.

10. Know your job description. Make sure your job description accurately describes your role and establishes boundaries of duties; recommend and make changes as your job develops over time.

11. Operate within the scope of your professional license, practice act, and code of professional conduct/ethics standards.

12. Don't just say, "No!" If you must be the bearer of bad news (i.e., a service is not covered), remember you are only the messenger and should not make financial and contractual decisions as a case manager. Inform the patient and family of the right to appeal and help them through the process if appropriate. This is one aspect of the patient advocacy role in action.

13. Use proper consent forms before releasing information to avoid breach of patient confidentiality or HIPAA violation (http://www.cms.hhs.gov/hipaageninfo).

14. Purchase your own professional liability insurance, even if your employer tells you that you are covered under its policy. Its policy is just that and if your employer can find a reason to carve you out of its coverage, it may. This is a low-cost way to avoid high-priced headaches.

15. Establish, review, and/or revise all policies and procedures, protocols, marketing materials, contracts, consent forms, and case management manuals on a regular basis. REMEMBER,
   a. HIPAA requires at least annual documented policy review/update.
   b. HIPAA requires at least annual in-service regarding policies and procedures.
   c. The days of dusty policy and procedure books on the shelf are over.
   d. Policies and procedures become part of the employment contract, so make sure they are up-to-date and relate to the manner in which you are currently practicing.

16. Apply utilization review and quality assurance criteria consistently, objectively, and in a nondiscriminatory manner.

17. Avoid contradictory and inconsistent inclusions in the medical records and case management notes.

18. Listen and be responsive to your patient/client. An angry patient/client is a potential plaintiff. It has been reported that the number one reason people bring malpractice lawsuits is because they feel neglected and abandoned.

STUDY QUESTIONS

1. Describe a risk management case you are aware of whether from published literature or your own experience. What are the circumstances that made the case a risk management one? Evaluate if the situation meets negligence criteria. Why?

2. Describe a utilization management case that resulted in denial of treatment. Was the denial based on negligent or inappropriate utilization review? What could you do in this case to prevent a negligent utilization review?

3. Share a situation where you were involved in a medical record review where documentation was incomplete or subjective. What could you do to remedy the situation?

4. What can a case manager do to safeguard a patient's privacy and confidentiality? How can a case manager handle a situation where a patient does not want the family to know his or her diagnosis and the family is asking for the diagnosis and the prognosis?

5. You were preparing a patient's discharge and suddenly you got a call from the payor-based case manager denying the transfer of the patient to a subacute care facility. How would you handle the situation?

6. You arrived at work one morning and found during report that one of the patients you were case managing had been intubated despite the fact that it was clear in the patient's living will or advance directives that the patient did not desire such intervention. What would you do? How would you go about disclosing the situation to the patient's healthcare proxy? What are the legal implications of such an act?

7. While you were discussing the surgical procedure with the patient and family, you found out that the patient had signed the consent without a clear understanding of the procedure, the risks and benefits, or the postsurgical care. What would you do? You informed the surgeon of the situation and the surgeon dismissed it, claiming that he explained everything to the patient already. How would you handle such a response?

▶ REFERENCES

American Association of Colleges of Nursing. (1999). *Position statement: Violence as a public health problem.* Washington, DC: Author.

Andrews, M., Goldberg, K., & Kaplan, H. (Eds.). (1996). *Nurse's legal handbook* (3rd ed.). Springhouse, PA: Springhouse Corp.

Banja, J. (1998). Advance directives and the do-not-resuscitate order. *The Case Manager, 9*(2), 30–33.

Bosek, M.S.D., & Fitzpatrick, J. (1992). A nursing perspective on advance directives. *MEDSURG Nursing, 1*(1), 33–38.

Case Management Society of America (CMSA). (2002). *Standards of practice for case management.* Little Rock, AR: CMSA.

Commission for Case Manager Certification (CCMC). (2005). Code of Professional Conduct for Case Manager with Disciplinary Rules, Procedures and Penalties. Available on-line: http://www.ccmcertification.org/.

Employee Retirement Income Security Act (ERISA) Available on-line: http://www.dol.gov/compliance/laws/comp-erisa.htm where e-tools, compliance information and a wealth of related links and information are available.

Feutz-Harter, S.A. (1991). *Nursing and the law.* Eau Claire, WI: Professional Education Systems Inc.

Franklin County Probate Court, State of Ohio. (1998). (accessed 5/2/2009). Living Will Declaration, 1998. [Online]. Available: http://www.franklincountyohio.gov/probate/PDF/Living_Will_Only.pdf.

Gammage & Burham. (1997). *Legal Issues Surrounding Managed Care and Case Management.* Phoenix, AZ: Gammage & Burham.

Joint Commission on Accreditation of Healthcare Organizations. (1985). *Accreditation manual for hospitals* (pp. 98–99). Oakbrook, IL: Author.

Keeton, W., Dobbs, D., Keeton, R., & Owne, D. (1984). *Prosser and Keeton on torts. Student handbook* (5th ed.). St. Paul, MN: West Publishing Co.

Mellette, P., & Kurtz, J. (May 1993). Corcoran v. United Healthcare, Inc., Liability of utilization review companies in light of ERISA. *Journal of Health & Hospitals Law, 26*(5), 129–132, 160.

Ovando, L., & Thies, L. (1997). Emerging liability risks. *Case Review, 3*(3), 68–73.

Perin, R.L. (1992). *Arizona statutes affecting nursing practice.* Eau Claire, WI: Professional Education Systems Inc.

Powell, S., & Tahan, H. (2008). *CMSA's core curriculum for case management* (2nd ed.). Philadelphia: Lippincott Williams & Wilkins.

Prosser & Keaton on Torts, §§ 1- 4, 5th ed. 1984

Robbins, D. (1998). *Integrating manage care and ethics.* New York: McGraw-Hill.

Sturgeon, S. (1997). Legal risks in the operation of referral and utilization review systems. *Managed Care Interface, 10*(12), 66–70.

Transplant Speakers International, Inc. www.transplant-speakers.org 4.20-27.2008 UNOS

United Network for Organ Sharing (UNOS). (2008). (accessed 4/27/2008). *Donate Life America.* [Online]. Available: http://www.unos.org/news/myths.asp.

United Network for Organ Sharing (UNOS). (accessed 5/1/209). Waiting list conditions. [Online]. Available: http://www.unos.org.

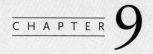

CHAPTER 9

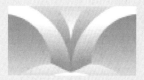

Ethical Issues in Case Management

"The pessimist complains about the wind; The optimist
expects it to change; The realist adjusts the sails."

WILLIAM ARTHUR WARD

LEARNING OBJECTIVES

Upon completion of this chapter, the reader will be able to:

1. Describe the process of ethical decision making.
2. Recognize ethical dilemmas in case management practice.
3. List four ethical principles important to case management practice.
4. Differentiate between clinical and organizational ethics.
5. Identify five strategies for the effective management of ethical dilemmas.

ESSENTIAL TERMS

Advance Directives • Assisted Suicide • Clinical Ethics • Code of Ethics • *Code of Professional Conduct for Case Managers* • Ethical Dilemma • Ethics • Ethics Committee • Gag Orders • Gatekeeper • Guide for the Uncertain in Decision-Making Ethics (GUIDE) • Medical Necessity • Organizational Ethics • Patient Advocate • Patient Self-Determination Act of 1990 • Rationing of Healthcare • *Standards of Professional Performance* • Unnecessary Treatment • Withdrawing Treatment • Withholding Treatment

Like a fork in the road, managed care intersects with the scarcity of resources, over 40 million uninsured Americans, and 76 million well-informed baby boomers who are on the verge of turning 65 years of age. This is certainly fodder for complexity and ethical dilemmas. Ethical issues shift as society, technology, and professional practice patterns change. Step back in time to 1950. Few of the prominent ethical issues of today were discussed then: abortion, euthanasia (assisted suicide), genetic experimentation, or rationing of healthcare. At the time, genetic research was not advanced far enough to cause major concern, and healthcare was basic enough—with little high-tech equipment—to be affordable. Healthcare decisions were made almost exclusively by physicians. For example, the 1950 American Nurses Association (ANA) code of ethics stated that a nurse's obligation was to carry out the physician's orders and to protect the physician's reputation (Wright, 1987). This code left

little motivation for a nurse to assess an ethical dilemma concerning a physician's poor treatment choices or practice patterns, if it were to come up. Case managers today cannot run away from dealing with these issues—in fact, addressing ethical issues is part of the case manager's job description and responsibilities. Professional life appeared more clear-cut than it does now, but not necessarily more ethical.

A relationship between law and ethics clearly exists; however, the relationship is often nebulous. We know there is a relationship, although sometimes it is difficult to say whether an issue is mostly legal or mostly ethical. One thing experienced case managers have found out is that the bridge between the two issues is patient advocacy. This is a key to remember when ethical dilemmas arise. Delivering care (including making decisions about what treatments should be implemented) that is patient-family-centered is the best way to avoid or prevent ethical concerns.

Ethics in healthcare is about choices, morals, and the basic rights of free choice, self-determination, and autonomy. Ethical dilemmas arise in situations where the ethically correct course of action is unclear, such as when one is not certain about which ethical principle to apply or when multiple ethical principles are in conflict. Ethical dilemmas are challenging; one must select a course of action while in most cases there is more than one choice available. Often each choice holds a potential for an undesirable outcome. Case managers are frequently confronted with ethical dilemmas during the course of a day's work. Each ethical dilemma can present a new twist. Like the turn of a kaleidoscope, each case necessitates a new perspective on the issue. The perspective we see is also influenced by our values, beliefs, and morals, both personal and professional; these are what shape our choices, helping to resolve conflict and come to a point of resolution.

Each case manager has a portfolio of ethical issues and dilemmas. Some are generic, others are similar, and still others are situation specific. A case manager who works in the neonatal intensive care unit (NICU) grapples with issues that are different from those of a pediatric case manager, an oncology case manager, or a rehabilitation case manager. Following are some classic examples.

▶ A family member will not consent to do not resuscitate (DNR) status for a patient. The patient has multisystem failure, and a Code Blue is imminent. The code occurs, the patient survives, and the rest of the story is a "nightmare." This scenario has been played out in thousands of hospitals.

▶ A patient, mentally competent to make decisions, insists on being discharged home—to a clearly unsafe situation. He has the right to self-determination and you know well that the home environment will jeopardize his health condition.

▶ A patient reveals her dread of being discharged because she will return to serious abuse perpetrated by her husband on their young daughter. She has told you to keep this secret. What about confidentiality? What about the legal aspect? Isn't child abuse a reportable event? Can you put aside the judgment about a mother failing to protect her child? A choice—to tell or not to tell—must be made in this case.

▶ A husband makes it clear that he does not want to be placed on a respirator. His medical condition destabilizes and he becomes unconscious, but his wife insists on intubation.

▶ A patient with a medical condition incompatible with pregnancy refuses to have an abortion. Her condition deteriorates daily. In the seventh month, the baby dies in utero. Two days later, the mother dies.

▶ A 75-year-old man had cardiac bypass surgery in 1983 that necessitated several blood transfusions. He is admitted with a perplexing diagnosis. Tests show that he is positive for the HIV virus and has full-blown AIDS. He wants to know what is wrong, but his wife insists that no one tell him the diagnosis.

Some ethical dilemmas end up in the courtroom and often are the theme on which future laws are made. Even court decisions may leave more ethical challenges than the original case appeared to have. They may resolve some aspects but do not always solve all the aspects or the original dilemma. Consider the case of Nancy Cruzan, whose parents were aware of her wishes about not wanting to remain in a persistent vegetative state. Still, they waited several years, from 1983 to 1990, for her to regain even basic awareness of the world. When the parents finally asked the courts to allow withdrawal of artificial food and hydration, the court ruled that there was no clear and convincing evidence of Nancy's desires (Kolodner, 1992). Nancy *telling* her family and friends that she would never want to be a "vegetable" was not enough.

Other cases never make it to the courtroom but have overtones that are more ominous. In Chicago, when a father's pleas to have his brain-dead child removed from the ventilator were met with hospital insistence that he obtain a court order, he held the medical staff at gunpoint and discontinued the ventilator himself (Fiesta, 1992).

These two heartbreaking cases did not go by unnoticed and without consequence. The impact of Nancy Cruzan's case resulted in the Patient Self-Determination Act of 1990 (Kolodner, 1992). Every patient in every hospital in America is affected by this. Had Nancy written her own advance directive, no court would have questioned her wishes. The impact in the second case is more subtle, but the message is clear. Should we hold human beings on the threshold of death just because we have the technology to do so? Fewer hospitals are now resisting removal from life support if the family agrees to it when a patient is declared brain dead.

As case managers, we play important roles in helping the patient understand what advance directives are all about and his or her choices concerning them. We are often privy to verbal statements about "no heroic measures," but without written, signed documents, the patient's wishes may go unfulfilled. Advance directives are about a patient making his or her own life choices. Explaining these important documents and helping to explore feelings about these life-directing decisions and life (or death) goals may be important advocacy roles. Remember that advance directives, including health-care proxy, are of great help in situations like this. Documenting the individual's wishes when he or she is alert and competent is important in preventing situations similar to Nancy's and her family's.

▶ WITHHOLDING AND WITHDRAWING CARE

Both of the preceding cases brought up the dilemma of withdrawing some treatment that the patient was receiving: food and hydration in one case and respiratory support in the other. Withholding and withdrawing some aspect of care is a recurrent theme in many ethical dilemmas and is the reason for much debate, both ethically and legally.

The public values on withdrawing or withholding treatment have changed throughout the years. From 1976 to 1991, when conflicts over these issues landed in court, almost every family wanted the treatment stopped or not started. Then, partially due to mistrust of the intentions of managed care (and the large amount of negative press about underutilization of services), conflicts arose that turned the attention to fighting for healthcare and demanding "everything be done" for the patient. John Banja tells of a case not uncommon during that period. An elderly woman with a long history of chronic obstructive pulmonary disease (COPD) was admitted to the hospital in critical condition. In the next 2 days, she also suffered two myocardial infarctions and a major stroke; the stroke left her with a silent electroencephalogram. When the family was approached by the pulmonologist, who protested the family's wishes that she be ventilated and kept in the intensive care unit (ICU), the son pointed a finger at the physician saying, "If Momma dies, you die" (Banja, 1996, p. 37).

In 1983, the President's Commission for the Study of Ethical Problems in Medicine and Biomedical and Behavioral Research discussed the withdrawing and withholding of treatment as follows:

> The distinction between failing to initiate and stopping therapy—that is, withholding versus withdrawing treatment—is not itself of moral importance. A justification that is adequate for not commencing a treatment is also sufficient for ceasing it (President's Commission, 1983).

The last sentence, written in 1983, has caught on. However, these are ethical recommendations—not legal precedents—and they lead to further questions. Is withdrawing or withholding life-saving treatment a form of assisted suicide? Is there a difference between actively causing death (withdrawing) and allowing it to occur by not intervening (withholding)? Asking tough questions can lead to a resolution that lies somewhere between right and wrong yet is neither—it is merely a best choice, hopefully made in good faith.

As in the Nancy Cruzan case, withholding or withdrawing nutrition and hydration is still being debated, and legal and medical people often have differing viewpoints. Case managers play a pivotal role in helping patients and their families clarify and articulate their views in these difficult cases. Many medical conditions lend themselves to an inability to feed a patient orally. Often the placement of a permanent feeding tube is a very difficult decision for a family to make, even if the patient is alert.

One case involved an 84-year-old nursing home resident who came in with pneumonia (probably aspiration pneumonia) and complaints that he was hungry. He was alert but very confused and managed to pull out every line the physicians and nurses could get into him. Because he had a recent history of several bouts of pneumonia, a modified barium swallow was performed to evaluate his swallowing ability. The results showed a high probability for aspiration if fed orally, so the recommendation was for placement of a permanent feeding tube.

The patient's daughter was distressed by this option. Unquestionably caring, she did not want to prolong her father's life "in this state." The case manager discussed with her the fact that although her father was frail, he was not showing signs of impending death. He had no end-stage organ diseases, and his vital signs were stable. In addition, he was telling the facility staff that he was hungry. After much deliberation the daughter agreed to the feeding tube. What if this patient had been imminently dying? Would not feeding him be ethically appropriate? What about hydration with intravenous (IV) fluids? Is this a form of withholding life support?

Leah Curtin stresses the distinction between withdrawal of life support and withdrawal of nutritional support: "It is one thing to decide not to resuscitate a terminally ill patient, it is quite another to starve a person to death whether or not he has some hope for survival" (Curtin, 1994, p. 14). To lump the question of withdrawal of nutritional support under the same classification as the withdrawal of medical life support measures confuses the issue (Curtin, 1994). The aforementioned patient died suddenly and unpredictably soon after the insertion of the feeding tube, but the decision was sound for this set of circumstances.

Suppose death is imminent. Whether to initiate feeding depends on the patient's medical and mental condition as well the cultural values, beliefs, interests, and social support system. Simple hydration may be appropriate in some cases. A more alert patient should be able to choose. Consider that:

> In the face of inevitable death from some other source, nutrition is used to provide comfort—not to sustain life. Any means of feeding that produces more discomfort than comfort can be eliminated from an ethical perspective. In some cases, the patient can tell us clearly what he wants. In other cases, we must rely on our own assessment and judgments. In all cases, the goal is comfort not adequate nutrition (Curtin, 1994, p. 15).

▶ ETHICS COMMITTEES

The kaleidoscope turns. Look at another case about nutritional dilemmas, similar to the last case but with a different perspective, which required the assistance of an ethics committee.

Mrs. Norris is a 79-year-old patient most recently hospitalized for pneumonia (probable aspiration pneumonia). Her medical history includes a cholecystectomy, hysterectomy, several surgeries for metastatic intestinal cancer (including resections for small bowel obstructions), multiple strokes, congestive heart failure, end-stage cardiomyopathy, and most recently, frequent bouts of pneumonia. Mrs. Norris was alert and oriented until 1 year ago. At that time she filled out an advance directives form stating her wishes not to be kept alive through artificial measures; this specified and included intubation and mechanical ventilation, food, and hydration as artificial measures that she did not want if her condition became irreversible and her quality of life was poor. After signing her wishes, a series of strokes occurred. Mrs. Norris is now cognitively poorly responsive. She opens her eyes and has reflexes, but does not respond meaningfully. Her present bout of pneumonia is clearing up. Swallowing studies confirmed that Mrs. Norris has severe esophageal reflux and is a firm candidate for further aspiration pneumonia if fed orally. Nasal feeding tubes have been unsuccessful because they have been coughed up or repeatedly pulled out. Due to multiple intestinal resections and complicated by severe esophageal reflux, a permanent feeding tube could be a rather tricky procedure requiring general anesthesia. The medical team is leaning toward comfort care measures only. Mrs. Norris is an extremely poor surgical risk, but attempts at feeding her without an intestinal feeding tube could lead to further aspiration pneumonia, which could also cause her demise.

Mrs. Norris's daughter Marion is furious with the doctors' suggestions of comfort care and states, "If you let my mother starve to death, I'll sue you!" No other family member voiced an opinion.

▶ Case Discussion

This case leaves several options open for the medical team:

- ▶ Opt for comfort care only on the guidance of the family's own judgment and Mrs. Norris' advance directives.
- ▶ Call for a family (case) conference.
- ▶ Attempt a feeding tube.
- ▶ Ask for judicial intervention.
- ▶ Ask the institution's ethics committee for assistance.

For the purpose of illustration, let us say that the last option was chosen, that is, calling the ethics committee for assistance. Almost all institutions today have organized ethics committees to guide them and their healthcare professionals (including case managers) through the quandary of ethical decision making and problem resolution. The core membership of these committees may include physicians, nurses, administrators, clergy/pastoral care, an attorney, an ethicist, and a patient advocate. Today, case managers and social workers are common active participants—in fact, they often coordinate an ethics committee meeting when one is needed. At times these committees appear to have some kind of magical ethical compass.

First, the ethics committee needs the medical facts, including a medical history, the present status of the patient, the plan of care (case plan), and a realistic prognosis. All possible treatment options and alternatives are then explored, including the possible outcomes for each modality. Brainstorming for unthought-of treatment alternatives may occur in the hopes that another answer may relieve the ethical dilemma. A psychosocial assessment is also pertinent. Often conflicting morals and values of family members are a main cause of ethical problems. In the case of Mrs. Norris, the patient's directions were challenged by the daughter, and the physician's attempts at explanations did not seem to clarify the medical problems and concerns. Mrs. Norris was not in a condition that would allow her to speak for herself.

When dealing with ethical dilemmas, it is important to distill any legal issues. In Mrs. Norris' case, the advance directives form was an important document to consider. Nevertheless, judicial resolution has its consequences: it is expensive; it is time-consuming, which can disrupt patient care; it can cause a strained relationship between the medical team and the surrogate decision makers; and it can turn a private matter into a media circus. Treading carefully is wise when dealing with sensitive and ethical issues.

Next, the ethics committee may apply various ethical decision-making "tools." The following are six examples case managers must become familiar with and use when needed.

1. Use of various schools and theories of ethical thought, which may help bring the case to a point of resolution. (Although this chapter will not analyze the various theories, several excellent books have been written on the subject. Additional resources are available on the Internet.)
2. Some feel it is important to use humor to gain or maintain a sense of perspective. Care must be taken not to "make fun" of the situation at the expense of anyone, especially the patient/family. However, a moment of shared laughter did occur when one of Marion's sisters quipped, "That Marion, even as a child she had trouble following Mom's directions!"
3. Consider contemporary thought on a particular issue. Expert opinions on the subject of withholding or withdrawing artificial food and hydration are as follows:
   ▶ *Unconscious, imminently dying patient (progressive and rapid deterioration).* The dying process will (most likely) not be reversed, and therefore nutrition and hydration are an unreasonable burden.
   ▶ *Conscious, imminently dying patient.* The patient is conscious and can make the decision, but artificial nutrition and hydration may be an unreasonable burden.
   ▶ *Conscious, irreversibly ill, not imminently dying patient.* Again, the patient can ultimately decide because he or she is conscious. The disease process may not be reversible or curable, but nutrition and hydration to sustain life are useful. As long as the patient wants it and does not feel it is an unreasonable burden, then it has use.

   ▶ *Unconscious, nondying patient.* Nutrition and hydration should be supplied to this patient. In this case, if no provisions were made to feed and hydrate the patient, the physician could be a party to starving the patient to death. Unless there are other indications to the contrary, nutrition and hydration are not an unreasonable burden and are justifiable.
4. Use effective communication skills. The art of listening and well-placed questioning punctuated with a caring attitude can often defuse difficult situations.
5. Use honesty. It has been said that, "Ethics is honesty in action." This basic human value is especially important in the final stage—deciding on recommendations. These recommendations will be born out of all the tools, personal values and morals, and judgments of the committee.
6. Balance the various opinions and perspectives associated with the ethical situation being dealt with. Know your own values. Know the patient's/family's values. Know your organization's policies and any laws that apply to the situation. Balance the three.

▶ Patient, Clinical, or Organizational Ethical Dilemmas

Case managers increasingly face ethical issues that are either clinical in nature, encompassing the medical and treatment needs of patients (e.g., dealing with end-of-life concerns such as in the case of Mrs. Morris); financial (e.g., concerns of the uninsured who also requires an expensive treatment, or denials of services by insurance companies); conflict between the patient and family regarding desired course of action; or conflict between patient/family and the healthcare team about the best treatment option. When faced with any of these issues, it is best for case managers to understand the facts and views of the various parties involved; gather all necessary and relevant information; identify the key dilemma(s); and seek the advice of supervisors and/or the ethicist in the organization regarding the course of action. It is customary today for healthcare organizations to have a designated individual ethics expert or an ethics committee the case manager can defer to for assistance in resolving an ethical dilemma.

Often times, case managers are dealing with ethical dilemmas that involve a challenge of balancing the needs and interests of patients and their families and those imposed by the healthcare organization and the insurance company (i.e., the payor). When case managers communicate to patients and/or their families decisions of insurance companies denying certain services and treatments (for example, an extended length of hospital stay, surgical procedure does not require inpatient stay, postdischarge services such as home care, or transfer to an acute rehabilitation facility), case managers are perceived by the patients and/or families to be taking the side of the organization or the payor. As a result, case managers may be perceived as being more concerned with cost than quality of care and therefore no longer are viewed as patient advocates. Issues of distrust and lack of confidence arise and complicate the situation. Such issues have led to a new type of ethical dilemma that was absent when managed care organizations were unpopular or uncommon. Ethical issues today are no longer limited to those that are clinical or medical in nature; therefore healthcare organizations have implemented the use of organizational ethics committees in addition to the traditional clinical ethics committees.

Case managers must be aware of the difference between a clinical and an organizational ethical issue. They also should know when to seek advice from a clinical ethics committee and when it is necessary to involve the organizational ethics committee. To clarify the difference, generally speaking, one may describe the main focus of clinical ethics committees as dealing with decisions regarding treatment options or the patient's right to withdrawing treatment such as in the case of terminal/end-of-life care. Organizational ethics committees, however, focus on utilization management issues, including resource allocation, delays in care (or system variance management), and appropriateness of the level of care. Other organizational ethics issues may deal with things that are not specific to an individual patient care situation such as false advertisement of outcomes of a certain treatment modality, public disclosure of errors, and business practices concerning vendors of pharmaceuticals and medical device companies.

One main difference between clinical and organizational ethics committees relates to type of experts needed as members. Clinical ethics committees include members who are experts in clinical care issues. Organizational ethics committees include members who are experts in utilization management, codes of professional conduct, and corporate compliance.

ETHICAL DECISION MAKING

Making ethical decisions, even on a day-to-day basis, requires a complex set of skills. Sometimes it helps to break down the various factors in each issue, thus lending more clarity to the situation. Clarify the following:

▶ The options or courses of action that are available in the situation.
▶ The options or courses of action that seem to be unavailable in the situation.
▶ The consequences, both good and bad, that can occur with the possible options.
▶ The rules, regulations, laws, protocols, standards, and values that will direct the choice.
▶ Who should make the choice?
▶ Exactly what is the desired outcome (Andrews et al. 1996)?
▶ Who can assist in resolving the situation or offer advice?

The communication skills required in evaluating and assisting the resolution of ethical problems is perhaps the most important talent a case manager can bring to the table. Some communication considerations include (Andrews et al. 1996):

▶ Follow the appropriate code of professional ethics specific to your profession. In addition, adhere to the code of professional conduct for case managers.
▶ Act within your bounds during the ethical process.
▶ Seek expert counsel and advice from other wise professionals; this is too important to "go it alone." An ethics expert can be very helpful.
▶ Validate information. Do not base ethical decisions on rumors, innuendoes, hearsay, or first impressions.
▶ If religious faith and spiritual values are important to any of the key people, consider suggesting prayer in the decision-making process.
▶ Avoid judgment or subjectivity and remain patient-/family-centered.

The case manager can also use aspects of the case management process to further examine the situation: assessment and problem identification, planning, implementation, and evaluation (Andrews et al. 1996).

1. Assessment and Problem Identification
   ▶ Gather all the facts, opinions, and perceptions about the situation.

▶ Identify key players and their roles, responsibilities, and decision-making abilities.

▶ Identify available resources: ethics committees, chaplain, rabbi, policies, laws, patient advocates, etc.

▶ Identify the problem(s), conflict(s), disagreement(s), or issue(s) to be addressed.

▶ Be a patient advocate. Assist the decision makers in a clarification of their own values and what constitutes quality of life, priorities, freedom, and dignity.

2. Planning

▶ Identify types of moral dilemmas that are involved, such as autonomy, self-determination, impartiality, justice, confidentiality, or veracity.

▶ Identify possible courses of action, along with their potential risks and benefits.

▶ List goals and objectives of the people involved in the situation; then assign priorities to the list.

▶ Determine the ethical obligations of those involved.

3. Implementation

▶ Develop an ethical goal that maximizes the most benefits and good in the situation. Do this collaboratively with the key people and ethics experts.

▶ Determine the course of action that will produce results most like the ethical ideal.

▶ Determine if that course of action violates legal or ethical principles. If it does, change or modify the actions.

▶ Implement the plan.

4. Evaluation

▶ Do the results bring the situation closer to the ethical ideal?

▶ Do the outcomes satisfy the parties involved, especially the patient and family?

▶ If not, have any new moral dilemmas been created?

▶ If necessary, go back to the assessment phase, revise your plan and attempt again to resolve additional moral dilemmas.

Resolving ethical dilemmas requires a shared decision-making approach. This is even more so because the context of the case manager's role is an interdependent one and case management outcomes are best realized in a team-based approach to case planning and management. The traditional approach of individualistic ethical decision making therefore no longer achieves the best possible outcomes. As stated earlier, with increased availability of managed care health plans, the ethical dilemmas case managers commonly encounter in their practice are of an "organizational ethics" nature. Those are best resolved applying a deliberative framework that focuses on two main components (Jansen, 2003):

1. Shared decision making is necessary to arrive at decisions that satisfy all parties directly or indirectly involved in the ethical dilemma being addressed (patient/family, provider, organization, and payor). It emphasizes that all affected parties are given the opportunity to express their views and interests and ultimately participate in making the final decision. Participants must also view each other as equal deliberative partners and avoid thinking in hierarchical terms or use the influence of their positions in the organization. For example, case managers should not always defer to the administrators for the ultimate say about the situation; they should be active and equal contributors to the discussion and decision.

2. The nature and purpose of the deliberation which, as a rule of thumb, should always be the need to reach ethically responsible decisions or solutions that are, and are seen to be, legitimate by the parties involved. This means that participants in the deliberative process should keep open minds, believe it possible that they will learn something new during deliberation, and anticipate that they may change their minds about the issue at hand.

▶ GUIDE FOR THE UNCERTAIN IN DECISION-MAKING ETHICS

Our present ability to sustain life or prolong dying almost indefinitely is the basis for many painful ethical situations. Medical personnel know that a fairly healthy heart plus a ventilator—maybe with the addition of hemodialysis treatments—can keep a human body alive for a long time; even if the brain is fatally damaged. Fewer and fewer people are seeing the glory in this scenario, and Americans are changing their ideas about dying. In quick succession, Jacqueline Onassis and Richard Nixon both said "no" to futile care that merely postponed the inevitable. Several articles about technology, death, and dying followed. A landmark study found that most dying patients or their families now decide against resuscitation efforts (Knox, 1994). Even with more public awareness and new attitudes, medical professionals—especially physicians and case managers—are often asked to referee disagreements between the patient/family and the healthcare team. This is a difficult task. Some believe the Guide for the Uncertain in Decision-Making Ethics (GUIDE) (Display 9-1) to be concrete help, especially when an ethics committee is not readily available.

The GUIDE, along with its companion algorithm, takes into consideration advance directives, proxy decision makers, and healthcare teams' preferences in their recommendations (Levenson & Pettrey, 1994). These guidelines contain nine scenarios, each defining key issues and conflicts between the patient/family and medical team. The recommendations use logically sequenced questions about the patient's competency, advance directives, treatment options, benefits and burdens of the treatment options, patient and family preferences, and patient prognosis. The case manager should be cautioned that this GUIDE and algorithm are not intended to take the place of legal or risk management advisement, nor that of an ethics committee or an ethicist. However, it is consistent with applicable law and good risk management. It should also be noted that it was written in Virginia with its legislation in mind. Similar laws and guidelines are available in other states. Case managers should be knowledgeable of such laws in their own state of practice. As stated in Chapter 8, case managers should also know the statutory regulations pertinent to healthcare in their state, not just those with ethical implications. Finally, the GUIDE is essentially for adult patients and perhaps for legally emancipated adolescents.

▶ ETHICAL PUBLIC OPINION: POLLS AND STUDIES

Ethical questions about life-sustaining treatments and about healthcare reform in the 1990s have been in the news almost daily. In the spring of 1992, St. Joseph's Hospital and Medical Center in Phoenix, Arizona, conducted a nationwide Delphi study on ethics and healthcare. Both consumers and experts were polled, with some interesting results:

▶ Both consumers and experts felt it was appropriate for people who engage in unhealthy lifestyles to pay more for healthcare.
▶ On administering or withholding medical treatment:
   1. Both groups felt it was appropriate to base the decisions on the chance for survival.
   2. Both groups were not as eager to base decisions on patient age, cost of treatment,

or a patient's expected contribution to society.
▶ 53% of the consumers placed individual rights over societal rights; 53% of the experts placed higher priority on the good of society as a whole.

The following statistics are taken from "expert" polls. These experts include ethicists, hospital administrators, doctors, and insurance administrators.

▶ 76% felt rationing of healthcare to the poor is not ethical.
▶ 74% felt that healthcare should not be treated as a commodity.
▶ 72% agreed that setting a monetary capitation ceiling is ethical.
▶ 55% were concerned that in healthcare reform individuals are not encouraged to take personal responsibility for their health.
▶ 34% felt concerned that healthcare reform would lead to more rationing based on sets of criteria.

As an adjunct to opinion polls, research studies have been done in an attempt to clarify how much America would save in healthcare dollars if policies were written disallowing futile care (other than comfort care) to terminally ill people. In a landmark $28 million study (is it ethically correct to spend $28 million for this information?), the following was discovered (Knox, 1994):

▶ Only $1 out of every $8 spent for medical care could be saved by a strict policy that ruled out life-prolonging care. The study found that this is because most dying patients or their families decide in advance against being coded. Most of that $1 savings comes from withholding care from relatively young, critically ill patients. (Consider the major diagnoses for this category of patient.)
▶ Only 14% of the 2,150 critically ill patients who died during the study had an attempted resuscitation. Therefore, it was estimated that reducing aggressive life-sustaining treatment would save "at most" 3.3% of the total U.S. healthcare expenditures. (Note that 3.3% of the more than $900 billion spent in 1993 was more than $30 billion.)
▶ Past projects to identify guidelines for withholding or withdrawing treatment based on objective criteria have not been very accurate. Newer prognostic criteria with very narrow criteria margins—in this case less than 1%

GUIDE FOR THE UNCERTAIN IN DECISION-MAKING ETHICS

Scenario	Guidelines
1. Healthcare team favors treatment, patient/family opposed to treatment	• Review options carefully to ensure that patient has complete understanding of prognosis and treatment options; a competent adult patient has right to refuse medical treatment if patient has adequate understanding of information. • If patient has executed an advance directive, it should be reviewed. In Virginia (and in almost all states today) the Health Care Decisions Act provides an optional formal advance directive procedure, which can be written or oral, that applies when the patient's death is imminent or the patient is in a persistent vegetative state. • Discussions and patient's decision(s), should be completely documented in chart.

2. Healthcare team favors treatment/patient not competent, family opposed	• Need to identify primary decision maker among involved family/significant others.*
	• Review information carefully to ensure that family/significant others have full understanding of patient's prognosis, condition, and options and can make an informed decision. This should include any advance directives made by the patient.
	• If other family member disagrees with primary decision maker, see Scenario 5.
	• May consult ethics committee.
	  * Surrogate Decision Maker: Virginia law (similar laws are available in other states) recognizes the authority of a Surrogate Decision Maker to make treatment decisions for an individual who is incompetent or incapable of making an informed decision. If patient previously made an advance directive appointing someone as "agent to make healthcare decisions" for him/her, that individual is empowered as the proxy (equivalent to durable power of attorney for healthcare). In the absence of any advance directive, Virginia law establishes the following order of priority for proxies:
	  1. A legal guardian, if one already had been appointed
	  2. The spouse
	  3. An adult son or daughter
	  4. A parent
	  5. An adult brother or sister
	  6. Any other relative in descending order of blood relationship

3. Patient and family in disagreement concerning treatment decisions	• An adult patient has the right to refuse or consent to any intervention if he or she has adequate understanding of all information and is competent to make an informed decision. • Family should be included in all discussions but final decision about resuscitation and other interventions is made by the competent adult patient. • Patient should consider an advance directive. • Provision for family support may be needed.
4. Healthcare team does not favor treatment/patient (or family if incompetent patient) does favor treatment.	• Healthcare team is not required to undertake interventions that cannot help. Engage in further conversation with patient/family; ensure that they have received adequate information about futility of treatment. Reinforce that intervention(s) in question is not being offered because no benefit (either cure or comfort) exists. • Encourage/arrange second opinion. • Give patient/family option to transfer patient's care to another physician/hospital. • May consult hospital ethics committee.
5. Patient is incompetent/ family in disagreement concerning treatment	• Attempt to identify primary decision-maker (see Scenario 2 for statutory priority). Under Virginia law, if two or more persons of same priority level (e.g., adult children of patient) disagree, the physician may rely on authorization of a majority. • However, every effort should be made to bring family to agreement. Attempt to have family/significant others focus on what the patient's wishes would be. Ask questions such as: "What would the patient tell us himself if he could speak?" and "Has he ever discussed what he would want if this happened?" Any advance directive made by the patient should be reviewed with the family. • May consult ethics committee.

(continued)

GUIDE FOR THE UNCERTAIN IN DECISION-MAKING ETHICS *(Continued)*

6. Healthcare team in disagreement concerning treatment (i.e., physician vs. nurse, attending physician vs. medical director)	• Attempt to reconcile through discussion and justification of viewpoint. • Seek guidance from chief of service, nurse manager, or other appropriate administrative pathway. • If patient favors treatment, seek second opinion about appropriateness of treatment. If treatment is judged to be futile (offering no benefit), see Scenario 4.
7. Healthcare team and family favor treatment/incompetent patient not objecting	• See Scenario 2 for guidance. Should identify primary decision maker, but parties essentially in agreement in this scenario.
8. Healthcare team and family favor treatment/incompetent patient objecting to treatment	• Under Virginia law, if an incompetent patient actively refuses treatment, a surrogate decision-maker cannot be used without judicial review. This may take the form of seeking the appointment of a legal guardian, or a judicial order allowing involuntary medical treatment. • Contact hospital superintendent, legal advisor, and/or ethics committee.
9. Not clear if (a) patient is competent, and/or (b) patient is in favor of or opposed to treatment.	• Reassessment of patient's capacity for decision making and/or of patient's preferences by primary physician. If possible, the source of the patient's ambivalence should be identified. • Psychiatric consultation if competence still unclear or if patient continues to express contradictory preferences. • If still unresolved, consult ethics committee.

Reprinted with permission of *American Journal of Critical Care*, March 1994, 3[2].

chance of survival for 60 days—were more accurate. In this study, 75% of patients died in 5 days, 98% died within 1 month, and 1 patient survived 10 months with a good quality of life.

The study concluded that the prognostic criteria would be acceptable to most people and "would sacrifice very few patients who might have lived" (Knox, 1994, p. A26).

In a 1996 study about evidenced-based guidelines for withdrawing life support, the results of 865 bone marrow transplant patients were examined. The goal of the study was to identify "evidenced-based" factors that could predict when further life support would be absolutely futile, due to almost certainty of death. The study results demonstrated that if patients had a combination of symptoms—lung deterioration coupled with either a specific level of hemodynamic instability or hepatic failure—the likelihood of survival was extremely low. Of the 398 of the 865 patients who were this ill, there were no survivors, and of 467 patients who developed 2 complications, only 1 survived (Robbins, 1998).

This study attempted to demonstrate, on a day-by-day basis, when it is reasonable to withdraw life support. There is nothing inherently wrong with this study; if it was reliable and valid, the study holds some interesting considerations. In fact, this and other outcomes studies may help paint a picture of what is actually "futile" versus what healthcare workers feel might be futile intuitively. It is how this information will be used that will tell the ethical tale. If families use the percentages to prevent further suffering to their loved ones, it poses different dilemmas than if utilization management uses these statistics for their purposes.

▶ CODES OF ETHICS

Codes of ethics are established to protect the public interest by guiding professionals about what constitutes ethical conduct and how one can ensure acceptable behavior. Case managers may be held accountable by one (or more) of several codes of ethics depending on the professional background of the case manager (e.g., nursing, socialwork). Nurse case managers (NCM) must adhere to the *American Nurses Association's Code of Ethics* and the *Standards of Professional Performance*. Vocational rehabilitation case managers who also hold a Certified Rehabilitation Counselor (CRC) credential are accountable to the *Commission on Rehabilitation Counselor Certification's Code of Professional Ethics*. Social work case managers must adhere to the *National Association of Social Workers Code of Ethics*. Every certified case manager (CCM) must also comply with the *Code of Professional Conduct for Case Managers* as adopted by the Commission for Case Manager Certification (CCMC). The *Statement of Ethical Case Management Practice* is the umbrella statement under which all case managers fall.

▶ Statement of Ethical Case Management Practice

Although not all case managers have the comfort of an ethics committee to call on when needed, more institutions are forming these important links to quality healthcare. All case managers have their pet list of ethical doubts and difficulties. The names and faces change, as do some of the medical and psychosocial details, but often the dilemmas have common roots. Realizing the need for ethical support for case managers, the Case Management Society of America (CMSA) formed an ethical task force and created the *Statement of Ethical Case Management Practice*. This document provides a basis for identifying ethical decision making while maintaining quality of care for patients. Case managers should obtain, read, understand, and apply this document. The document is available at CMSA's Web site at http://www.cmsa.org.

▶ American Nurses Association's Code of Ethics/Standards of Professional Performance

Nurses are held liable to perform nursing duties responsibly, legally, and ethically. In addition to adhering to the *Statement of Ethical Case Management Practice,* NCMs must adhere to both the *American Nurses Association Code of Ethics for Nurses with Interpretive Statements* and the *Standards of Professional Performance. The Standards of Professional Performance* state that the nurse is guided by the Code of Ethics for Nurses; maintains client confidentiality; acts as a client advocate; delivers care in a nonjudgmental, nondiscriminatory manner that is sensitive to cultural diversity; delivers care in a manner that preserves and protects client autonomy, dignity, and rights; and seeks available resources to help formulate ethical decisions. The *American Nurses Association Code of Ethics* is one of the oldest codes developed for healthcare professionals and has undergone several revisions since it was established; it was most recently revised in 2008.

▶ The American Nurses Association Code of Ethics

The code is accessible at the ANA Web site (http://www. nursingworld.org/MainMenuCategories/ThePracticeof ProfessionalNursing/EthicsStandards.aspx).

1. The nurse in all professional relationships, practices with compassion and respect for the inherent dignity, worth, and uniqueness of every individual, unrestricted by considerations of social or economic status, personal attributes, or the nature of health problems.
2. The nurse's primary commitment is to the patient, whether an individual, family, group, or community.
3. The nurse promotes, advocates for, and strives to protect the health, safety, and rights of the patient.
4. The nurse is responsible and accountable for individual nursing practice and determines the appropriate delegation of tasks consistent with the nurse's obligation to provide optimum patient care.
5. The nurse owes the same duties to self as to others, including the responsibility to preserve integrity and safety, to maintain competence, and to continue personal and professional growth.
6. The nurse participates in establishing, maintaining, and improving healthcare environments and conditions of employment conducive to the provision of quality healthcare and consistent with values of the profession through individual and collective action.
7. The nurse participates in the advancement of the profession through contributions to practice, education, administration, and knowledge development.
8. The nurse collaborates with other health professionals and the public in promoting community, national, and international efforts to meet health needs.
9. The profession of nursing, as represented by associations and their members, is responsible for articulating nursing values, for maintaining the integrity of the profession and its practice, and for shaping social policy.

▶ Code of Professional Conduct for Case Managers

All CCMs must adhere to the *Code of Professional Conduct for Case Managers* and the professional code of ethics for their specific profession (such as nursing, social work, etc.). One of the underlying principles in the *Scope of Practice for Case Managers,* developed by CCMC, is that case managers are guided by the principles of autonomy, beneficence, nonmaleficence, justice, and veracity (CCMC, 2008). These definitions are not everyday language, so here they are further explained based on CCMC's *Code of Professional Conduct for Case Managers*:

▶ Autonomy is a form of personal liberty whereby the individual possesses sufficient mental capacity to determine his or her course of action in accordance with a plan chosen and developed by him- or herself.

▶ Beneficence is the obligation or duty to promote good, to further another's legitimate interests, and to actively prevent harm or diminish its impact as much as possible.

▶ Nonmaleficence is refraining from harming others, or if harm is inevitable, insuring that as little harm occurs as possible.

▶ Justice is achieving a fair distribution of benefits and burdens.

▶ Veracity is simply being honest and truthful.

The *Code of Professional Conduct for Case Managers* was first published in 1996 and has gone through multiple revisions, most recently in 2005. In addition to the ethical principles published in the Code, CCMC requires case managers to adhere to six other standards of professional conduct (CCMC, 2008). These are:

1. Advocacy, which focuses on the role of the case manager as a client advocate, explaining to the client their options for necessary treatments, and facilitating access to needed services.

2. Professional responsibility, especially in the areas of representation of practice, competence, representation of qualifications, legal and benefit systems requirements, use of CCM designation, conflict of interest, reporting of misconduct, and compliance with proceedings.

3. Case manager/client relationship, which emphasizes description of services to clients, relationships with clients, termination of services, and objectivity.

4. Confidentiality, privacy, and record keeping, which describe the role of the case manager in legal compliance, disclosure, client identity, records (including maintenance, storage and disposal), electronic recordings, and reports.

5. Professional relationships, which addresses testimony, dual relationships, unprofessional behaviors, fees, advertising, and solicitation.

6. Research, which focuses on legal compliance and subject privacy.

CCMC takes ethical complaints against case managers very seriously, and the review process is extensive. For copies of the *Scope of Practice for Case Managers,* the *Code of Professional Conduct for Case Managers,* or information about case management certification,

refer to CCMC's Web site (http://www.ccmcertification.org). Although CCMC's *Code of Professional Conduct* is written specifically for case managers who are certified by the Commission (i.e., hold the CCM credential), over time, application of the *Code* has expanded to those who are not certified as well. When a legal or ethical issue is being addressed, authorities (including legal, ethical, employers, and others) have used the *Code* as a standard against which they examined the issue. As a result, case managers are better off adhering to the *Code*, regardless of certification status. Therefore, they should be familiar with the *Code* and abide by it in their practice at all times.

▶ Consumer Bill of Rights and Responsibilities/Patient Bill of Rights

In November 1997, the Presidential Advisory Commission on Consumer Protection and Quality in the Health Care Industry released its *Consumer Bill of Rights and Responsibilities* in healthcare; because this is not in the form of law, it has been included in the chapter on ethics. This bill is an effort to give back to patients some empowerment in their healthcare. Many states have similar clauses, and the Centers for Medicare & Medicaid Services (CMS) have had a Patient Bill of Rights for Medicare beneficiaries for many years. Various levels of care have *Patient Bills of Rights:* hospitals, hospices, skilled nursing facilities (SNFs), and long-term care facilities. Bills of rights issued by healthcare institutions are not legally binding unless there are state laws to back them up; however, federal funding for those who are regulated by the CMS or accreditation of those accredited by The Joint Commission (TJC) may be jeopardized if the bills of rights are not enforced.

When reading the bill of rights (and patient responsibilities), keep in mind that these are the types of issues case managers have always dealt with. The stated goals of the *Consumer Bill of Rights and Responsibilities* include:

▶ To strengthen consumer confidence by ensuring the healthcare system is fair and responsive to consumers' needs, provides consumers with credible and effective mechanisms to address their concerns, and encourages consumers to take an active role in improving and ensuring their health.

▶ To reaffirm the importance of a strong relationship between patients and their healthcare professionals.

▶ To reaffirm the critical role consumers play in safeguarding their own health by establishing both rights and responsibilities for all participants in improving health status.

The *Consumer Bill of Rights and Responsibilities* includes eight areas (President's Advisory Commission on Consumer Protection and Quality in the Health Care Industry, available at http://www.hcqualitycommission.gov/final/append_a.html):

1. Information Disclosure
   Consumers have the right to receive accurate, easily understood information to make informed healthcare decisions about their health plans, professionals, and facilities. Such information includes:
   ▶ Health plan information. Covered benefits, cost-sharing, and procedures for resolving complaints; licensure, certification, and accreditation status; comparable measures of quality and consumer satisfaction; provider network composition; the procedures that govern access to specialists and emergency services; and care management information.
   ▶ Health professional information. Education, board certification, and recertification; years of practice; experience performing certain procedures; and comparable measures of quality and consumer satisfaction.
   ▶ Healthcare facility information. Experience in performing certain procedures and services; accreditation status; comparable measures of quality and worker and consumer satisfaction; and procedures for resolving complaints.
   ▶ Information about consumer assistance programs. Programs must be carefully structured to promote consumer confidence and to work cooperatively with health plans, providers, payors, and regulators. Sponsorship that ensures accountability to the interests of consumers and stable, adequate funding are desirable characteristics of such programs.
2. Choice of Providers and Plans
   Consumers have the right to a choice of healthcare providers that is sufficient to ensure access to appropriate high-quality healthcare. To ensure such choice, the Commission recommends the following:
   ▶ Provider network adequacy. All health plan networks should provide access to sufficient numbers and types of providers to ensure that all covered services will be accessible without unreasonable delay. This includes access to emergency services 24 hours a day, 7 days a week. If a health plan has an insufficient number or type of providers to provide a covered benefit with the appropriate degree of specialization, the plan should ensure that the consumer obtains the benefit outside the network at no greater cost than if the benefit were obtained from participating providers.
   ▶ Women's health services. Women should be able to choose a qualified provider offered by a plan (such as gynecologists, certified nurse midwives, and other qualified healthcare providers) for the provision of covered care necessary to provide routine and preventive women's healthcare services.
   ▶ Access to specialists. Consumers with complex or serious medical conditions who require frequent specialty care should have direct access to a qualified specialist of their choice within a plan's network of providers. Authorizations, when required, should be for an adequate number of direct access visits under an approved treatment plan.
   ▶ Transitional care. Consumers who are undergoing a course of treatment for a chronic or disabling condition (or who are in the second or third trimester of a pregnancy) at the time they involuntarily change health plans, or at a time when a provider is terminated by a plan for other than just cause, should be able to continue seeing their current specialty providers for up to 90 days (or through completion of postpartum care) to allow for transition of care.
   ▶ Choice of health plans. Public and private group purchasers should, wherever feasible, offer consumers a choice of high-quality health insurance plans.
3. Access to Emergency Services
   Consumers have the right to access emergency healthcare services when and where the need arises. Health plans should provide payment when a consumer presents to an emergency department with acute symptoms of sufficient severity—including severe pain—such that a "prudent layperson" could reasonably expect the absence of medical attention to result in placing that consumer's health in serious jeopardy, serious impairment to bodily functions, or serious dysfunction of any bodily organ or part.

4. Participation in Treatment Decisions
Consumers have the right and responsibility to participate fully in all decisions related to their healthcare. Consumers who are unable to participate fully in treatment decisions have the right to be represented by parents, guardians, family members, or other conservators.

Physicians and other health professionals should:

▶ Provide patients with sufficient information and opportunity to decide among treatment options consistent with the informed consent process.

▶ Discuss all treatment options with a patient in a culturally competent manner, including the option of no treatment at all.

▶ Ensure that persons with disabilities have effective communications with members of the health system in making such decisions.

▶ Discuss all current treatments a consumer may be undergoing.

▶ Discuss all risks, benefits, and consequences to treatment or nontreatment.

▶ Give patients the opportunity to refuse treatment and to express preferences about future treatment decisions.

▶ Discuss the use of advance directives, both living wills and durable powers of attorney for healthcare, with patients and their designated family members.

▶ Abide by the decisions made by their patients and/or their designated representatives consistent with the informed consent process. Health plans, providers, and facilities should:

▶ Disclose to consumers factors—such as methods of compensation, ownership of or interest in healthcare facilities, or matters of conscience—that could influence advice or treatment decisions.

▶ Ensure that provider contracts do not contain any so-called "gag clauses" or other contractual mechanisms that restrict healthcare providers' ability to communicate with and advise patients about medically necessary treatment options.

▶ Be prohibited from penalizing or seeking retribution against healthcare professionals or other health workers for advocating on behalf of their patients.

5. Respect and Nondiscrimination
Consumers have the right to considerate, respectful care from all members of the healthcare industry at all times and under all circumstances. An environment of mutual respect is essential to maintain a quality healthcare system. To ensure that right, the Commission recommends the following:

▶ Consumers must not be discriminated against in the delivery of healthcare services consistent with the benefits covered in their policy, or as required by law, based on race, ethnicity, national origin, religion, sex, age, mental or physical disability, sexual orientation, genetic information, or source of payment.

▶ Consumers eligible for coverage under the terms and conditions of a health plan or program, or as required by law, must not be discriminated against in marketing and enrollment practices based on race, ethnicity, national origin, religion, sex, age, mental or physical disability, sexual orientation, genetic information, or source of payment.

6. Confidentiality of Health Information
Consumers have the right to communicate with healthcare providers in confidence and to have the confidentiality of their individually identifiable healthcare information protected. Consumers also have the right to review and copy their own medical records and request amendments to their records.

7. Complaints and Appeals
Consumers have the right to a fair and efficient process for resolving differences with their health plans, healthcare providers, and the institutions that serve them, including a rigorous system of internal review and an independent system of external review.

8. Consumer Responsibilities
In a healthcare system that protects consumers' rights, it is reasonable to expect and encourage consumers to assume reasonable responsibilities. Greater individual involvement by consumers in their care increases the likelihood of achieving the best outcomes and helps support a quality improvement, cost-conscious environment. Such responsibilities include:

▶ Take responsibility for maximizing healthy habits, such as exercising, not smoking, and eating a healthy diet.

▶ Work collaboratively with healthcare providers in developing and carrying out treatment plans.

▶ Disclose relevant information and clearly communicate wants and needs.

▶ Use the health plan's internal complaint and appeal processes to address concerns that may arise.

▶ Avoid knowingly spreading disease.

▶ Recognize the reality of risks and limits of the science of medical care and the human fallibility of the healthcare professional.

▶ Be aware of a healthcare provider's obligation to be reasonably efficient and equitable in providing care to other patients and the community.

▶ Become knowledgeable about their health plan coverage and health plan options (when available) including all covered benefits, limitations, and exclusions; rules regarding use of network providers; coverage and referral rules; appropriate processes to secure additional information; and the process to appeal coverage decisions.

▶ Show respect for other patients and health workers.

▶ Make a good-faith effort to meet financial obligations.

▶ Abide by administrative and operational procedures of health plans, healthcare providers, and government health benefit programs.

▶ Report wrongdoing and fraud to appropriate resources or legal authorities.

▶ National Association of Social Workers' Code of Ethics

According to NASW, social workers promote social justice and social change with and on behalf of *clients*

NOTE

Free copies of the *Consumer Bill of Rights and Responsibilities* are available from:

White House Web site (http://www.whitehouse.gov) or the Commission's Web site (http://www.hcqualitycommission.gov). Copies can also be obtained from
Consumer Bill of Rights
P.O. Box 2429
Columbia, MD 21045-1429
Telephone: (800) 732-8200

(a term generically used to refer to individuals, families, groups, organizations, and communities). The association also believes that professional ethics is the core of social work. The *NASW Code of Ethics* offers a set of values, principles, and standards to guide decision making and everyday professional conduct of social workers. The *Code* was approved by the NASW Delegate Assembly in 1996 and last revised in 1999. It is currently used by most social work licensing boards. The *Code* sets forth the values, principles, and standards that guide social workers' conduct. It serves six purposes (NASW, 2008):

1. To identify core values on which social work's mission is based.

2. To summarize broad ethical principles that reflect the profession's core values and establish a set of specific ethical standards that should be used to guide social work practice.

3. To help social workers identify relevant considerations when professional obligations conflict or ethical uncertainties arise.

4. To provide ethical standards to which the general public can hold the social work profession accountable.

5. To socialize social workers who are new to the field to social work's mission, values, ethical principles, and ethical standards.

6. To articulate standards that the social work profession itself can use to assess whether social workers have engaged in unethical conduct.

NASW emphasizes the following six ethical principles. Case managers who are social workers must be familiar with and adhere to the principles at all times to ensure ethical practice. For more information on *NASW's Code of Ethics*, refer to the association's Web site (http://www.socialworkers.org).

1. Service. Social workers' primary goal is to help people in need and to address social problems. They elevate service to others above self-interest.

2. Social Justice. Social workers challenge social injustice and pursue social change, particularly with and on behalf of vulnerable and oppressed individuals and groups of people.

3. Dignity and Worth of the Person. Social workers respect the inherent dignity and worth of the person and treat each person in a caring and respectful fashion, mindful of individual differences and cultural and ethnic diversity. Social workers promote clients' socially responsible self-determination. Social workers

seek to enhance clients' capacity and opportunity to change and to address their own needs.

4. Importance of Human Relationships. Social workers recognize the central importance of human relationships and understand that relationships between and among people are an important vehicle for change. Social workers engage people as partners in the helping process. Social workers seek to strengthen relationships among people in a purposeful effort to promote, restore, maintain, and enhance the well-being of individuals, families, social groups, organizations, and communities.

5. Integrity. Social workers behave in a trustworthy manner and are continually aware of the profession's mission, values, ethical principles, and ethical standards, and practice in a manner consistent with them. Social workers act honestly and responsibly and promote ethical practices on the part of the organizations with which they are affiliated.

6. Competence. Social workers practice within their areas of competence and develop and enhance their professional expertise. They continually strive to increase their professional knowledge and skills and to apply them in practice.

▶ ETHICAL DILEMMAS IN CASE MANAGEMENT

▶ Balancing Advocacy Versus Cost-Containment Roles

Ethical dilemmas are a consequence of our contemporary healthcare climate, and they continue to haunt us. The issues are not static, and more will be revealed as healthcare reform unfolds. As case managers, we may be subject to ethical discomfort from the very roles we must perform: as gatekeepers of resources versus patient advocates, and as coordinators-facilitators of multidisciplinary teams. One common thread that appears over and over, sometimes in subtle disguises, is the issue of healthcare rationing.

The very idea of rationing healthcare is extremely distasteful to many Americans. However, like any budget, healthcare's is finite—and it continues to spiral out of control. Consider the following statistics according to the National Coalition on Health Care (2008):

▶ Healthcare spending reached $2.3 trillion in 2007. It is projected to reach $4.2 trillion by 2016.

▶ Healthcare spending constituted 16% of the gross domestic product (GDP) in 2007. It is projected to reach 20% by 2016.

▶ Nearly 47 million Americans are uninsured.

▶ We spend more on healthcare than other industrialized nations such as Canada, France, Germany, Switzerland, and the United Kingdom; and these countries provide health insurance to all their citizens.

▶ Premiums for employer-based health insurance rose by 6.1% in 2007. Small employers saw their premiums, on average, increase 5.5%. Firms with fewer than 24 workers experienced an increase of 6.8%.

▶ The annual premium that a health insurer charged an employer for a health plan covering a family of four averaged $12,100 in 2007. Workers contributed nearly $3,300 or 10% more than they did in 2006.

When most people think of rationing healthcare, they have visions of cutting off life-saving, high-cost procedures to a defined population. Perhaps people older than 80 years will not be allowed coronary bypasses; or anyone older than 65 years would not be allowed organ transplants or hemodialysis; or heroic measures would not be started on premature babies younger than 22 weeks' gestational age. The truth is that America already rations healthcare. The present discussions on newer, more stringent sets of criteria are for the purpose of rationing it further. Some feel that this is in order to serve a larger population (i.e., the currently uninsured). Others believe it is for reasons of financial benefit to the payor agency. The rationing fire is also being fueled by the media (Internet, print, broadcast, and so on), Congressional debates on healthcare reform (Medicare and Medicaid reform), and presidential debates.

Americans are grappling with the question of whether healthcare is a right or a commodity, which is another subtle way to evaluate whether healthcare should be rationed. Many of today's questions cross-examine whether healthcare is a right and how far the rights of individuals should go. Should noncompliant people who engage in unhealthy lifestyles be covered? Some question whether rationing or limiting of healthcare should be imposed on noncompliant persons. Should ceilings be placed on their medical care dollars? Should those who can afford to pay have higher premiums? What is legal and what is ethical? Consider the Delphi study responses mentioned earlier in this chapter.

Even the definition of noncompliance does not consider all the ethical ramifications. Noncompliance is a failure of the patient to cooperate with the medical plan by not carrying out needed procedures or lifestyle changes. The very concept of noncompliance betrays the professional's concern about patient autonomy; in other words, that patients are free to make life-directing decisions. Care must be taken not to label all those who do not follow a prescribed medical plan of treatment as noncompliant. Cultural beliefs are deeply ingrained in people's basic humanity. Food, health, and religious ritual practices will not be changed simply because a Western health practitioner dictated a prescription. Also, children and incapacitated adults who are in the care of noncompliant guardians may be penalized if society rations healthcare to noncompliant people. The kaleidoscope turns and the perspective changes.

Case managers deal with rationing on a daily basis. For example, two women have breast cancer. Both could die. Both have families and young children. One is allowed a bone marrow transplant by her insurance carrier; the other is not. Insurance companies ration their healthcare dollars through allowed benefits all the time: who is allowed benefits such as organ transplants, bone marrow transplants, extended care benefits, or experimental treatments. Subtle rationing of benefits takes many forms, and the case manager must be alert to a denial of services based on an interpretation of benefits that may be erroneous.

> One case involved a cancer patient with stomach, esophageal, and intestinal tumor involvement. Surgically, there was little to be done for the patient and her prognosis was poor, although death was not imminent. She was alert and oriented and chose hospice care, as she was no longer trying to cure the cancer with medical treatment. She was receiving total parenteral nutrition (TPN) as her only possible source of nutrition and was receiving radiation for palliative, not curative, purposes. Her case manager was told that the TPN was disallowed because hospice does not cover services that are merely for prolonging life. Not feeling that basic nutrition falls under the "not prolonging life" umbrella in this case, any more than eating food would in a lung cancer hospice patient, the case manager argued. The patient received hospice and TPN. The bottom line is that TPN is an expensive treatment option and difficult to budget for, so it is not routinely considered a covered service.

Some insurance companies cloak their rationing under terms such as medical necessity or unnecessary treatments. These vague terms must be treated with care, as they are arbitrary and prone to personal judgments when used as a measuring stick for insurance guidelines. Clarifying the implications and use of medical necessity sometimes requires semantic analysis, but it is not merely a semantic exercise. Confusion, conflict, and refractory dilemmas inevitably emerge when the intertwined layers of meaning(s) inherent in the concept remain hidden. The case manager—as a patient advocate—must be alert to vague interpretations of benefits. In addition, a payor inappropriately interpreting benefit language to cut its losses to the detriment of the claimant is courting malpractice.

In a positive sense, case managers help to ration healthcare. Through astute case planning and attention to detail, case managers avoid duplication and overutilization of finite resources. This is done through their gatekeeper role. As a gatekeeper, the case manager's job responsibilities may include monitoring resources, allocating and authorizing resources, and introducing incentives to improve the quality of care provided. In essence, the gatekeeper controls and rations limited resources in a world where there appears to be unlimited need. When the case manager superimposes the role of patient advocate on that of gatekeeper, role conflict and ethical dilemmas may result. Many feel that the combined patient advocate-gatekeeper role of a case manager is an impossible marriage. A gatekeeper controls entry to services and uses them economically; an advocate strives to gain all the services the patient needs for a safe, efficient, and effective case plan. Is it possible for one person to be both a patient advocate and a gatekeeper of healthcare resources? Can the case manager maintain quality while cutting costs? It is a challenge. There are factors that play into how effectively this merger can be accomplished.

The type and definition of the individual case management position may weight one role more heavily than another. A case manager for a Medicaid plan may feel that allocation of resources for her population of many thousands of patients (the whole) supersedes the needs of the individual (the part); therefore, her gatekeeping role may be stressed. A case manager in an oncology unit may feel that her patient's needs are the most important factor; this case manager may practice 75% patient advocacy and 25% gatekeeper. Potentially serious conflicts of interest are possible when the agencies that provide services send their case managers to do the assessment of need and make the case plans. If the company's objective is to increase business, overutilization may be practiced; if the company's objective is to control utilization of services, underutilization may be the result. The case manager may be placed in the unfavorable position of asking, "How can I really advocate for this patient when it means fighting with the person paying my salary?"

Perhaps the most important factor in how effectively the merger is accomplished is your own personal style and ability to balance the two roles so that everyone wins. Although this is not always possible, you should strive for it. Whenever it is not possible, err on the side of patient advocacy. A case manager misinterpreting his or her role to be primarily that of a provider or payor *employee* and secondarily that of a *patient advocate* will truly cause divisiveness regarding case management. Consumers of healthcare services will perceive the case manager as an "unethical" person.

▶ The Coordinator/Facilitator Role

Another case management role that at times is the cause of ethical discomfort is that of a coordinator/facilitator. Case managers are often asked to facilitate consensus of a large multidisciplinary team when a case is soaring out of control. A forum such as a case conference is held for this purpose. It may include any or all of the following: the patient, the family, the attending physician, physician specialists, residents or interns, respiratory therapists, speech therapists, occupational therapists, physical therapists, staff nurses, hospital administrators, risk management specialists, social workers, insurance company liaisons, insurance utilization review nurses or case managers, nutritionists, finance officers, or anyone else essential to that individual's case. Case managers deal with so many people making decisions on each case that it is dizzying. Ethicist John Banja likens this facilitator role to an air traffic controller who must coordinate flight patterns so that everyone is not crashing into one another (Boling, 1991).

At times, it feels as though some team members are on a collision course. Most case managers have been in situations in which the payor (insurance company) was found to have a different agenda from the physician. The payor felt that the patient could be safely provided for at a lesser level of care. The physician felt that the patient was not stable enough for a step-down change. The payor felt that it must make wise and strict use of resources, because it has a very large population to manage and must ration the funds carefully. The physician was focused on the best care for this patient at this time.

Sometimes the biases come from opposing viewpoints about the best treatment for a particular patient. One physician believes that a patient needs a lower extremity amputation; another physician believes that care should be "comfort only" at this point. The physical therapist believes it is unsafe for the patient to go home alone; the patient insists that he will go home. A patient refuses care for a gangrenous foot; the family threatens to sue if the patient dies of a gangrenous foot. As the air traffic controller/case manager gathers a meeting and allows each dissenting opinion time on the runway to air views on the best way to handle this situation, he or she should not forget to state the heart of the case management agenda—that of patient advocacy.

▶ Gag Clauses

This section is for the purpose of "case manager—beware." Gag clauses are provisions in managed care contracts that prevent physicians (and potentially other employees) from being fully open with their patients. This issue is so potent that it is even addressed in the *Consumer Bill of Rights and Responsibilities*. Issues that have been under gag clauses include:

- ▶ Discussing with patients treatment options that are not covered by the managed care plan;
- ▶ Referring a patient to specialists outside the plan, even if the physician feels it is in the patient's best interests to see a particular specialist;
- ▶ Discussing financial relationships between the physician and the managed care plan with the patient, especially if there are financial incentives for the physician to earn more by providing less care.
- ▶ Most beneficiaries have the periodic opportunity to choose their health plans. As part of that selection process, many consult with their physician to determine which plans the physician accepts and how a certain plan's payment practices compare with other plans. Gag orders interfere with this decision-making process.
- ▶ Gag orders prevent physicians from informing patients about any decision to terminate a physician's contract with a plan. Plans, on the other hand, often retain the authority not only to communicate such changes, but to arbitrarily assign a new physician to a patient.
- ▶ Arguing with a health plan on behalf of a patient's medical needs is time-consuming and frustrating. The result of such disputes is often interpreted as damaging to a health plan's reputation. Gag orders effectively limit a physician's freedom of speech, while making the physician appear unsympathetic to the patient.

The American Medical Association (AMA) took a strong stand against these gag clauses several years ago. Although many managed care companies have, one-by-one, removed them from contracts, they still exist, and case managers need to be aware of the implications. Of all the ethical issues these clauses attack, none is more important than the issue of trust between a patient and the healthcare team. Healthcare professionals are obliged to discuss treatment alternatives with patients so that patients cannot be subject to making decisions with inadequate information, as this would be a violation of informed consent requirements.

Pressures to soften these clauses also have been surfacing. The *Consumer Bill of Rights and Responsibilities* mentions accreditation as one possible method of ensuring consumer protections in the healthcare system; for example, certain accreditations require that financial incentives be revealed. Others, although for good intentions, place physicians between two differing paradigms. On one hand, physicians have to deal with gag clauses. On the other hand, CMS bars physicians who work with Medicare and Medicaid patients from withholding information on treatment options.

State legislation has been very active. For example, Massachusetts enacted the Patient Confidentiality Bill that would bar HMOs from including gag orders in their provider contracts. In California, legislation has been enacted that prevents retaliation against physicians who advocate on behalf of patients despite contractual prohibitions. Laws in Arizona and Indiana require organizations to disclose financial incentives or penalties that are intended to encourage the minimalization of services provided. Likewise, similar bills have been considered in all other states.

▶ Organ Donation

Effective in late 1999, CMS-certified facilities are required to report all deaths to the organ procurement organization (OPO) in their city, county, or state. The intent of this is to increase the availability of organs for people who cannot live without them. There are at least two ethical dilemmas with regard to organ donation:

1. Who gets the scarce organs?
2. What is legal and ethical when harvesting suitable organs?

Perhaps someday organs will not be scarce; humans appear to have the ability to clone living things at will, and certainly human organs are on the agenda. This will likely bring up additional ethical problems. For the purposes of case management at this time, let us assume that organs will remain scarce for a few more years.

For example, in 2007 about 26,400 transplants were performed, but more than 96,600 people were waiting for transplantation of a single or multiple organs; more than 7% died before transplantation occurred (OPTN, 2008). Then the question arises: who will get the first chance at scarce resources?

The government has ordered that life-saving organs be given to the sickest first. Under the previous system, organs went to the patients living closest to the donor, even if there was someone more critical elsewhere. In March 1998, Donna Shalala, Secretary of Health and Human Services, declared that people are dying simply because of where they live. A regulation was issued governing the United Network for Organ Sharing that included a mandate that the network devise a new allocation scheme for organ distribution. The network and the government have had more than a few problems ever since. As with many of life's events, no answer will make everyone happy. As case managers, many of us have watched our patients die while awaiting an organ; who could have needed it more, we wondered?

The ruling stated at the beginning of this section may increase the chances of more successful organ transplantations. However, there are other, less ethically clear-cut, methods being examined to increase the organ pool. Organ cloning or "personal pigs" are the lesser of the dilemmas. Prisoners are being targeted as a potential answer to organ scarcity. In 1996, Arizona rejected the Death Row Inmate Organ Donor Bill (HB 2271) (Johns, 1996). This would have effectively harvested the organs of inmates. One major problem is how a prisoner can be executed and still have useable organs. A lethal injection of a fatal chemical is not conducive to organ recycling. Who knows what electricity does to livers or cardiac tissue? One entrepreneurial legislator in Georgia introduced a bill to use the guillotine method; this would not harm the organs and therefore facilitate organ extraction.

Arizona's bill would have allowed the prisoner to have his choice between lethal injection or dying on the operating table. This leaves one more "quirky medical ethical issue" (Johns, 1996). Can a physician take a person's organs before that individual is brain-dead? What about first causing no harm?

▶ Assisted Death and the Right to Die

Assisted suicide, doctor-assisted suicide, euthanasia, mercy killing, legalized killing, managed death, terminal sedation, end-of-life care, murder—assisted death has been called by many names. Case managers will likely continue to be affected by its ethical and legal implications. Withholding or withdrawing life support or food/fluids is the tip of the iceberg, as that is more like passively assisting death. What physician-assisted suicide does is actually end life at a given moment in time and through intentional actions. In November 1998, his first "euthanasia" was broadcasted publicly on national television.

Regardless of what the process is called, the result is the same: a patient's death. The difference between assisted suicide and euthanasia appears to be the degree to which assistance is provided. Consider this: the American Hospital Association states that approximately 70% of the deaths in hospitals happen after a decision has been made to withhold treatment, another degree to which assistance for the dying is provided. Other patients die when pain medications depress their breathing, or medications to maintain blood pressure are discontinued. Nurses have witnessed these events for decades. Less information is known about SNF deaths and those in private homes.

Like many healthcare issues, it is difficult to separate the legal issues from the ethical ones pertaining to assisted death. Like abortion, the debate will go on for decades; the difference being that one ends life at the beginning, while the other focuses on the end of life. Those who want physician-assisted suicide state that it allows terminally ill people, who so desire, the ability to die peacefully and with dignity. Those against it feel it is a radical departure from existing medical and legal tradition and risks fallible judgments and irreversible errors; needless to say, opposition is strong on many fronts. It is also clear that there are no absolutes in life. Einstein did not intend for atomic energy to be used as a weapon of mass destruction. Assisted suicide laws should not be used for anything except relief of suffering. There are no answers at the back of a book on ethics. There are no assurances that the choice one makes is the best choice. However, for decisions to be truly ethical ones, they must be uncontaminated by personal gain, fear of reprisal, or other ulterior motives. The kaleidoscope changes colors and shapes again, but only history will tell what is (or should have been) the right thing to do.

▶ SUMMARY

Regardless of the ethical issues faced, if case managers act based on ethical principles and professional codes of conduct, keeping the patient/family interests above all others, they can ensure the achievement of desired outcome(s)—those that please all parties: patients and their family members, providers of care, healthcare organizations they work for, payors, and regulatory or accreditation agencies. Ethically competent case

managers protect their patients and advance what is in the patients' best interest (patient advocacy); are accountable for their own practice; effectively mediate ethical conflicts when they arise; and abide by their professional code of conduct and related ethical principles.

STUDY QUESTIONS

1. What do ethics mean to you? What constitutes an ethical dilemma? What constitutes ethical case management practice?

2. Would Nancy Cruzan's case be resolved differently today than in the 1980s? Why?

3. Recall and discuss an ethical dilemma that occurred with one of your cases.

4. For each of the nine scenarios in the GUIDE presented in Display 9-1:
   ▶ Discuss a real case that matches the scenario.
   ▶ Discuss the recommendations given for the case scenario.

5. If an ethics committee has ever been consulted on one of your cases, discuss the case, the ethical dilemma, and the committee's recommendations. Were the issues organizational or clinical in nature? How did you go about organizing an ethics committee meeting to deliberate the issue? Discuss what worked and what did not. Could you have done anything differently?

6. In your opinion, is there an ethical difference between withholding and withdrawing life-sustaining treatment? Describe cases from your own practice that are examples of these issues.

7. When does ordinary treatment become extraordinary? Provide one or more examples from your practice where ordinary treatment became extraordinary. How did it change? Who was involved? How could you have avoided or prevented the situation?

8. Is withholding or withdrawing nutritional support from a person ethically justifiable? When, if ever? What criteria could be used? What about hydration?

9. Are nutritional support and hydration different from other forms of life support? If so, how are they different? Is discontinuing nutritional

support active euthanasia? Is it passive euthanasia?

10. Discuss differences between a patient who is terminally ill and one who is imminently dying. Would the case plans differ? What are the ethical implications for the care of each patient?

11. Discuss your views on the points mentioned in the Delphi poll.

12. Discuss a case that you felt had an ethical twist to it concerning rationing healthcare. How did

you address the situation? What ethical principles did you apply?

13. Discuss a case in which you felt your patient advocate role was compromised by your gatekeeper role.

14. Discuss a case in which your gatekeeper role was influenced by your patient advocate role.

15. Discuss a case in which you felt medical necessity was misused.

▶ REFERENCES

American Nurses Association. (accessed 9/18/2008). *Code of Ethics for Nurses with interpretive statements.* [Online]. Available: http://www.nursingworld.org/MainMenuCategories/ThePracticeofProfessionalNursing/EthicsStandards.aspx.

Andrews, M., Goldberg, K., & Kaplan, H. (1996). *Nurse's legal handbook* (3rd ed.). Springhouse, PA: Springhouse Corp.

Banja, J. (1996). If Momma dies, you die. *The Case Manager, 16*(1), 37–39.

Boling, J. (1991). Profile—John Banja. *The Case Manager,* 76–81.

Commission for Case Manager Certification. (accessed 9/18/2008). *Code of professional conduct for case managers with standards, rules, procedures, and penalties.* [Online]. Available: http://www.ccmcertification.org/pages/13frame_set.html.

Commission on Consumer Protection and Quality in Health Care. (1998). *President's advisory commission releases consumer bill of rights and responsibilities.* [Online]. Available: www.hcquality-commission.gov.

Curtin, L. (1994). Ethical concerns of nutritional life support. *Nursing Management, 25*(1), 14–16.

Fiesta, J. (1992). Refusal of treatment. *Nursing Management, 23*(11), 14–18.

Jansen, L. (2003). Ethical Decision making in case management. In T. Cesta & A. Tahan, *The case manager's survival guide: winning strategies for clinical practice* (2nd ed., pp. 324–335). St. Louis, MO: Mosby.

Johns, C. (1996, February, 18). Should prisons be organ farms: "harvesting" bills raise scary implications. *The Arizona Republic,* H3.

Knox, R. (1994, May 27). Noted deaths reflect attitude shift: most patients and families oppose resuscitation efforts, study finds. *The Phoenix Gazette,* A26.

Kolodner, D. (1992). Advance medical directives after Cruzan. *MEDSURG Nursing, 1*(1), 56–59.

Levenson, J., & Pettrey, L. (1994). Controversial decisions regarding treatment and DNR: an algorithmic guide for the uncertain in decision-making ethics (GUIDE). *American Journal of Critical Care, 3*(2), 87–91.

National Association of Social Workers. *Code of ethics.* Available online: http://www.socialworkers.org. Accessed September 18, 2008.

National Coalition on Health Care. *Facts on health care costs.* Available online: http://www.nchc.org/facts/cost.shtml. Accessed September 18, 2008.

Organ Procurement and Transplantation Network. *Data reports.* [Online]. Available: http://optn.org. Accessed September 18, 2008.

President's Advisory Commission on Consumer Protection and Quality in the Health Care Industry. (accessed 9/18/2008). *Consumer Bill of Rights and Responsibilities.* [Online]. Available: http://www.hcqualitycommision.gov/final/append_a.html.

President's Advisory Commission on Consumer Protection and Quality in the Health Care Industry. (1998). President's Commission releases consumer bill of rights and responsibilities. [Online]. Available: http://www.hcqualitycommision.gov.

President's Commission for the Study of Ethics Problems in Medicine and Biomedical and Behavioral Research. (1983). *Deciding to forego life-sustaining treatment.* Washington, DC: U.S. Government Printing Office.

Robbins, D. (1998). *Integrating managed care and ethics.* New York: McGraw-Hill.

Wright, R.A. (1987). *Human values in health care: the practice of ethics.* New York: McGraw-Hill.

PART 4

Practical Applications

"To laugh often and much, to win the respect of intelligent people and the affection of children; to earn the appreciation of honest critics and endure the betrayal of false friends; to appreciate beauty; to find the best in others; to leave the world a bit better, whether by a healthy child, a garden patch or a redeemed social condition; to know even one life has breathed easier because you lived. This is to have succeeded."

RALPH WALDO EMERSON

CHAPTER 10

Case Management Credentials, Organizations, and Standards

LEARNING OBJECTIVES

Upon completion of this chapter, the reader will be able to:

1. Identify professional organizations or societies that are important to case management.
2. Describe accreditation and accreditation agencies affecting case management responsibilities and processes.
3. Identify the various case management credentials and certifications.
4. List the eligibility criteria and examination content for organizations and agencies that provide case management certifications and credentials.
5. Describe case management standards, guidelines, and protocols.
6. Define accreditation.

ESSENTIAL TERMS

Accreditation • Case Management Adherence Guidelines • Case Management Practice Guidelines • Case Management Standards • Case Management Society of America • Certification • Commission for Case Manager Certification • Credentialing • National Association of Healthcare Quality • National Association of Social Workers • National Committee of Quality Assurance • National Transitions of Care Coalition • Standards of Practice for Case Managers • The Joint Commission • The Joint Commission International • Utilization Review Accreditation Commission

As the healthcare industry strives to monitor and demonstrate accountability to the population it serves, professional specialty certifications, standards, and accreditations have become an important part of the overall picture. Case management is no exception. Further, the certifications and accreditations are no longer just medals on a uniform, but are considered by some employers, businesses, and governmental agencies to be mandatory. The Joint Commission's (TJC) seal of approval has been mandatory for many years for facilities that provide care to Medicare beneficiaries. Now, regulatory agencies and quality improvement organizations are weaving outcomes management into the mix. Outcomes are being addressed by a number of accountability-oriented initiatives, including the National Committee for Quality Assurance (NCQA) utilizing the Health Plan Employer Data and Information Set (HEDIS); TJC utilizing the core measures program (previously known as ORYX); and the Centers for Medicare & Medicaid Services (CMS) using core measures for specific diagnoses such as heart failure and pneumonia.

Many of these different quality initiatives appear to be duplicative. In some respects, that is true. Nevertheless, they are also complementary and are providing a service that, as yet, cannot be fully realized. Managed care quality assessments have been evolving. A challenge lies in the fact that unmanaged care is more difficult to assess. Further, comparing managed care and unmanaged care plans has not yet been completely worked out. The evolution of assessing quality in healthcare is in its infancy. One thing is clear: case managers contribute to quality care and safety in more ways than perhaps any other single strategy. Case managers are more than an asset to any organization; during these times of regulatory monitoring and accountability, they are critical.

This chapter will discuss the following:

▶ Professional organizations or societies important to case management;
▶ Guidelines, protocols, and case management standards;
▶ Credentials germane to case management, utilization management, and quality management; and
▶ Regulatory agencies and accreditations affecting case management responsibilities and processes.

▶ ORGANIZATIONS
▶ The Case Management Society of America and CMS International

The Case Management Society of America (CMSA) is an international nonprofit organization that was founded in 1990 to promote and support the development of professional case management through educational forums, networking opportunities, and legislative involvement. CMSA's membership has grown to more than 11,000 individuals and companies. CMSA members belong to over 70 affiliated and prospective chapters based in the United States, Australia, Hong Kong, and London. CMSA

> envision[s] case managers as pioneers of healthcare change...key initiators of and participants in the health-care team who open up new areas of thought...research and development...leading the way toward the day when every American will know what a case/care manager does and will know how to access case and care management services. [CMSA aims to] positively impact and improve patient wellbeing and healthcare outcomes (CMSA, 2008).

To execute this mission, CMSA bases its efforts on the following three ideologies:

1. To inform consumers about the services case and care managers provide.
2. To educate physicians and other providers about improved patient outcomes through the services case and care managers provide.
3. To educate payors and regulators about improved patient outcomes that case and care management services can provide (CMSA, 2008).

CMSA sponsors annual conferences and educational forums, promotes international networking among case managers, and participates in legislative involvement. It developed the *Standards of Practice for Case Management* and the *Ethics Statement on Case*

Management Practice, both released in 1995. In addition, CMSA has organized several critical task forces to enhance research and knowledge pertinent to the case management profession. These include the Communities of Practice; the Council for Case Management Accountability (CCMA), which was formed to research and develop case management outcomes, evidence-based guidelines, and accountability; and the Government Affairs Committee, which focuses on legislative and public policy issues relevant to case management practice and healthcare delivery. CMSA has established special interest groups to serve its diverse membership and is currently working on a case management curriculum (CMSA, 2008).

With healthcare costs rising around the world, case management has been the focus of international attention; other countries wanted to know how the United States was containing costs and sustaining quality of care and turned to CMSA for leadership and collaboration. The next logical step for CMSA was the development of the Case Management Society International (CMSI). Members live in Australia, New Zealand, Canada, the United Kingdom, Puerto Rico, South Africa, and Germany. Interested groups have formed in China, Japan, Singapore, and Spain. Australia has formed CMSAustralia, which is CMSA's first international affiliate.

CMSA has members in various disciplines and with a diversity of professional licenses. This diversity is responsible for much of CMSA's success. With the complexity of the healthcare system, each profession adds a different perspective. Only by looking at the magnitude of the challenges from a 360-degree perspective, can case managers affect healthcare to the degree that has been accomplished thus far.

CMSA members are offered two publications. The first is *Professional Case Management: The Leader in Evidence-Based Practice.* This peer-reviewed journal is published by Lippincott Williams & Wilkins and features best practices and industry benchmarks for the professional case manager. It focuses on coordination of patient care, efficient use of resources, improving the quality of care, data and outcomes analysis, research in case management, ethical and legal practices, and patient advocacy, among many other topics.

The second publication is *Case in Point*, a magazine published by Dorland Healthcare Information. It is a contemporary, nationally focused magazine designed to meet the professional, personal, and lifestyle needs of today's case managers. The magazine offers cutting-edge clinical information to address challenges that confront healthcare professionals and covers the latest issues, resources, trends, tools, technology, and news in healthcare, enabling case managers to stay up-to-date and promoting professional growth and development. *Case in Point* also provides all of CMSA's members with the latest news and information from the Association by including the *Case Report* in every issue of the magazine.

Both publications offer a wealth of case management information to keep case managers and other readers on the cutting edge of the profession. The CMSA Web site is an updated source of information, healthcare links, and communication forums. Although CMSA strongly supports the concept of credentialing case managers, it is not the credentialing body.

NOTE

For information on the Case Management Society of America (CMSA), contact:

Case Management Society of America
6301 Ranch Drive
Little Rock, AR 72223
Telephone: (501) 225-2229
Fax: (501) 221-9068
E-mail: cmsa@cmsa.org
Web site: http://www.cmsa.org

▶ The Disease Management Association of America

The Disease Management Association of America (DMAA), also known as The Care Continuum Alliance, is an organization that represents more than 200 corporate and individual stakeholders, including wellness, disease, and care management organizations; pharmaceutical manufacturers and benefits managers; health information technology innovators; biotechnology innovators; employers; physicians, nurses and other health care professionals; researchers; and academicians. Its primary goal is population health improvement through health and wellness promotion, disease management, and care coordination. DMAA promotes the role of population health improvement in raising the quality of care, improving health outcomes, and reducing preventable health care costs for individuals with chronic conditions and those at risk of developing chronic conditions. DMAA activities in support of these efforts include advocacy, research, and the promotion of best practices in care management (DMAA, 2008).

The DMAA believes that the highest health status is attained through the promotion and alignment of population health improvement through the following activities (DMAA, 2008):

- Promoting a proactive, patient-centric focus across the care continuum.
- Convening health care professionals to share and integrate care models.
- Emphasizing the importance of both healthful behaviors and evidence-based care in preventing and managing chronic conditions.
- Promoting high quality standards that address wellness, disease, and, where appropriate, case management and care coordination programs, as well as support services and materials.
- Identifying, researching, sharing, and encouraging innovative approaches and best practices in care delivery and reimbursement models.
- Establishing consensus-based outcomes measures and demonstrating health, satisfaction, and financial improvements.
- Supporting delivery system models that ensure appropriate care for chronic conditions and coordination among all health care providers. This may include strategies such as the Chronic Care Model, the physician-led medical home concept, and the disease management model.
- Encouraging the widespread adoption and interoperability of health information technologies.
- Advocating the principles and benefits of population health improvement to public health officials, including state and federal government entities.
- Underscoring the level of commitment to population health improvement and timeframes necessary to realize the full benefits.

The DMAA provides healthcare professionals with vehicles for information sharing that help them in the development, implementation, assessment, and improvement of disease prevention and management strategies. It also provides its members with information on current research, partnerships, and processes that underscore the delivery of cost-effective, quality care. *Population Health Management*, the official journal of DMAA, is a member benefit, peer-reviewed journal published on a bimonthly basis. It comprehensively covers the clinical and business aspects of the field of disease management. The journal features peer-reviewed clinical research and case studies, papers on the practical aspects involved in implementing disease management initiatives, and perspectives and insights from professionals involved in disease and care management (DMAA, 2008).

NOTE

For information on the Disease Management Association of America (DMAA): The Care Continuum Alliance, you may contact:

Disease Management Association of America
701 Pennsylvania Avenue NW, Suite 700
Washington, DC 20004-2694
Telephone: (202) 737-5980
Fax: (202) 478-5113
E-mail: dmaa@dmaa.org
Web site: http://www.dmaa.org

❱ Case Management Practice Guidelines

Early on, case managers realized that quality of life improved, patient and family satisfaction increased, and costs of healthcare decreased, on a case-by-case basis. Measuring case management outcomes began with measuring details specific to the individual patient. Next, case managers pooled total caseloads and disease-specific populations to assess factors across larger groups of patients. With the assistance of CCMA, these pooled outcomes will grow in statistical significance (power in numbers) and can eventually become the core ingredients of which guidelines are made. Guidelines are not static entities; they are dynamic statements that must change when improved methods of care delivery and practice are discovered.

Aetna Health Plans and the Individual Case Management Association (ICMA) collaborated on the development of *The Case Management Practice Guidelines* (Coeur, 1996). The ICMA has since merged with CMSA, and the name CMSA is used. The guidelines were published in 1996 as an effort to move case management from a predominately intuitive model to one of a more concrete nature (i.e., one in which disease management/case management could originate, and outcomes measurement studies could be initiated).

Several disease-specific guidelines are outlined, including dealing with AIDS/HIV, brain injury, high-risk neonate/pregnancy, low back injury, oncology, pediatrics, workers' compensation, spinal cord injury, transplants, amputations, asthma, cystic fibrosis, renal failure, substance abuse, and gerontology. Within each

guideline the following attributes are discussed: primary diagnosis, referral triggers, goals, medical considerations, special considerations, long-term care/life-care planning, patient/family teaching, psychosocial issues, vocational issues, patient and family issues, resources/support groups, barriers to effective outcomes, and case management outcomes effectiveness (Coeur, 1996). One important consideration with any disease-specific condition is that the knowledge and the treatment options of the disease are dynamic. As with any guidelines, even the Agency for Healthcare Research and Quality (AHRQ) guidelines, they must be periodically updated or they may become less useful. The case manager must be aware of changes and check current, credible information.

An example of practice guidelines is CMSA's medication adherence tool, known as a *Case Management Adherence Guideline* (CMAG). Launched in 2004, it was developed based on key concepts including patient information, motivation, and behavior skill needs. This guideline has received positive feedback and ratings from the case management community. CMAG is now recognized as the "best standard" and set of tools ever developed to assist case managers in working effectively with their patients to improve their adherence to taking prescription medications. Specifically, the purpose of the CMAG guidelines is to help case managers in the assessment, planning, facilitation, and advocacy of patient compliance. The guidelines include an interaction and management algorithm for use in the assessment and improvement of the patient's knowledge and his or her motivation to take medications as they are prescribed. They are flexible enough to allow case managers to incorporate a patient's individual needs (CMSA, 2008). For more information on the CMAG guidelines, refer to CMSA's Web site (http://www.cmsa.org/PROGRAMSEVENTS/CaseManagementAdherenceGuidelinesCMAG/tabid/90/Default.aspx).

❱ Standards of Practice for Case Management

The literature often cautions professions against writing standards of care that are too idealistic—this would put an impossible burden on the one who must perform under those standards. It is recommended that standards represent the safe, minimum level that the profession must follow; therefore, it is expected that, at this level, the standards must be followed explicitly. Standards can and do end up in courts of law. To that end, it is essential that case managers know the recommended standards that pertain to case management practice.

The *Standards of Practice for Case Management* were developed and released by CMSA in 1995. They were revised in 2002; as of this writing, the standards are undergoing a third revision. The standards are generic and provide a framework for case managers in a variety of settings and specialties. They can be translated into working tools for preparation, management, and evaluation of all case managers. The standards were developed as guidelines for practice excellence, with the intent that they were to be the forerunner for establishing formal guidelines from a variety of settings.

Some have questioned whether these standards put an impossible burden on case managers. It is not so much due to the way they are written; rather, case management is a tremendously pervasive specialty with multiple roles and responsibilities. Not all case managers are required to perform every case management role or responsibility addressed in CMSA's case management practice standards. However, it is important that case managers follow those portions that correspond to their job descriptions.

The CMSA *Standards of Practice for Case Management* is divided into four parts as described below (CMSA, 2002).

I. Introduction. This section describes the concept of case management, its history, definition, philosophy, purpose, and goals, as well as roles of case managers.
II. Standards of Care. This section addresses the case management process and explains its steps, which include client identification and selection for case management services, problem identification, planning, monitoring, evaluating, and outcomes. As each step is described, the relevant standards of care required for safe and effective case management services are defined.
III. Performance Indicators. This section discusses quality of care; qualifications of a case manager, including the knowledge, education, and preparation required for the role; collaboration with others; legal, ethical, and advocacy issues; resource management stewardship; and research utilization.
IV. Definitions. This section describes several pertinent definitions such as evidence-based criteria, case management plan of care, predictive modeling, and risk stratification.

The full text of CMSA's *Standards of Practice for Case Management* can be obtained from CMSA (see previous section on CMSA in this chapter).

▶ National Transitions of Care Coalition

The National Transitions of Care Coalition (NTOCC) was formed in 2006 by CMSA and Sanofi-Aventis. It brought together thought leaders, patient advocates, and healthcare providers from various care settings across the continuum for the main purpose of improving the quality of care coordination and communication when patients are transferred from one level of care to another. Today, NTOCC has more than 30 participating associations, professional societies, and organizations. All share a common goal: "addressing the critical issues surrounding transitions of care." NTOCC views transitions of care as a major challenge to health care delivery and acknowledges that this concern can only be addressed by breaking down the existing silos and barriers between the various healthcare settings. As a result, NTOCC is working collaboratively for the good of the patient to provide key information and tools to patients, caregivers, healthcare professionals, policy makers, and media representatives to assist them to better understand and improve transitions of care challenges (NTOCC, 2008).

Transitions of care, as described by NTOCC, are the movements of patients from one care setting or provider to another. During these transitions, poor communication and coordination between professionals, patients, and caregivers can lead to unsafe and serious events, wasting of healthcare resources, or frustration of healthcare consumers and providers. NTOCC was formed to define solutions addressing these gaps that impact safety and quality of care for transitioning patients. Its work is carried out by an Advisory Task Force and four other groups (NTOCC, 2008).

▶ The Advisory Task Force includes an invited group of leading organizations who discuss ways to create and implement solutions and resources to benefit patients during transitions of care. The Task Force is joined by associate members, that is, organizations that wish to support this important work and are in a position to advance transitional care awareness and solutions.
▶ Education and Awareness Group works to address awareness and general knowledge about the problems associated with transitions of care and to provide the necessary information to various stakeholders—patients, caregivers, health care professionals, and government officials.
▶ Tools and Resources Group identifies practical tools and resources that can be used by healthcare professionals, caregivers, and patients

to improve communication in a consistent manner between care settings and providers, and to reduce risk associated with care transitions.

▶ Policy and Advocacy Group assesses ways to improve care through enhanced communication tools, collaborative partnerships, and improved reimbursement for transitional care support and technical medical information shared between care settings.

▶ Performance and Metrics Group assesses and defines appropriate performance measurement frameworks to demonstrate the impact of interventions on reducing risk associated with transitional care.

▶ As of this writing, NTOCC is planning to launch a Health Information Technology Group and a "consensus" panel to develop transitions of care guidelines.

On its Web site, NTOCC shares key information and several tools healthcare providers, including case managers patients, and families, can access, download, and use for free. These tools are useful for case managers to incorporate in their work with patients, especially to encourage adherence to medications intake and to educate regarding safety and self-care. The tools include the following:

▶ My Medicine List (consumer-focused).
▶ Taking Care of My Health (consumer-focused).
▶ Transitions of Care Checklist.
▶ Medication Reconciliation and Essential Data Specifications.
▶ Informational brochure about transitions of care.
▶ Information slides that describe the issue of transitions of care and NTOCC's work in this regard.

NOTE

For information about the National Transitions of Care Coalition (NTOCC), contact

Transitions of Care Coalition
6301 Ranch Drive
Little Rock, AR 72223
Web site: http://www.ntocc.org

NTOCC Project Coordinator
Case Management Society of America (CMSA)
Telephone: (501) 673-1113.

▶ Policy paper that in essence is a white paper describing the state of transitions of care and recommended actions that can be taken to improve transitions.
▶ Framework for Measuring Outcomes of Transitions of Care.
▶ Improving on Transitions of Care: How to Implement and Evaluate a Plan.

▶ CREDENTIALS
▶ Case Management Credentials
CERTIFIED CASE MANAGER

The Certified Case Manager (CCM) is one of the premiere case management certifications. Since the first CCM examination in 1993, an estimated 30,000 case managers have earned the CCM credential. To take the examination, an applicant must meet acceptable standards with regard to work experience and hold a recognized license or certification in a field that promotes client physical, psychological, or vocational well-being. The Commission for Case Manager Certification (CCMC) is an independent credentialing agency that sponsors and oversees the CCM credentialing process. CCMC is accredited by the National Commission for Certifying Agencies (NCCA).

While researching the necessity of this credential in 1991, the National Case Management Task Force realized that no single profession could "own" case management; rather, it was the coordinating and advocacy approach to healthcare that case managers brought to the table. Therefore, CCM is not a primary credential. It is a secondary credential as an adjunct to a licensed professional in a recognized health and human services field (i.e., RN, LCSW, RPT, MD, and so on).

The CCM certification examination focuses on six core domains of case management knowledge. These core domains evolved from a large survey of CCMs and represent an aggregate view of the most important roles, responsibilities, and spheres of knowledge required for case managers to perform their case management functions. It is an extensive list; however, CCMC is testing for case management knowledge, skills, and experience—a broad and comprehensive set of responsibilities. (Note: Details of the core domains are from *The CCM Certification Guide*, published by the CCMC, and available for free on CCMC's Web site). The domains covered on the certification examination are described below (CCMC, 2008).

I. Case Management Concepts
This domain addresses the process associated with case management practice and methods for

establishing quality measures and parameters of practice.

- Accreditation standards and requirements.
- Case management models.
- Case management process and tools.
- Case recording and documentation.
- Goals and objectives of case management.
- Program evaluation and research methods (e.g., outcomes, satisfaction).
- Quality and performance improvement concepts.

II. Case Management Principles and Strategies
This domain considers professional practice behaviors and the impact of external influences upon those behaviors.

- Confidentiality.
- Conflict resolution strategies.
- Negotiation.
- Ethics (including issues relating to advocacy, experimental treatments, protocols, end-of-life/ refusal-of-treatment services, benefit limits, professional conduct).
- Healthcare and disability-related legislation (e.g., Americans with Disabilities Act, Health Insurance Portability and Accountability Act).
- Interpersonal communication (e.g., group dynamics, relationship building, interviewing).
- Legal and regulatory requirements.
- Risk management.
- Standards of practice.

III. Psychosocial and Support Systems
This domain discusses specific interventions, family and cultural issues and resources that must be integrated into case management practice.

- Behavioral health and psychiatric disability concepts.
- Psychological and neuropsychological assessment.
- Management of clients with substance use/ abuse/addiction.
- Wellness and illness prevention strategies.
- Community resources (e.g., elder services, fraternal/religious organizations, governmental resources, Meals on Wheels).
- Support programs (e.g., support groups or resources provided by professional organizations such as the American Heart Association).
- Multicultural issues as they relate to health behavior.
- Psychosocial aspects of chronic illness and disability.
- Spirituality as it relates to health behavior.

- Management of complementary alternative medicine (CAM) practices.
- Concepts related to working with clients who have been abused (emotionally, psychologically, physically, financially).
- Crisis intervention strategies.

IV. Healthcare Management and Delivery
This domain includes knowledge of various healthcare delivery systems and associated collaboration with other providers. Case management activities across practice settings are emphasized.

- Management of acute and chronic illness and disability.
- Assessment of physical functioning.
- Assistive technology.
- Continuum of care.
- Critical pathways, standards of care, practice guidelines (including average duration of treatment associated with various disabilities).
- Healthcare delivery systems.
- Levels of care.
- Management of medications use.
- Rehabilitation service delivery systems.
- Roles and functions of other providers.
- Healthcare providers (including vendors available in the community).
- Roles and functions of case managers in various settings.

V. Healthcare Reimbursement
This domain addresses case management responsibilities in relation to funding for healthcare services.

- Managed care concepts.
- Cost containment principles.
- Healthcare insurance principles.
- Managed care reimbursement concepts.
- Prospective payment system.
- Private benefit programs (e.g., pharmacy benefits management, indemnity, employer-sponsored health coverage, individual-purchased insurance, home care benefits).
- Public benefit programs (e.g., SSI, SSDI, Medicare, Medicaid).
- Utilization management.
- Cost-benefit analysis.

VI. Vocational Concepts and Strategies
This domain includes topic areas related to disability and workplace issues and strategies for work as a life activity.

- Ergonomics.
- Job analysis, modification and accommodation, and vocational assessment.

▶ Disability compensation systems (e.g., workers' compensation, auto insurance, short-term disability, accident, and health).
▶ Job development and placement.
▶ Vocational aspects of chronic illness and disability.
▶ Work adjustment and work transition.
▶ Workers' compensation principles.
▶ Work-hardening resources and strategies.

These six domains are further clarified through the following attributes:

▶ The case manager must perform all of eight essential activities, including assessment, planning, implementation, coordination, monitoring, evaluation, outcomes, and general (e.g., privacy, advocacy, and adherence to ethical, legal, and accreditation standards).
▶ The case management activities must be performed in at least five of the six domains of practice described above.
▶ Case management services must be provided across the continuum of care, beyond a single episode, and must address the ongoing needs of the patient.
▶ The domains require that the case manager interact with all relevant people in the patient's care team.
▶ The domains require that the case manager must work with the whole universe of the patient's needs (rather than direct patient care).

The CCMC does not endorse or approve any CCM preparation courses. CCM is a voluntary credential. However, its influence in case management should not be underestimated; every year, more advertised case management positions require this credential. Those interested in applying for the case management certification, requesting

The CCM Certification Guide, or in need of information on continuing education credits for recertification should contact CCMC.

CERTIFIED PROFESSIONAL IN UTILIZATION REVIEW

The Certified Professional in Utilization Review (CPUR) is sponsored by InterQual and is the only comprehensive utilization review certification. To date, more than 5,000 healthcare professionals have been certified. Case managers do not need to be InterQual licensees to attend the course; anyone involved in the utilization review/utilization management field can take the accreditation examination. The program takes 2 days and includes course work and the CPUR certification examination. CPUR was created to educate healthcare professionals about the value and challenges of utilization review and management. It provides a thorough and current background in topics such as:

▶ Key historical healthcare legislation and regulations.
▶ Effective resource management tools and strategies.
▶ Current healthcare delivery systems.
▶ Legal issues surrounding utilization review and management.

After successful completion of the examination, a CPUR credential is awarded, which is valid for 2 years. An updated study guide is published annually. Thirty contact hours are required for certification.

NOTE

Commission for Case Manager Certification (CCMC)

CCMC Certification Center
P.O. Box 17009
St. Paul, MN 55117
Telephone: (651) 789-3744
Fax: (800) 648-1828
E-mail: support@ccmchelp.org
Web site: http://www.ccmcertification.org

NOTE

Certified Professional in Utilization Review (CPUR)

McKesson Corporation
One Post Street
San Francisco, CA 94104
Telephone: (415) 983-8300
E-mail: Education@McKesson.com
Web site: http://www.mckesson.com

THE AMERICAN NURSES ASSOCIATION: NURSING CASE MANAGEMENT CREDENTIAL

The Nursing Case Management (RN, CM) credential is provided by the American Nurses Credentialing

Center (ANCC), the credentialing arm of the American Nurses Association (ANA). Candidates must meet the following criteria to qualify for the certification exam:

▶ Hold an active RN license and a baccalaureate or higher degree.
▶ Have practiced the equivalent of 2 years full time as a registered nurse.
▶ Have a minimum of 2,000 hours of clinical practice in case management within the last 3 years.
▶ Have completed 30 hours of continuing education in case management within the last 3 years.

The framework for the Nursing Case Management credential includes eight components: clinical practice, management of data, resource management, processes of quality management, legal and ethical considerations, principles of education/learning, tools for case management practice, and professional development. (The following is from the *Modular Certification Examination Catalog* of the ANCC, 2008).

I. Clinical Practice
  a. Nursing case management concepts
    i. Definition
    ii. Role functions and principles of case management
  b. Nursing process
    i. Assessment
      1. Physical/clinical
      2. Psychosocial (including support systems/ family dynamics)
      3. Developmental
      4. Financial (e.g., insurance, personal funds)
    ii. Planning (e.g., individualized health care options, plan of care development)
    iii. Implementation and coordination
      1. Goal setting
      2. Negotiation skills (with insurance provider, suppliers, healthcare providers, etc.)
      3. Contracting (with patient, vendor/ provider)
    iv. Monitoring and evaluation
      1. Outcomes measurement
      2. Patient compliance with plan of care
      3. Services (e.g., services authorized by payor, community services; are the services working?)
    v. Interaction
      1. Collaboration
      2. Consultation and referrals

      3. Communication skills (e.g., interpersonal communication, conflict resolution, facilitation)
  c. Management of disease
    i. Pathophysiology
    ii. Psychosocial conditions (e.g., support systems, financial resources, living conditions)
    iii. Cultural/religious influence on disease
    iv. Clinical standards of care (e.g., American Diabetes Association, American Cancer Society, American Heart Association)
    v. Health education (e.g., theory, readiness)
  d. Wellness promotion and illness prevention
    i. Physical characteristics of wellness (including symptom control)
    ii. Psychosocial characteristics of wellness
    iii. Cultural/religious perspective of wellness
    iv. Readiness for change (e.g., lifestyle changes)
II. Management of Data (paper and electronic data)
  a. Individual data
    i. Collection
    ii. Analysis (e.g., cost-benefit)
    iii. Evaluation
    iv. Reporting
    v. Application
  b. Aggregate data
    i. Collection
    ii. Analysis (e.g., predictive modeling, stratification of data)
    iii. Evaluation
    iv. Reporting
    v. Application
III. Resource Management
  a. Support services
    i. Emergency assistance (e.g., food, clothing, medications, housing, transportation)
    ii. Voluntary/charitable/religious organization services
    iii. Social services (e.g., adult/child protective services, food stamps, financial counseling)
    iv. Public health services (e.g., reporting communicable diseases)
    v. Educational services
    vi. Vocational services
    vii. Legal services
  b. Level of care options
    i. Acute care (e.g., hospital, long-term acute care, acute rehabilitation)
    ii. Home care (e.g., hospice, skilled care, private duty, infusion)
    iii. Subacute care (e.g., skilled nursing facility, subacute rehabilitation)
    iv. Custodial long-term care

v. Assisted living facility/home
vi. Outpatient treatment facilities (e.g., infusion, rehabilitation, wound care)
c. Medical supplies
i. Medical disposable supplies
ii. Pharmaceuticals
iii. Durable medical equipment (DME)/maintenance
d. Utilization management
i. Benefit design/coverage
ii. Authorization and certification
1. Preauthorization
2. Concurrent review
3. Retrospective review
iii. Contract interpretation and negotiation
iv. Discharge planning
v. Denial and appeals process
e. Payor and reimbursement methods
i. Payor and reimbursement methods
ii. Government (e.g., Medicare, Medicaid, U.S. Department of Veterans' Affairs [VA], Tricare)
iii. Private (e.g., preferred provider organization [PPO], health maintenance organization [HMO], point-of-service provider [POS], self-insured)
iv. Forms of payment (e.g., fee for service, capitation, diagnosis-related groups [DRG], prospective payment, subrogation, stop loss)
v. Disability insurance (e.g., short-term disability/long-term disability, Social Security Disability Insurance)
vi. Workers' compensation
IV. Processes of Quality Management
a. Benchmarking
b. Peer review (organizations/ombudsman)
c. Best practice profiling/evidence-based practice
d. Variance tracking/outlier analysis
e. Continuous quality improvement/performance improvement
f. Core measures
g. Risk management
h. Health Plan Employer Data and Information Set (HEDIS)
i. Accreditation (e.g., National Committee for Quality Assurance [NCQA], URAC, The Joint Commission)
V. Legal and Ethical Considerations
a. Confidentiality (e.g., Health Insurance Portability and Accountability Act [HIPAA])

b. Patient rights (e.g., Bill of Rights, patient self-determination)
c. Documentation
d. Advanced directives
e. Legal responsibilities (e.g., negligence, malpractice, abandonment, reporting of abuse, informed consent, guardianship)
f. Conflict of interest
g. Access to care
h. Government policies and regulations (e.g., related to occupational safety and health, workers' compensation, Americans with Disabilities Act, Emergency Medical Treatment and Active Labor Act [EMTALA])
i. Quality versus cost
VI. Principles of Education/Learning (as pertaining to educating patients, families, communities, staff, providers, and payors)
a. Learner readiness
b. Learning style
c. Cultural influences
d. Shared responsibility for learning
e. Interpreter services/materials
VII. Tools of Case Management Practice
a. Standards of practice
b. Review criteria (e.g., InterQual, Milliman Care Guidelines)
c. Screening tools (e.g., SF-36, risk screening)
d. Clinical guidelines
e. Clinical pathways/care practice algorithms
f. Satisfaction surveys
VIII. Professional Development
a. Mentorship and preceptorship
b. Staff development
c. Self-evaluation/peer review
d. Professional activities (e.g., continuing education, publishing, presentations, research)

NOTE

For information about the RN, CM credential, contact:

American Nurses Credentialing Center
8515 Georgia Avenue, Suite 400
Silver Spring, MD 20910-3492
Telephone: (800) 284-4378 or (301) 628-5000
Fax: (301) 628-5004
Web site: http://www.nursecredentialing.org

▶ Quality Credentials

NATIONAL ASSOCIATION FOR HEALTHCARE QUALITY AND CERTIFIED PROFESSIONAL IN HEALTHCARE QUALITY

The National Association for Healthcare Quality (NAHQ) was founded in 1976 and is one the largest and leading organizations for healthcare quality management professionals. Its mission is to empower healthcare quality professionals from every specialty by providing vital research, education, networking, certification and professional practice resources, as well as acting as the strong voice for healthcare quality. It currently is made up of more than 5,000 individual and 100 institutional members. Its goal is to promote the continuous improvement of quality in healthcare by providing educational and development opportunities for professionals at all management levels and within all healthcare settings (NAHQ, 2008). NAHQ is the parent organization of the Healthcare Quality Certification Board (HQCB). HQCB oversees the Certified Professional in Healthcare Quality (CPHQ) examination program and establishes policies, procedures, and standards for certification in healthcare quality management. NAHQ also provides an educational foundation through the Healthcare Quality Educational Foundation (HQEF) (NAHQ, 2008).

The Journal for Healthcare Quality (JHQ) is the bimonthly official journal of NAHQ. The journal addresses professionals who are responsible for promoting and monitoring quality, safe, cost-effective healthcare, and provides practical applications and tools for its delivery. The focus of the journal is on quality improvement, risk management, case/utilization review, and the latest regulations from TJC, peer review organizations, and payment systems. More information about the *JHQ* is available at http://www.nahq.org/journal.

The CPHQ is a voluntary credential that recognizes professional and academic achievement of individuals in healthcare quality management. The examination's focus is on performance improvement and includes quality improvement and management, case management, utilization management, and risk management at all employment levels and in all healthcare settings. More than 11,000 professionals have taken the examination, which was first introduced in 1984. The CPHQ examination is accredited by NCCA and the accrediting arm of the National Organization for Competency Assurance (NOCA).

The 1998 CPHQ examination was changed to include more emphasis on case management activities. This change occurred after test writers and statistics showed that hospitals were using case managers more

than ever, regardless of their managed care penetration. Resource case management is listed separately from clinical case management. Resource case management emphasizes cost-effective ways to deliver care, financial issues, and identification of available resources for patients; this may include home health versus skilled nursing facility settings, or hospice versus home health choices. Clinical case management focuses on patient treatment, particularly in terms of pre- and postoperative care, preventative teaching, and posthospital follow-up. Questions about risk management, quality management, and utilization management are also included in the examination.

HQCB recognizes that to survive, institutions must be data driven; therefore, information management comprises one-fourth of the examination. Case managers taking this examination will need to understand data management; what constitutes valid, reliable data; data analysis; continuous quality improvement principles, tools, and techniques; and cross-functional teams.

In 2003, more changes to the certification exam took place. The HQCB Board of Directors voted to eliminate the minimum education and experience criteria previously required to apply for and take the CPHQ examination. The decision, effective January 1, 2004, removed perceived subjective barriers to certification. However, with elimination of the previous minimum education and experience requirements, each candidate must now take the time to assess and judge his or her own readiness to apply to take the CPHQ examination, particularly if the candidate has not worked in the field for at least 2 years. A careful review of all available information about the tasks covered in the CPHQ examination content outline, the sample examination questions, reference list, and any other available data is essential before one makes the decision to apply for the examination. The following are the main domains upon which the certification exam is built (NAHQ, 2008).

1. Management and Leadership
   i. Strategic
      a. Facilitate development of leadership values and commitment
      b. Facilitate assessment and development of the organization's quality culture
      c. Participate in organizationwide strategic planning
      d. Identify internal customer/supplier relationships
      e. Identify external customer/supplier relationships
      f. Participate in developing an organizational vision statement

g. Participate in developing an organizational mission statement

h. Develop goals and objectives

i. Develop and use performance measures (e.g., balanced scorecards, dashboards, core measures)

j. Determine lines of authority/accountability

k. Evaluate applicability of performance improvement models (e.g., FOCUS, PDCA, Six Sigma)

l. Evaluate applicability of national/international excellence standards/quality models

m. Facilitate evaluation and/or selection of appropriate voluntary accreditation process(es)

n. Develop a performance improvement plan

o. Link performance improvement activities with strategic goals

p. Demonstrate financial benefits of a quality program

q. Facilitate change within the organization

ii. Operational

a. Facilitate establishment of a performance improvement oversight group (e.g., Quality Council, Steering Council, QM Committee)

b. Identify the need for a performance improvement team or teams

c. Identify the appropriate team structure (e.g., cross functional, self-directed)

d. Identify champions (e.g., process owners, quality, patient safety)

e. Monitor the activities of consultants (e.g., quality and patient safety)

f. Assist in developing objective performance measures/indicators

g. Contribute to development and revision of a written plan for a risk management program

h. Contribute to development and revision of a written plan for a case/care/disease/utilization management program

i. Coordinate survey processes (i.e., accreditation, licensure, or equivalent)

j. Participate in cost analysis

k. Participate in developing and managing a budget for a department

2. Information Management

i. Design and Data Collection

a. Maintain confidentiality of performance improvement activities, records, and reports

b. Organize information for committee meetings (e.g., agendas, reports, minutes)

c. Assess customer needs/expectations (e.g., surveys, focus groups, teams)

d. Perform or coordinate data inventory listing activities (i.e., what is available from which sources?)

e. Perform or coordinate data definition activities

f. Perform or coordinate data collection methodology

g. Assist with the evaluation of computer software applications

h. Evaluate computerized systems for data collection and analysis

i. Implement computerized systems for data collection and analysis

j. Use epidemiological theory in data collection and analysis

k. Collect qualitative and quantitative data

l. Aggregate/summarize data for analysis

ii. Measurement

a. Use or coordinate the use of process analysis tools to display data (e.g., fishbone, Pareto chart, run chart, scattergram, control chart)

b. Use basic statistical techniques to describe data (e.g., mean, standard deviation)

c. Use or coordinate the use of statistical process control components (e.g., common and special cause variation, random variation, trend analysis)

d. Use the results of statistical techniques to evaluate data (e.g., t-test, regression)

iii. Analysis

a. Use comparative data to measure or analyze performance

b. Interpret benchmarking data

c. Interpret incident/occurrence reports

d. Interpret outcome data

e. Interpret data to support decision making

iv. Communication

a. Interact with medical staff and support personnel regarding individual patient management issues

b. Promote organizational values and commitment among staff

c. Compile and write performance improvement reports

d. Integrate quality concepts within the organization

e. Coordinate the dissemination of performance improvement information within the organization

f. Ensure accuracy in public reporting activities (e.g., organizational transparency, Web site content)

g. Facilitate communication with accrediting and regulatory bodies

3. Performance Measurement and Improvement
   i. Planning
      a. Facilitate establishment of priorities for process improvement activities
      b. Facilitate development of performance improvement action plans and projects
      c. Facilitate development or selection of process and outcome measures
      d. Facilitate evaluation or selection of evidence-based practice guidelines (e.g., for standing orders or as guidelines for physician ordering practice)
      e. Participate in the development of clinical/critical pathways or guidelines
      f. Aid in evaluating the feasibility to apply for external quality awards (e.g., Malcolm Baldrige, Magnet)
   ii. Implementation
      a. Coordinate the performance improvement process
      b. Lead performance improvement teams
      c. Facilitate performance improvement teams
      d. Participate on performance improvement teams
      e. Participate in the credentialing and privileging process
      f. Coordinate or participate in quality improvement projects
      g. Participate in the processes of medication usage review, medical record review, infection control, peer review, service-specific review (e.g., pathology, radiology, pharmacy, nursing), patient advocacy (e.g., patient rights, ethics)
      h. Perform or coordinate risk management activities: risk prevention, risk identification, mortality review, failure mode and effects analysis
      i. Collaborate with quality department
   iii. Education and Training
      a. Develop organizational performance improvement training (e.g., quality, patient safety)
      b. Provide performance improvement training
      c. Evaluate effectiveness of performance improvement training
      d. Facilitate change within the organization through education
      e. Develop/provide survey preparation training (e.g., accreditation, licensure, or equivalent)
   iv. Evaluation/Integration
      a. Evaluate team performance
      b. Analyze/interpret performance/productivity reports
      c. Analyze patient/member/customer satisfaction
      d. Conduct or coordinate practitioner profiling
      e. Perform or coordinate complaint analysis
      f. Incorporate performance improvement into the employee performance appraisal system
      g. Incorporate findings from performance improvement into the credentialing/appointment/privilege delineation process
      h. Integrate results of data analysis into the performance improvement process
      i. Integrate outcome of risk management assessment into the performance improvement process
      j. Integrate outcome of utilization management assessment into the performance improvement process
      k. Integrate quality findings into governance and management activities (e.g., bylaws, administrative policies, and procedures)
      l. Integrate accreditation and regulatory recommendations into the organization
4. Patient Safety
   i. Strategic
      a. Facilitate assessment and development of the organization's patient safety culture
      b. Identify applicability of patient safety goals (e.g., The Joint Commission, Joint Commission International [JCI], National Quality Forum [NQF], Institute of Healthcare Improvement [IHI])
      c. Facilitate development of a patient safety program
      d. Link patient safety activities with strategic goals
      e. Integrate patient safety concepts within the organization
      f. Integrate patient safety findings into governance and management activities (e.g., bylaws, administrative policies, and procedures)
   ii. Operational
      a. Contribute to development and revision of a written plan for a patient safety program
      b. Coordinate a patient safety program
      c. Assess how technology can enhance the patient safety program (e.g., computerized physician order entering [CPOE], barcode medication administration [BCMA], electronic medical record [EMR])
      d. Integrate technology to enhance the patient safety program
      e. Integrate patient safety goals into organizational activities (e.g., Joint Commission, JCI, NQF, IHI)

f. Participate in the process of patient safety goals review
g. Perform or coordinate risk management activities: incident report review, sentinel/unexpected event review, root cause analysis

---

NOTE

National Association for Healthcare Quality (NAHQ)
4700 W. Lake Avenue
Glenview, IL 60025
Telephone: (800) 966-9392
Fax: (877) 2198-7939
Web site: http://www.nahq.org

Case managers interested in seeking the CPHQ certification can contact the Healthcare Quality Certification Board (HQCB).

NOTE

Healthcare Quality Certification Board (HQCB)
P.O. Box 19604
Lenexa, KS 66285-9604
Street Address:
18000 W 105th Street
Olathe, KS 66061-7543
Telephone: (913) 895-4609
Fax: (913) 895-4652
E-mail: info@cphq.org
Web site: http://www.cphq.org

AMERICAN BOARD OF QUALITY ASSURANCE AND UTILIZATION REVIEW PHYSICIANS

The American Board of Quality Assurance and Utilization Review Physicians (ABQAURP) was established in 1977 and has evolved to become one of the largest organizations of interdisciplinary healthcare professionals in the United States. Through its goal to improve the quality of healthcare, it provides healthcare education and certification for physicians, nurses, and other professionals. The ABQAURP is the only healthcare quality and management organization to offer a certification examination that is developed, administered, and evaluated through the National Board of Medical Examiners' (NBME) testing expertise. The certification is called the International Certification in Health Care Quality and Management (HCQM). An eligible candidate must be a licensed MD, DO, DDS, DMD, DPM, RN, or other healthcare-licensed professional. The certification is based on work experience and work-related activities in the area of healthcare quality and patient safety. Other eligibility criteria include 20 continuing education hours approved by ABQAURP and a license to practice in one's specialty where applicable. ABQAURP certifications have been given to more than 8,200 Diplomates to date, making it one of the largest interdisciplinary healthcare professional credentials (ABQAURP, 2008).

The examination contains factual material, application of concepts, and realistic vignettes. Key concepts covered in the examination include (ABQAURP, 2008):

1. Accreditation Organizations. NCQA and HEDIS, TJC, URAC, ABQAURP.
2. Pay for Performance. Leapfrog Group, Bridges to Excellence, Integrated Healthcare Association.
3. Insurance and Managed Care. Consumer Directed Health Care, Tricare, Indemnity, HMO, Medicare, Medicaid, PPO, Point of Service, EPO, Case Management.
4. Workers' Compensation, Compensability, Independent Medical Exams, Return To Work, Safety Programs, Impairment, Second Opinion.
5. Clinical Resource Management. Utilization Review, Predictive Modeling/Management, Medicare Audits, Demand & Disease Management.
6. Credentialing and Privileging. Core Concepts, Re-credentialing.
7. Quality Improvement, Management, and Assurance: Quality Improvement Organizations, Best Practices, Pathways, Peer Review, Statistical Process Control, CQI (Continuous Quality Improvement), TQM (Total Quality Management), and Theories in Quality.
8. Risk Management. Stark Laws, Anti-Kickback Statutes, Anti-Referral Laws, Safe Medical Devices, ADA, Tort Reform, Informed Consent, Patient Bill of Rights, Patient Safety, Root Cause Analysis (RCA), Computer Physician Order Entry (CPOE).
9. Regulatory Environment. ERISA (Employee Retirement Income Security Act), COBRA (Consolidated Omnibus Budget Reconciliation

Act), PPS, DRGs, Health Care Quality Improvement Act, HIPAA.

The ABQAURP certification examination includes case management scenarios and questions relating to case management, including history and philosophy; case manager profile; and elements of a case management plan.

NOTE

American Board of Quality Assurance and Utilization Review Physicians (ABQAURP), Inc.
6640 Congress Street
New Port Richey, FL 34653
Telephone: (800) 998-6030
Fax: (727) 569-0195
Web site: http://www.abqaurp.org

▶ Certified Social Work Case Manager and Certified Advanced Social Work Case Manager

The National Association of Social Workers launched its specialty certification program in early 2000 to help its members attain enhanced professional and public recognition and increased visibility as specialized, professional social workers. NASW specialty certifications provide a vehicle for recognizing social workers who have met national standards and possess specialized knowledge, skills, and experience. NASW is committed to assisting in the process of certifying social workers, and is working to emphasize the importance of employing social workers who have specialized training and experience. NASW's specialty certifications and other professional credentials provide recognition to those who have met national standards for higher levels of experience and knowledge, and are not considered by the association as a substitute for required state licenses or certifications (NASW, 2008).

NASW's specialty certifications in case management examination are based on the seven core functions of case management delineated by the association. These are listed below with examples (NASW, 2008).

1. Engagement. Outreach, working alliance, screening, consent (release) forms, initial intake, and receiving referrals
2. Assessment. Needs (functional and/or psychosocial), strengths, challenges,

opportunities, biopsychosocial, comprehensive intake, sociocultural, and resource/financial.
3. Planning. Service, intervention, treatment, care, direction, rehabilitation, strategic, support, and crisis prevention.
4. Implementation/coordination. Resource/service brokering, monitoring service delivery, service provision, project implementation, client support, and crisis management.
5. Advocacy. Working for systems improvement, promoting client wellbeing and/or client functioning, liaison, and mediation.
6. Reassessment and evaluation. Monitoring, efficacy, effectiveness, appropriateness, efficiency, review/revise, plan, data collection and analysis.
7. Disengagement. Termination, transfer, and discharge planning.

Eligibility criteria for the Certified Social Work Case Manager (C-SWCM) are a current NASW membership; a Bachelor's of Social Work (BSW) degree from an institution accredited by the Council on Social Work Education (CSWE); 1 year and 1,500 hours of paid, supervised, post-BSW work experience; evaluation from an approved supervisor; a reference from a BSW or MSW colleague; and either NASW/ACBSW (Academy of Certified Baccalaureate Social Workers) credential, current state BSW-level license, or a passing score on the ASWB Basic exam. Candidates also must agree to adhere to the NASW Code of Ethics, the NASW Standards for Social Work Case Management, and the NASW Standards for Continuing Professional Education. Eligibility criteria for the Certified Advanced Social Work Case Manager (C-ASWCM) are the same as

NOTE

For information about the Certified Social Work Case Manager (C-SWCM and C-ASWCM), refer to the National Association of Social Workers:

National Association of Social Workers
P.O. Box 98272
Washington, DC 20077-7343
Telephone: (202) 408-8600, ext 409 or (800) 638-8799, ext 409
E-mail: credentialing@naswdc.org
Web site: http://www.socialworkers.org/credentials/specialty/c-swcm.asp

those of the C-SWCM except for the requirement of a Master's in Social Work degree (NASW, 2008).

▶ The Case Management Administrator Certification

The case management administrator certification (CMAC) is sponsored by The Center for Case Management (CFCM) and offered to individuals who have responsibility for the administration function of case management services in any venue of practice. CFCM identifies case management administrators as those who supervise case management employees in various areas of the health continuum and environments (payors, providers, private, or community) with the understanding that these employees perform the following functions (CFCM, 2008):

- ▶ Case finding.
- ▶ Comprehensive assessment of client situation.
- ▶ Evaluation and coordination of the plan of care.
- ▶ Matching client resources to client need.
- ▶ Monitoring delivery of services.
- ▶ Critical thinking, appropriate prioritization, and time management.
- ▶ Measurement and evaluation of financial, clinical, functional, and satisfaction outcomes.
- ▶ Accountability for financial, clinical, functional, and satisfaction outcomes.
- ▶ Effective leadership and communication.
- ▶ Evaluation and response to the learning needs of clients, clinicians, and community.

Individuals are eligible to take the examination for CMAC who meet any one of the three broad categories listed below (CFCM, 2008):

1. General Criteria
   - ▶ Master's degree and one (1) year experience in case management administration or,
   - ▶ Bachelor's degree and three (3) years' experience in case management administration or,
   - ▶ Master's degree and three (3) years' experience as a Case Manager or,
   - ▶ Bachelor's degree and five (5) years' experience as a Case Manager.
2. Equivalent Certification Criteria
   Active certification in one or more of the following organizations (evidence of certification must be supplied upon application):
   - ▶ A-CCC from the National Board of Certification in Continuity of Care.

- ▶ CRRN from the Rehabilitation Nursing Certification Board.
- ▶ CCM from the Commission for Case Manager Certification.
- ▶ CDMS from the Certification of Disability Management Specialists Commission.
- ▶ C-SWCM (Certified Social Work Case Manager) and C-ASWCM (Certified Advanced Social Work Case Manager) from the National Association of Social Workers.
- ▶ RN, C (Modular Certification in Nursing Case Management) from the American Nurses Credentialing Center.

3. Faculty Criteria
   Faculty in academic settings teaching graduate level courses in case management and/or case management related content will be admitted to the certification examination. Length of experience teaching case management and /or case management content must be:
   - ▶ Minimum of two consecutive academic semesters within a 24-month period, or
   - ▶ Two academic semesters within a 24-month period.

The CMAC certification examination focuses on leadership, management, case management, and systems thinking principles. The following are the content areas covered (CFCM, 2008):

- ▶ Identification of at-risk populations.
- ▶ Assessment of clinical systems components.
- ▶ Development of strategies to manage at-risk populations.
- ▶ Leadership for change.
- ▶ Market assessment and strategic planning.
- ▶ Human resource management.
- ▶ Program evaluation through outcomes management.

NOTE

For information about the Case Management Administration Certification, refer to:

The Center for Case Management
6 Pleasant Street
South Natick, MA 01760
Telephone: (508) 651-2600
Fax: (508) 655-0858
Web site: http://cfcm.com/resources/certification.asp

▶ REGULATORY AGENCIES AND ACCREDITATIONS

Accreditation is a process of verifying that an organization meets a certain set of nationally recognized standards. It is a voluntary and formal review process to certify that an organization has the necessary structures and processes to provide quality healthcare services and preserve the rights of patients and providers. According to TJC, standards for accreditation are statements of expectation set by a competent authority concerning a degree or level of requirement, excellence, or attainment in quality or performance.

Whether in a hospital setting or a health maintenance organization, accreditation standards enhance quality and consistency. More specifically, accreditation efforts provide the following benefits:

▶ Establish quality benchmarks.
▶ Ensure accountability.
▶ Increase reliability.
▶ Create national standards.
▶ Reduce costs.
▶ Offer more specialized reviews.
▶ Demonstrate to the public that an organization is concerned about the public's safety.
▶ Identify the next generation of improvements.
▶ Enhance an organization's reputation and credibility.

An ever-growing challenge to all those who provide healthcare services is that all regulatory and accreditation agencies require different measures using various time frames and their own brand of measurement.

▶ CMS and QISMC

The Centers for Medicare & Medicaid Services (CMS) is the regulatory agency responsible for overseeing and monitoring all health plans that provide care to Medicare and Medicaid beneficiaries. As the nation's largest purchaser of healthcare, CMS developed an approach to measure quality and improvement in the Medicare/ Medicaid population. The Quality Improvement System for Managed Care (QISMC) initiative is a system created for managed care organizations contracting with Medicare and Medicaid; audits on performance determine if a managed care organization is eligible to enter into a Medicare or Medicaid contract. The ultimate goal of QISMC is to establish objective and measurable standards that will improve the health and satisfaction of the Medicare/Medicaid population enrolled in a managed care plan. QISMC looks beyond whether an organization's infrastructure has the capacity to improves care to whether an organization actually improves care. It defines, in advance for health plans, what is acceptable, demonstrable, and measurable improvement. One thing is certain: *QISMC is another managed care component that pushes case management into the limelight.*

QISMC standards are composed of four domains:

1. Quality assessment and performance improvement (QAPI).
2. Enrollee rights.
3. Health services management.
4. Delegation.

The basic requirements of health plans include:

▶ Plans must operate an internal QAPI program with demonstrable improvements in enrollee health, functional status, or satisfaction.
▶ Plans must collect and report data of standardized measures of health outcomes and enrollee satisfaction, and meet minimum performance levels.
▶ Plans must comply with administrative structure and process requirements.

The QISMC system for Medicare uses CMS as the oversight organization, and compliance with QISMC is mandatory for managed care organizations covering Medicare beneficiaries. The Medicaid system uses the Medicaid state agencies as the oversight organization; managed Medicaid compliance with QISMC is, at this time, up to the Medicaid state agencies.

This regulatory accreditation is important for any case manager who works with Medicare or Medicaid beneficiaries covered under a managed care plan; the requirements will affect case management activities. Furthermore, case management is important to those who provide services to managed Medicare or managed Medicaid patients. The four domains of the QISMC standards include multiple case management interventions and processes:

I. QAPI
   This domain includes three distinct but related strategies:
   a. Performance levels: Case managers are key players when addressing:
      ▶ How well the care provided by an organization meets established standards for preventive care or the care and treatment of certain health conditions.
      ▶ How well an organization ensures access and appropriate utilization of services.

▶ Measures of beneficiaries' satisfaction with the care provided.

b. Performance improvement projects: Case managers are key players when addressing:

▶ Any component of a quality improvement project that is also chosen to comply with QISMC regulatory requirements.

▶ Both clinical and nonclinical conditions must be addressed in QISMC quality improvement projects. Clinical conditions include primary, secondary, and tertiary prevention of acute and chronic conditions; care of acute and chronic conditions; high-volume and high-risk services; and continuity and coordination of care. Nonclinical focus areas include availability, accessibility, and cultural competency of services. This almost sounds like a case management job description.

▶ Other areas that can be addressed in QISMC projects include "the management of social and psychological interaction between client and practitioner" and projects relating to appeals, grievances, and complaints.

c. Attributes of performance improvement projects: Case managers are key players when addressing many of the interventions that can be chosen to improve quality of care.

II. Enrollee Rights

Case managers are key players when addressing:

a. Communication with beneficiaries related to policies, procedures, appeals, grievances, submitting complaints, changing primary care physicians (PCPs), enrollment issues, billing issues, how to obtain services, federal and state laws affecting beneficiary rights.

b. The implementation of patient confidentiality policy and procedures.

c. Assurance that the beneficiaries receive services that are meaningful to them. Services must be accessible to those with limited English proficiency or reading skills, those with diverse cultural and ethnic backgrounds, the homeless, and those with physical and mental disabilities.

d. Patient autonomy. QISMC requires that patients participate in decision making regarding their healthcare, treatment decisions and options, and advance directive decisions. Patients must receive information on accessibility of their medical records.

III. Health Services Management

Case managers are key players when addressing:

▶ Availability and accessibility of services for beneficiaries, without impedance from cultural barriers, geographical barriers, or undue waiting periods for obtaining care.

▶ Identifying patients with complex needs, thoroughly assessing these patients, and providing and monitoring appropriate medical treatment. This includes access to specialists when needed. QISMC expects that within 90 days of a patient becoming a new enrollee, an attempt at an initial assessment will be made; the assessment is not mandatory (thus, the word "attempt" because of possible patient variables/resistance that may preclude the assessment from taking place).

▶ Continuity and coordination of care, which emphasize the role of the primary care provider as a gatekeeper and the case manager as coordinator and facilitator of care for enrollees with complex health conditions.

▶ That mechanisms are in place to ensure consistent application of review criteria (the utilization management part of the case management-hybrid role).

▶ The appeals process (all phases) and the specific time frames that must be honored.

▶ Completeness of the medical record, which must include identifying information about the enrollee; identification of all providers involved in the enrollee's care and information on the services they provided; a problem list; presenting complaints, diagnoses, and treatment plans; prescribed medications, including dosages, dates, refills; information on allergies and adverse reactions; information on advance directives; medical history; physical examination results; and risk factors.

▶ The confidential exchange of information among those treating the patient; this includes the standard that, when an enrollee changes PCPs, his or her medical record must transfer as well.

IV. Delegation

The fourth domain addresses the oversight of "carve outs" and "carve ins."

Case management skills are interwoven into every aspect of the QISMC standards. It is clear from this brief overview that case managers are of critical value to monitoring and improving care to Medicare and Medicaid beneficiaries.

NOTE

The Centers for Medicare & Medicaid Services (CMS)

7500 Security Boulevard
Baltimore, MD 21244
Telephone: (410) 786-3000 or (877) 267-2323
Web site: http://www.cms.hhs.gov

▶ URAC

The Commission/URAC is an independent, not-for-profit organization, founded in 1990, and known as a leader in promoting healthcare quality through accreditation. It was originally known as the Utilization Review Accreditation Commission (URAC) and focused on utilization review activities. This agency has since expanded its accreditation activities to include other aspects of managed care, health plans and networks, and preferred provider organizations, and changed its name to URAC. URAC's mission is to promote continuous improvement in the quality and efficiency of healthcare management through processes of accreditation and education (URAC, 2008). URAC uses a modular approach to accrediting organizations. What this means is that organizations can seek accreditation through several interlocking and complementary sets of standards; each addresses different components of managed care operations. The modular approach allows flexibility so an organization can tailor its accreditation process to the particular services it offers. URAC offers accreditation and certification programs in 22 areas of healthcare. Some of these programs are related to case management practice, such as those listed below (URAC, 2008).

- ▶ Utilization management and claims processing.
- ▶ Health plans and networks.
- ▶ Worker's compensation utilization management.
- ▶ Healthcare practitioner credentialing.
- ▶ Credentials verification organizations.
- ▶ Disease management.
- ▶ Medicare Advantage Deeming.
- ▶ Vendors.
- ▶ Case management.
- ▶ Call centers.
- ▶ Pharmacy benefit management.

Within each set of standards, the agency monitors several organizational processes. The different accreditation and certification programs have different monitoring expectations; however, the following areas are examples of the processes URAC monitors:

- ▶ Network or organizational structure.
- ▶ Quality assurance and performance improvement program.
- ▶ Utilization management services.
- ▶ Licenses, credentialing and certification.
- ▶ Confidentiality, privacy and patient protections procedures and practices including management of complaints.
- ▶ Continuing education and training activities.
- ▶ Corporate/managerial leadership.
- ▶ Appropriate clinical oversight.
- ▶ Job descriptions and performance appraisals.
- ▶ Performance measures.

URAC's accreditation and certification programs examine written policies and procedures and also ensure that the written policies have actually been implemented during the on-site portion of the accreditation process. This is a rigorous review process, and the organization must demonstrate compliance with the applicable accreditation standards.

NOTE

For more information about URAC's accreditation programs in utilizations management or case management, refer to:

Utilization Review Accreditation Commission/URAC
1220 L Street NW—Suite 400
Washington, DC 20005
Telephone: (202) 216-9010
Fax: (202) 216-9006
E-mail: businessdevelopment@urac.org
Web site: http://www.urac.org

▶ Case Management Organization Standards

In the spring of 1998, URAC and CMSA formed a partnership to develop accreditation standards for case management. A Case Management Advisory Committee was developed to address the multiple challenges a new accreditation program must face. One of the largest challenges was to create standards that addressed the range of case management practice patterns in use. This is one reason that the initial accreditation reviews were focused primarily on utilization management organizations, networks, and managed care organizations. The Case Management Advisory Committee included case management experts, the CMSA, the CCMC, the ANCC, and the American Medical Association (AMA). The case management accreditation standards were developed through collaborative efforts by major constituents affected by managed care. In addition to the broad-based advisory committee, the standards were circulated for public comment and in draft format. Since then they have undergone multiple revisions; the public forum gave interested parties an opportunity to present their ideas for targeting these national benchmark standards. The standards were revised most recently in 2008.

According to URAC, important benefits can be obtained for managed care and other organizations that undergo the case management accreditation process. Case management program accreditation may:

- Assist companies in transitioning from the utilization management model to the case management model.
- Establish a system to measure and assess services provided by case managers with appropriate feedback loops.
- Require high performance standards and public accountability.
- Provide an educational forum to help accredited companies keep pace with best practices.
- Mitigate the need for state-specific case management regulations (utilization management regulations are enforced on a state-by-state basis).
- Highlight the benefits of case management services to many types of healthcare stakeholders.
- Create a forum to identify future improvements in the case management profession.

URAC's case management accreditation standards require managed care and other organizations to establish processes to assess, plan, and implement case management interventions. They also address approaches for ensuring that appropriate patient protection has been established, such as policies for confidentiality of patient information, informed consent, dispute resolution, and other issues. Case management processes and functions considered in the accreditation standards include several critical operational categories as described below (URAC, 2008):

- Staff structure and organization including policies, procedures, and communications practices.

- Staff management and development including qualifications, performance evaluations, clinical oversight, caseloads, credentialing and certifications, and training/education. Information management, including interdepartmental coordination and relationships.
- Quality improvement and management, including improvement projects, consumer safety, consumer satisfaction, and medical errors reduction.
- Case management process, including identification of individuals for case management services, informed consent, documentation, assessment, plans of care, monitoring and evaluation of progress, and termination of case management services.
- Oversight of delegated functions, including delegation criteria and contracts with other organizations or entities.
- Organizational ethics, including regulatory compliance, financial incentives, and consumer protection.
- Complaints, including appeals management and reporting.

▶ TJC and the ORYX/Performance Measures Initiative

TJC, formerly known as the Joint Commission on Accreditation of Health Care Organizations, was founded in 1951 and is the oldest and largest accrediting agency in healthcare. Its mission is to continuously improve the safety and quality of care provided to the public through the provision of healthcare accreditation and related services that support performance improvement efforts in healthcare organizations (TJC, 2008). TJC evaluates and accredits nearly 20,000 facilities and programs, including hospitals, home health agencies, laboratories, skilled nursing facilities, long-term care facilities, behavioral health facilities, health plans, ambulatory care, and integrated delivery networks. Generally, the TJC accreditation standards measure the following functional areas (TJC, 2008):

- Ethics, rights, and responsibilities.
- Provision of care, treatments, and services.
- Medication management.
- Surveillance, prevention, and control of infections.
- Improving organizational performance.
- Leadership.
- Management of the environment of care.
- Human resources management.
- Management of information.
- Medical staff.

▶ Nursing.

▶ Sentinel events.

▶ National Patient Safety Goals.

▶ Performance measurement and the ORYX initiative/performance measures/core measures.

TJC is developing a performance measures library (The Joint Commission Measures Reserve Library) that will provide healthcare providers with access to measures that are already tested and considered evidence based. This will be a comprehensive quality indicator library with performance measures judged by national experts to be valid for use in various types of healthcare organizations.

The ORYX initiative was launched by TJC in 1997 to integrate an organization's outcomes with accreditation requirements. Organizations are required to collect and report performance data on specific core measure sets to TJC as part of the accreditation process. These include heart failure, acute myocardial infarction, pneumonia, pregnancy and related conditions, and surgical infection prevention. Intensive care units, children's asthma, and hospital-based inpatient psychiatric services measure sets are being considered for future implementation. The goals for ORYX include the following:

▶ To increase the relevance and value of TJC accreditation.

▶ To serve as a support system for quality improvement efforts in accredited organizations.

▶ To allow the comparison of patient outcomes between organizations.

Facilities have been applying the ORYX initiative in their preparation for TJC accreditation. It is important that case managers who are in TJC-accredited healthcare organizations understand the quality indicators/performance measures/ORYX/core measures. Often, these indicators pertain to case management roles and responsibilities. Again, case managers are critical for gaining accreditation in their organizations. Information on TJC and ORYX can be found on the same Web site.

NOTE

The Joint Commission (TJC)
One Renaissance Boulevard
Oakbrook Terrace, IL 60181
Telephone: (630) 792-5000
Web site: http://www.jointcommission.org

▶ The Joint Commission International

The Joint Commission International (JCI) is a subsidiary of TJC and was founded in 1997 as a division of Joint Commission Resources, Inc., as a private, not-for-profit entity to extend TJC's mission globally. Like CMSI, JCI recognized that commitment to improve healthcare must occur worldwide. Since 1994, JCI has provided consultation services to governments, hospitals, and other healthcare organizations in numerous countries in Western Europe, the Middle East, Africa, Latin America, the Caribbean, Central and Eastern Europe, Asia and the Pacific Rim. International standards and principles were developed by an international task force composed of physicians, nurses, administrators, and public policy-makers. This task force ensured that the standards apply worldwide, and that they accommodate cultural differences. As of 1999, JCI has been accrediting international organizations (JCI, 2008).

NOTE

The Joint Commission International (JCI)
1515 22nd Street, Suite 1300W
Oakbrook, IL 60523
Telephone: (630) 268-7400
Fax: (630) 268-7405
E-mail: jciaccreditation@jcrinc.com
Web site: http://www.jointcommissioninternational.org/

▶ NCQA and HEDIS

NCQA, founded in 1990, is a private, nonprofit accreditation agency, widely recognized as the leader in the effort to assess, measure, and report on the quality of care provided by managed care organizations. NCQA's original accreditation efforts focused on HMOs. It has since expanded to include the accreditation of behavioral health organizations, physician credential verification organizations, and physician organizations. NCQA accreditation is voluntary; however, a growing list of large corporate employers require contracted health plans to be NCQA accredited.

The accreditation standards fall into several broad categories. Except for physician credentials, case managers have responsibilities that directly affect each segment of the NCQA testing grounds.

▶ Quality improvement: Does the plan examine the quality of care it provides to its members? What is done to improve quality?

▶ Physician credentials: Does the plan meet the requirements for investigating and educating physicians?

▶ Member rights and responsibilities: Are members educated on how to access healthcare, choose or change physicians, or make a complaint?

▶ Preventive health services: Does the plan educate and encourage members to have preventive tests and immunizations?

▶ Utilization management: Does the plan have reasonable and consistent processes for utilization management, denials, and appeals?

▶ Medical records: Are physician office medical records in compliance with the standards? Do they demonstrate follow-up for abnormal results? (Morris & Eppler, 1998).

NCQA realized that although the day-to-day care rendered to patients was administrated by the health plans, it was provided primarily in physician offices and institutional settings. To measure the quality of care effectively, physicians and provider organizations who participate in health plans must be evaluated. NCQA is the accreditation agency that administers HEDIS, which is the forum for this evaluation.

HEDIS is a set of standardized performance measures designed to assist purchasers of healthcare and consumers to select managed care plans based on proven performance, rather than solely on cost. The measures were also developed with the intent of holding managed care plans accountable for the competent care of their enrollees. Each indicator outlines the data collection methodologies to enhance comparability and consistency across the health plans.

HEDIS measures address a range of health issues. Prevention and early detection (i.e., immunizations and mammograms) are emphasized for various age groups (children, adolescents, adults, and seniors). Acute and chronic care evaluate conditions such as AIDS, breast cancer, smoking addiction, heart disease, and diabetes.

The eight HEDIS evaluation categories and example performance measures are:

1. Effectiveness of care. Does the health plan meet the needs of sick enrollees and prevent illness in well members? Example performance measures:
   ▶ Childhood immunizations.
   ▶ Comprehensive diabetes care.
   ▶ Advising smokers to quit.
   ▶ Beta blocker treatment after myocardial infarction.

2. Access/availability of care. Can the member obtain services in a timely manner and without unnecessary burden? Example performance measures:
   ▶ Availability of PCPs.
   ▶ Annual dental visit.
   ▶ Adult's access to preventive/ambulatory health services.

3. Satisfaction with the experience of care. What do the enrollees think about the healthcare services and the HMO? Example performance measures:
   ▶ Member satisfaction survey.
   ▶ Survey descriptive information.

4. Cost of care. This category evaluates the resource utilization and charges to an enrollee: coinsurance, deductibles, premiums, etc. Example performance measures:
   ▶ Rate trends, especially for chronic illnesses.
   ▶ Relative resources use by illness.

5. Informed healthcare choices. Does the health plan involve their members in healthcare choices through use of education? Example performance measures:
   ▶ New member orientation.
   ▶ Language translation services.

6. Use of services. This category documents enrollees' rates of use of healthcare services. Example performance measures:
   ▶ Ambulatory visits.
   ▶ Outpatient drug utilization.
   ▶ Inpatient utilization and average length of stay.

7. Health plan descriptive information: This category evaluates the structure and strategies of the health plan: networks, utilization management strategies (case management strategies), physician compensation/incentives, and quality improvement processes. Example performance measures:
   ▶ Board certification and compensation of providers.
   ▶ Recredentialing.

8. Stability of the health plan: This category evaluates the change in member size or network of providers, the organization structure, and the financial status. Example performance measures:
   ▶ Disenrollment.
   ▶ Provider turnover.

HEDIS is a dynamic standard set. The current HEDIS standards include a significant change by replacing the original member satisfaction survey with the AHRQ's Consumer Assessment of Health Plans Study (CAHPS). For those case managers who work in health plans, this tool should be used as a guide for patient satisfaction. More specifically, health plans using HEDIS are required to submit results on the following measures based on consumer surveys. Case management is a key to success in managed care plans.

▶ Access to needed care.
▶ Getting care quickly.
▶ Physician's ability to communicate.
▶ Courteous and helpful office staff.
▶ Ease in locating a physician or nurse.
▶ Claims processing.
▶ Customer service.
▶ Rating of personal physician, nurse, and specialist.
▶ Rating of care provided.
▶ Overall rating of health plan.

NOTE

National Committee for Quality Assurance (NCQA) and Health Plan Employer Data and Information Set (HEDIS)

1100 13th Street, NW, Suite 1000
Washington, DC 20005
Telephone: (202) 955-3500
Fax: (202) 955-3599
Web site: http://www.ncqa.org

Future versions of the HEDIS standards will continue to focus on outcomes and other measures of clinical quality; however, the effectiveness of care—not merely the provision of care—will continue to be targeted.

STUDY QUESTIONS

1. Do you hold a certification in case management? What type? How does it differ from the others available?

2. What is the difference between accreditation and certification? Give examples of each.

3. Describe a situation where you were engaged in a case management program accreditation survey. What was your experience? What did you learn? What went well? What were the things that need improvement?

4. What preparation activities can one perform to get ready for a case management certification exam? Why do you consider them valuable?

5. What preparation activities can an organization perform to be ready for case management accreditation? Why do you consider them valuable?

6. Does the practice environment of case management matter when it comes to accreditation? Certification? Why?

▶ REFERENCES

American Board of Quality Assurance and Utilization Review Physicians. (accessed 9/29/2008). *International certification in health care quality and management.* [Online]. Available: http://www.abhcqurp.com.

American Nurses Credentialing Center (ANCC). (2008). (accessed 9/27/2008). *Certification examinations catalog: Case management.* [Online]. Available: http://www.nursecredentialing.org/NurseSpecialties/CaseManagement.aspx.

Case Management Society of America (CMSA). (2002). *Standards of practice for case management.* Little Rock, AR: CMSA.

Case Management Society of America (CMSA). (2008). (accessed 9/18/2008). *CMSA's strategic vision.* [Online]. Available http://www.cmsa.org.

Coeur, M. (Ed.) (1996). *Case management practice guidelines.* St. Louis: Mosby.

Commission for Case Manager Certification (CCMC). (2008). (accessed 9/28/2008). *The CCM certification guide.* [Online]. Available: http://www.ccmcertification.org.

Disease Management Association of America (DMAA)/The Care Continuum Alliance. (2008). (accessed 9/18/2008). *Mission.* [Online]. Available: http://www.dmaa.org/about_our_mission.asp.

Morris, L., & Eppler, A. (Eds.) (1998). *Quality improvement strategies in managed care.* Sacramento, CA: Sierra Health Foundation.

National Association for Healthcare Quality (NAHQ). (accessed 9/28/2008).*Certified professional in health care quality.* [Online]. Available: http://www.nahq.org.

National Association of Social Workers. (accessed 9/28/2008). *Certified social work case manager.* [Online]. Available: http://www.socialworkers.org/credentials/specialty/c-swcm.asp.

National Transitions of Care Coalition (NTOCC). (2008). (accessed 9/28/2008).

National Transitions of Care Coalition (NTOCC). (2008). (accessed 9/18/2008). *About us.* [Online]. Available: http://www.ntocc.org.

The Joint Commission. *Facts about the Joint Commission.* [Online]. Available: http://www.jointcommission.org/AboutUs/Fact_Sheets/joint_commission_facts.htm.

The Joint Commission International. (accessed 9/28/2008). *Facts about the Joint Commission International.* [Online]. Available: http://www.jointcommissioninternational.org.

The Center for Case Management (CFOM). (accessed 9/28/2008). *Case management administrator certification.* [Online]. Available: http://cfcm.com/resources/certification.asp.

Utilization Review Accreditation Commission (accessed 9/28/2008). *Accreditation programs in utilization management.* [Online]. Available: http://www.urac.org/healthcare/accreditation/.

CHAPTER 11

Job Stress and Success Factors in Case Management Practice

> "FAITH. When you have come to the edge of all the light you know, and are about to step off into the darkness of the unknown, Faith is knowing that one of two things will happen: There will be something solid to stand on, or you will be taught how to fly."
>
> PATRICK OVERTON

LEARNING OBJECTIVES

Upon completion of this chapter, the reader will be able to:

1. List three strategies for avoiding role conflict.
2. Describe the five steps of problem solving.
3. Recognize subtle approaches to effective time management.
4. Explain the importance of self-care.
5. Illustrate five strategies for effective communication.
6. Recommend four techniques for enhancing emotional intelligence skills.
7. Name three effective approaches to multidisciplinary collaboration.

ESSENTIAL TERMS

Change • Collaboration • Communication • Early Intervention • Emotional Intelligence • Grief • Humor • Hunch • Intuition • Judgment Daze • Multidisciplinary Collaboration • Problem Solving • Resources Manual • Role Clarification • Role Conflict • Role Confusion • Role Perception • Role Relationships • Self-Care • Stimuli • Stress • Support System • Time Management • Time Robbers

All "helping" professionals can succumb to job stress and burn-out, and case managers are certainly no exception. This chapter focuses on success factors that can considerably reduce stress associated with case management practice. It highlights specific areas case managers must pay closer attention to if they desire to succeed in their role and overcome, reduce, or prevent job-related stress. The reader is advised to refer to Chapter 2 for more information on effective skills for case managers.

Stress is the perception of threat or an expectation of future discomfort that arouses, alerts, or otherwise activates the individual's affect or behavior in an undesirable way. Stress itself is not harmful. However, the way you react to stress or cope with it may result in untoward consequences. It is even more

important for case managers, compared to other healthcare professionals, to be aware of their reactions to stressful stimuli because it is inherent in their roles that they handle delays in care or treatment, prevent undesirable outcomes (both organizational or patient related), resolve conflict, negotiate solutions, address ethical dilemmas or risk-management events, and advocate for what is in the best interest of patients and their families.

Too little stress can leave you listless and apathetic, whereas a small dose of stress can provide an edge, a positive boost to action. Volumes have been written on the havoc stress imposes on physical, psychological, emotional, social, and mental health. An optimal level of stress is the perfect motivator and is essential for success. Finding this optimal level is an individual matter and entails being able to read your own personal stress meter. Through self-awareness, it is possible to notice when the reading gets close to the stress overload level. The actual red flag indicators are different for various people: poor judgment, bursts of anger or frustration, depression, forgetfulness, preoccupation with worrying, nonproductive time, isolation, feeling the urge to quit your job immediately, or an inability to make decisions. On the other hand, feeling good about outcomes achieved, content with what you do every day, satisfied with your job, and energized to come back to work the next day, among other positive things, are signals that stress is under control. Recognizing these reactions not only in yourself but in others allows you the opportunity to anticipate how to interact with them as well as recognize when it is appropriate to act as their support system if needed. We all have been in the situation when our coworkers exhibit certain subtle cues that signal to us how they feel (sad, angry, or happy), and based on these cues, we decide how to approach them. For example, a coworker whose voice gets quieter and her handwriting larger when she is approaching "stressed out"—her response to feeling overloaded—indicates that it is time to step in and ask if you can help. However, someone else who exhibits the same cues may signal to us "leave me alone," and we know that is not the opportune time to offer assistance.

How one handles perceived insurmountable stress is also an individual matter. Scarlet O'Hara would affirm, "Fiddle dee-dee. I'll think about it tomorrow." Some call on a peer to help process stress; others may seek spirituality. Others quit or find other nursing positions, as in the following case.

Consider this story from Biller (1992):

> In the early 1990s administrators at a 350-bed, nonteaching hospital in southern California decided to make some changes at their facility. Their goals were to decrease lengths of stay, improve quality of care, and escalate nursing retention. They felt that instituting nursing case management could best accomplish these goals. Three case managers were selected and told they would be in charge of decreasing the lengths of stay and ensuring that patients received high-quality care. At first, the nurses felt privileged and excited in their new roles. Within 2 months, they felt overworked, unprepared, unheard, and unsupported. They all abandoned their case manager roles because of unrelieved frustration and burn-out.

That the administration goals were positive really did not matter. Because these nurses were essentially thrown into their new roles with little preparation, education, or support from staff or management, they were doomed to fail. Unfortunately, similar events still happen today despite the existing expansive knowledge base and evidence of case management practice; there seems to be a lack of preparation of case managers for success in their roles.

▶ ROLE CONFLICT, CONFUSION, AND CLARIFICATION

No matter how much clinical expertise a new case manager has, the role requires many new skills, knowledge areas, associated competencies, and learning curves. It is essential that a case manager has support from the facility's upper management, nursing staff, physicians and other professionals, and most importantly, from fellow case managers. It is also imperative that the novice case manager receive some training (both in the classroom and on-the-job with a mentor/experienced case manager). The hospital administration in the case example above learned the hard way that case management support and training are important for the case manager and essential for meeting the goals of case management. This chapter offers usable suggestions that will assist in a successful case management career.

When designing and implementing a case management program, it is necessary to clearly define the case manager's role, including its reporting structure. Often, healthcare leaders mistakenly assume that the role of the case manager is clear just by virtue of implementing one; or that the role will become clearer over time as case managers practice their roles, interact with other professionals, and build their role relationships. This is an erroneous assumption that sometimes may cost an institution its case management program as well as unnecessarily waste resources (funds and staff), efforts, and reputation, and create resistance to having case management.

Each job has certain key roles; these roles include accountabilities and responsibilities with which come authority. Responsibilities, on the other hand, involve multiple activities that are usually required to satisfy the assigned responsibility. Each activity, in turn, involves specific behaviors for its effective execution. When implementing the case manager's role, it is important to clarify the level of authority you assign to the role. To accomplish this, the job description should explicitly describe the role responsibilities and accountabilities, stated in a simple manner, preferably in the form of functions, activities, role relationships and behaviors. Job descriptions also should include required educational background, knowledge, skills, and competencies that make up the qualifications for the role. The role descriptions and qualifications are essential for overcoming role confusion or conflict.

For example, in a practice environment where the level of authority assigned to the case manager role is not well defined and the case manager identifies delay in a radiology test result, he or she naturally would call radiology to investigate the situation and attempt to expedite the report/resolve the issue. The radiology department most likely would not be responsive to the case manager due to lack of awareness that the case manager had been given the authority (i.e., responsibility and accountability) to follow-up on any delay in care. In contrast, in an environment where the case manager's authority was clearly communicated to the various departments and staff, the radiology department would most likely expect and welcome the case manager's action. Completion of the process results in a common understanding across a working team of the roles and responsibilities of other team members and the critical interactions that need to take place among the group. Role clarification in this case makes all the difference in effective implementation of the case manager's role and ultimately satisfaction in the role.

Role clarification is often required for a team's productivity, especially when new members are added (e.g., case managers), or many changes have occurred (e.g., introduction of case management into the practice environment). Effective role clarification can help avoid redundancies in jobs, empower staff, foster effective relationships among staff, increase productivity, enhance job satisfaction, and improve outcomes. One strategy we found helpful in case manager role clarification is periodically setting aside time to give and receive feedback. This can be done either in an individual meeting between the case manager and the case management program leader or during a regularly scheduled staff meeting. Either way, during the session the case manager can describe how he or she is executing the role, using clear and concrete examples of activities or behaviors. Based on the examples shared, the leader can then suggest to the case manager which role statements he or she should perform more and which ones less. Avoid labeling the role statements "good" or "bad" as such an approach may result in resentment and role dissatisfaction. The ultimate goal of this session should be validation of what the case manager should be doing; that is, activities, behaviors, and relationships.

There is no question that the case manager's role is an interdependent one. It is executed best when there is clearly communicated authority and in an environment where teamwork and cross functional/departmental relationships are effective. Role confusion and conflict surface when the case manager's role, including authority, responsibility, and accountability, is not clearly defined and it is left to members of the healthcare team to interpret the existence of the role as they rightly or wrongly understand it. A prerequisite to role clarification is role perception. An organization can have the clearest and best written job descriptions but continues to experience role conflict or confusion. The reason for this most likely lies in the case manager's perception of his or her role. Case managers will exercise their roles the way they understand and perceive them. If their perception is faulty, the result is either role confusion, conflict, or both.

During the preparation period (i.e., training and education) of case managers for their roles, it behooves an organization to spend ample time discussing role perception and expectations with the case managers in practical and concrete terms. A favorable approach is the use of role play, case-based scenarios, and problem-based learning techniques. These sessions provide an opportunity for case management leaders to clarify what the case manager's role is all about, correct misconceptions, explain what authority means, demonstrate how one can best execute case management activities, and evaluate whether the case managers clearly understand their role and related expectations.

▶ Role confusion occurs when case managers perceive their role to be one thing while the defined role is something else; that is, when there is a mismatch between role definition and role perception. For example, the case manager identifies a variance/delay in care, enters the variance in the log but does not manage the variance or institute action to resolve it, assuming that it is someone else's role to manage variances.

▶ Role conflict occurs when case managers execute their role one way while the defined role is something else; that is, when there is a mismatch between role definition and role acceptance. For example, the case manager conducts a root cause analysis for a significant event when such responsibility is clearly that of the risk manager or quality-improvement specialist. Conducting a root cause analysis may result in conflict with the risk manager.

To avoid role confusion or conflict, communicate with all members of the healthcare team and with all departments affected by the implementation of the case management program and the case manager's role. This should be done as a training and education session, in newsletters, as well as in departmental or organization-wide reports. Regardless of the format, the communication should, at a minimum, include model design, goals and expectations, table of organization, job description (e.g., role responsibilities, concrete examples of activities, and qualifications for the role), impact on the healthcare team, and how each staff member can assist in the success of the case management program.

▶ AN UNDERSTANDING OF CASE MANAGEMENT AND MANAGED CARE

The nonteaching hospital highlighted in the case example earlier finally came to the conclusion that "preparation is the key to success" (Biller, 1992, p. 146). To understand the ramifications of a diagnosis-related groups' (DRGs) reimbursement method compared with a per diem reimbursement; to know the utilization review and management modalities; to grasp the goal of holistic, quality care for an ill person and his or her family—all that is covered in this book. The unique knowledge and skills needed for your type of case management practice are essential for you to be a confident and successful case manager.

Maintaining the most current knowledge base in your area of clinical expertise allows intelligent discussion with physicians and managed care representatives, which increases the case manager's credibility. The mental and emotional preparation also ensures a proper case plan for the patient. It may take some homework time to do this but, as former stellar UCLA basketball coach John Wooden says, "It's what you learn after you know it all that counts."

Ideally, you will be service based and working with patients in your area of clinical expertise. Knowledge of evidence-based standards/treatments and expected outcomes allows the case manager to anticipate the patient's length of stay and facilitate an appropriate course of treatment. This gives the case manager a handle on how much time is needed to manage the case. Keeping current on ever-changing tests, medications, and medical breakthroughs gives the case manager the sharp clinical edge.

At times, case managers may deal with other types of patients. An adult medical-surgical case manager may feel a little stressed if asked to cover the neonatal intensive care unit. Sincere questions to specialty nurses or attending physicians usually elicit enough information to allow the case manager to speak to families and insurance company representatives and to plan alternative levels of care. If you are routinely asked to cover an area with which you are less familiar or knowledgeable, time spent in learning more about it will be time saved in apprehension and questions, ultimately experiencing less stress or lack of confidence.

An at-your-fingertips knowledge of resources available to your patients is a good confidence builder. Visiting other facilities (e.g., skilled nursing facilities, acute or subacute rehabilitation, or group homes) to see firsthand the layout and what is offered often allows you to speak with your patients and their families from a position of knowledge, credibility, and confidence. This makes you better able to demonstrate that the choice you are recommending is a better match for the patient's needs. In addition, it allows you to be able to answer their questions as they come up. A vast world of different services is offered among various extended care facilities, rehabilitation units, hospices, home care agencies, and acute care hospitals.

Perhaps the best resource that a case manager can have is a knowledgeable social worker. Social workers are trained to match the psychosocial issues with the community resources available. An up-to-date resource book specifically written for the particular community or state may be an added comfort for the case manager's office in case a social worker is unavailable. Having a resource book readily available seems to be the trend in most case management programs today. Some organizations have these resources available in paper/manual format; others have them online. In any case, if you do not have one, you may begin to build your own. Take some time to identify your individual case management assets and limitations. Accept both while you turn your limitations into strengths. When developing the resource manual, assemble the following information in an organized manner:

▶ Names, addresses, and Web sites of community resources in your region. List all those that exist in your catchment area or market share. If you have patients from outside your immediate region, include those regions as well. Most of the time it is the exception that presents potential problems and delays in care.

▶ Make sure that the information on the community resources you make available includes home care agencies, nursing homes/skilled nursing facilities, acute/subacute rehabilitation, group homes, day care centers, durable medical equipment agencies, transportation agencies (both ground and air), child and elder protection agencies, crisis intervention teams, police and fire departments, other hospitals and emergency departments, charitable agencies, Meals on Wheels, and so on.

▶ Include information about insurance companies (Medicare, Medicaid, and commercial insurance companies). This information should include addresses and contact information for the managed care case manager, quality improvement organizations, and important contact numbers in case of a denial, complaint, or appeal.

▶ The resources manual should contain procedures to be followed in communicating utilization review and management information, including names of representatives, phone numbers, fax numbers, e-mail addresses, and so on.

▶ Since you cannot be as comprehensive as you desire to be initially, you should update the resources manual over time and on an ongoing basis. Add new information as it becomes available, especially information for agencies outside of your routine catchment area. Revise the resources as the information of the agencies you deal with changes.

▶ Use the resources manual for training new case managers. The manual should provide an invaluable source of knowledge for those newly hired. In most instances, it reduces apprehension, anxiety, and stress. It also acts as a source of comfort and boosts confidence.

▶ EARLY INTERVENTION

You may have noticed that early intervention in cases has been emphasized repeatedly throughout this book. This is because it is so important to the formulation of a good case plan and to the mental health and satisfaction of a case manager. If you were the type in high school who waited until the day before the term paper was due to start it and are still a last-minute type of person, use caution. Crisis case management—cases that need intervention *now*—occurs all too frequently anyway. With too many of these, you run the risk of work and stress overload, poor judgment, inability to prioritize competing demands, and possibly suboptimal case plans. Avoid procrastination and mismanagement of time.

During this early phase, you are free to assess a possible discharge or transfer plan without pressure and time constrictions. Unless a case is very strong for the first plan assessed, we suggest that you have and "try on" a Plan B. Although this approach is not in vogue, if allows you to remain ahead of the "game"

and to avoid surprises or events you are not otherwise prepared to handle. Evaluate Plan A, looking for possible areas of failure, and solve problems in advance. If Plan A does fail—as in the "worry" scenario—then Plan B is already considered and ready to be put into action; 98% of the time one of these plans, or a modification, is usable. This alleviates scrambling for ideas on the day before or the day of discharge or at the last minute when an unforeseen change in your patient's condition occurs that warrants modification in the case plan or the discharge plan.

Early medical coordination is an important case manager responsibility. With complicated surgical or trauma patients, this may mean fewer surgical procedures, tests, or delays. This coordination makes the physicians and the insurance companies happy, and usually the patient and family are more satisfied with the overall hospital or care experience. For those using clinical pathways, they should be initiated as early as possible and followed daily. When milestones are not met, Plan B should be executed.

Early intervention and communication with the insurance company also are useful. First, prove yourself to be a good contact person; this makes your facility or your company more user-friendly than organizations in which it is sometimes difficult to elicit information about members for authorization-of-treatments purposes. Second, find out early in the illness process what outpatient services are covered. This is essential before Plan A or Plan B can be truly considered. It is a real sore spot (and stressor) when a case manager puts together a wonderful case plan only to find out that there is no payor source. If the patient or family has already agreed to the case plan, this can leave them feeling disappointed, dissatisfied, and less than confident in your abilities. It is best to know the strengths and limitations in the case as early as possible.

▶ DEVELOP AND MAINTAIN A SUPPORT SYSTEM

Maintaining a positive and healthy attitude is not always easy when working with difficult or tragic human predicaments each day. Add to that an insurance atmosphere that is squeezing us tighter with every new idea or criteria that managed care can throw at us—sometimes it feels downright unmanageable.

Remember the three case managers mentioned at the beginning of this chapter? They were placed in the role of case manager lacking more than knowledge about managed care and the case management process or clear role responsibilities—they lacked support from upper management and their peers. Upper management gave them no specific role definition to work with, and hard feelings emerged between the case managers and the other primary nurses on the units because the staff felt as if they were losing their autonomy (Biller, 1992). No one in the organization acted as support or mentors for these fledgling case managers, and this hospital's initial attempt at case management failed swiftly and miserably. This would have been easily prevented if the case managers' support was evident from the start and the needed resources, knowledge, and training were made available to them. Wasted time and effort would have been saved.

There are few case managers, no matter how new, who do not have an area of expertise that makes them worthy of being called mentor to one less knowledgeable in that area. Each of us came to the case management profession with a pocketful of information that others may lack. We frequently call on our peers for ideas on cases in which we are insufficiently knowledgeable about clinical areas or resources, and we are grateful that there is someone to whom we can turn. Sometimes we just need a sounding board to vent frustration. Reciprocally, we are mentors to others in our specific areas of expertise. This mutual support system is a fortunate and effective means of reducing stress and enhancing a positive attitude.

▶ PROBLEM-SOLVING TECHNIQUES

There are times when a case seems to be "stuck," and no amount of rational thinking produces the magic answer to the tenacious problem. When a case has a serious variance (or delay) from the expected milestones or goals included in the clinical pathway, a case conference may be indicated. There are two types of case conferences case managers are involved in: a multidisciplinary team-based case conference and a patient-/family-focused case conference. The team conference can include any or all of the multidisciplinary staff members working on the case. The latter includes the family and/or even the patient. They are necessary participants in the conference, depending on the problem being addressed. The case conference should be planned at as convenient a time as possible, with a time limit specified in advance—15 to 20 minutes is usually sufficient.

The multidisciplinary team-based conference is needed when disagreements exist about the plan of care, the discharge plan, or when the payor denies (lack of authorization) certain treatment options or procedures that the healthcare team views as otherwise

necessary. The main focus of the case conference in this instance is on resolving conflict, on ensuring that members of the healthcare team are all on the same page regarding the patient's plan of care, or on strategizing how to appeal the denial. A patient-/family-focused case conference is needed when the patient is in agreement with the plan of care proposed by the healthcare team but the family is not, or vice versa; or when both the patient and family are in disagreement with the healthcare team. The main purpose of the case conference in these situations is reaching agreement or consensus on the plan of care.

Guidelines for problem solving when variance or disagreement exists include the following steps: (1) performing variance analysis, (2) focusing on desired outcomes, (3) brainstorming alternative strategies or approaches, (4) finding the next best intervention, and (5) evaluating the plan (Zander, 1989).

▶ Step 1: Performing Variance Analysis

The first step in problem solving is to identify the problem. It is important to have a clear idea of what you are solving before you can solve it. If possible, break it down into smaller issues or concerns. This strategy makes resolution more manageable. When more than one problem is identified, assess whether there may be a common denominator at the root of the problem or problems. This may require further data collection; it will certainly require gathering all the facts. Using a case conference or a multidisciplinary team meeting to discuss variances, delays in care, or other problems encountered is essential for identifying how best to proceed and to ensure the collaboration of other healthcare professionals in resolving the problem. Sometimes it may be important to interview other healthcare professionals or team members to gather the facts and understand the problem from every possible angle.

▶ Step 2: Focusing on the Desired Outcomes

Identifying the type of data needed to understand the problem is necessary for effective handling of the problem. As the case manager, it is important to focus your data collection first on those data that are directly related to the problem or outcome, then on those that are indirectly related to it. For example, identify what contributed to the variance or delay in treatment. Was it a medical error committed by a healthcare team, member? Was it a patient refusal? Or was it a denial of the treatment/procedure from the payor? To be more focused in your approach, it is necessary to seek the opinions of other members of the healthcare team, whether formally in a case conference forum or informally by discussing the situation one on one. When you develop a satisfactory understanding of the problem at hand, you can then begin to effectively develop your goals for resolving the problem. What do you, as a group, feel would be the best end result to the problem or problems assessed in step 1? What short-term goals are possible? What long-term goals are possible? Are there limitations that must be overcome (e.g., limited social, financial, or insurance support; limited desire from the patient to manage the illness; limited mental capacity to learn and handle self-care; or denial from the payor). Can the limitations be overcome successfully or at least diminished? Can a thorough and detailed utilization review activity take care of the problem?

▶ Step 3: Brainstorming Alternative Strategies or Approaches

Brainstorming is a strategy often used by case managers during a case conference to resolve a problem and reach agreement, decide how best to approach a conflict, or tackle denial of service. Anything goes during brainstorming sessions. Participants are encouraged to be as creative as possible to explore new ideas and ways of looking at the problem, potential resources, and possible interventions (Zander, 1989). The primary rule during a brainstorming session is that all suggestions are acceptable and all judgment is withheld until all suggestions are squeezed out (the stage of brainstorming that our peers sometimes refer to as "brainstemming"). Judgment often arrests the creative flow, and many potentially useful suggestions may never be spoken.

When all the participants have brainstemmed (i.e., have no further suggestions) options, the ideas can be listed in order of feasibility. Those that have the greatest potential to provide the solution are discussed.

▶ Step 4: Finding the Next Best Intervention

The brainstorming session often elicits potentially workable interventions (or strategies and approaches) that may be attempted. This intervention must be realistic and take into consideration all the strengths and weaknesses of the individual case. If no promising intervention is found, ask whether the problem needs to be redefined (Zander, 1989)/. It is likely that the focus was inappropriate; perhaps issues that are indirectly related to the problem were being handled first instead of those that were directly related. If that is the case, do not worry; just modify your approach accordingly, refocus, and try again.

▶ Step 5: Evaluating the Plan

Sometimes, you may not be certain that you have identified the best strategy to resolve the problem. In such an event, try it out and evaluate its effect on the situation. Some problems may require testing more than one strategy until one works. If your first attempt does not work, try your other alternative solutions. Your brainstorming session must have resulted in identifying at least a few relevant alternative solutions. Usually at the close of the case conference, it is hoped that a new, realistic, individualized plan for the problem or case has been defined. This plan compensates for weakness and fills in needed gaps. The case's strengths are assessed and used to their fullest capacity. Occasionally, a case comes along that remains tenaciously difficult; the solutions to the problem remain elusive. Then the case conference may serve as a support system for the dejected case manager, who will realize that he or she is not alone, uncreative, or incompetent. The good news is that although some cases seem basically unresolvable, we have never had a case that did not eventually come to closure. As Will Rogers said, "Things will get better despite our efforts to improve them." The support system around you is essential; seek the assistance or guidance of another case manager who has experienced similar situations in the past or who has more experience than you. No case is worth burning-out a good case manager—too many other patients need your expertise.

▶ TIME MANAGEMENT

There is a story about a strapping young man who wanted to be a lumberjack. On his eighteenth birthday, he set out to get a job in the logging industry. Being young, strong, and healthy, he quickly got his wish. He was given his axe and set out to work. On the first day, he single-handedly felled 12 trees. The boss was very pleased and commended him on his energy and strength. On the second day, the young man seemed to work just as diligently but cut down only 10 trees. On the third day, he cut 7 and on the fourth day, still trying very hard, only 3 trees came down. By the fifth day, with all the effort he could muster, no trees were cut.

The boy went to his boss, feeling terrible, and explained he had not cut one tree that day. The boss asked why. "I am working as hard as I can. I'm really trying, sir," was the reply. Then the boss asked, "Have you taken the time to sharpen your axe?" The boy had not. He had been working so hard that he did not take the time to work smart.

Sharpening your axe, or your time management skills, saves time and effort. Time is a limited commodity, and case managers usually have much to do in their allotted time frame. Some people seem to be naturally disorganized, but like any skill, time management can be learned. Articles, books, seminars, and college courses are available on this subject. The time spent sharpening the axe—learning organizational skills—will be rewarded many times over in reduced stress and frustration. Here are some work efficiency tips.

▶ Assess the Time Robbers

The time robbers include anything that stops us from reaching our objectives most efficiently (Charlesworth & Nathan, 1984). Each person has individualized robbers that they allow, ranging from minor distractions and problems with attitudes to the inability to make basic decisions in a reasonable amount of time. Once these problem areas have been recognized, the next step is to work to make them strengths.

▶ Make Lists

Lists are security blankets. After a task goes on your list, do not waste energy worrying that you might be forgetting something. Lists are the perfect tool for the essential time management skill of prioritizing. They can be labeled, starred, numbered, and crossed out, and details can be added to the main subject—whatever works for the individual case manager. Lists also help you make sure that you are not forgetting any important tasks, activities, follow-ups, and so on. Coupled with time management savers, you should be able to manage keeping your list at an appropriate length. You should be crossing out completed tasks as you add new ones to the list.

Using lists is not enough for managing your time effectively. Examine your progress periodically; if you find that you are adding more to your list than crossing out, it means that having a running list of tasks to help manage your time better and be more organized is not working. Look in other places and see why is it that you are unable to get your tasks done. Perhaps you are not focused on the right thing; you are not delegating to others; or you are assuming others' responsibilities. If you are taking on more than your time allows, you should look for ways to engage other members on your team. For example, instead of assuming responsibility for patient and family education yourself, have the registered nurse participate. You can supervise instead of completing the actual task.

▶ Sharpen Prioritizing Skills

Establish clear-cut goals, both short-term and long-term. Ask what has to be done this hour, this morning, this afternoon, this day. Do those first (in that order). "This hour" priorities may include a meeting, finalizing a priority case that will be picked up very soon, or the unexpected "now" situation that suddenly occurs. A Code Blue on one of your patients is a priority; other priorities fall a step below. "This day" priorities may include insurance calls, confirming tomorrow's discharges, or finding resources for patients who will need them in a few days.

Making the priority list is the first thing you should do in the morning; it is how you can plan your day. Refrain from assigning item numbers indicating the order of priorities because this can be too rigid. Order of priorities changes throughout the day; you should be flexible in shifting gears as the need at that moment in that moment in time demands. Stars are put on the most pressing cases, but often new situations arise and cases not on the original list are put on and starred. This may include situations such as a new patient who needs attention immediately or an unexpected need for a family meeting or case conference.

▶ Be Succinct

If you ask certain people what time it is, they will tell you how to make a watch. Rambling and going off on tangents are major time-wasters and are annoying to the busy recipient of the verbosity. This is not the same as small talk, which in measured doses adds to camaraderie and job satisfaction. When you are on the phone with a managed care organization-based case manager sharing a concurrent review, be clear, to the point, and succinct in your delivery of information. Be prepared and certain of the message you deliver. If you ramble on and go in circles, your inability to be clear in your information may result in a denial of service. Additionally, a few minutes interaction may result in a half-hour question and answer. Being well-prepared cuts down on the time you need to complete a task such as a concurrent review.

▶ Be Efficient

One way to be efficient is to plan ahead. Case managers spend a great deal of time on the telephone and on hold. In this instance, you can make a choice: (A) bring something to do in case you are placed on "eternal hold" (this might be a case to review or your list to go over and possibly reprioritize); or (B) use the time to take a breath and recharge. Choice A eliminates the frustration of wasting valuable time when so much needs to be done. Choice B is useful and necessary for reduced stress and increased production. The important point is that by planning ahead you have made a conscious choice of how you will use your time; you are in control of the situation. No "terminal hold" stress reaction will be initiated.

Efficient use of time also includes not wasting time pursuing avenues that have been closed or are in need of major reconstruction work. For example, if you feel a patient needs a special piece of equipment that you cannot negotiate from the insurance company, take another route. Know when persistence may work or when to look elsewhere. Know the limitations of a case early on, and use your time and energy on more viable possibilities.

▸ Delegate

Some individuals try to be all things to all people. Not only is this impossible, it is a time robber and is often not in the best interests of your patient. If the patient needs a minister, rabbi, social worker, or any variety of ancillary services, provide that person. Initial processing may be needed to ascertain what is needed, but then it is time to delegate. Some people see delegation as a loss of power and control (Charlesworth & Nathan, 1984). Be conscious of this possibility and put your patient's needs first. Some simply do not trust others to do the job correctly (Charlesworth & Nathan, 1984); they live by the credo that if you want something done correctly, do it yourself. If this is true and back-up people cannot be relied on to do a good job, then that issue should be addressed. If you happen to see delegation as loss of power or control, you need to start now to change your perception; remind yourself that delegating to others does not mean that you are no longer involved, or even that you have relinquished your responsibility. You are still accountable for following up on the outcome. You will need to make sure that the delegated activity has been completed and the expected outcome or goal has been achieved. An effective delegator is someone who does not feel tangential to a delegated task; on the contrary, someone who feels intimately involved, in control, and responsible for ensuring the desired outcome has been achieved regardless of who physically completes the actual activity.

It is important to distinguish your own job responsibilities, which are the case manager's responsibilities, from those responsibilities that can or should be delegated. The best interests of the patient should always be the deciding factor. Some case managers feel a legal liability when delegating responsibility. This is not without merit, but there are a few delegation standards that will minimize risk:

1. Always act in a reasonable and prudent manner.
2. Assign tasks that are within the person's scope of training, practice, and responsibility.

3. Provide proper supervision to the person to whom the task was delegated.
4. Use job descriptions as a guide to delineate who on your team can do what.
5. Follow up on the delegated tasks and evaluate the outcome achieved.
6. Keep the delegated task on your list of things to do, indicating that you are to go back and oversee the outcome achieved.
7. Provide to the person to whom you delegate a time frame when you expect him or her to report back to you on the outcome. This is essential in keeping the delegated person closer to you. Over time, it builds effective relationships.

Some accreditation surveys look at delegation with a serious eye. A nonlicensed person taking demographic information is acceptable, according to The American Accreditation HealthCare Commission/URAC; however, anything more clinical will require a "script," and only for simple information such as primary and secondary diagnosis. Therefore, what is delegated and how it is delegated must be given careful attention. Consider the following recommendations for effective delegation, whether you are working as a supervisor or as a team leader:

▸ Stress results, not details. Make it clear that you are more concerned with the final outcome than all the day-to-day details. This provides autonomy to the one who is responsible for the results.

▸ Do not always become the solution to everyone's problems. Teach others how to solve problems, rather than just providing the answer. Again, this builds confidence and independence, and provides autonomy.

▸ When an employee or coworker comes to you with a problem and a question, ask him or her for possible solutions. Be there to brainstorm when needed.

▸ Establish measurable and concrete objectives. Make them clear and specific. This is the road map that others can follow.

▸ Develop reporting systems. Obtain feedback from written reports, statistical data, and planned face-to-face meetings. This does not always work in case management if a particularly tough problem arises; teach employees when to come to you with details, and when to come to you after exhausting other avenues.

▸ When appropriate, give strict but realistic deadlines. This gives the task credibility and gives the person accountability.

▶ Keep a delegation log. This is especially important for very busy people or those with many employees.

▶ Recognize and utilize the talents and personalities of the people you work with. Being a good delegator is very much like being a good coach.

▶ Trust Your Hunches/Intuition

Let's move from the left, logical side of the brain to the right side for a moment. Balancing the logical and intuitive sides of your personality can prevent all types of headaches. Nurses have cultivated "nurse's intuition" since the days of Florence Nightingale. As staff nurses, we could sense that a patient's condition was going to deteriorate. That intuition should still be used when negotiating an additional hospital day from an insurance company or when you have a "gut feeling" that the discharge plan you put in place is going to fail and resort to "Plan B" instead. You are there with the patient and can see subtle changes that sound alarms in your data bank. Once, a case manager did not listen to her intuitive feeling, and the patient was back in the emergency department in 3 hours with pulmonary emboli.

Perhaps your hunch says that the discharge plan may fail in whole or in part. Try to put your finger on the disconcerting feeling and have a modified Plan B available for use. This action most likely will avoid an impending disaster from happening. It may also prevent being caught off guard at the last minute when "Plan A" did not work.

Sometimes it behooves the case manager to listen to the patient's intuitions and not waste valuable time making elaborate discharge plans that will never come to pass. Do not underestimate the power of a patient to predict the timing of his or her death. One 92-year-old asked for help to the bedside commode early one morning, then promptly said, "Oh, please help me back to bed. I'm going to die now." Within minutes, she was unresponsive; within 30 minutes, she had died.

It is surprising how often hunches become reality. Listening to that small voice called intuition can be a truly efficient time management ally. In a recent editorial, Powell stated:

> Intuition is a component of our healthcare life— whether yours or the patient's/family's. When we receive intuitive information from any source, check it for validity, use your decision-making skills, and above all use common sense. We cannot simultaneously talk about "activating patients" in their own care and disregard what they are feeling or telling us about their experiences (Powell, 2008, p. 192).

Intuitive knowing is knowledge about a fact (past, present, or future) without the conscious knowing why it surfaces to consciousness at that moment in time. One may not be certain that it is a fact; however, one perceives it as a truth. When a case manager experiences such knowing, it is advisable not to dismiss it, rather investigate deeper what might be going on, identify whether parts of the truth were missed in the first round, and act on it by revising a plan, offering more teaching, or reassessing and monitoring the patient's and family's responses to the implemented actions (case plan).

To summarize: be efficient; work smarter, not harder; and keep your case management tools (including your intuitive thinking skills) sharpened.

▶ JUDGMENT DAZE

Critical thinking and use of critical judgment are essential when matching laboratory data, radiology results, and the patient's symptoms to the case plan. No case manager should leave home without them. However, being critically judgmental when it refers to a patient's life choices has little place in our profession. A large number of hospitalized patients or patients in rehabilitation facilities are there because of their life choices: alcohol, poor diet, noncompliance (watch judgment on this one!), illegal drugs, high-risk sexual practices, and smoking. We have seen excellent clinical nurses, utilization review nurses, and case managers burnout through excessive condemning and sitting in judgment. They became so miserable (and made others miserable) that they felt they needed to change jobs. We all can share stories of watching individuals (particularly critical nurses) go through multiple job changes; unfortunately, they took their judgmental attitude with them and were no happier with the changes. In the end a miserable person is miserable no matter which job they hold or pursue. It is the personality and attitude, not the job, that needs changing.

Being judgmental seems to be a universal human trait. When you find yourself criticizing someone else, take the time to remind yourself that you have no right to do so because you have no way of knowing the whole story. Someone wrote to Ann Landers once, angry that taxpayers' dollars in the form of food stamps were being used frivolously. It seems this writer was a cashier at a grocery store when she observed a woman purchasing a $32 bag of shrimp and a $17 birthday cake with her Food Stamps. The grocery clerk railed against this use of food stamps for luxury items, and in support of her stance an onslaught of angry letters ensued applauding the courageous complainer. Then came another letter from the "perpetrator of the crime." The shrimp and cake purchaser remembered the withering look of the store clerk. What the clerk did not know was that the expensive birthday cake and the shrimp (a favorite food) was for her little girl who had terminal bone cancer. She was not expected to live out the year; this birthday would be her last. Judging without having access to all the details is problematic; it is similar to identifying a problem when assessing a patient before you complete your assessment and gather all the necessary data. It leads to a faulty case plan and case managers do not have the time or efforts to waste. Minimizing judgmental behavior will definitely lower the incidence of "foot-in-mouth" disease and burnout.

▶ HUMOR

Not far from the Ann Landers column, there is a picture of a disgruntled-looking little guy saying, "God put me on this earth to accomplish a certain number of things. Right now I am so far behind I will never die." We suspect most case managers will live a long, long time. Taking oneself lightly certainly lifts burdens, but what about the use of humor with patients, families, physicians, and peers? Are "needling" patients and going for the "jocular" vein in good taste?

Like other treatments, humor can be assessed using the "rights" learned in nursing school; assess the right timing, the right recipient, and the right dose (not too much). Some patients and families relish a lighter perspective and a break in the focus on illness and anxiety.

> Mrs. Farris' esophageal cancer had progressed to the point where she needed a permanent feeding tube. After an 8-day hospitalization with a variety of medical complications, she had become quite confused. Because this was her third visit on the same unit, the staff and family had become well acquainted with each other. As yet another day ended with Mrs. Farris still confused, her husband pleaded with the charge nurse to give her something for sleep so that he could get some rest. "She's been calling me every 15 minutes from Las Vegas asking for money," he related. The charge nurse, deadpan, asked, "Tell me something, Mr. Farris, has she won anything?" "No!" he responded. "That's why she keeps calling me for money!"

After the mutual laughter, the walls tumbled down. The laughter allowed Mr. Farris a moment of release, and he was able to share his fear about his wife being so ill; explained that in 50 years of marriage he had never seen her in such a state. The ability to laugh during bleak times sends a message that life is tolerable, even now. Often the family needs that healing message as much as the patient.

Studies have shown that humor and that universal means of communication, laughter, have a wonderful array of positive benefits when used judiciously. Humor and laughter can:

▶ Help keep stressful situations in perspective.
▶ Reduce stress and tension. Some educators rely on humor and games during the teaching process, feeling it allays fear and anxiety related to serious diseases.
▶ Help facilitate more serious communication and in some situations neutralize conflicts.
▶ Build and maintain group morale and bonding by promoting a sense of affiliation and cohesion.
▶ Provide a catharsis and release pent-up energy.
▶ Increase heart rate, increase oxygenation to rates seen in aerobic activity, release endorphins (the morphine-like biochemical responsible for "runner's high"), and exercise hundreds of muscles throughout the body.

Humor and laughter are not just for patients. We laugh every chance we get. No matter how stressful the day is, laughter and humor cut through the stress like a laser and make the job worth doing again. Laughing at our own profession also levels the playing field. The following are actual medical documentations gathered by an unknown source, but likely a professional who can laugh at him- or herself. It is difficult to know if these were typographical errors, exhaustion, stress, or anatomically incorrect medical terminology, but they are fun:

▶ "While in the emergency department, she was examined, X-rated, and sent home."
▶ "M.D. at bedside attempting to urinate. Unsuccessful."
▶ "The baby was delivered, the cord clamped and cut and handed to the pediatrician, who breathed and cried immediately."
▶ "Patient passed fetus…two short, one long."
▶ "Discharge status: alive, but without permission."
▶ "Patient complains of indigestion since last night when he ate a stake."
▶ "Rectal examination revealed a normal-size thyroid."
▶ "She is numb from her toes down."

▶ "The patient lives at home with his mother, father, and pet turtle, who is presently enrolled in day care three times a week."

▶ "Patient has chest pains if she lies on her left side for over a year."

▶ "The patient had waffles for breakfast and anorexia for lunch."

▶ "Examination reveals a well-developed male lying in bed with his family in no distress."

▶ "By the time she was admitted to the hospital, her rapid heart had stopped and she was feeling much better."

▶ "The skin was moist and dry."

▶ "When she fainted, her eyes rolled around the room."

▶ "Healthy appearing, decrepit 69-year-old female, mentally alert, but forgetful."

▶ "Examination of genitalia reveals that he is circus-sized."

▶ "On the second day, the knee was better, and on the third day, it had completely disappeared."

▶ "The patient was to have a bowel resection. However, he took a job as a stockbroker instead."

▶ "The patient was alert and nonresponsive."

▶ "Both breasts are equal and reactive to light and accommodation."

▶ "I saw your patient today, who is still under our car for physical therapy."

▶ "The test indicated abnormal lover function."

▶ "If he squeezes the back of his neck for 4 or 5 years, it comes and goes."

▶ "Indwelling urinary catheter draining large amount of urine the color of American beer."

▶ "Patient was in his usual state of good health until his airplane ran out of gas and crashed."

▶ "Patient was seen by the physician who felt we should sit tight on the abdomen and I agreed."

▶ "She stated that she had been constipated most of her life until 1989, when she got a divorce."

▶ "Skin somewhat pale, but present."

▶ "Examination of genitalia was completely negative except for the right foot."

▶ "Bleeding started in the rectal area and continued all the way to Los Angeles."

The Norman Cousins story about how he managed a rare disease with vitamin C and laughter is common knowledge. A lesser-known study shows what happened in a burn unit. An enterprising physician created a humor room and filled it with comedy tapes, funny books, and funny toys. The burn patients were encouraged to recall humorous moments in their lives and to laugh as often as possible. The result: a 13% to 33% increase in cell regeneration over the average (Braverman, 1993).

The Hawaiian Hunas have a saying: "Where your attention goes, energy flows." In essence, this is because joy and sadness pathways cannot operate simultaneously (White & Howse, 1993). Humor and anger, for example, are antithetical; try holding onto anger during a prolonged belly laugh!

Although some nurses have difficulty with the use of light-heartedness when it comes to patients, consider the following story about a young mother of four who was dying of cancer.

> Once, in a workshop she was attending, the woman asked the group how they felt about a 28-year-old mother with four young children who was dying of cancer. The participants responded with a barrage of joylessness, anger, pity, sadness, and horror. Then she asked, "How would you feel if you were that 28-year-old mother and everyone who came to visit you felt that way?" (Braverman, 1993).

For everyone to focus constantly on illness does not always serve the patient. As a patient advocate and a human being, try to maintain a balanced perspective that includes joy, hope, support, and whenever possible, the gift of laughter.

▶ EMOTIONAL INTELLIGENCE

Emotional intelligence (EI) is one of the necessary skills for successful leaders. Those who possess EI characteristics make better leaders. Because case managers also are leaders in their organizations, EI skills are necessary for their success, too. These skills are even more important given that the case manager's role is built on the notion that to be effective, one must be an excellent communicator—better yet, an outstanding communicator. EI skills ensure this quality of communication. As you may have thought, the term has something to do with the effective management of emotions. EI is the case manager's ability to sense, understand, control, steer, and use one's and others' emotions (both whether verbally or nonverbally expressed) as sources of information for the purpose of effective communication, decision making, negotiation, building relationships, resolving conflict, and instituting actions (Tahan, 2000).

Feelings and emotions, whether negative, positive, or neutral, influence the case managers' thoughts, opinions, perceptions, and experiences about a situation, which ultimately influences their decisions, actions, and behaviors in response to the situation. They also affect how the case manager connects with him- or herself and others when developing relationships. The case managers' success in establishing effective relationships with other healthcare professionals, patients, and families depends on three essential things (Tahan, 2000):

1. Perception and awareness of one's feelings and emotions.
2. Perception and awareness of others' feelings and emotions.
3. Perception and awareness of the effect of these feelings and emotions on the situation at hand.

Self-awareness of emotions and feelings raises a case manager's consciousness to his or her strengths, capabilities, and challenges. This allows the case manager to have better control over actions, reactions, and interactions (Tahan, 2000). Control can best be demonstrated when, for example, the hospital-based case manager knows that the payor-based case manager is "annoying," "dismissive," or always "late" to respond, but does not allow these negative emotions to interfere in his or her relationship and still continues to communicate with the payor-based case manager in a respectful or courteous manner, share information as needed, and negotiate resolution on denied services. He or she controls any destructive impulses, regulates his or her mood in effort to prevent stress, and maintains focus on the needs and interests of the patient and family.

Awareness of others' feelings and emotions means that the case manager is attuned to the subtle signals others send through their verbal communication, body language, written words, actions, and behaviors. Such awareness allows the case manager to better understand others' needs, emotions, and perspectives; this is empathy in action. It also enhances understanding, teamwork, decision making, and satisfaction (Tahan, 2000). In the example above, the hospital-based case manager could have easily confronted the payor-based case manager, argued about the exhibited behavior, or expressed concern that such behavior is not acceptable; however, he or she chose not to escalate the situation and remained focused on the goal of quality patient care. Such empathy ensures better outcomes. The hospital-based case manager must have recognized that the timing was not right to discuss the disruptive behavior and thoughtfully ignored the behavior at that time.

Being aware of the effects of feelings and emotions on the situation at hand is essential for their effective management and for preventing their negative impact on the situation, including the relationships between the case manager, the patient or family, and other healthcare professionals. To be successful at managing the effects of emotions and feelings, the case manager must possess social skills that enhance his or her ability to build influential relationships. Social skills include making others feel welcome, part of the team, and at ease, especially during stressful events; controlling one's own emotions and feelings; adeptness at inducing desirable responses in others; interpersonal effectiveness; having a nurturing attitude toward oneself and others; group work and synergy; and thinking "outside the box" and looking for nontraditional approaches to solving problems (Tahan, 2000). In the example above, the hospital-based case manager demonstrated social skills that allowed him or her the ability to control the situation, focus on the task, and manage the issue without compromising the existing relationship with the payor-based case manager.

Emotional intelligence allows the case manager to establish effective role relationships. These can be demonstrated through a relationship with the patient and/or family, oneself, and with others such as team members. Getting along well with the patient and family can best be achieved through careful attention and understanding of their needs, interests, desires, and goals. In addition, developing a case plan that is patient-/family-centric and culturally sensitive demonstrates that the case manager listened to them, has their interests "at heart," and works as their ally and advocate. Examples of how a case manager develops a successful relationship with the patient and family may include respect for their values and beliefs, right to self-determination, and safeguarding their dignity and well-being. Not being able to understand and manage one's and others' emotions and feelings could lead to an ineffective relationship that ultimately may trigger deviation from the case plan or delays in achieving the desired outcomes.

Developing an effective relationship with yourself is as important as the relationship with the patient/family. In your role as case manager, it allows you to recognize when you feel sad, happy, angry, or anxious; with such recognition comes the ability to control these emotions and prevent them from interfering with your ability to work well with the patient/family and fellow healthcare professionals. An example of building relationships with yourself is knowing yourself and taking the time to engage in self-care activities such as engaging in long walks, deep breathing exercises, or listening to relaxation music (especially when under stress) to re-energize or re-vision yourself.

Establishing effective relationships with others is essential to achieving desired case management outcomes and being satisfied in the case manager role. Examples of behaviors that demonstrate the ability to develop relationships with others are expressing respect and appreciation for team interdependence and the uniqueness of each team member, and recognizing that team achievements are dependent on every member's contribution. Others include building a culture of learning, mutual support, respect, and creative problem solving. Case managers with effective relationships with others inspire those others and make them comfortable in social situations, especially when conflict or disagreements exist.

▶ CASE MANAGEMENT SELF-CARE

Case managers give, and problem solve, and give some more. It is like always breathing out and never breathing in. If that sequence continues, there will be a point at which the case manager is all used up (usually referred to as burnt out); it is as detrimental to life as never breathing in. We teach self-care to our patients but we do not always practice what we preach.

▶ Just ask. In work, if lack of training is causing stress, ask for what you need. Be specific with requests to supervisors: If you specialize in medical case management and receive a case that requires workers' compensation expertise, you would probably feel unsure and stressed. You may ask your supervisor, "Can I attend a seminar for this specialty or can you suggest good reading material?" If requests are denied, find out why. Were they unrealistic or was the timing wrong? Is there another way to obtain what you feel you need that can be supported? If ethical situations are more than you can bear, find a support team—even if it is online. If every diplomatic attempt to improve working conditions has failed, consider updating your resume; sometimes, it is a cue to move forward.

▶ Get a life! This is not meant colloquially but rather literally. Every case manager must have priorities outside the stressful world we work in. This is not always easy; everyone is well aware of what it takes to survive. However, finding something that is enjoyable to you—no matter how small—is critical to your health. One case manager comes home from work, makes a cup of tea, and listens to her favorite musician for 15 minutes; she is recharged. It is a small thing, but to her it is essential and she looks forward to it.

A case manager with interests outside of case management and beyond caregiving, who can find joy and excitement in life, has a gift to give to patients. Instead of a tired and weary plan, we bring vitality and creativity. Make self-care a priority in your life.

▶ COMMUNICATION AND INFORMATION-GATHERING TECHNIQUES

Communication is critical in every aspect of the case management process; good communication and interpersonal skills are required to perform effective case management. Without these skills, case management job responsibilities will certainly become extremely stressful. Within the case management process is the need at times to conduct an interview for the purpose of gathering data. This activity has been elevated to the form of "art" and has made several talk show hosts a healthy living. Like any skill, it takes practice. Asking sensitive, personal, and sometimes disturbing questions cannot always be avoided in case management, but there are some basic steps to take and some paths to follow to make it less intimidating and more productive.

▶ Introduction. Introduce yourself and explain why you will be asking so many questions. Reasons may include helping the patient to regain independence and assisting him or her by providing a safe treatment and discharge plan. Ask permission to proceed.

▶ Empowerment. Let the patient do most of the talking. Be patient if he or she has a memory block or an inability for self-expression. Allow the patient to finish all sentences.

▶ Trust. Establishing trust is not always easy in sensitive or vulnerable situations, especially if this is a first meeting. However, trust is essential to best help the patient. Using layman's terminology avoids a language barrier and puts the patient more at ease. Self-disclosure (in small doses) often makes you appear more human. Reassurances that you are capable of managing this case and conveying commitment to it are necessary.

▶ Respect. Maintain a level of respect and empathy. Being judgmental can be picked up in nonverbal body language.

▶ Body language. Observe the patient for general appearance: nervousness, withdrawal, avoidance, congruence. Use all the senses. Body language is a form of communication and should not be ignored during your interaction with a patient. Sometimes body language cues are more telling than spoken words.

▶ Active listening. Listening, in contrast to hearing, is an active cognitive process requiring sensitivity and focused attention. Hearing is what adolescents do with their parents; it does not require paying attention and not much sinks in. Active listening requires real participation and uses attending behaviors such as facial gestures, head nodding, and reflecting back what is said.

▶ Data collection. Use a pad and pencil as a tool to prevent omissions, but avoid taking too many written notes during the interview, because it is distracting and can promote suspicion about what you are writing. If you decide to take notes during the interview, ask permission and explain what you will be jotting down and why.

▶ Questioning. Ask about the major problem first (if appropriate). The more detailed, delicate questions may be answered without asking as the patient talks about other topics. Use open-ended questions whenever possible; these require more than a "yes" or "no" answer. Too many "why" questions may sound accusatory. Attempt to combine several questions into one, so that you are not "firing" short questions at the patient. Example: "Tell me about your family, employment, and what you do to relax and enjoy yourself." However, be careful how you do that. With some patients, combining several questions into one may be distracting, a source of anxiety, or a stressful task. Some patients may have problems remembering a lengthy question. If they forget the details, they may be embarrassed to share that with you or may feel upset about it. Be sensitive during questioning. Understand your patient and act accordingly.

▶ Testing discrepancies. Sometimes patients' words do not match their body language. In general, words are easier to change than the way they are expressed. If the words are positive but the expression is not, consider the message negative. If the words are negative but the expression is positive, consider the message positive. When you notice discrepancy, it is best to clarify your observation with your patient. Be sensitive, objective, and nonjudgmental in the way you clarify.

Close the interviews with a verbal summary that captures the essence of the interview. This allows the patient to add or correct the summary and also shows that you were listening. Interviews are influenced by both internal factors, such as anxiety, and external factors, such as noisy rooms. For some case managers, the interview can take place in the patient's home. This is often ideal because the patient usually feels less anxious. Some patients reside in a skilled nursing facility or are temporarily in a hospital, making privacy more difficult. If the patient does not have a private room, interview him or her while the roommate is having a procedure done or is out of the room for some other reason. Attempt to have as few distractions as possible. Let the staff know you will be conducting an interview and time it for between medications or tests. Turn off the television or radio and close the doors or curtains. Make sure the patient is as comfortable as possible. Always ask permission first. For example, asking the patient's permission to turn off the TV or radio is necessary to show that you are courteous and respectful. Such gestures allow you to establish trust and build effective relationships.

▶ PERCEPTIONS IN COMMUNICATION

Perhaps one of the most essential components to understand when communicating with others (be it a patient, your boss, members of the multidisciplinary team, your children, or your spouse) concerns perception. Consider the definition of stress at the beginning of this chapter: stress is the perception of threat or an expectation of future discomfort that arouses, alerts, or otherwise activates the individual. Perception is also discussed in relation to pain in Chapter 6. What is stressful or painful to you may be no problem to another. Perceptions are totally subjective, and true communication cannot occur unless the case manager at least understands "where the person is coming from"; stated another way, how the person perceives the situation.

Dr. Stephen Covey and his seven habits of highly effective people can be very helpful to the case manager (Covey, 1989). One of the habits is to "seek first to understand, then be understood." It sounds so simple; however, underneath it, is one of the most difficult of skills. Most people seek first to be understood, then maybe, to understand. To truly understand another's perception—which is often the cause of the problem, misunderstanding, or behavior—the case manager must listen and determine the perceptions behind the words; we must be able to see through that person's eyes. One of Dr. Covey's methods for doing this is to give the person "emotional air." Essentially, this means let the person talk! Just as humans require the exchange of oxygen to live, they require the exchange of emotions—the giving and the receiving. The case manager may find a different definition of health, or success, or grief, or hope than the definitions they harbor. Because venting often precedes rational discussion, giving "emotional air" is critical to getting to the deeper issues. Therein lies the key to the goal of matching the patient's perceptions to the plan of care. By doing this, the case manager may observe greater compliance because the other person's perceptions and capabilities have been acknowledged and respected. Understanding the patient's and/or family's perceptions is essential for establishing a case management plan that reflects their interests, wishes, problems, and goals.

▶ CHANGE

We seem to be living in an age of instability. The face of healthcare is changing so rapidly that in a few years we may scarcely recognize it. Although some people embrace change, most find it intimidating; it is change that is at the core of stress. Case management is more important than ever before to manage these changes in the best interests of the patients; case managers are "change agents." New and fast-changing financial constraints must also be managed to keep necessary institutions fiscally healthy. Staff nurses feel squeezed from unrelenting downsizing, and many physicians cannot play by the new rules; they want the "good old days" back. The situation will not go back to the way it was. We cannot change that. Nevertheless, "strangely enough, this is the past that somebody in the future is longing to go back to" (Ashleigh Brilliant). When looking at change from that future perspective, perhaps the state of healthcare today is worthy of another assessment. Compare your job duties to the nurses of 1887 (Figure 11.1).

Collaborative Consulting, Inc. expresses the eight truths of change. There is wisdom in each one.

1. To gain, you must first give up. Every transition begins with an ending. We have to let go of the old before we can take up the new…not just outwardly, but inwardly too.
2. Every transition is an ending that prepares the ground for new growth and new beginnings. The curtain drops so the stage can be set for a new scene.
3. The more you leave behind, the more room there is to discover something new.
4. Distress is not a sign that something is wrong but a sign that a transition is taking place.

5. The lesson in all experiences of transitions is when we are truly ready to make a beginning, an opportunity will come.
6. The only way to get rid of the fear of change is to go directly into the change. "The doing it" comes before the fear goes away. Fear of change situations dissolves when they are confronted.
7. You are not the only one to experience fear when in unfamiliar territory. Feeling inadequate is a universal response to change.
8. Living through the fear of change takes far less effort than living the emotional turmoil and negative consequences of resistance.

Change gets a bad rap. People are suspicious of change. Substitute the word "change" for the word "truth" in the first line to reveal a recurring phenomenon:

> Every truth passes through three stages before it is recognized:
> First it is ridiculed.
> Then it is opposed.
> And finally, it is regarded as self-evident.

Physicians washing their hands before assisting in childbirth; the earth is round; women are smart enough to vote–these were once blasphemous beliefs, but everything changes, even death and taxes. Fifty years ago we did not have the technology to hold human beings on the threshold of death, and taxes change every year. We cannot do much about the fact that change happens. We can do quite a bit about our response to change. Because of the unpredictable nature of change, some people respond to it with fear. Others, realizing that inherent in change is the need to give up something (exchanging one thing for another), react with anger. More positively, still others choose to reframe the situation. Changing how you look at the situation mentally often changes how you respond to it. Here are some ideas to bear in mind when changes occur that may have you feeling frustrated or off-balance.

▶ Sometimes the dragon wins. You have worked hard with the case and used the clinical pathways. Then it seems the case is falling off the path at every turn, and variances (or dragons) are winning. The magnetic resonance imaging (MRI) machine breaks down; there is still barium in the patient's colon necessitating another bowel preparation before proceeding with the test; the family refuses to pick up Mom

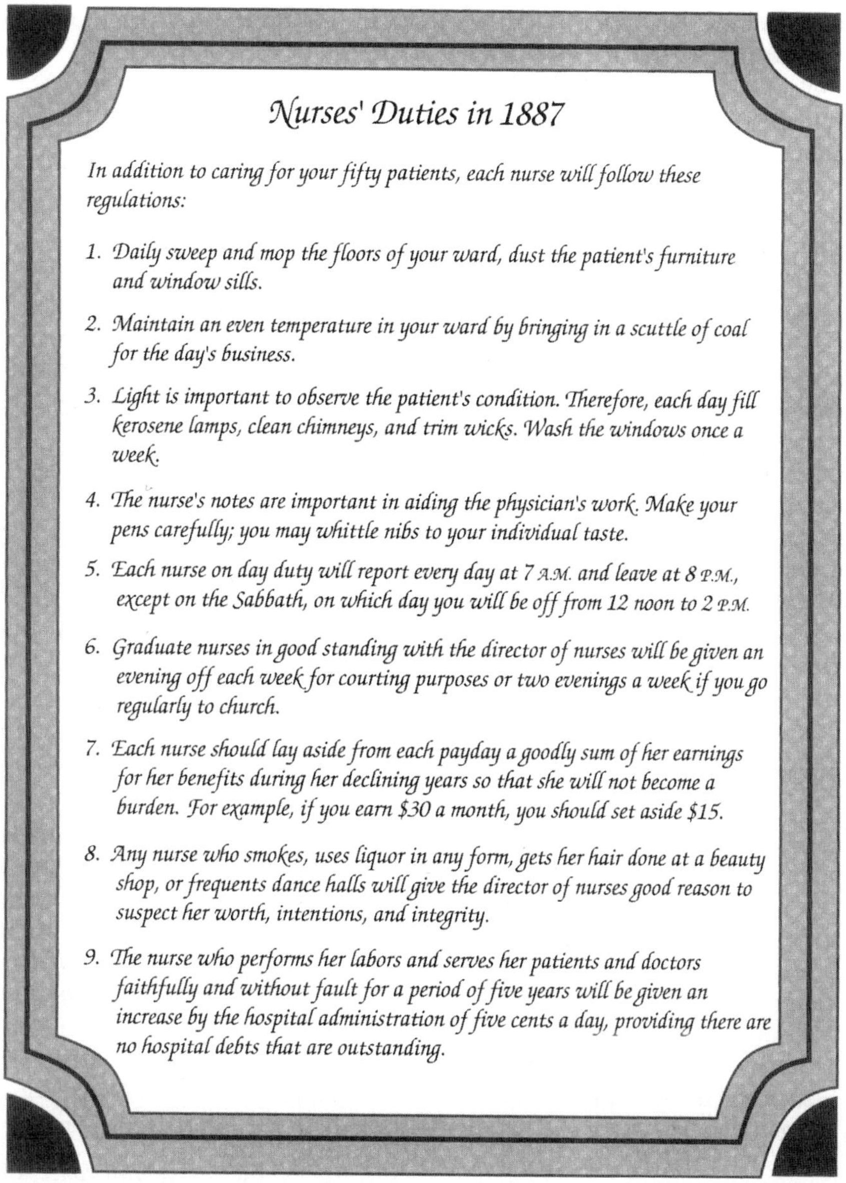

Nurses' Duties in 1887

In addition to caring for your fifty patients, each nurse will follow these regulations:

1. *Daily sweep and mop the floors of your ward, dust the patient's furniture and window sills.*
2. *Maintain an even temperature in your ward by bringing in a scuttle of coal for the day's business.*
3. *Light is important to observe the patient's condition. Therefore, each day fill kerosene lamps, clean chimneys, and trim wicks. Wash the windows once a week.*
4. *The nurse's notes are important in aiding the physician's work. Make your pens carefully; you may whittle nibs to your individual taste.*
5. *Each nurse on day duty will report every day at 7 A.M. and leave at 8 P.M., except on the Sabbath, on which day you will be off from 12 noon to 2 P.M.*
6. *Graduate nurses in good standing with the director of nurses will be given an evening off each week for courting purposes or two evenings a week if you go regularly to church.*
7. *Each nurse should lay aside from each payday a goodly sum of her earnings for her benefits during her declining years so that she will not become a burden. For example, if you earn $30 a month, you should set aside $15.*
8. *Any nurse who smokes, uses liquor in any form, gets her hair done at a beauty shop, or frequents dance halls will give the director of nurses good reason to suspect her worth, intentions, and integrity.*
9. *The nurse who performs her labors and serves her patients and doctors faithfully and without fault for a period of five years will be given an increase by the hospital administration of five cents a day, providing there are no hospital debts that are outstanding.*

Figure 11.1 Nurses' duties in 1887. (Source: Cobb Memorial Hospital, Phoenix City, AL.)

after she has been discharged (why did they not mention anything on the telephone this morning?); the patient refuses every other test and there is still no definitive diagnosis; the patient who insisted on going home rather than to an extended care facility is back in the emergency department within 24 hours. Every case manager can add his or her own story. There is no shortage of dragons. First, assess whether you could have done anything differently for a better outcome. If so, learn from it. If not, realize that sometimes the dragon wins.

- Choose your battles. Once, during an extremely frustrating case, a wise physician counseled a case manager with this pearl of wisdom. Many aspects of case management are completely out of the case manager's realm of control. Assess whether the problem is something on which you can have an effect. If not, save your battle energy for more productive endeavors.

▶ Remember this wise adage. Dr. Robert Eliot, a cardiologist at the University of Nebraska, developed two rules for keeping things in perspective (Charlesworth & Nathan, 1984):
1. Don't sweat the small stuff.
2. It's all small stuff.

▶ Although it is not meant for us to take our responsibilities lightly, from a cardiologist's perspective the present problem is probably not worth having a coronary over. Then you are in the hospital with a case manager managing you!

▶ Change is risk. According to Ray Bradbury, the alternative to never taking risks is not very appealing. "If we listened to our intellect, we'd never have a love affair. We'd never have a friendship. We'd never go into business, because we'd be cynical. Well, that's nonsense. You've got to jump off cliffs all the time and build your wings on the way down." Instead of spending time and energy fighting change, build your wings and plan how you can succeed within the changing environment. Remember, control is overrated; trying to control a situation that is generally not controllable is a waste of effort.

▶ It is OK to disagree. Not everyone has to be in agreement to move forward. One continuous quality improvement technique (consensus) is built on this assumption.

▶ Anticipate changes. Do not wait for changes to happen. This has been said in many different ways. Be proactive. Have a Plan B ready when a change in the patient's condition or the family's attitude occurs. By anticipating changes, you remain poised and alert for them. This allows you to refocus quickly, often without missing a step, rather than becoming flustered. This rapid refocusing necessitates a certain degree of flexibility and spontaneity. Here you stand at the crossroads between what is and is not in your control. You could not control the change in plans, but you could quickly redirect the case in a new direction.

We cannot direct the wind…
But we can adjust the sails. (Author Unknown)

▶ CHANGE AND GRIEF

The insecurity and fear associated with change may be one of the greatest causes of stress. In fact, change reactions have been likened to the reactions one has to grief. In "The Ten Stages of Change," the phases of change are compared to Elisabeth Kübler-Ross's grief stages from her famous book, *On Death and Dying* (Pearlman & Takacs, 1990). The ten stages of change include (Pearlman & Takacs, 1990, p.30):

1. Equilibrium. Here the staff, employer, or manager is comfortable and content with the organization. Balance is the keynote of this stage.
2. Denial. Pressures become strong, and the ability to maintain equilibrium is no longer on solid ground. Personal energy is used to resist change.
3. Anger. There is blaming taking place as well as demands that someone "fix" what is going on.
4. Bargaining. The staff and employees attempt to prevent the inevitable from happening. Often, negotiations demonstrate unrealistic solutions and little concrete data.
5. Chaos. Diffuse energy, insecurity, and feelings of powerlessness appear. Nothing seems to make sense, and people feel like there is no direction.
6. Depression. Self-pity and sorrow characterize this stage.
7. Resignation. Acceptance of reality starts to occur.
8. Openness. Growth in new directions occurs.
9. Readiness for the change.
10. Reemergence. Energy increases to the point that the individual becomes more proactive and willing to take chances. There is a more realistic sense of what can be controlled.

Change does cause grief. Life will never be the way it was, which often leads to fear and insecurity. However, life always remaining exactly the same does not leave room for growth and anticipation (which is oftentimes the most fun part of looking forward). Deepak Chopra puts it another way and guides us through some of these stages:

The search for security is an illusion. In ancient wisdom traditions, the solution to this whole dilemma lies in the wisdom of insecurity; or the wisdom of uncertainty. This means that the search for security and certainty is actually an attachment to the known. And what's the known? The known is our past. The known is nothing other than the prison of past conditioning…Without uncertainty and the unknown, life is just the stale repetition of outworn memories….Relinquish your attachment to the known, step into the unknown, and you will step into the field of all possibilities. In your willingness to step into the unknown, you will have the wisdom of uncertainty factored in. This means that in every moment of your life, you will have excitement, adventure, mystery. You will experience the fun of life—the magic, the celebration, the exhilaration, and the exultation of your own spirit...- When you experience uncertainty, you are on the right path—so don't give up. You don't need to have a complete and rigid idea of what you'll be doing next week or next year, because if you have a very clear idea of what's going to happen and you are rigidly attached to it, then you shut out a whole range of possibilities (Chopra, 1994, pp. 86–88).

Building a safe harbor to cope with job (and life) stresses is no easy task. As Grace Hopper so eloquently worded it, "A ship in port is safe, but that's not what ships are built for." The healthcare field is constantly changing and shows few signs of slowing down. Change is the force that creates, destroys, and recreates. Remember that stress is often "in the eye of the beholder," and how one *perceives* occurrences in their lives can determine whether it is an adverse venture or an adventure. The Chinese symbol for change consists of two symbols: danger and opportunity. Change *is* dangerous; it often destroys systems and structures. Change also recreates, and therein lies the opportunity.

STUDY QUESTIONS

1. Take a moment to remember when you first became a case manager. Describe your perception of your role then. Compare it to your perception of your role today. Did role confusion or conflict exist then? Do they exist today? What do you attribute this to? (Note: if you are about to assume this role use your perception of the role to answer these questions.)

2. Picture a recent day where you had too much to do and not much time to achieve it all, describe how you went about prioritizing your day/ activities? How did you use time management to effectively complete your tasks? How did you feel at the end of the day? Could you have done anything differently?

3. Describe a recent event where you either supported a fellow case manager or a fellow case manager supported you. How did it feel? Describe another where support was lacking. How did it feel? What lessons did you learn from both encounters?

4. Describe a situation of conflict where too many feelings and emotions were exhibited. How did you handle the situation? Did your behavior reflect emotional intelligence skills? Why? How could you have handled the situation if you were emotionally intelligent?

5. Describe a situation where you did not follow your intuition and there was a negative patient consequence/outcome. What made you not listen to your intuition? How could you have acted differently?

▶ REFERENCES

Biller, A.M. (1992). Implementing nursing case management. *Rehabilitation Nursing, 17*(3), 144–146.

Braverman, T. (1993, August). Warning: humor may be hazardous to your health. *The Arizona Light,* p. 14.

Charlesworth, E. & Nathan, R. (1984). *Stress management: A comprehensive guide to wellness.* New York: Atheneum.

Chopra, D. (1994). *The seven spiritual laws of success.* San Rafael, CA: Amber-Allen Publishing.

Covey, S.R. (1989). *The 7 habits of highly effective people.* New York: Simon and Schuster, Inc.

Pearlman, D., & Takacs, G. (1990). The ten stages of change. *Nursing Management, 21*(4).

Powell, S. (2008). Intuition: believe it or not...but place in your toolbox. *Professional Case Management, 13*(4), 191–192.

Tahan, H. (2000). Emotionally intelligent case managers make a difference. *Lippincott's Case Management, 5*(4), 162–167.

White, C. & Hows, E. (1993). Managing humor: When is it funny—and when is it not? *Nursing Management, 24*(4), 80–92.

Zander, K. (1989). Case consultation: Determining the next action. *Definition, 4*(1), 3841.

CHAPTER 12

Practicing Case Management by Proxy

LEARNING OBJECTIVES

Upon completion of this chapter, the reader will be able to:

1. Describe the problem-based learning approach to practicing case management by proxy.
2. Demonstrate the ability to apply the problem-based learning method to the practice of case management.
3. Identify the strengths found in each case study.
4. Recognize the weaknesses or concerns found in each case study.
5. Determine effective approaches to addressing the issues identified in each of the case studies.

ESSENTIAL TERMS

Action Plan • Active Learning • Case Study • Educator • Facilitator of Learning • Issue-Centered Instruction • Knowledge • Learning • Learning Group • Mentor • Performance • Problem-Based Learning

Issue-centered instructional methods are effective strategies used to prepare case managers for their roles and enhance their performance. They help individuals to expand their knowledge, acquire necessary skills and competencies, increase productivity, and ensure success. This chapter focuses on the problem-based learning (PBL) method and its application in case management. We include this chapter to assist case managers, case management leaders, and educators in the application of the various key concepts discussed in this book to the practice of case management. We recognize that such a strategy will be effective because it is learner-centered rather than educator-driven. It allows an "adult learning" approach to building one's knowledge for practice, improving existing skills and competencies, and developing necessary new ones. We consider it a valuable approach because case managers will find it flexible and easy to apply, whether formally in a classroom setting or informally during a round table discussion, conversation, or reflective thinking session.

Problem-based learning is simply the gaining of new knowledge and information through working with problems in groups wherein members reflect on their past experiences. It is a form of instruction where learning is driven by challenging, open-ended questions;

learners work in small, collaborative groups; and teachers assume the role of "facilitators" of learning. In PBL, learners confront contextualized, ill-structured problems and strive to find meaningful solutions by utilizing prior knowledge, experiences, and skills, or constructing new ones through literature reviews or consulting with experts (Duch, 2008; Gallo, 2008; & Wikipedia, 2008a,b).

Active, experiential learning applies a "minds-on, hands-on" strategy and takes place in a group dynamic setting whereby through social interactions (e.g., discussions, knowledge sharing, questioning, and brainstorming) case managers probe deeply into issues searching for meaning and connections, grappling with complexity, and using prior (or new) knowledge to fashion suitable solutions. During the learning process each member of the group of learners (i.e., case managers) may assume a specific role; that is, either a patient, another healthcare professional, administrator, payor, or vendor. The roles assumed by group members are usually relevant to the problem being addressed. In any case, one of the learners would need to assume the case manager's role. When roles are not assigned, group members will need to consider all aspects of the problem (from the perspectives of the various individuals involved in the problem) to effectively come up with a reasonable recommendation to solving the problem.

Beginning the learning process using the PBL method puts learners in the driver's seat: to learn as they attempt to address the problem and at their own pace. They can use and explore what they already know, their hunches, and their wildest ideas to try for a solution. During this thinking process they can develop an inventory of their already existing knowledge areas and at the same time identify what they need to know. Once the learners get a sense of what they need to know, they can set off to question the facilitator of learning (e.g., educator, mentor, case management leader, or expert) and/or their groupmates; plunder the library; or surf the Internet seeking information and potential solutions to the problem (Wikipedia, 2008a,b; Study Guides and Strategies, 2008). What makes the PBL approach desirable by most learners is that they are not expected to simply memorize knowledge; rather, they apply knowledge to real situations. This approach to learning allows case managers a better understanding of what is being taught, instead of just the ability to restate facts.

When applying the PBL method to case management, before case managers learn new information, you (the individual who is assuming the role of educator or facilitator of learning) should present the group of learners (case managers) with a problem you have structured based on a real-life situation, in a way that allows them to apply their experiential knowledge and/or seek to acquire new knowledge and skills. As a rule of thumb, present them with some—not all—of the facts; enough to spur them to engage in a lot of talking—stating impressions, thoughts, and ideas; defending propositions; and criticizing possible solutions. To enhance the potential for learning you must design and use problem scenarios that raise the bar for thinking and searching, and prompt the case managers who are learning to pursue the knowledge with which you would like them to become familiar. As a result of PBL, case managers should become effective problem solvers, skilled practitioners, outstanding communicators, and successful managers of time, projects, and meetings.

The benefits of the PBL method are numerous. During the PBL group discussion and learning activities, case managers are be able to (Duch, 2008; Gallo, 2008; Wikipedia, 2008a,b):

❱ Act as if they were practitioners in real-life situations.
❱ Interact with peers.
❱ Examine and try out what they know.
❱ Discover what they need to learn.

❱ Pursue new knowledge that is needed to handle the problem (e.g., literature review, consult with an expert).
❱ Develop people skills necessary for achieving higher performance.
❱ Experiment with different leadership styles and discover how they react to successes and disappointments.
❱ Improve communication, teamwork, critical thinking/judgment, and problem-solving skills.
❱ State and defend positions (thoughts about plan of action) with evidence and sound argument.
❱ Become more flexible in processing information and meeting obligations.
❱ Practice skills needed for handling similar situations in the future.

The following is a description of seven key steps in the PBL process (Study Guides and Strategies, 2008). Although they are listed in a particular order, steps one through five are iterative and can be repeated any time the learning case managers feel the need to. The seven steps described herein are a guide for those interested in applying PBL to case management. We suggest that you apply them to the case studies shared in this chapter.

1. **Introducing the problem and exploring the issues.** As the educator and facilitator of learning, you begin PBL by an introduction of a "contextualized, ill-structured" problem to the group of learning case managers. You then discuss the problem statement and list its significant parts. The case managers may feel they don't know enough to solve the problem. Assure them that this is normal—that is the challenge and impetus for learning! The feeling of unknowing should prompt the case managers to generate hypotheses, identify the facts, gather information, and learn new concepts, principles, or skills as they engage in the problem-solving and learning process. Guide them in these activities.

2. **Developing and writing down the problem statement in their own words.** A problem statement should be formulated based on each member's opinion, the group's analysis of what is already known, and consideration for what new knowledge or information may be needed to solve the problem. Ask the learning case managers to write the problem statement as they understand and agree on it as a group. When done drafting their statement, they should seek feedback on it from you, (the educator or the facilitator of the learning

experience). The problem statement is often revisited and edited as new information is discovered, or "old" information is discarded. Inform the case managers that it is part of the PBL process to revise the problem statement, especially when they gain more knowledge about the problem being addressed.

3. Listing possible solutions and actions. At this time, the group of case managers has gathered what the problem is and are ready now to start to develop an action plan for resolving the problem. They first would brainstorm possible solutions to the problem, then order those possibilities from strongest to weakest. The group may use a consensus-building strategy to rank-order the possible solutions. Next, the group would choose the best one, or the most likely to succeed, as the most desired action. The following is a set of questions that would help the case managers to design the action plan and to identify their learning needs.
   ▶ What do we have to know and do to solve the problem?
   ▶ What outcomes do we expect to achieve?
   ▶ What are possible solutions?
   ▶ How do we rank the possible solutions?
   ▶ How do the solutions relate to the problem statement?
   ▶ Do we agree as a group on the solutions and their ranking?
   ▶ What modifications do we need to make?

4. Identifying already existing knowledge. In this step, the learning case managers identify the knowledge areas they already possess that they consider helpful in solving the problem. This includes both what they actually know and what strengths and capabilities each group member has. Encourage the case managers to consider or note everyone's input, no matter how familiar or strange it may appear; it could hold a great possibility for managing or solving the problem. This step in the PBL process prompts the case managers to engage in reflective thinking and sharing of knowledge and as a result, it guides them in identifying their knowledge gaps.

5. Determining the need for new knowledge. The group members' already existing knowledge may not always result in generating an appropriate action plan for solving the problem. As a result, they would be required to research additional or new information and gather data/evidence to support their solution. These

activities are necessary to fill in missing knowledge gaps. In this step, case managers are expected to identify what possible additional resources are needed; they may interview experts, review books, surf Web sites, and so on, aiming to develop the most effective action plan. They also are expected to acquire the new knowledge. In some situations, additional knowledge may not be needed; in these cases such activities are necessary to provide evidence that supports the action plan.

6. Presenting and defending the plan of action. Ask the learning case managers to share their plan of action in writing (e.g., prepare a report). An alternative, depending on the formality of the learning session (classroom or roundtable discussion), is a presentation of the findings and recommendations for action to other learning groups. The report or presentation must always include the problem statement, questions raised, data/information gathered, action plan, knowledge areas applied, and support/evidence for solutions or recommendations: in short, the process and outcome of learning. The learning case managers should consider the following tips when they share their learning with others.
   ▶ State clearly both the problem and conclusions.
   ▶ Summarize the process used, options considered, and difficulties encountered.
   ▶ Convince others; do not overpower them.
   ▶ Help others learn, as you have learned.
   ▶ If a challenge arises that you cannot respond to, accept it as an opportunity to be explored. If challenged, present your answer clearly. If you do not have an answer, acknowledge it and refer it for more consideration.

7. Reviewing performance. An integral aspect of PBL is the opportunity to debrief about the process and its outcomes when a problem has been completely addressed. Part of concluding the process of learning is providing to and receiving feedback from those who participated in the PBL session(s). The facilitator of learning should dedicate ample time for a review of performance and debriefing, which should apply both to individuals and to the group. This exercise provides an opportunity for the learning case managers and the facilitator of learning to take pride in what they have done well; learn from what they have not done well; and discuss possible options for improvement.

▶ CASE STUDIES/PROBLEM-BASED LEARNING SCENARIOS

The following case studies reflect real life situations and dilemmas. In case management, answers are neither right nor wrong; the case management field is a fluid, creative process tailored to the immediate, individual, and changing needs of the patient. No two patient situations are alike; each patient is a kaleidoscope of medical, financial, and psychosocial components. Therefore, no "answers" will be given at the end of this chapter. These cases are included for the purpose of discussion, teaching, and practicing case management by proxy, especially for applying the PBL method, whether formally in a classroom setting or informally in a round table discussion.

Not a day goes by in which we lack interesting or challenging situations. Sometimes the outcomes are so well orchestrated that everyone is satisfied. At other times, our hands have been so tied by the magnitude of needs and lack of financial, social, or insurance support that the outcomes cause sleepless nights. Although these instances are rare, most case managers (CMs) with any longevity have had their share of them.

Consider the case of Chuck. All the nurses were fond of Chuck, nicknamed Chuckles because of his bright and positive attitude. Chuck, in his twenties, suffered from a form of leukemia that seemed intractable to all therapies attempted. The only hope for his survival was bone marrow transplantation.

In the mid-1980s, his state's Medicaid plan did not include bone marrow transplantation in its list of covered services. Nonetheless, his case manager delivered a barrage of telephone calls over a 6-month period, and physicians wrote several letters to Medicaid on Chuck's behalf. However, Medicaid's stance was firm—no bone marrow transplantations. Suddenly a letter was received from Medicaid stating that, in 3 months' time, autologous bone marrow transplantations would be added to their list of covered services. Chuck's case manager quickly made all arrangements and scheduled Chuck's appointment so that on the first allowable day Chuck would be ready to go.

On the day preceding his appointment, Chuck went into grand mal seizures. His disease had spread, and he had central nervous system involvement. The transplantation procedure was postponed. An Ommaya reservoir, chemotherapy, and two further bone marrow transplantations were planned, but each time Chuck was too ill to attempt the surgery. He died a short time later.

This experience with Chuck was his case manager's first big revelation about the inequities in the healthcare system, and for a time she felt somewhat bitter that Chuck was denied timely access to a procedure for a possible cure.

The CM can have an impact—positively—on a case-by-case basis. Although it was too late for Chuck, the case manager could not help feeling that all the telephone calls and letters helped to identify a major problem and eventually to change Medicaid policy. Therefore, as you manage your cases, broaden your scope and look for ways that CMs can effect future changes in the healthcare system. To further illustrate the benefit of CMs, the case of Mr. Travers described next demonstrates how case management intervention can change the course of a person's illness curve. The patient in this case was readmitted into the acute hospital level of care within 2 weeks of discharge. This case was selected for case management for the following three reasons:

1. The condition of the patient on admission indicated poor care at home.
2. The home health agency liaison reported that the patient's significant other felt exhausted and totally overwhelmed with the care required.
3. The diagnosis included a recent tracheostomy with a fistula formation, pneumonia, and malnutrition—all red-flags.

Mr. Travers (58 years old) was admitted to a medical floor with a primary diagnosis of cancer of the larynx (squamous cell) with metastases to the lymph nodes and neck. His admitting diagnoses included right lower lobe pneumonia, a fistula leaking into his tracheobronchial tree, extreme swelling of the neck, and malnutrition. On hospital day 2, the home health liaison referred this case for case management, stating that Mr. Travers' mate was exhausted and overwhelmed with his care. Afraid of "causing more damage," she wanted the patient placed in an extended care facility. However, Mr. Travers, being alert and oriented, did not want to be placed in a nursing home; he wanted to maintain his independence at home.

A review of the patient's history revealed that approximately 3 weeks before this admission, Mr. Travers had gone to the doctor's office with a 2-month history of hoarseness. He underwent endoscopy; a massive tumor was found; and a tracheostomy was immediately placed to relieve airway compromise. The following day, the surgeons performed a total laryngectomy, partial pharyngectomy, and a left radical neck dissection. His postoperative course included fever and major swelling of the neck after the removal of two Jackson-Pratt drains, necessitating a reopening of the neck wound and reinsertion of one drain.

Mr. Travers remained in the hospital for 10 days. During this time, a home health agency was consulted and met with him and his mate. A speech therapist referred him to the American Cancer Society for support and a "loaner" electrolarynx; she also conducted a brief session on stoma care and recommended one or two speech therapy visits at home. However, the electrolarynx was not obtained, and Mr. Travers health insurance plan would not pay for home speech therapy visits; stating that "he is ineligible and did not meet criteria."

During the first hospitalization, nurses performed all stoma care, changing of inner cannulas, and tube feeding care. The day before discharge, a nurse reported that Mr. Travers' mate refused to learn tracheostomy care. This was the first time anyone had broached the subject, and the mate was fearful, stating that she preferred an extended care facility stay. On the day of discharge, the physician's orders were the following:

▶ Discharge home with Jackson-Pratt bulb suction.
▶ Discharge to home health or extended care facility.
▶ Needs: tracheostomy care, tube feeding, empty Jackson-Pratt bulb each day, and office visit in 4 to 5 days.

On the day of discharge, the discharge nurse instructed the patient and his mate in the following:

▶ Various aspects of tracheostomy care.
▶ How to change the inner cannula.
▶ How to clean the stoma.
▶ How to redress the stoma.
▶ How to flush the feeding tube with water.
▶ How to empty the Jackson-Pratt drain.

Written instructions were given and a home health nurse was authorized for two to three visits for tube feeding purposes. No equipment other than a feeding pump and oxygen was obtained for this patient and no social services were requested.

Mr. Travers received no teaching. He did not know how to suction himself, clean and dress his tracheostomy, or set up his tube feedings and pump. He did not even know how to cough correctly; he covered his mouth (as was his habit since childhood), and sputum was expelled out of his tracheostomy. Although his mate was very supportive, she was unsure of herself and needed more help.

Mr. Travers was readmitted to the hospital with the tracheostomy grossly infected; suctioning revealed significant amounts of bloody sputum with clots. Treatment included intravenous antibiotics, frequent suctioning every 2 to 4 hours, intravenous fluids, chest percussion therapy, and small volume nebulizer (SVN) treatments every 2 to 4 hours, and tube feedings for malnutrition. A social service consult was placed.

This time the nurse case manager assessed Mr. Travers' needs and self-care capabilities with the medical staff, the social worker, the patient, and the patient's mate. They came to agreement that the hospital days would be used for intensive teaching in addition to healing the fistula and treating the pneumonia. If Mr. Travers could become independent in self-care, his mate might not feel so overwhelmed.

After the infection started subsiding, orders were written for respiratory therapists to teach all aspects of self-suctioning. Mr. Travers quickly became proficient at suctioning, along with tracheostomy cleaning and redressing. Another order was written for nurses to teach the patient to administer his own tube feeding independently; again, Mr. Travers quickly learned to do this.

The speech therapist requested that a barium swallow study be performed near the day of discharge, which showed only one questionable, tiny fistula remaining and little or no aspiration. Puréed foods were added, which the patient had no difficulty swallowing. The dietary department helped him by teaching nutritious combinations and incorporated some of his favorite foods in puréed form. Because Mr. Travers had lost about 30 pounds before his initial surgery, the physician chose to continue tube feedings at 75 mL/hour from 9:00 P.M. to 7:00 A.M. each day, in addition to his puréed diet. Again, Mr. Travers was encouraged to obtain the electrolarynx from the

American Cancer Society, because his Medicaid plan would not cover the cost of one for him. Home health visits were reinstated.

During the hospitalization, a catheter was inserted into the fistula and placed to suction. The fistula gradually closed, allowing the discontinuation of that catheter before discharge. Mr. Travers' pneumonia cleared up, and he was discharged with liquid antibiotics. The following items were set up or ordered for Mr. Travers on discharge:

- A hospital bed.
- A bedside commode (from the American Cancer Society).
- A shower chair (from the American Cancer Society).
- Feeding bags, tubing, and feeding solution were ordered. Mr. Travers was given his new feeding schedule. A tube feeding pump was already in the home.
- A portable oxygen tank to allow more mobility and an aerosol set-up for the tracheotomy wound to reduce the chance of infection and bleeding from dryness. (Oxygen was already in the home.)
- A suction machine and catheters were ordered because Mr. Travers still required intermittent suctioning.
- Tracheostomy and stoma supplies including dressings, tracheostomy ties, peroxide and normal saline solutions, and cleaning brushes. (Mr. Travers' type of tracheostomy was changed during this admission, and he no longer required inner cannulas.)

This time, when Mr. Travers was discharged, both he and his mate were comfortable doing the tasks required. Because Mr. Travers was independent in his self-care, his mate did not feel solely responsible. In addition, Mr. Travers felt more in control of his situation and less depressed.

At a certain point in Mr. Travers' disease process, a short stay in an extended care facility was needed for strengthening and finishing up a course of intravenous antibiotics. At this point, a hospice referral was initiated because of his advanced stage of cancer. Through the care of the hospice attendants, Mr. Travers was able to return home, as was his wish. He died shortly after, with hospice and loved ones present.

Without case management, Mr. Travers and his family experienced exhaustion, frustration, and a preventable deteriorating condition. Case management added the element of self-care and independence to his life, allowing the remainder of his life to be lived at home, which was his wish. This patient received quality care. Because the family and patient provided the remainder of his care at home with intermittent home health and finally hospice visits, his care was also cost effective.

We have seen many patients who were not provided with the skills of a case manager. In general, these patients stay in the hospital too long because the diagnostic and treatment portions of their care are drawn out; they often contract nosocomial infections, which further extend their stays.

Examples of poorly managed care—in hospitals and extended care facilities or in the community—are common. For example, patients may be subjected to two operations (one for a foot and bone debridement and one for a long-term intravenous access) when one operation may suffice. Perhaps home healthcare is ordered when the skills and emotional support of hospice case management are more appropriate. Conversely, perhaps more support is ordered than was required merely because a thorough psychosocial assessment was not performed. This assessment might reveal a strong formal and informal patient support system, which could easily have met all the unskilled needs that the patient required. Subjecting the patient to professional agencies, often at a high premium for the patient, may not be in the patient's best interests.

An analysis of cases that received case management, compared with those that have been poorly managed, reveals that quality care *is* cost-effective care. A case that has been skillfully assessed and creatively planned should translate into the two main goals of case management and managed care: quality of patient care and the wise use of healthcare resources.

❯ DIRECTIONS FOR PRACTICING CASE MANAGEMENT BY PROXY

The remainder of this chapter contains a number of case studies that can be used for further training and education purposes and for practicing case management by proxy. We suggest that the case management expert facilitating the learning experience modify the case studies as necessary to meet the desired learning objectives as well as the needs of the learning case managers group involved in PBL. Although it may not be necessary, we also suggest that the expert facilitating learning develop a set of case-study–specific questions based on the case circumstance to be used, in addition to the general questions listed below under seven main areas of case management practice.

We advise you to approach each case study as a PBL opportunity. Discuss the case study in a group and apply the seven key steps of PBL described earlier, as well as attempt to answer, to the degree they are applicable, the questions listed in the following seven major aspects of learning case management.

1. Look at role definitions, skills, and knowledge.
   - What might the case manager do in this situation?
   - What value might the social worker be in this circumstance?
   - What might the case manager–social worker team share or do together?
   - What value might other health professionals be in this circumstance?
   - What knowledge and skills are necessary to effectively manage the situation?
   - Do you already possess the knowledge and skills required to solve the problems?
   - What new knowledge and skills might you need to effectively handle the situation?
   - Where and how will you make sure you acquire the new knowledge and skills?

2. Assess strengths in each case study.
   - Is there a strong support system? This may include family, significant others, friends, neighbors, and any informal support that can be tapped.
   - Are the patient and/or family able to handle the situation?
   - Does the patient or family have the financial ability to provide the patient with the optimal circumstances?
   - Is the insurance policy adequate to meet the needs assessed for medical care and discharge or transitional planning?
   - Are the patient's own emotional, mental, social, psychological, and spiritual resources positive?

3. Consider the limitations in each case.
   - Assess any knowledge deficit, in the patient, family, and in any caregivers.
   - Assess the limitations of insurance coverage.
   - Assess limitation or lack of social support.
   - Assess housing or homelessness.
   - Assess limitations due to poor medical status that cannot be changed or improved.
   - Consider the limitations resulting from nonadherence to the medical regimen.
   - Assess limitations from poor financial status.
   - Assess which limitations might be improved and how this can be best accomplished.

4. Think about the case management plan during hospitalization.
   - Actualize a comprehensive case management/medical plan.
   - Determine appropriate utilization of resources.
   - Evaluate the patient's financial status. including presence of health insurance.
   - Examine the appropriateness of the level of care based on acuity of patient's condition and healthcare resources needed.
   - Determine whether authorizations, by payor for services, were obtained. Discuss the necessity of authorizations.
   - Actualize a tight transitional/discharge plan.
   - Assess for quality of care and use of standardized medical guidelines.
   - Assess the status of advance medical directives.

5. Consider the patient's needs for posthospital care.
   - Determine placement and discharge needs.
   - Determine the need for authorization by the payor for services, level of care, transitions, and so on.
   - Assess availability of insurance coverage, either private insurance or Medicaid/Medicare.
   - Assess availability of public community resources.
   - Determine the level of rehabilitation needed. This may range in scope from in-home physical, speech, or occupational therapies to acute (inpatient) or subacute rehabilitation.
   - Assess the home environment for safety.

6. Consider other miscellaneous issues.
   - Are there any psychological issues, such as mental capacity/competency, grave disability, danger to self, and danger to others?
   - Are there any substance abuse issues?
   - Are there any adult or child abuse issues?
   - Assess the need for ethics committee involvement.
   - Determine any legal and risk management issues that need attention.
   - Finally, ask the question, "Is this a case in which everything that could be done was attempted but still failed?" If so, do not be discouraged. Remember that sometimes the dragon wins.

7. Take time to evaluate and reflect.
   ▶ Examine whether the interventions worked; if not why? if yes, offer rationale.
   ▶ Explain your views of the situation. What would you have done differently? Provide a rationale for your actions.
   ▶ Think about what you already know that is applicable to the case study and what areas for additional learning were brought out by the case study.

CASE STUDIES

CASE STUDY 1: MR. TIMMER

Mr. Timmer, age 76, arrived at the emergency department on a Thursday evening complaining of chest and abdominal pain. Although generally a poor historian, he did manage to convey to the staff that he had suffered gunshot and bayonet wounds and malaria as a POW during World War II. He also stated that he has had pneumonia.

The electrocardiogram (ECG) taken in the emergency department showed an acute anterolateral myocardial infarction (MI). Since he was not eligible for a primary angioplasty, tissue plasminogen activator was immediately started with effective results. His chest radiograph revealed cardiomegaly and questionable congestive heart failure. His breath sounds were described as tubular; no pedal pulses could be appreciated.

In questioning Mr. Timmer, emergency department personnel found his living situation to be transient; currently, he was residing in a motel. He had two children but did not know where they were or how to get in touch with them. They had not spoken for a few years.

Mr. Timmer was admitted to the intensive care unit (ICU), where tissue plasminogen activator was continued, along with heparin, Tridil, and lidocaine drips as well as IV methylprednisolone (Solu-Medrol). An echocardiogram, abdominal ultrasonography, and cardiac catheterization were ordered.

On hospital day 2, the ultrasound examination showed cholelithiasis. On day 3, Mr. Timmer was moved to a telemetry floor level of care. A cardiac catheterization, originally scheduled for Monday (day 5), was rescheduled for Tuesday (day 6) because of catheterization laboratory scheduling conflicts.

The cardiac catheterization revealed the need for a triple coronary artery bypass graft (CABG X 3). Surgery was performed the following day, day 7.

Mr. Timmer was on an intra-aortic balloon pump until day 9 (postoperative day 2) and went to the telemetry floor on day 11 (postoperative day 4).

Day 12. Mr. Timmer complained of being too weak to ambulate; cardiac rehabilitation was ordered. His oxygen was increased from 2 to 4 L per nasal cannula. Small volume nebulizer treatments were added for diminished breath sounds and egophony in the left base.

Day 13. Mr. Timmer again refused to leave his room to ambulate.

Day 14. Mr. Timmer still refused to work with cardiac rehabilitation staff. A social service consultation was ordered.

Day 15. Complaints of weakness continued. A chest radiograph revealed atelectasis and small pleural effusions. A multigated acquisition (MUGA) scan was performed.

Day 16. Arterial blood gases with patient on 2 L of oxygen showed an oxygen saturation of 97%; therefore, Mr. Timmer's oxygen was discontinued. He still refused to leave his room for cardiac rehabilitation.

Day 17. The MUGA scan taken 2 days previously was read and revealed an adequate ejection fraction of 48%. A transfer for the following day to a skilled nursing facility (SNF) was requested. Social service personnel saw the patient and began working on a transfer to a veterans' facility.

Day 18. On the planned day of transfer, Mr. Timmer complained again of chest pain. Because of the patient's sedentary postoperative course, physicians felt the need to rule out pulmonary emboli and ordered a ventilation/qualification (V/Q) scan.

Day 20. V/Q scan was negative. An adenosine Cardiolite stress test was performed; it showed no MI or ischemia. Still, the patient complained of chest pain. The chest radiograph showed atelectasis without any change from the last radiograph. Mr. Timmer began to ambulate 40 feet with a minimum assistance of two people. He was told he would be transferred the next day. On hearing this news, the patient expressed suicide ideation but refused to speak to a psychiatrist for a consult.

Day 21. Patient was transferred to a respite center.

CASE STUDY 2: JIMMY

Twelve-year-old Jimmy was normal and healthy until 3 years ago. At that time, Jimmy developed a severe, unsubsiding headache. Magnetic resonance imaging (MRI) scanning performed 3 months later showed carotid and basilar aneurysms. Several months after that, Jimmy suffered a brain-stem stroke. A basilar aneurysm clipping was performed, but the basilar artery remained thrombosed postoperatively.

A long and stormy course followed surgery, with vocal cord paralysis and pneumonia manifesting as complicating factors. Jimmy worked tirelessly in an inpatient rehabilitation unit and was eventually able to return to school, where he was a well-liked "A" student. Nearly 2 years later, Jimmy suddenly developed seizure activity. A residual right-sided weakness in this right-handed adolescent was disconcerting. A computed tomography (CT) scan again revealed the carotid aneurysm. A carotid repair and bypass were performed. According to records, Jimmy did well postoperatively and was discharged home.

The day after discharge, a fever and recurrent seizure occurred. An electroencephalogram (EEG) and MRI were both abnormal. Herpes viral titers proved to be high; Jimmy was treated with the appropriate medication, acyclovir, and restarted on dexamethasone for presumed herpes encephalitis. Urinary tract infections and gastrointestinal (GI) problems were also identified. Inpatient rehabilitation was again provided, and soon Jimmy "graduated" to a day rehabilitation unit. Because of constant GI upsets and frequency of urination, the day hospital could not continue to provide care.

Multiple urinalysis cultures, with occasional exceptions, were negative. Jimmy responded well to an oral antibiotic prescribed for the presumed urinary tract infection.

Jimmy's GI symptoms persisted. GI workups were performed several times, with few conclusive returns. An esophagogastroduodenoscopy (EGD) showed mild gastroparesis. Jimmy showed a low iron level on laboratory tests, but his mother stopped his iron at home because of GI complaints.

Jimmy is now readmitted 3 months after his last cranial surgery. The mother's stated concerns for her son are his persistent nausea, abdominal pain and vomiting, fevers to 102° F, urinary frequency every 3 minutes, constant seizures (low voltage), blackouts, head deviation, and facial twitching.

Another thorough workup is performed. Jimmy's Dilantin level is low and intravenous Dilantin is started. On hospital day 4, his potassium level drops to 2.9 mEq/L (normal levels, 3.5 to 5.5 mEq/L) requiring intravenous boluses. He is afebrile much of the time, with low-grade fevers to 101° F noted. Occasional small emesis (75 ml) is charted, although Jimmy is frequently complaining of nausea. Urinary frequency every 3 minutes has not been noted. His iron level remains low at 14 mg/dL (normal level, 36 to 150 mg/dL).

Neurologic findings are nystagmus, perhaps a little more than Jimmy's chronic state, which is consistent with his old brain-stem stroke. Cognitively, Jimmy remains stable, according to neurologists. He does have a significant short-term memory loss.

Following are the hospital tests and their results for this admission:

❯ MRI—no acute changes; some atrophy that may be from the recent herpes infection.
❯ 24-hour Holter EEG—no acute changes; essentially negative for anything new.
❯ Urinalysis—one of four was positive for leuko esterase.
❯ UGI-SBFT (upper GI, small bowel follow-through)—negative.
❯ Barium enema—negative.
❯ CT of abdomen and pelvis—normal.
❯ Lumbar puncture—negative, no growth of cultures.

There are many unresolved issues between Jimmy's mother and the physicians. According to the physicians, these range from unreasonable demands by the mother to nonpayment of medical bills. Doctors claim that insurance reimbursement checks sent to the mother were never paid to the physicians. The nursing staff states that they are under attack from Jimmy's mother for not charting mental status changes that she deems are occurring (and for not noticing them) and for not knowing all details about Jimmy when she asks.

Jimmy's mother is angry because she feels that no one is in charge. Her request for one doctor to give her overviews has been granted; however, she is displeased with him. The same day she requested two more specialists: a hematologist and an endocrinologist. The request is carried out, although it is explained to the mother that this type of consultation can be provided on an outpatient basis because the patient is stable.

The mother now demands a multidisciplinary team meeting immediately, and the social worker sets it up quickly—with only 2 hours' lead time. The mother has announced that she will be tape recording the session and clearly states, "This is not just a threat but a promise that everyone involved in this case will be going to court."

During the 1.5-hour meeting that follows, Jimmy's mother demands a diagnosis for all of Jimmy's problems before discharge or she will refuse to pick up her son and take him home. She also wants to know why her son was like his "old self" after a lumbar puncture.

CASE STUDY 3: MICHAEL

Michael is 24 years old with an extensive history of suicide attempts and substance abuse. Methods of suicide gestures have included one attempted hanging, one self-inflicted knife wound of a superficial nature, and several drug overdoses, some of which he claimed were accidental. His use of drugs includes alcohol, LSD, marijuana, cocaine, and amphetamines.

Precipitating factors focus on dysfunctional relationships and episodes of major depression. Each admission has lasted 2 to 3 days, because Michael quickly stabilizes medically and each time renounces any further plans to harm himself.

Michael is now readmitted after ingesting a handful of cold medicine tablets and the remainder of his prescription for fluoxetine (Prozac), about 22 pills. The precipitating event is a date with a man, which occurred 1 week ago. He enjoyed the experience and is feeling immensely distressed because of it.

After 24 hours in the ICU, Michael is medically stable and ready for another level of care. He has again been diagnosed with major depressive episodes and multidrug abuse. Because Michael's condition is now stable and he has been eager to go home for 2 days, discharge orders have been written. Discharge will occur pending a social service referral to appropriate outpatient counseling and support groups. (Outpatient care is limited for this patient because of inadequate psychiatric insurance coverage, which includes only 72 hours of emergency inpatient care for episodes such as suicide attempts.)

The social worker has assessed available options and is discussing with Michael the appointments that have been made and the support groups available. In a surprising turn of events, Michael now states that he wants to remain in the hospital and that if he cannot be an inpatient, he will do further harm to himself when he leaves.

The discharge is being held to allow psychiatrists to reevaluate the patient. While waiting for his psychiatric interviews, Michael again turns the tables, announcing that he wants to leave the hospital immediately, before any additional evaluation has taken place.

CASE STUDY 4: ETHICS

As a case manager for a large Medicaid plan, you feel ethically imbalanced as you perform your gatekeeper role in the following two cases.

Case Study A: Mrs. Varo

Mrs. Varo is 46 years old with advanced metastatic breast cancer. She finished a course of chemotherapy that left her with intractable nausea and vomiting. She has not vomited for 24 hours but is very weak and nauseated. She lives alone with little social support. She has no intensity of service with which to authorize any further hospital days. The physician advisor of the insurance plan felt that she could be managed at home.

Later the same day, you perform an initial review on the following case.

Case Study B: Mr. Ciro

Mr. Ciro's admitting diagnosis was suicide attempt. He was placed in an ICU bed for close observation. Mr. Ciro had called 911, saying he had just swallowed most of a bottle of diazepam (Valium) and had drunk a fifth of whiskey. His toxic screen showed very little drugs or alcohol. However, it did test positive for cocaine. Later that day, Mr. Ciro told a social worker that he had spent his last dollar on cocaine and that he considered the weather to be too hot (it was August in Phoenix) to sleep outside, so he feigned suicide. On physical examination, the physician finds cellulitis on both of his legs from cocaine injections. His hospitalization is authorized for initiation of IV antibiotics for bilateral cellulitis.

CASE STUDY 5: MRS. BROWNELL

Mrs. Brownell, age 77 and widowed, lives in a supervisory care setting where she has her own room and bathroom. The minimum requirement for living in this setting is the ability to get to and from the bathroom and dining room independently. Before this admission, Mrs. Brownell was alert and oriented and able to ambulate independently with a walker.

Mrs. Brownell's history includes gastrointestinal bleeding from ulcers, non–insulin-dependent diabetes mellitus, hypertension, breast cancer with bilateral mastectomies 12 years earlier, atrial fibrillation, a cerebral vascular accident 5 years earlier, and alcohol abuse with hepatic cirrhosis and hepatic encephalopathy. She now presents to the hospital with a cough with brown sputum, diarrhea, mental status changes, and a decreased ability to ambulate because of weakness, falling at home, and anorexia. A left facial droop and right-sided weakness are also noted.

Mrs. Brownell was admitted with bilateral pleural effusions noted on chest radiograph, specifically *Klebsiella* pneumonia found by sputum culture. Her blood urea nitrogen (BUN) was 50 mg/dL and her white blood cell count was 19.5 TH/UL. She was immediately hydrated and given intravenous (IV) antibiotics. A computed tomography (CT) scan of the head revealed no irregularities except for some ischemic small vessel disease. Radiographs revealed the possibility of metastases; therefore, a bone scan was ordered. Uptake was noted in the thoracic and lumbar areas, but these findings were more consistent with degenerative or osteoarthritic changes.

During the course of hospitalization, Mrs. Brownell's mental state and weakness improved. Physical therapy was instituted.

It is the anticipated day of discharge, because all antibiotics are oral and Mrs. Brownell's temperature has remained normal for 24 hours. She is eating 100% of her diet, and her laboratory values are within normal limits. She can walk 20 to 40 feet with minimum assistance but cannot get up and out of bed independently, secondary to severe back pain.

CASE STUDY 6: MR. COLLINS

Mr. Collins, age 52, has been a diabetic since 1973. In 1989, he had a left below-knee amputation at ankle level. His history includes retinal macular degeneration, which has rendered him nearly blind. He also has pulmonary edema from severe valvular insufficiency.

Mr. Collins is admitted with multiple bilateral leg ulcers; one of them is huge with foul-smelling drainage. He states that this condition, along with a steadily increasing abdominal girth, has been on-going for nearly 4 months. A physical examination reveals anasarca. Bilateral above-knee amputations may also be necessary.

Mr. Collins has several nonmedical problems: a recent nasty divorce, impending loss of his private insurance, and current unemployment. He also recently lost his home. Mr. Collins has five sons, none of whom he feels he can turn to for help. They have not been in contact for more than 5 years. Mr. Collins refuses to contact any of his sons and insists that he can handle his situation and states he does not need any help.

Although Mr. Collins is very ill and facing the possibility of losing both legs, he is fixated on nonhealth matters. His physician feels that Mr. Collins is in maximum denial of his illness (as evidenced by his waiting 4 months to seek medical assistance) and has some "paranoid ideation."

CASE STUDY 7: MR. LUBER

Mr. Luber, age 31, disappeared from his girlfriend's home 4 days before admission. On his return he was shaking, seemed disoriented, and then fell in a parking lot. Paramedics were called. Emergency department doctors found Mr. Luber to be agitated, combative, and verbally inappropriate. The emergency department assessment showed blood pressure, 130/86 mm Hg; pulse, 130 beats/min; respirations, 40 breaths/min; and temperature, 103.3° F (39.6°C). A toxicology

screen was positive for cocaine and marijuana. This patient also has a history of alcohol abuse.

A chest radiograph revealed a left lobe infiltrate; Mr. Luber was admitted for pneumonia (probably aspiration), fever, and confusion, and to rule out meningitis. The results of a lumbar puncture proved unremarkable, and Mr. Luber was given appropriate IV antibiotic therapy for pneumonia.

Mr. Luber claims he has had amnesia for the past 2 years; physicians have conflicting opinions about this. Mr. Luber says he remembers driving a truck cross-country 3 years ago but does not remember that he has lived with his girlfriend for the past 18 months. The neurologist on the case feels his amnesia is "fictitious," whereas the psychologist feels that it is a possible dissociative state or psychoactive substance-induced organic mental disorder.

Mr. Luber's girlfriend says that he currently makes a living making bottles at a manufacturing plant. Mr. Luber lost both parents when he was 12; they died 6 months apart. His mother may have had amnesiac states. He has two children who live 800 miles away. He has served several jail sentences for driving under the influence and assault and battery. Mr. Luber has no support system other than his girlfriend and no medical insurance.

CASE STUDY 8: MR. QUINLAN

This is the third admission in 6 weeks for 46-year-old Mr. Quinlan, who is developmentally delayed and living in a training center. Each admission diagnosis has been for dehydration, acute renal failure (BUN 50 mg/dL, creatinine greater than 3.0 mg/dL), thrombocytopenia, anemia, and mental status changes. His history also includes seizures.

During the first two admissions, dehydration, renal failure, and mental status changes returned to normal by the time of discharge. It was believed that his seizure medication was causing the thrombocytopenia, and it was changed to another agent. Still, his problems returned and compounded.

Mr. Quinlan had been independent in self-care and living in a cottage on the center's grounds with other "high-functioning" persons. Because his condition began to deteriorate, he was moved to the center itself, where more care could be provided. The training center attendants reported that Mr. Quinlan's condition had been going downhill for the past 4 months. Recently, he started refusing food and was losing a considerable amount of weight. When questioned, the attendants said they believed this behavior to be related to a temper tantrum reaction.

The patient had many bruises on admission. The caregiver told the clinicians that the patient had fallen against a railing. The staff nurses were aware of Mr. Quinlan's thrombocytopenia and knew that he bruised easily. The staff nurses also reported fearful cries of, "Don't hit me," when the patient was incontinent. When asked who was hitting him, Mr. Quinlan consistently named the training center attendants.

This time, the hospital course has been very complex and without clear answers as to a cause of his symptoms. It started much like the previous two hospitalizations, with the symptoms of renal failure and dehydration resolving quickly.

IV medications were needed, but no IV access could be obtained because of the patient's poor vein status. Because a percutaneous endoscopic gastrostomy (PEG) feeding tube placement was believed to be in the patient's best interests, a central line was to be inserted at the same time. The patient was at times wildly agitated, so the procedures were obtained under general anesthesia. Mr. Quinlan did not resume spontaneous breathing, and a postoperative chest radiograph showed right-sided "whiteout" with questionable pleural effusions versus aspiration. Two IV antibiotics were initiated while the patient remained ventilated. A nasogastric tube insertion produced a heme-positive return, and his anemia deteriorated to a hemoglobin of 6.7 gm/100 mL and a hematocrit of 19.0, requiring transfusions. Three days later, Mr. Quinlan masterfully extubated himself and was able to resume spontaneous respirations.

Mr. Quinlan was sent to floor status with IV antibiotics, a nasogastric tube (still draining bile-colored secretions), and orders to start physical therapy. Tube feedings were initiated after 5 days of attempts because of intolerance and vomiting of the formulas. Several competent physicians, including pulmonary, gastrointestinal, and neurology specialists, are still unsure of the cause of the patient's diagnosis.

CASE STUDY 9: MR. VAQUERO

Mr. Vaquero, age 26, has a history of insulin-dependent diabetes mellitus. Consistently non-compliant with his medical care for most of his life, Mr. Vaquero developed retinopathy, neuropathies, several diabetic foot ulcers, and chronic renal failure. He is now legally blind. A year ago, Mr. Vaquero's renal function became so impaired that hemodialysis was initiated.

Mr. Vaquero lives in the country, almost 50 miles from the nearest hemodialysis unit. His parents live next door, but his mother is also blind and his father has advanced Alzheimer disease. He has only one friend, and this friend is unable to help. There is no public or volunteer transportation to help him get to and from hemodialysis three times each week, and no other social support is acknowledged.

Mr. Vaquero has been in the acute care setting many times in diabetic ketoacidosis (DKA) and with dangerously elevated BUN, creatinine, phosphorus, and potassium from being inadequately dialyzed. He also has been hospitalized for several foot problems, resulting from carelessness and not wearing shoes. His injuries include nonhealing cuts and cellulitis and second-degree burns from hot pavement. Mr. Vaquero has private insurance but the policy has no long-term care or SNF benefits.

CASE STUDY 10: MRS. OLIVER

Mrs. Oliver is 58 years old. She has a medical history that includes lupus erythematosus, insulin-dependent diabetes mellitus, diabetic neuropathies, neurogenic bladder requiring an indwelling Foley catheter, chronic bladder yeast infections, chronic renal failure, congestive heart failure with cor pulmonale, and frequent episodes of shortness of breath resulting in frequent emergency department visits. Mrs. Oliver also has gained hundreds of pounds over the past several years, making her morbidly obese. She now weighs approximately 550 pounds. This raises the question of Pickwickian episodes. The abdominal skin folds frequently break down, making abdominal cellulitis another recurring problem.

Two months earlier, Mrs. Oliver was able to get out of bed and use her walker to get to a bedside commode or chair. Now she is totally bedbound and requires the maximum assistance of two physical therapists to "stand" her for 5 seconds.

Mrs. Oliver habitually requires a lengthy hospitalization every few months, often on a telemetry unit. Her first hospitalization of the current year was in February for congestive heart failure and pneumonia in addition to her other chronic problems. Her husband, age 70 and 135 pounds, is very supportive but is finding it almost impossible to care for his wife at home any longer. Nevertheless, each time the issue of a SNF is broached, Mrs. Oliver bursts into tears and begs her husband to take her home. To complicate matters, at the end of a previous hospital stay (after discharge orders were written), the home health agency previously helping with her care declined her case on the grounds of serious safety issues. No other home health agency could be found to take the case.

There seems to be only one alternative now, and Mr. Oliver convinces a protesting and teary Mrs. Oliver to go to a SNF for physical therapy in an effort to get her back to baseline.

Two weeks later, Mr. Oliver is calling the case manager. He said that Mrs. Oliver insisted on leaving the SNF. A home health agency was found to take her case. Unfortunately, the agency is not providing enough help. Mrs. Oliver is on a waiting list for a SNF with an excellent reputation for rehabilitation/physical therapy, but while waiting for a bed to become available, Mr. Oliver finds himself at his outermost limits. He does not feel that he can handle his wife's care any longer.

The bed in the SNF did not manifest soon enough. After two more emergency department visits for shortness of breath, Mrs. Oliver was readmitted with pneumonia. The long-awaited SNF bed became available, and Mrs. Oliver was transferred while finishing her last days of IV antibiotics.

Six weeks later, Mrs. Oliver is still not making progress in physical therapy at the SNF. Her insurance company will pay for up to 50 skilled home health nurse visits and 100 days of SNF skilled care for 1 year. Mrs. Oliver has too many assets to qualify for the state's long-term care and too few assets to privately pay for all the care she requires. No one else in the Oliver family will help.

By June, Mrs. Oliver has been bounced from the SNF to the hospital several times with severe respiratory distress, congestive heart failure, and pulmonary edema. Her CO_2 has reached the middle 70s and BiPAP ventilation has been tried. She now has 3 weeks of SNF coverage remaining.

CASE STUDY 11: MS. SIMMS

Seventy-two-year-old Ms. Simms has a history of schizophrenia and chronic obstructive pulmonary disease. The emergency department report states that she has been extremely schizophrenic, delusional, and paranoid for the past week. Her chief complaint is shortness of breath. Her physical examination reveals some expiratory wheezes after a small volume nebulizer treatment, but no respiratory distress, rales, or rhonchi and no use of accessory muscles. She is speaking in full sentences. Ms. Simms is afebrile; blood pressure, 143/90 mm/Hg; pulse, 96 beats/min; and respirations, 26 breaths/min. The emergency department diagnoses rule out paranoid schizophrenia and chronic obstructive pulmonary disease. She is admitted to a medical floor.

Ms. Simms is very frightened. She feels the Vietnamese, the Chinese, and the Germans are out to get her and her family. She believes she is not safe anywhere and will not make it out of the hospital alive. The Asian resident assigned to the case had to make himself scarce because Ms. Simms exhibited severe fright, accusing him of following her and planning to transfer her out of town to be tortured.

Ms. Simms wishes to go to the state hospital, although she is sure the staff will rape her and put her into a machine that will crush her.

Ms. Simms never married. She lived in a convent many years ago, but her bizarre behaviors made it impossible for her to become a nun. She trusts the Catholic priests and states that God has talked to her.

Ms. Simms has a twin. When her sister is out of town, as she is during this admission, the schizophrenic exacerbations intensify. Her niece and grandnephew are sympathetic and willing to help, but when they visit they are physically attacked by their aunt.

Ms. Simms has been taking appropriate psychotropic medication, but there is some question about her compliance. A transfer to an inpatient mental health unit has been arranged, but she refuses to sign the conditions of admission forms.

CASE STUDY 12: MRS. LING

Seven years ago, Mrs. Ling, who was on hemodialysis, received a kidney from her son, one of her 10 children. The kidney transplantation was a success, and for many years under the meticulous care of her husband, she maintained a serum creatinine level of 0.8 mg/dL. Mr. Ling closely monitored his wife's complicated medical requirements for diabetes, chronic urinary tract infections, anemia, coronary artery disease, hypertension, and medications to maintain the kidney. She also had a history of a left cerebral vascular accident and underwent laser surgery to her eyes because of diabetic complications.

About 6 months ago, Mr. Ling suffered a cerebral vascular accident and was no longer able to care for his wife. The adult children took over the care of both parents, but their care proved to be haphazard. Cyclosporine was not listed among Mrs. Ling's medications, and azathioprine was being given incorrectly.

Mrs. Ling was admitted to the hospital with intractable nausea and vomiting; she was unable to keep down food and was intolerant of any medications. Her critical admission laboratory values included the following:

BUN, 178 (normal, 5–25),

Creatinine, 17.5 (normal, 0.7–1.5),

Potassium, 7.8 (normal, 3.5–5.5), and

Phosphorus, 12.3 (normal, 2.5–4.5).

The degree of kidney failure indicated that the rejection was not acute. Mrs. Ling's physicians had not seen her in more than 6 months; this was in contrast to the careful way Mr. Ling made and kept physician appointments. It is difficult to say how long the rejection had been occurring. After 10 days of receiving heavy IV methylprednisolone (Solu-Medrol) doses and frequent hemodialysis, the creatinine was still around 6.5 mg/dL. Outpatient hemodialysis was set up. The patient has Medicaid and although only 61 years of age will soon be eligible for Medicare because of hemodialysis.

CASE STUDY 13: MS. JOHNSON

Ms. Johnson is a 36-year-old divorced woman with a long history of multiple hospital admissions for medical and psychiatric problems. She lives with her 15-year-old daughter. Her mother had bipolar disorder, and her father was schizophrenic. Her insurance coverage is Medicare and Medicaid. She is unemployed and on disability.

She also hospital-hops, so that it is difficult to assess true hospital admission numbers. In 1 year, Ms. Johnson entered one hospital 18 times—six times in 1 month. It is not known how many times she was also admitted to various other hospitals during the same period. Medically, Ms. Johnson's history includes asthma with frequent exacerbations, bowel obstructions, seizures, bladder incontinence, and an appendectomy. Psychiatrically, Ms. Johnson meets criteria for chronically mentally ill, with the diagnoses of borderline personality and psychotic depression. She has had several inpatient hospital stays at five different mental health facilities.

Ms. Johnson's behaviors include superficially slashing her wrists (at one point three times in 1 week), overdosing on carbamazepine and other pills, hallucinating, consuming excessive amounts of alcohol, and manipulation. Her "usual" admission can be psychiatric, medical, or a combination of both and is very short. If presented with a plan that Ms. Johnson finds distasteful, she leaves against medical advice (AMA). She often shows up in an emergency department within 1 or 2 days of the AMA episode.

After several such events, one psychiatrist deemed Ms. Johnson severely mentally ill, and a petitioning process was initiated. She was court-ordered into treatment (she fired that particular psychiatrist). After her court-ordered "incarceration," she resumed her previous behaviors of multiple suicide gestures, asthma exacerbation admissions, and leaving AMA.

Ms. Johnson has learned that it is easier to leave AMA when she "voluntarily" agrees to a psychiatric admission than when the involuntary "court order" is initiated, so now she rarely, if ever, refuses a psychiatric admission.

CASE STUDY 14: MS. PAINE

Thirty-two-year-old Ms. Paine was diagnosed with HIV 5 years ago. Three of her eight children have died of AIDS. The remaining five children, the youngest of whom is 3 months old, live with relatives or are in foster care. Ms. Paine earns her living through prostitution. This supports her polysubstance abuse habit, which includes the use of cocaine (inhaled and injected), alcohol, and whatever else will keep her "drugged out." She practices no regular birth control and does not practice "safe sex." She is currently homeless. Her mental status is assessed as lethargic, alert, and oriented, but she is inconsistent in her answers to different examiners. For example, she changes her occupation from prostitute to burglar when the issue of "safe sex" is broached.

Ms. Paine has a history of being admitted to hospitals and leaving AMA (against medical advice)—she actually "disappears" when specific issues are raised. She is savvy about the system and knows she cannot be deemed incompetent or incarcerated involuntarily in a mental health unit unless she "threatens her own life or the life of someone else in this state."

On her first admission to a particular local hospital, Ms. Paine appeared cachectic, ill-kempt, and disheveled. She had not had anything to eat or drink for 3 days, secondary to frequent smoking of crack during this time. Her left foot had obvious cellulitis. She was admitted for dehydration, cellulitis (rule out osteomyelitis), and electrocardiographic T-wave abnormalities and bradycardia. She has a history of severe oral thrush and pneumonia. On this admission, Ms. Paine's thrush was severe and her chest radiograph was clear, but she had a persistent dry cough. IV antibiotics, IV fluids, and supportive care were initiated.

In addition to treating Ms. Paine's obvious physical problems and checking her toxicology screen (positive for cocaine during the hospitalization) and pregnancy test (negative), the attending physician used the time to address the many psychosocial needs and issues of this case. The attending physician felt that Ms. Paine was definitely a public health concern and ordered a psychiatric evaluation.

The psychiatrist deemed Ms. Paine competent with antisocial tendencies. The recommendation was to explore petitioning on the grounds that she showed definite judgment impairment, that she was "acutely and persistently disabled," and that she was unable to safely care for herself. However, this psychiatric status could not be court-ordered, because the patient knew of alternative options for taking care of herself (she can live with relatives) and she had no previous documented psychiatric history.

Hint: Ethical and legal issues define and also limit the possibilities and probable outcomes for this case.

CASE STUDY 15: MR. JENSEN

Mr. Jensen was a pleasant but persistently noncompliant patient known to every hospital emergency department in the metropolitan area. He was an unstable diabetic (even during hospital admissions) with a lifetime of poor diabetic control. His blood sugar levels would routinely register "HHH" or "LLL" on the glucose monitors, and yet he was able to sit up and carry on a full conversation with a blood glucose level of 18 mg/100 mL. It is no surprise that Mr. Jensen suffered from every diabetic "-opathy" in the medical literature.

In his late thirties, Mr. Jensen underwent several angioplasties to his lower extremities for severe artery disease. He had chronic, extensive leg ulcers and partial foot amputations, but he managed to maintain self-care with the use of a wheelchair.

Mr. Jensen had an impressive IV drug abuse habit, and after injecting a large amount of cocaine one day, suffered a myocardial infarction necessitating an emergency four-vessel coronary artery bypass. Mr. Jensen's drug use did not decrease, and many more hospital emergency department visits and admissions were needed to treat his congestive heart failure, chest pain, diabetic ketoacidosis, pneumonia, endocarditis, and out-of-control diabetes. Most emergency department visits included the complaint of chest pain; he knew just how to manipulate the nurses and doctors at these emergency departments. Although Mr. Jensen's assessment revealed drug-seeking behaviors, it is also likely that he did have pain and that his tolerance for pain medications was high.

Mr. Jensen's insurance coverage was fairly thorough; he had both Medicare and Medicaid. Nevertheless, with all his extensive hospital utilization, he was dipping heavily into his Medicare lifetime reserve days. When not residing in the hospital, emergency department visits would range from few times per week to daily.

Mr. Jensen has lived with his girlfriend for many years. She is much healthier than he physically, but several times she had to be escorted off hospital units for abusive behavior toward the staff. She was also an "aider and abettor" during several episodes when Mr. Jensen went "downstairs for a smoke." A two-pack-a-day guy, Mr. Jensen often returned to the floor glassy-eyed and with positive toxicology screens.

Mr. Jensen received maximum social service, psychiatric, and case management attention but never followed through on medical or community suggestions and referrals.

Discharge planning was complicated by several factors. Although home IV therapy would have shortened hospital lengths of stay, no physician could safely send Mr. Jensen home with an easy IV access because of his IV drug abuse. Home nurses were ruled out because those who visited him at home refused to go back, scared because of all the drug paraphernalia and hard-core addicts hanging around his apartment. Eventually, no home health agency would touch his case.

Extended care facilities soon became out of the question, too. When sent to a SNF for endocarditis, which required several weeks of IV antibiotics, Mr. Jensen would (as in the hospital) go outside where someone would meet him, and he would come back stoned. He was even caught trying to sell drugs to other SNF residents. Nips of alcohol would be supplied freely to these residents. SNFs, like home health agencies, are no longer an option for Mr. Jensen.

▶ REFERENCES

Duch, B. (2008). *Problems: a key factor in PBL.* Available online: http://www.udel.edu/pbl/cte/spr96-phys.html. Accessed October 20, 2008.

Gallow, D. (2008). *What is problem-based learning?* Available online: http://www.pbl.uci.edu/whatispbl.html. Accessed October 20, 2008.

Study Guides and Strategies. *Techniques and strategies for learning with problem-based learning.* Available online: http://www.studygs.net/pbl.htm. Accessed October 20, 2008.

Wikipedia. (2008a). *Problem-based learning: problem solving and cognitive load.* Available online: http://en.wikipedia.org/wiki/Problem-based_learning. Accessed October 20, 2008.

Wikipedia. (2008b). *Problem-based learning: presenting problems to learners.* Available online: http://en.wikipedia.org/wiki/Problem-based_learning. Accessed October 20, 2008.

INDEX

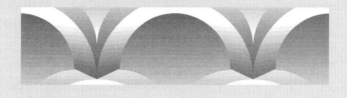

Numbers followed by t indicate table. Numbers in italics indicate figures.

A

AACN. *See* American Association of Colleges of Nursing (AACN)
ABQAURP. *See* American Board of Quality Assurance and Utilization Review Physicians (ABQAURP)
Abuse
    child, mandatory reporting of, 294, 296
    elder, mandatory reporting of, 296–297
Accountability, of case manager, 53
Accreditation
    described, 342
    regulatory agencies and, 342–348
Active, experiential learning, described, 368–369
Activities of daily living (ADLs)
    assessment of, in case management process, ad, 215
    defined, 27
Acupuncture, knowledge of, 52
Acute care, 172–174
    case management related to, 12–14
Adequate patient education, defined, 27
ADLs. *See* Activities of daily living (ADLs)
Admitting office case management, 13–14
Advance directives, legal issues related to, 291–292
Advanced Directive for Healthcare or Living Will for a Do Not Resuscitate Order, 297–298
Adverse determination, 105
Adverse patient outcome (APO), described, 245, 247
Advocacy
    by case managers, examples of activities, 44
    cost-containment roles vs., ethical issues related to, 318–320
    family, optimal vs. inadequate outcomes of, 37–38
    patient, optimal vs. inadequate outcomes of, 37–38
Advocate(s), patient, case manager as, 41–43
AFDC. *See* Aid to Families with Dependent Children (AFDC)
Affidavit of Merit, 269
Agency for Healthcare Research and Quality (AHRQ), 329
Aggressive model
    strengths of, 51
    weaknesses of, 51
Aggressive negotiator, 50–51
Aging With Dignity, 291
AHCA. *See* American Health Care Association (AHCA)
AHRQ. *See* Agency for Healthcare Research and Quality (AHRQ)
Aid to Families with Dependent Children (AFDC), 70
Air ambulance, transferring patient by, 202
Alternative healing therapies, 211

Ambulance(s)
    air, transferring patient by, 202
    transferring patient by, 202
American Accreditation HealthCare Commission/URAC, to NCQA, 55
American Association of Colleges of Nursing (AACN), on mandatory reporting, 294
American Board of Quality Assurance and Utilization Review Physicians (ABQAURP), 339–340
American Dietetic Association, 212–213
American Health Care Association (AHCA), on subacute care, 175
American Hospital Association (AHA), on transfer DRGs rule, 190
American Nurses Association (ANA), 4, 41, 303
    on mandatory reporting, 294
American Nurses Association's Code of Ethics, 313
American Nurses Credentialing Center (ANCC), 333–335
ANA. *See* American Nurses Association (ANA)
Anatomical gifts, legal issues related to, 298–299
ANCC. *See* American Nurses Credentialing Center (ANCC)
Antibiotic(s), intravenous, Medicare coverage of, 163
APO. *See* Adverse patient outcome (APO)
Appeal(s), 106, 275–278
    defined, 275
    expedited, 276
    procedures related to, reducing need for, 277–278
    standard, 276
    who may request, 277
Assertiveness skills, of case manager, 55–56
Assessment, in case management process, 210–219
Assessment tools, in case management process, 218–219
Assisted death, ethical issues related to, 321–322
Assisted living/custodial care, level of care of, 176t–177t
Attitude, caring, of case manager, 59
Authorization
    concurrent, 105
    insurance, 105–106
    precertification, 105
    retrospective, 105
Autopsy(ies), legal issues related to, 299–300
Avoided costs, 48

B

Background checks, 293
Balanced Budget Act (BBA), 188
Basil v. Wolf, 275
BBA. *See* Balanced Budget Act (BBA)

Behavior(s), caring, of case manager, 59
Belief(s)
    personal, case management model matched with, 10–11
    religious, in case management process, 217–218
    spiritual, in case management process, 217–218
Benefit(s), coordination of, 77–78
Billing(s), terminology related to, 94
Brainstorming alternative strategies, 355
Brick wall syndrome, 216–217
Bundling, 76

C

California Civil Code Section 3428, 279–280
CAM. *See* Complementary and alternative medicine (CAM)
Canada, case management in, 31–33
Canada Health Act, 31
CAP, 71–72
Capitation, 75
Care
    acute, 172–174
        case management related to, 12–14
    custodial, 170–171
    defined, 27
    important aspects of, described, 247
    intermediate, 171
        level of care of, 176t-177t
    lack of, 27
    managed. *see* Managed care
    nonskilled, vs. skilled care, 27
    postacute, 174–188
    shared, 29
    skilled, vs. nonskilled care, 27
    skilled nursing. *See* Skilled nursing care
    skin, skill vs. nonskilled services related to, 186t
    subacute. *See* Subacute care
    transmural, 29
Care coordination, in transitions of care, 199
Care management, case management vs., 5
Care planning activities, in case management process, 218
Caregiver, defined, 296
CARF. *See* Commission on Accreditation of Rehabilitation
            Facilities (CARF)
Carve-out plan, insurance, 72
Case closure, 239
Case evaluation, in evaluation and follow-up, 229–230
Case in Point, 327–328
Case management. *See also specific components, models, and
            types*
    in Canada, 31–33
    care management vs., 5
    community-based, optimal vs. inadequate outcomes of, 38
    confusing terms related to, 25–28
    defined, 2, 101
        by consumer, 5
    described, 4–5
    documentation of, "paper and pencil" approach to, 20
    ethical issues in, 303–323
    evolution of, milestones in, 6
    goals of, 35–38
        unmet, 35–39
    historical perspective on, 5–6

hospice case management, 15
hospital-based, responsibilities of, 7
information technology and, 20–21
intermittent services in, 26–27
international perspectives on, 28–31
introduction to, 1–97
job responsibilities and skills, 35–68
key concepts in, 241–323
large, 14
legal issues in, 267–302
models of, 11–17
    acute care case management, 12–14
    admitting office case management, 13–14
    case management firms, 16
    changing of, steps in, 19–20
    described, 11–12
    disease management, 14
    emergency department case management, 13
    entrepreneurial case management, 16–17
    evaluation of, 17–19
    factors impacting, 13
    home health case management, 15
    hospitalists, 17
    insurance case management, 14–15
    large case management, 14
    matching personal goals and beliefs with, 10–11
    on-site case management, 15
    palliative care case management, 15
    perioperative services case management, 14
    physician groups, 15
    public health/community-based case management, 16
    rehabilitation specialists, 16
    selection of, steps in, 19–20
    skilled nursing facility case management, 15–16
    telephonic case management, 15
    vocational case management, 16
    workers' compensation, 16
nursing, opportunities in, 9–10
on-site, 15
outcomes of, in evaluation and follow-up, 230–231
outpatient, optimal vs. inadequate outcomes of, 38
overview of, 2–34
patient safety and, 254–258, 255t-257t
perioperative services, 14
process, 99–240
public health/community-based, 16
QI and RM with, 249–253
telehealth and, 21
telephonic, 15, 105
trends in, 25–33
understanding of, in case management practice, 352–353
UR, UM and, relationship among, 101–103
Case management academia, 63–67
Case Management Administrator Certification (CMAC), 341
Case Management Advisory Committee, 344–345
Case management by proxy, 368–382
    case studies, 375–382
    directions for practicing, 373–375
    PBL, 368–382. *See also* Problem-based learning (PBL)
Case management code of professional conduct, 8–9
Case management firms, 16
Case Management Leadership Coalition (CMLC), 5
Case management plan(s) (CMPs), in UM, 115–120

Case management plan/clinical pathway, example of, 138–153
Case management practice, interstate, legal issues related to, 278–279
Case management process, 205–240
  introduction to, 205–206
  stages of, 206
    assessment/problem identification, 210–219
      ADLs assessment in, 215
      care planning activities in, 218
      cultural diversity in, 217–218
      current medical status in, 211–212
      environmental factors in, 214–215
      financial assessment in, 214
      functional assessment in, 214–215
      home environment assessment in, 214–215
      medication assessment in, 213–214
      nutritional assessment in, 212–213
      patient's history and demographics in, 211
      psychological assessment in, 215–217
      religious diversity in, 217–218
      screening and assessment tools in, 218–219
    case closure and termination of case management services, 239
    case plan implementation, 222–226
      case managers outside facilities, 224–226
      case managers within facilities, 223–224
    case selection, 206–210
      psychological indicators in, 208–209
      socioeconomic indications in, 209–210
    continuous monitoring, reassessing, and reevaluating, 231–239, *234, 235, 236t, 237t, 238*
      evolving educational needs, 233
      family satisfaction, 238–239
      goals, 239
      medical status, 232
      pain management, 233–238, *234, 235, 236t, 237t, 238.* See also Pain management, in continuous monitoring, reassessing, and reevaluating
      patient satisfaction, 238–239
      quality of care, 232
      social stability, 232
    development and coordination of case plan in, 219–222
      goals in
        establishing of, 220
        prioritizing of, 220–221
      needs in, prioritizing of, 220–221
      service planning and resource allocation, 221–222
    evaluation and follow-up, 226–231
      case evaluation in, 229–230
      case management outcomes, 230–231
      familial
        needs in, 226–229
Case management protocol, admission as, 123–124
Case management services, termination of, 239
Case Management Society International (CMSI), 28
Case Management Society of America (CMSA), 4, 25, 41, 278, 327
  on Standards of Practice for Case Management, 230–231
Case Management Standards of Practice, 287
Case manager(s). *See also specific types and duties*
  ability to read poor penmanship by, 58
  accountability of, 53
  advocacy activities of, examples of, 44
  assertiveness skills of, *55–56*
  in assessing and reassessing, 45
  attention to detail by, 58
  in basic vs. advanced case management skills, 61–62
  caring attitude and behavior of, 59
  as case presenter, 60
  as case screening expert, 44
  as clinical expertise disease management expert, 51–52
  as coach, 57
  commitment and desire to be, 57
  as competent professional, 53
  on concurrent coding, DRG assignments, ICD-9-CM coding issues, 60–61
  confidence of, 58
  as conflict resolution expert and referee, 57
  as coordinator of care, 44–45
  as cost-benefit analyst, 47–51. *See also* Cost-benefit analyst, case manager as
  in CQI and outcomes management, 55
  creativity of, 58
  as crisis intervention/grief counselor, 59
  criteria for, 6–8
  as critical thinker and problem solver, 52–53
  defined, 2
  as devil's advocate, 61
  diplomacy of, 58
  as discharge planner and facilitator in level of care changes, 45
  as documenter of plans and report writer, 57–58
  education of, 64
  as educator, 60
  external, reimbursement changes related to, 196–197
  as facilitator of multidisciplinary patient care rounds, 54
  within facilities, in case plan implementation, 223–224
  flexibility of, 58
  in follow-up and follow-through, 45–46
  functions of, domains of, 43
  hospital-based, responsibilities of, 7
  in identification and anticipation of potential problems, 250
  information guide for, 59
  as insurance benefit analyst, 47
  as integrator, 59
  in knowledge and use of legal and quality issues and standards of practice, 53
  knowledge of complementary and alternative medicine of, 52
  as liaison between payor and patient, 60
  management and leadership skills of, 56
  nurses as, 7–8, 21–25
  organizational skills of, 57
  outside facilities, in case plan implementation, 224–226
  as patient advocate, 41–43
  in physician support, 54
  prioritization skills of, 57
  as protector of privacy and confidentiality, 44
  resourcefulness of, 58
  respect and trust by peers of, 58
  responsibilities of, 41–62
  risk-taking by, 58
  roles of, 41–62
    domains of, 43
  in selecting and monitoring clinical pathways, 61
  self-directedness of, 58
  self-esteem of, 58

sense of humor of, 59

skills and personality traits of, 62–63

in staff development and informational resource, 59–60

strong interpersonal communication skills of, 55

as team player, 54

as technology user, 61

training for, 64

   core competence, 64–67

as utilization manager, 46–47

Case Manager Certification (CCMC), Code of Professional Conduct for Case Managers of, 9

Case manager liability, 269–270

Case manager/patient—family unit, 39, *40*

Case mix groups (CMGs), 73

Case plan

   development and coordination of, in case management process, 219–222

   implementation of, in case management process, 222–226

Case presenter, case manager as, 60

Case screening expert, case manager as, 44

Case selection, in case management process, 206–210

C-ASWCM. *See* Certified Advanced Social Work Case Manager (C-ASWCM)

CCM. *See* Certified Case Manager (CCM)

CCM credential. *See* Certified Case Manager (CCM) credential

CCMA. *See* Center for Case Management Accountability (CCMA)

CCMC. *See* Commission for Case Management Certification (CCMC)

CDACs. *See* Clinical data abstraction centers (CDACs)

CDE. *See* Certified Diabetes Educators (CDE)

Center for Case Management (CFCM), 341

Center for Case Management Accountability (CCMA), 25, 53

Centers for Medicare & Medicaid Services (CMS), 9, 107–108, 342–344

   on NONCs, 164, 166

Centers for Medicare & Medicaid Services (CMS)—related measures, described, 247–249, 248t

Certification, lack of, 105

Certified Advanced Social Work Case Manager (C-ASWCM), 340–341

Certified Case Manager (CCM), 331–333

Certified Case Manager (CCM) credential, 4

Certified Diabetes Educators (CDE), 7

Certified Professional in Healthcare Quality (CPHQ), 336–339

Certified Professional in Utilization Review (CPUR), 333

Certified Social Work Case Manager (C-SWCM), 340–341

CFCM. *See* The Center for Case Management (CFCM)

CHAMPUS. *See* Civilian Health and Medical Program of the Uniformed Services (CHAMPUS)

Change, in case management practice, 364–366, *365*

   grief and, 366–367

Charge(s), potential, 48–49

Child abuse, mandatory reporting of, 294, 296

Civilian Health and Medical Program of the Uniformed Services (CHAMPUS), 89

Claims administrators, 94

Claims categories, used by RM departments, 265–266

Clarification, role-related, job stress related to, 350–352

Clinical data abstraction centers (CDACs), 95

Clinical expertise disease management expert, case manager as, 51–52

Clinical Guidelines for Subacute Units, 117–118

Clinical indicators, 259–262

Clinical pathways

   case management plans and, 115–120

   selection and monitoring of, case manager in, 61

   in UM, 115–120. *See also* Utilization management (UM), clinical pathways in

Clinical pathways/case management plan, example of, 138–153

CMAC. *See* Case Management Administrator Certification (CMAC)

CMGs. *See* Case mix groups (CMGs)

CMLC. *See* Case Management Leadership Coalition (CMLC)

CMPs. *See* Case management plans (CMPs)

CMS. *See* Centers for Medicare & Medicaid Services (CMS)

CMSA. *See* Case Management Society of America (CMSA)

CMSI. *See* Case Management Society International (CMSI)

Coach, case manager as, 57

COBRA. *See* Consolidated Omnibus Budget Reconciliation Act (COBRA)

Code of professional conduct, case management, 8–9

Code of Professional Conduct for Case Managers, 313–314

   of CCMC, 9

Codes of ethics, 312–319

Coinsurance, 71

Commission for Case Manager Certification (CCMC), 4, 41, 269, 331

Commission for the Study of Ethical Problems in Medicine and Biomedical and Behavioral Research, 305

Commission on Accreditation of Rehabilitation Facilities (CARF), on subacute care, 175

Communication

   in case management practice, 362–363

      perceptions in, 363–364

   with physicians, UM-related, 106

Communication skills, interpersonal, of case manager, 55

Community standards, in UM, 279–281

Competence, core, in case management training, 64–67

Competency, of case manager, 53

Complementary and alternative medicine (CAM), knowledge of, 52

Concurrent authorization, 105

Concurrent review, 103–104

Concurrent review nurses, role of, 102

Condition Code 44, 124

Confidence, of case manager, 58

Confidentiality

   case manager as protector of, 44

   legal issues related to, 289–290

Conflict, role-related, job stress related to, 350–352

Conflict resolution, case manager in, 57

Confusion, role-related, job stress related to, 350–352

Consent, informed, legal issues related to, 287–289

Consolidated Omnibus Budget Reconciliation Act (COBRA), 77, 273

Consumer Bill of Rights and Responsibilities, 314–317

Continuous QI (CQI), 242–243

Continuous QI efforts, case manager in, 55

Cooperative method

   strengths of, 51

   weaknesses of, 51

Coordination of benefits, 77–78

Coordinator/facilitator of care

   case manager as, 44–45

   ethical issues related to, 320

Copayment, insurance, 71
Corcoran v. United Healthcare, Inc., 274
Core competence, in case management training, 64–67
Core measures, described, 247–249, 248t
Cost(s)
    avoided, 48
    potential, 48–49
Cost-benefit analyst, case manager as, 47–51
    hard savings, 48
    negotiation skills, 49–50
    soft savings, 48–49
Cost-containment roles, advocacy vs., ethical issues related to, 318–320
Cost-sharing strategies, for insurance companies, 71
CPHQ. *See* Certified Professional in Healthcare Quality (CPHQ)
CPUR. *See* Certified Professional in Utilization Review (CPUR)
CQI. *See* Continuous QI (CQI)
Creativity, of case manager, 58
Credentials, 331–341
    ABQAURP, 339–340
    ANCC, 333–335
    C-ASWCM, 340–341
    CCM, 331–333
    CCMC, 331
    CMAC, 341
    CPHQ, 336–339
    CPUR, 333
    C-SWCM, 340–341
    NAHQ, 336–339
    NASW, 340
    Nursing Case Management (RN, CM), 333–335
    quality, 336–340
Crisis intervention/grief counselor, case manager as, 59
Critical thinker, case manager as, 52–53
C-SWCM. *See* Certified Social Work Case Manager (C-SWCM)
Cultural diversity, in case management process, 217–218
Current Procedural Terminology (CTP) codes, 94
Custodial care, 170–171

D

Days per thousand, described, 95
Death
    assisted, ethical issues related to, 321–322
    legal issues related to, 298–299
Decision making, ethical, 308–309
Decision-making ethics, guide for, 309–310
Deductible, insurance, 71
Deferred liability, insurance, 72
Deficit Reduction Act of 2005, 197
Delegate, in time management, 357–358
Demographics, in case management process, 211
Denial, 105, 275–278
Deposition, 270–271
Diabetic supplies, home health changes related to, 192
Diagnostic-related groups (DRGs), 73–74
    transfer, 190–191
Diagnostic-related groups (DRGs)/Prospective Payment System, 3
Diet(s), skilled vs. nonskilled services related to, 186t
Diplomacy, of case manager, 58
Discharge, premature, legal issues related to, 284–287

Discharge planner, case manager as, 45
Discharge planning
    adequacy of, 285–287
    defined, 161
    early, 164
    legal issues related to, 284–287
    Medicare on, 166–167
    TJC on, 161–162
Disclosure of information, in informed consent, 287–288
Discounted fee-for-services, 76
Disease management, 14
Disease Management Association of America (DMAA), 328
Disenrollment, described, 76
Diversity, cultural, in case management process, 217–218
DMAA. *See* Disease Management Association of America (DMAA)
DME. *See* Durable medical equipment (DME)
DNR law. *See* Do Not Resuscitate (DNR) law
Do Not Resuscitate (DNR) law, 298
"Do not resuscitate—no code blue," legal issues related to, 297–298
Documentation, 271–272
    legal issues related to, 281–283
    TJC on, 282
    UM, 106–110
Domestic violence, mandatory reporting of, 294
DRGs. *See* Diagnosis-related groups (DRGs)
Dunn v. Praiss, 275
Durable medical equipment (DME), 79
    changes related to, 197–198
    in home environment, insurance coverage for, 183–184

E

Educational needs, evolving, in continuous monitoring, reassessing, and reevaluating, 233
Educator, case manager as, 60
Efficiency, in time management, 356–357
Elder abuse, mandatory reporting of, 296–297
Elimination, skilled vs. nonskilled services related to, 186t
E-mail, legal issues related to, 290–291
Emergency department case management, 13
Emotional intelligence, in case management practice, 360–362
Employee Retirement Income Security Act (ERISA), 92–93, 273–274
Employer groups, 94
Employer health insurance plans, self-funded, 92–93
Enrollee, described, 76
Enrollment, described, 76
Entrepreneurial case management, 16–17
Entrepreneurial characteristics, 17
Environment, home
    assessment of, in case management process, 214–215
    skilled nursing care in, part-time or intermittent, 182
Environmental factors, in case management process, 214–215
ERISA. *See* Employee Retirement Income Security Act (ERISA)
Ethic(s)
    codes of, 312–319
    decision-making, guide for uncertain in, 309–310
Ethical issues, 303–323
    assisted death, 321–322
    balancing advocacy vs. cost-containment roles, 318–320

in case management, 318–322
codes of ethics, 312–319
coordinator/facilitator role and, 320
decision making, 308–309
ethics committees, 306–308
gag clauses, 320–321
organ donation, 321
public opinion, 310, 312
right to die, 321–322
withdrawing care, 305–306
withholding care, 305–306
Ethical public opinion, 310, 312
Ethics committees, 306–308
Ethics Statement on Case Management Practice, 327
Evaluation, in case management process, 226–231
Exceptional Medical Expenses Act, 29
Expert witness, 269
External case manager, reimbursement changes related to,
196–197

F

Familial needs, in evaluation and follow-up, 226–229
Family advocacy, optimal vs. inadequate outcomes of, 37–38
Family satisfaction, changes in, in continuous monitoring,
reassessing, and reevaluating, 238–239
Fee(s), global, 94
Fee schedule, 94
Fee-for-services, 75–76
discounted, 76
private, 91–92
Financial assessment, in case management process, 214
Fiscal responsibilities, optimal vs. inadequate outcomes of, 37
Five wishes, 291
Flexibility, of case manager, 58
Follow-up, in case management process, 226–231
From Novice to Expert, 53
Functional assessment, in case management process,
214–215
Functional changes, in continuous monitoring, reassessing, and
reevaluating, 232–233

G

Gag clauses, ethical issues related to, 320–321
Gatekeeper, in HMO, 91
Generic template LOS data reported based on participation in
national database, 129
Global fee, 94
Goal(s)
case management, 35–38
in continuous monitoring, reassessing, and reevaluating,
239
in development and coordination of case plan
establishing of, 220
prioritizing of, 220–221
personal, case management model matched with, 10–11
Grief, in case management practice, 366–367
Grievance
defined, 276
described, 95

GUIDE. *See* Guide for the Uncertain in Decision-Making Ethics
(GUIDE)
Guide for the Uncertain in Decision-Making Ethics (GUIDE),
310–312

H

Hard savings, 48
HCAHPS. *See* Hospital Consumer Assessment of Health care
Providers and Systems (HCAHPS)
HCEA. *See* Health Care Financing Administration (HCEA)
*HCFA Conditions of Participation for Medicare Hospitals—
HCFA Discharge Planning Regulations,* 162
Healing therapies, alternative, 211
Health Care Financing Administration (HCEA), 9
Health Insurance Portability and Accountability Act (HIPAA) of
1996, 44, 273
Health maintenance organizations (HMOs), 90–91
gatekeeper in, 91
models of, 90–91
primary care physician in, 91
specialist care provider in, 91
Health Plan Employer Data and Information Set (HEDIS), 326,
346–348
Health resources, minority, 218
Health Status Survey (SF-12 or SF-36), 219
Healthcare insurance. *See* Insurance
Healthcare team members/professionals, collaboration among,
optimal vs. inadequate outcomes of, 36
HEDIS. *See* Health Plan Employer Data and Information Set
(HEDIS)
Herbal medicine, knowledge of, 52
HHRGs. *See* Home health resource groups (HHRGs)
HINNs. *See* Hospital-Issued Notices of Noncoverage (HINNs)
HIPAA. *See* Health Insurance Portability and Accountability Act
of 1996 (HIPAA)
HIPAA of 1996, 44, 273
HMOs. *See* Health maintenance organizations (HMOs)
Home care services, 182–187, 186t-187t
insurance coverage for, 182–184
insurance criteria for, 182
services not covered by insurance, 184–187, 186t-187t
Home environment
assessment of, in case management process, 214–215
skilled nursing care in, part-time or intermittent, 182
Home health, changes related to, 191–192
benefits, 191–192
diabetic supplies, 192
venipuncture, 191–192
Home health aide services, insurance coverage for, 183
Home health care management, 15
Home health coverage, for postacute care, vs. hospice, 180
Home health resource groups (HHRGs), 73
Home infusions pumps, Medicare and, 80–83
Home social services, insurance coverage for, 183
Homebound, defined, 27
Hospice, for postacute care, 179–182
benefit periods, 181
coverage vs. home health coverage, 180
Medicare criteria for, 180–181
myths and realities, 181
palliative care, 181–182

Hospice case management, 15
Hospital(s), transitional, 174
Hospital Consumer Assessment of Health care Providers and Systems (HCAHPS), 249
Hospital managers, reimbursement changes related to, 196–197
Hospital Outcome of Care Measures, 249
Hospital-based case management, responsibilities of, 7
Hospital-Issued Notices of Noncoverage (HINNs), for traditional Medicare beneficiaries, 164, 166
Hospitalists, 17
Hughes v. Blue Cross of Northern California, 279
Humor
    of care manager, 59
    in case management practice, 358–359
Hunch(es), in time management, 358

I

Important aspects of care, described, 247
"Important Message from Medicare," 164–168
    highlights of, 167–168
    types of, 168–170
In timely manner, defined, 27–28
Incident, described, 247
Incident report, described, 247
Indemnity plans, 90
    managed, 90
Indicators, clinical, 259–262
Information gathering, in case management practice, techniques, 362–363
Information technology, case management and, 20–21
Informational resource, case manager as, 59–60
Informed consent
    disclosure of information in, 287–288
    legal issues related to, 287–289
    signing of, 288–289
Inpatient and Surgical Care Guidelines, 122–123
Inpatient rehabilitation centers, 173–174
Insurance, 69–97. *See also* Reimbursement
    billing-related terms, 94
    claims administrators, 94
    coordination of benefits, 77–78
    employer groups, 94
    ERISA, 92–93
    future prospects in, 97
    HMOs, 90–91
    home care services not covered by, 184–187, 186t-187t
    indemnity plans, 90
    for inpatient rehabilitation centers, 173–174
    LTC, 92
    malpractice, 292
    MCO, 90
    Medicaid, 87–89. *See also* Medicaid
    medical savings accounts, 92
    Medicare, 78–87. *See also* Medicare
    MIPs, 90
    models/systems of, types of, 77–94
    OWA, 92
    PHOs, 92
    POS, 91
    PPOs/PPAs, 91
    private fee-for-service, 91–92
    PSOs, 91
    reinsurance/stop loss personnel, 94
    special, enrollment terms and qualification for, 76–77
    third-party payor, 94
    Tricare, 89
    types of, 70–71
    workers' compensation, 89–90
Insurance authorizations, 105–106
    admission certification, 105
    appeal, 106
    concurrent authorization, 105
    denial, 105
    pended, 105
    precertification authorization, 105
    retrospective authorization, 105
    subauthorization, 105
Insurance benefit analyst, case manager as, 47
Insurance (third-party payor) case management, 14–15
Insurance companies
    cost-sharing strategies for, 71
    protective strategies for, 71
Insurance coverage, for home care services, 182–184
Insurance criteria
    for home care services, 182
    for skilled nursing facilities, 179
Integrated care delivery, 29
Integrator, case manager as, 59
Intelligence, emotional, in case management practice, 360–362
Intensity of service, criteria of, 114
Intensity of service and severity of illness (ISSI), 46
Intermediate care, 171
    level of care of, 176t-177t
Intermittent services, described, 26–27
International Classification of Diseases, 9th revision–*Clinical Modifications* (ICD-9), 94
Interpersonal communication skills, of case manager, 55
InterQual, 112–115
    criteria of, 113
        example of, 130–137
        intensity of service, 114
        severity of illness, 113–114
Interrogatories, 270
Intervention(s), next best, finding, 355
Intuition, in time management, 358
ISD criteria, 113
ISSI. *See* Intensity of service and severity of illness (ISSI)

J

JCI. *See* Joint Commission International (JCI)
Job(s)
    responsibilities and skills, 35–68
        essential, 39–41, *40*
    roles in, 350–351
        clarification related to, 350–352
        conflict related to, 350–352
        confusion related to, 350–352
Job stress, in case management practice, 349–367. *See also specific components and solutions, e.g.,* Time management
    change, 364–366, *365*

communication and information-gathering techniques, 362–363
develop and maintain support system, 353–354
early intervention, 353
emotional intelligence, 360–362
grief, 366–367
humor, 358–359
judgment daze, 358–359
perceptions in communication, 363–364
problem-solving techniques, 354–355
role clarification, 350–352
role conflict, 350–352
role confusion, 350–352
self-care, 362
time management, 355–358
understanding case management and managed care, 352–353
Joint Commission International (JCI), 346
Joint Commission on Accreditation of Healthcare Organizations (JCAHO). *See* The Joint Commission (TJC)
Journal for Healthcare Quality (JHQ), 336
Judgment daze, in case management practice, 358–359

L

Lack of certification, 105
Lag days, 108–110
Large case management, 14
Lawsuit(s), if you are named in, 270–272
Leadership skills, of case manager, 56
Learning
active, experiential, described, 368–369
problem-based, 368–382. *See also* Problem-based learning (PBL)
Legal issues, 267–302. *See also specific issues, e.g.,* Malpractice
advance directives, 291–292
anatomical gifts, 298–299
autopsy, 299–300
background checks, 293
commonsense safeguards, 301
community standards in UM role, 279–281
confidentiality, 289–290
death, 298–299
discharge planning, 284–287
"do not resuscitate—no code blue," 297–298
documentation, 281–283
e-mail, 290–291
ERISA, 273–274
informed consent, 287–289
interstate case management practice, 278–279
liability, techniques to minimize, 300–301
malpractice, 268–272
mandatory reporting, 294–297. *See also* Reportable events, mandatory
mandatory reporting guidelines of New Jersey Board of Nursing, 295–296
medical record, 283–284
negligence, 268
negligent referrals, 272–273
negligent utilization management/review, 274–275
organ donation, 299
premature discharge, 284–287

Privacy Rule, 283
protecting your license, 292
tissue donation, 299
Length of stay (LOS), 74–75, 111–112
data reported based on participation in national database, generic template, 129
Level of care changes, case manager as facilitator of, 45
Levels of care, 170–172
Liability
case manager, 269–270
deferred, insurance, 72
techniques to minimize, 300–301
third-party, insurance, 72
License(s), protecting, legal issues related to, 292
Limit(s), in health-insurance plan, 72
Limitations, statute of, 271
Line(s), during transport of patient, 202
List(s), in time management, 356
Long-term care (LTC), 92, 172
LOS. *See* Length of stay (LOS)
LTC. *See* Long-term care (LTC)

M

Magnetic therapy, knowledge of, 52
Malpractice, 268–272
Affidavit of Merit, 269
case manager liability, 269–270
expert witness, 269
summons and complaint, 270–272
Malpractice insurance, 292
Managed care
background of, 2–3
defined, 2–5
described, 2–5
understanding of, in case management practice, 352–353
Managed care contracts (MCCs), 95–97
Managed care organization (MCO), 90
Managed care systems, background of, 3
Managed indemnity plans (MIPs), 90
Management information system (MIS), 95
Management skills, of case manager, 56
MAPs. *See* Medicare Advantage Plans (MAPs)
MCCs. *See* Managed care contracts (MCCs)
MCO. *See* Managed care organization (MCO)
MDS assessment. *See* Minimum Data Set (MDS) assessment
Medicaid, 87–89
described, 87–88
eligibility for, 88–89
prescription needs covered by, 164
Medical necessity, defined, 26
Medical record, legal issues related to, 283–284
Medical savings accounts, 92
Medical status
changes in, in continuous monitoring, reassessing, and reevaluating, 232
current, in case management process, 211–212
Medical supplies, in home environment, insurance coverage for, 183
Medicare, 78–87, 80t–82t, 85t, 86t
beneficiaries of, 167–168
HINNs for, 164, 166

Conditions of Participation, 162–163
    described, 78
    on discharge planning, 166–167
    home infusion pumps, 80–83
    home intravenous antibiotics covered by, 163
    medications, 80–83
    Part A, 78–79, 80t, 81t
    Part B, 79–80, 82t
    Part C, 83–84
    Part D, 84–85, 85t
    QIO of, 164, 166–167
    review process of, 168–170
Medicare Advantage Plans (MAPs), 83–84, 185
Medicare hospice criteria, 180–181
Medicare observation status guidelines, 124–126, *125*
Medicare Payment Advisory Committee (MEDPAC), 249
Medicare Prescription Drug Plan (PDP), 84
Medicare SELECT, 87
Medication(s)
    in home environment, insurance coverage for, 184
    Medicare and, 80–83
    skilled vs. nonskilled services related to, 186t
Medication assessment, in case management process, 213–214
Medigap plans, 85–87, 86t
MEDPAC. *See* Medicare Payment Advisory Committee
    (MEDPAC)
Milliman Care Guidelines
    examples of, 154–160
    in UM, 120–123
Minimum Data Set (MDS) assessment, 193
Minority health resources, 218
MIPs. *See* Managed indemnity plans (MIPs)
MIS. *See* Management information system (MIS)
Mobility, changes in, in continuous monitoring, reassessing, and
    reevaluating, 232–233
Monitoring, case management, continuous, 231–239, *234, 235,*
    236t, 237t, *238*
Multidisciplinary patient care rounds, facilitator of, case
    manager as, 54

N

NAHQ. *See* National Association for Healthcare Quality
    (NAHQ)
NASW. *See* National Association of Social Workers (NASW)
National Advisory Council on Health Care, 29
National Association for Healthcare Quality (NAHQ), 336–339
National Association of Social Workers (NASW), 4, 41, 269,
    340
National Association of Social Workers' Code of Ethics, 317–318
National Association of Subacute/Postacute Care (NASPAC),
    117–118
    on subacute care, 175
National Committee for Quality Assurance (NCQA), 326,
    346–348
    American Accreditation HealthCare Commission/URAC to, 55
National Institutes of Health (NIH), 52
    on alternative healing methods, 211
National Patient Safety Goals (NPSGs), 254–258, 255t, 257t
National quality measures, 247, 248t
NASPAC. *See* National Association of Subacute/Postacute Care
    (NASPAC)

National Transitions of Care Coalition (NTOCC), 330
NCQA. *See* National Committee for Quality Assurance (NCQA)
Need(s)
    in development and coordination of case plan, prioritizing of,
        220–221
    familial, in evaluation and follow-up, 226–229
Negligence, 268
Negligent referrals, 272–273
Negligent utilization management/review, 274–275
Negotiation
    behaviors to avoid during, 52
    skills in, 49–50
Negotiator(s)
    aggressive, 50–51
    cooperative, 51
Neonatal intensive care unit (NICU), ethical issues related to,
        304
New Jersey Board of Nursing, mandatory reporting guidelines
        of, 295–296
NICU. *See* Neonatal intensive care unit (NICU)
NIH. *See* National Institutes of Health (NIH)
NODMAR. *See* Notice of Discharge and Medicare Appeal
        Rights (NODMAR)
Noncertification, 105
Noncoverage, notices of, 164–170. *See also* Notices of
        Noncoverage (NONCs)
NONCs. *See* Notices of Noncoverage (NONCs)
"Nondiscrimination in Post-Hospital Referral to Home Health
        Agencies and Other Entities," 185, 187
Nonskilled care, skilled care vs., 27
Notch group, described, 95
Notice of Discharge and Medicare Appeal Rights (NODMAR),
        164, 166–167
Notices of Noncoverage (NONCs), 164–170
    CMS on, 164, 166
NPSGs. *See* National Patient Safety Goals (NPSGs)
NTOCC. *See* National Transitions of Care Coalition (NTOCC)
Nurse(s)
    as case managers, 7–8
    duties in 1887, *365*
Nurse case manager
    actual day in life of, 22–24
    day in life of, 21–25
    discussion of, 24–25
    ideal day in life of, 22
Nurse case manager/social worker team, 7–8
    effectiveness of, 8
Nurse Licensure Compact, 278
Nurse Practice Act, 269, 278
Nursing, skilled. *See* Skilled nursing care
Nursing care management, opportunities in, 9–10
Nursing Case Management (RN, CM) credential, 333–335
Nutrition, skilled vs. nonskilled services related to, 186t
Nutritional assessment, in case management process, 212–213

O

OASIS. *See* Outcomes and Assessment Information Set (OASIS)
Occupational therapy (OT), reimbursement changes related to,
        194–197
Occurrence report, described, 247
OCR. *See* Office of Civil Rights (OCR)

Office of Alternative Medicine, 52
Office of Civil Rights (OCR), 273
Office of Minority Health Resource Center (OMHRC), 218
Office of Prepaid Health Care Operations and Oversight
    (OPCOO), 95
Older Americans Act of 2006, 296, 297
OMHRC. *See* Office of Minority Health Resource Center
    (OMHRC)
On-site case management, 15
OPCOO. *See* Office of Prepaid Health Care Operations and
    Oversight (OPCOO)
Open enrollment period, described, 76
OPO. *See* Organ procurement organization (OPO)
Organ donation
    ethical issues related to, 321
    legal issues related to, 299
Organ procurement organization (OPO), 321
Organization(s), 327–331. *See also specific organizations*
ORYX initiative, 346
OT. *See* Occupational therapy (OT)
Other weird arrangement (OWA), 92
Outcome(s), 242–258
    adverse patient, 245, 247
    described, 245
    desired, focusing on, 354–355
    optimal vs. inadequate, 35–39
Outcome measures, relevant to case management programs,
    examples of, 245, 246t
Outcomes and Assessment Information Set (OASIS), 73
Outcomes management, 245
    case manager in, 55
Outpatient services, 163
Outpatient/community-based care management, optimal vs.
    inadequate outcomes of, 38
OWA. *See* Other weird arrangement (OWA)
Oxygen, during transport of patient, 202

P

P4P. *See* Pay-for-performance (P4P)
Pain distress scales, 237, *238*
Pain management, in continuous monitoring, reassessing, and
    reevaluating, 233–238, *234, 235,* 236t, 237t, *238*
    approaches to, 234–235, 236t, 237t
    considerations in, 236–238, 237t, *238*
    inadequate pain relief, causes of, 233–234, *234, 235*
Palliative care, 15
    hospice, 181–182
PAS document, 200
PASAAR form, 200
Patient advocacy, optimal vs. inadequate outcomes of, 37–38
Patient advocate, case manager as, 41–43
Patient Bill of Rights, 314–317
Patient care rounds, tips for, 54
Patient education, adequate, defined, 27
Patient history, in case management process, 211
Patient safety, case management and, 254–258, 255t–257t
Patient satisfaction, changes in, in continuous monitoring,
    reassessing, and reevaluating, 238–239
Patient Self-Determination Act of 1990, 291, 304
Pay-for-performance (P4P), 76
PDP. *See* Medicare Prescription Drug Plan (PDP)

Pending review, 105
Per diem reimbursement, 75
Performance improvement (PI), 243
Perioperative services case management, 14
Personal beliefs, case management model matched with,
    10–11
Personal goals, case management model matched with, 10–11
PHOs. *See* Physician hospital organizations (PHOs)
Physical therapy (PT)
    in home environment, insurance coverage for, 183
    reimbursement changes related to, 194–197
Physician groups, 15
Physician hospital organizations (PHOs), 92
Physician support, case manager in, 54
PI. *See* Performance improvement (PI)
Plan(s), evaluation of, 355
PNCM. *See* Professional Nurse Case Manager (PNCM)
POA. *See* Power of attorney (POA)
Point of service (POS), 91
Population Health Management, 328
POS. *See* Point of service (POS)
Postacute care, 174–188. *See also* Transitional planning,
    postacute care
Postacute discharge/transfer rule, 190–191
Potential costs/charges, 48–49
Potential savings, 48–49
Potentially compensable event, described, 247
Power of attorney (POA), 291
PPOs/PPAs. *See* Preferred provider organizations (PPOs)/
    preferred provider arrangements (PPAs)
PPSs. *See* Prospective Payment Systems (PPSs)
Preadmission review, 103, 114
Precertification authorization, 105
Preferred provider organizations (PPOs)/preferred provider
    arrangements (PPAs), 91
Premature discharge, legal issues related to, 284–287
Premium, insurance, 71
Prescription needs, Medicaid coverage of, 164
Pre-trial, 270
Primary care physician, in HMO, 91
Prioritizing skills, in time management, 356
Privacy, case manager as protector of, 44
Privacy Rule, 273, 283
Private fee-for-service, 91–92
Private vehicles, transferring patient by, 200
Problem identification, in case management process, 210–219
Problem solver, case manager as, 52–53
Problem-based learning (PBL), 368–382
    in case management, described, 369
    case studies, 371–373, 375–382
    defined, 368
    steps in, 369–370
Problem-solving techniques, in case management practice,
    354–355
    brainstorming alternative strategies, 355
    evaluating plan, 355
    finding next best intervention, 355
    focusing on desired outcomes, 354–355
    variance analysis, 354
Process, case management, 205–240. *See also* Case management
    process
*Professional Case Management: The Leader in Evidence-Based
    Practice,* 327

Professional negligence, 268–272. *See also* Malpractice
Professional Nurse Case Manager (PNCM), 31
Professional practice, optimal vs. inadequate outcomes of, 38–39
Prospective Payment Systems (PPSs), 72–73, 188–190
Protecting your license, legal issues related to, 292
Protective strategies, for insurance companies, 71–72
Provider-sponsored organizations (PSOs), 91
PSOs. *See* Provider-sponsored organizations (PSOs)
Psychological factors
    assessment of, in case management process, 215–217
    in case selection in case management process, 208–209
Psychological nurse assistance, in home environment, insurance
        coverage for, 184
PT. *See* Physical therapy (PT)
Public health/community-based case management, 16
Public opinion, ethical, 310, 312

Q

QI. *See* Quality improvement (QI)
QIO. *See* Quality Improvement Organization (QIO)
QISMC. *See* Quality Improvement System for Managed Care
        (QISMC)
QM. *See* Quality management (QM)
Quality improvement (QI)
    case management and, RM with, 249–253
    goal of, 243
    regulation of, 242
    responsibilities of, 243–244
    RM vs., 244
    terminology related to, 245–249, 246t, 248t
Quality Improvement Organization (QIO), 164, 166–167
Quality Improvement System for Managed Care (QISMC),
        342–344
Quality indicators, 253–254
Quality management (QM), 242–258
    regulation of, 242
Quality of care
    in continuous monitoring, reassessing, and reevaluating, 232
    inadequate, circumstances signaling, 263–264
    issues related to, optimal vs. inadequate outcomes of, 36
Quality reviews, 250–251
    admissions concerns, 251
    delayed diagnoses, 251
    described, 250
    examples of, 250–251
Quality screens, generic, 263–264

R

Reasonable and necessary, defined, 26
Reassessing, case management, continuous, 231–239, *234, 235,*
        236t, 237, *238*
Recovery audit contractors, 126–127
Reevaluating, case management, continuous, 231–239, *234, 235,*
        236t, 237, *238*
Referral(s), negligent, 272–273
Refusal of Treatment Release Form, 288
Regulatory agencies, 342–348. *See also specific agency*
    CMS, 342–344
    HEDIS, 346–348
    JCI, 346
    NCQA, 346–348
    ORYX initiative, 346
    QISMC, 342–344
    TJC, 345–346
    URAC, 344
Rehabilitation, skilled vs. nonskilled services related to, 187t
Rehabilitation centers, inpatient, 173–174
    insurance for, 173–174
Rehabilitation services, 172–173
    subacute, categories of, 175, 176t-177t, 178
Rehabilitation specialists, 16
Reid v. Aetna Casualty & Surety Co., 275
Reimbursement, 69–97. *See also* Insurance
    changes related to
        for PT, OT, ST, and respiratory therapy, 194–197
        for SNFs, 191–192
    DRGs, 73–74
    ERISA, 92–93
    future prospects in, 97
    HMOs, 90–91
    indemnity plans, 90
    LTC, 92
    MCO, 90
    medical savings accounts, 92
    MIPs, 90
    OWA, 92
    PHOs, 92
    POS, 91
    PPOs/PPAs, 91
    PPS, 72–73
    private fee-for-service, 91–92
    protective strategies related to, 71–77
    PSOs, 91
    for transportation for transfer of patient, 203
    Tricare, 89
    types of, 72–76
        bundling, 76
        capitation, 75
        discounted fee-for-services, 76
        DRGs, 73–74
        fee-for-service, 75–76
        LOS, 74–75
        P4P, 76
        per diem reimbursement, 75
        PPS, 72–73
        unbundling, 76
    viatical settlements, 93–94
    workers' compensation, 89–90
Reinsurance, 72
Reinsurance/stop loss personnel, 94
Religious beliefs, in case management process, 217–218
Religious diversity, in case management process, 217–218
Reportable events, mandatory, 294–297
    child abuse, 294, 296
    domestic violence, 294
    elder abuse, 296–297
    New Jersey Board of Nursing guidelines for, 295–296
Resource, informational, case manager as, 59–60
Resource allocation, in development and coordination of case
        plan, 221–222
Resource utilization groups (RUGs), 73
    SNF payments by, 193

Resourcefulness, of case manager, 58
Respiratory system, skilled vs. nonskilled services related to, 186t
Respiratory therapy
  changes in, in transitional planning, 194–197
  reimbursement changes related to, 194–197
Retrospective authorization, 105
Retrospective review, 104
Review, concurrent, 103–105
  nurses in, role of, 102
Right to die, ethical issues related to, 321–322
Risk management (RM), 243
  case management and, QI with, 249–253
  goal of, 243
  QI vs., 244
  recommendations and prevention skills of, 251–253
  responsibilities of, 243–244
  terminology related to, 245–249, 246t, 248t
  traditional, 243–244
Risk management (RM) departments, claims categories used by, 265–266
Risk-adjusted, defined, 249
Risk-taking, by case manager, 58
RM. *See* Risk management (RM)
RUGs. *See* Resource utilization groups (RUGs)

S

Safety issues, patient-related, case management and, 254–258, 255t-257t
Sarchett v. Blue Shield of California, 275
Saving(s)
  hard, 48
  potential, 48–49
  soft, 48–49
Screening tools, in case management process, 218–219
Self-care, case management, 362
Self-directedness, of case manager, 58
Self-esteem, of case manager, 58
Self-funded employer health insurance plans, 92–93
Sense of humor, of care manager, 59
Service planning, in development and coordination of case plan, 221–222
Severity of illness, criteria in, 113–114
Shared care, 29
Skilled care, nonskilled care vs., 27
Skilled nursing care, 171–172
  level of care, 176t-177t
  part-time or intermittent, in home environment, 182
Skilled nursing facilities (SNFs)
  case management in, 15–16
  changes related to, 192–193
  coverage options, 179
  insurance criteria, 179
  for postacute care, 178–179
  reimbursement changes for PT, OT, ST, and respiratory therapy, 195–196
  RUGs' payment to, 193
  selection of, factors in, 178–179
Skilled services, nonskilled services vs., 186t-187t
Skin care, skilled vs. nonskilled services related to, 186t
SNFs. *See* Skilled nursing facilities (SNFs)

Social Security Act, Title XIX of, 87
Social Security Disability (SSD), 70
Social Security Income (SSI), 70
Social services, home, insurance coverage for, 183
Social stability, changes in, in continuous monitoring, reassessing, and reevaluating, 232
Social worker/nurse case manager, 7–8
  effectiveness of, 8
Socioeconomic factors, in case selection in case management process, 209–210
Soft savings, 48–49
Specialist care provider, in HMO, 91
Specialty pharmacy providers, 187–188
Speech therapy (ST)
  in home environment, insurance coverage for, 183
  reimbursement changes related to, 194–197
Spend down, described, 77
Spiritual beliefs, in case management process, 217–218
SSD. *See* Social Security Disability (SSD)
SSI. *See* Social Security Income (SSI)
ST. *See* Speech therapy (ST)
Staff development, case manager in, 59–60
Standards for Privacy of Individually Identifiable Health Information, 283
Standards of Practice for Case Management, 53, 327, 329–330
  CMSA on, 230–231
Standards of Practice for Case Management, Revised 2002, 278
Standards of Professional Performance, 313
Statement of Ethical Case Management Practice, 313
Statute of limitations, 271
"Stop loss," 72
Stress
  defined, 349
  job, in case management practice, 349–367. *See also* Job stress, in case management practice
  levels of, 349–350
Stretcher vans, transferring patient by, 202
Subacute care
  categories of, 175
  definitions of, 174–178, 176t-177t
  levels of, 176t-177t
  provision of, according to TJC, 178
Subacute rehabilitation services, categories of, 175, 176t-177t, 178
Subauthorization, 105
Success factors, in case management practice, 349–367
Succinctness, in time management, 356
Summons and complaint, 270–272
Support system, in case management practice, 353–354

T

Taxicab, transferring patient by, 200–201
Team player, case manager as, 54
Telehealth, case management and, 21
Telephonic case management, 15, 105
Telephonic review, 104–105
Telephonic utilization management, 104
The American Accreditation HealthCare Commission/URAC, on time management, 357–358
The American Nurses Association Code of Ethics, 313

The Care Continuum Alliance, 328
The Case Management Practice Guidelines, 329
The CCM Certification Guide, 331–333
The Conditions of Participation for Medicare Hospitals—CMS Discharge Planning Regulations, 12
The Joint Commission (TJC), 53, 95, 326, 345–346
  on discharge planning, 161–162
  on documentation, 282
  on nutritional assessment, 212–213
  provision of subacute care according to, 178
  in QI and QM regulation, 242
The Medicare Handbook, 168
Third-party liability, insurance, 72
Third-party payor, 14–15, 94
3-Rule Rule, 188
3-Midnight Rule, 188
Time management
  assess time robbers in, 356
  be efficient in, 356–357
  be succinct, 356
  in case management practice, 355–358
  delegate in, 357–358
  make lists in, 356
  sharpen prioritizing skills in, 356
  trust hunches/intuition in, 358
Tissue donation, legal issues related to, 299
TJC. *See* The Joint Commission (TJC)
Transcript, 271
Transfer DRGs, 190–191
Transfer note, information to be covered in, 201
Transferring patients, 198–203
  oxygen during, 202
  transfer note, information to be covered in, 201
  transitions of care, 198–200. *See also* Transitions of care
  transportation in, 200–203
    air ambulance, 202
    ambulances, 202
    considerations in planning, 202–203
    costs of, 202–203
    private vehicles, 200
    reimbursement for, 203
    stretcher vans, 202
    taxicab, 200–201
    wheelchair van, 201–202
  tubes and lines during, 202
Transitional hospitals, 174
Transitional planning, 161–204. *See also* Discharge planning
  acute care, 172–174
  defined, 161
  DME changes, 197–199
  home health changes, 191–192
  "Important Message from Medicare" in, 167–168
  incentives of change in, 188–191
  levels of care, 170–172
  long-term care, 172
  Medicare extended care benefit in, 188
  NONCs in, 164–170
  postacute care, 174–188. *See also specific types, e.g.,* Home care services
    home care services, 182–187, 186t-187t
    hospice, 179–182
    skilled nursing facilities, 178–179
    specialty pharmacy providers, 187–188

subacute care, 174–178, 176t-177t
  reimbursement changes in, PT, OT, ST, and respiratory, 194–197
  respiratory therapy changes in, 194–197
  review process in, 168–170
  SNF changes in, 192–193
  standards and expectations in, 162–163
  transferring patients, 198–203. *See also* Transferring patients
Transitions of care, 198–200
  care coordination, 199
  defined, 198
  described, 198–199
  PAS document in, 200
  patients at increased risk during, 199
  transfer packet components, 199–200
Transmural care, 29
Transplant Speakers International, Inc., 299
Transportation, in transferring patients, 200–203. *See also* Transferring patients, transportation in
Tricare, 89
Tube(s), during transport of patient, 202

U

UM. *See* Utilization management (UM)
Unbundling, 76
UR. *See* Utilization review (UR)
URAC. *See* Utilization Review Accreditation Commission (URAC)
U.S. Department of Health and Human Services, on emergency department visits, 10
Utilization management (UM), 100–160
  case management, and UR, relationship among, 101–103
  clinical pathways in, 115–120
    benefits of, 118–119
    chart, 116
    development of, 119–120
    goals of, 118–119
  CMPs in, 115–120
  communication with physicians about, tactics for, 106
  community standards in, 279–281
  defined, 101
  described, 110
  documentation in, 106–110
  historical background of, 101
  lag days, 108–110
  modalities of, 110–127, *125*
    admission as per case management protocol, 123–124
    Condition Code 44, 124
    InterQual, 112–115
    LOS, 111–112
    Medicare observation status guidelines, 124–126, *125*
    Milliman Care Guidelines, 120–123, 154–160
    present on admission, 125–126
    recovery audit contractors, 126–127
  services of, 103–106
    concurrent review, 103–104
    insurance authorizations, 105–106
    preadmission review, 103
    retrospective review, 104
    telephonic review, 104–105
  skills in, 106

telephonic, 104
variances, 108–110
Utilization manager
    case manager as, 46–47
    role of, 102
Utilization review (UR), 100. *See also* Utilization management
        (UM)
    defined, 101
    described, 102
    UM, case management and, relationship among, 101–103
Utilization Review Accreditation Commission (URAC), 344
Utilization Review Accreditation Commission (URAC)/American
        Accreditation HealthCare Commission, to NCQA, 55

V

Variance(s), 108–110
    causes of, 108
    characteristics of, 109
    community, 110
    described, 247
    identification of, 108
    institution/systems, 109–110
    patient/family, 109

practitioner, 109
Variance analysis, 354
Venipuncture, home health changes related to, 191–192
Viatical settlements, 93–94
Villizon v. PruCare, 274
Violence, domestic, mandatory reporting of, 294
Vital signs, skilled vs. nonskilled services related to, 186t
Vocational case management, 16

W

WCB. *See* Workers' Compensation Board (WCB)
Wheelchair van, transferring patient by, 201–202
White House Commission on Complementary and Alternative
        Medicine Policy, 52
Wickline v. State of California, 274
Wilson v. Blue Cross of Southern California, 274
Withdrawing care, ethical issues related to, 305–306
Withhold, 94
Withholding care, ethical issues related to, 305–306
Witness(es), expert, 269
Workers' compensation, 16, 89–90
Workers' Compensation Act, 32
Workers' Compensation Board (WCB), of British Columbia, 31

Continuing Education Enrollment Forms and Posttests

Case Management: A Practical Guide for Education and Practice, 3rd Edition

Directions

- There is a test and a mail-in enrollment form/answer sheet for each chapter.
- Take the test, recording your answers on the test answers section (Section B) of the CE enrollment form. Each question has only one correct answer.
- Complete the registration (Section A), course evaluation (Section C), and payment (Section D).
- Mail completed test with registration fee to: Lippincott Williams & Wilkins, CE Group, 333 7th Ave., 19th Floor, New York, NY 10001.
- Within 4-6 weeks after your CE enrollment form is received, you will be notified of your test results.
- If you pass, you will receive a certificate of earned contact hours and an answer key. If you fail, you have the option of taking the test again at no additional cost.

Questions? Contact Lippincott Williams & Wilkins: 800-787-8985.

Continuing Education Information for Certified Case Managers

This Continuing Education (CE) activity is provided by Lippincott Williams & Wilkins and has been pre-approved by the Commission for Case Manager Certification (CCMC)

This CE is approved for meeting the requirements for certification renewal.

Registration deadline: October 31, 2011.

Continuing Education Information for Nurses

Lippincott Williams & Wilkins (LWW) is accredited as a provider of continuing nursing education by the American Nurses Credentialing Center's Commission on Accreditation.

LWW is also an approved provider of continuing nursing education by the District of Columbia and Florida #FBN2454. LWW home study activities are classified for Texas nursing continuing education requirements as Type 1. This activity is also provider-approved by the California Board of Registered Nursing, Provider Number CEP 11749.

Your certificate is valid in all states.

Registration deadline for Nurses: October 31, 2011.

Disclosure Statement

The authors have disclosed that they have no significant relationship with or financial interest in any commercial companies that pertain to this educational activity.

CHAPTER 1

OVERVIEW OF CASE MANAGEMENT

GENERAL PURPOSE:

To provide case managers and nurses with information about case management models, definitions, and the history of the evolving role of case managers.

OBJECTIVES:

After reading this chapter and taking the test, you will be able to:

1. Define case management.
2. State the difference between case management and managed care.
3. List four milestones in the history and evolution of case management systems.
4. Name five models of case management.
5. Describe the role of the nurse versus the social worker in case management.
6. Recognize five strategies in ensuring the effectiveness of case management models.
7. Determine the value of telehealth and information systems in the practice of case management.

1. **Which is true about the case management definition?**
   a. There is more than one national definition of case management that is used.
   b. The American Nurses Association's definition is used the most.
   c. No consumer-friendly definition has been developed to date.
   d. There are numerous definitions created by many professionals and organizations.

2. **In 1990, Yee defined** *case management* **as**
   a. "the activities of monitoring patient care."
   b. "to limit patient care to a bare minimum to reduce costs."
   c. "the process of getting the right service to the right client."
   d. "reviewing patient charts for ways to decrease hospital lengths of stay."

3. **The differences between case management and managed care include**
   a. case management is people oriented, and managed care is system oriented.
   b. case management focuses on financial benefits and managed care focuses on patients.
   c. managed care negotiates to help patients, and case managers negotiate to limit care.
   d. managed care emphasizes quality care, and case managers focus on financial restraint.

4. **Definitions of managed care include**
   a. insurance benefit limitations and exclusions.
   b. hospital stay lengths determined by physicians.
   c. caring for patient needs and quality of service.
   d. patients have unlimited access to care and resources.

5. **Case management evolution includes the milestone**
   a. number of case mangers exceeded 100,000 in the mid-1980s.
   b. use of case managers in private physician offices in the 1970s.
   c. coordination of services for patients with polio in the 1920s.
   d. insurance companies coordinate services for soldiers post-World War II.

6. **During the late 1990s to early 2000s, case management was**
   a. considered a position only for social workers.
   b. practiced in every setting across the health care continuum.
   c. in jeopardy due to changes in the political structure in the United States.
   d. an ineffective position regarding managed care reimbursement.

7. **Which is** *not* **included in the "factors that impact models of case management"?**
   a. the patient population
   b. the reimbursement method
   c. the context of care setting
   d. the case manager training methods

8. **The "Acute Care Case Management Model"**
   a. utilizes mostly physicians as case managers.
   b. always provides management using one specific way.
   c. is usually episodic and time-limited care in the hospital setting.
   d. does not have case managers practicing hands-on care with any patients.

9. **Patients with chronic illness, disabilities, and catastrophic illnesses requiring short- or long-term management of services are included in the**
   a. "Large Case Management Model."
   b. "Admitting Office Case Management Model."
   c. "Emergency Department Case Management Model."
   d. "Palliative Care and Hospice Case Management Model."

10. **"Disease Management Model" case managers**
    a. apply evidence-based guidelines or protocols.
    b. are usually utilized in hospital settings.
    c. follow their patients for only a short amount of time.
    d. must be experts on all diseases to effectively manage care.

11. **For a foster child target population, the best choice for a case manager would be**
    a. a nurse.
    b. a social worker.
    c. a respiratory therapist.
    d. an occupational therapist.

12. **Social worker case managers differ from nursing case managers because they**
    a. focus more on the patient's complex discharge planning and financial needs.
    b. are more effective at meeting the patient's medical needs on a long-term basis.
    c. can anticipate needed medications better than nurse case managers.
    d. are better able to handle the case manager role than professional nurses.

13. For over five years, the nurse case manager-social worker team was used in healthcare settings, resulting in recommendations to
   a. place nurse case managers and social workers under one department.
   b. have the social worker and nurse work completely independently of each other.
   c. minimize in-service team programs, and concentrate on each case individually.
   d. overlap areas of the position for duplication of work to make sure it all gets done.

14. Strategies to ensure effectiveness of the case management model include all of the following *except*
   a. develop a list of goals that are important to your organization.
   b. evaluate future trends that will affect care and reimbursement in your population.
   c. adapt aspects of current case management models to your needs and requirements.
   d. prioritize goals from the patient's and family's points of view for reimbursement needs.

15. When a case management model is not adequate, it is important to evaluate the organization's
   a. geographic location.
   b. parking and transportation availability.
   c. numbers of patients seen within an 8-hour period.
   d. types of healthcare providers caring for the patients.

16. When collecting and analyzing data to evaluate case management model effectiveness for a given population,
   a. assess recidivism.
   b. evaluate one type of patient in the population.
   c. find out which diseases give the best financial reimbursement.
   d. decide which type of reimbursement program is easier to work with.

17. For evaluation of a model, metrics should be
   a. used for only one purpose (not multipurpose).
   b. used only if no other evaluation method is available.
   c. considered after implementation of the model evaluation.
   d. determined based on the goals and expectations of the model.

18. Telehealth is
   a. not recommended as a tool in case management.
   b. the provision and management of healthcare services from a distance.
   c. a concept used since the 1920s that reinforces healthcare provider services.
   d. a term used for patients who refuse to attend healthcare facilities for care.

19. Examples of telecase management includes all of the following *except*
   a. telephone triage.
   b. concurrent reviews of patient care.
   c. handling of reimbursement denials and appeals.
   d. providing direct patient care in an office or hospital setting.

20. Which is true about the use of current information systems with case management?
   a. Case managers use "paper and pencil" charting more than new technology.
   b. Increased medication errors are one problem with new information technology.
   c. McGonigle and Mastrian claim that information technology will provide solutions.
   d. Case management work is viewed as "top secret" and only case managers have access.

CHAPTER 2

ESSENTIAL CASE MANAGEMENT JOB RESPONSIBILITIES AND SKILLS

GENERAL PURPOSE STATEMENT:
To provide case managers and nurses with information about job responsibilities and essential skills needed for performing a case management position, and to describe educational programs for case management preparation.

LEARNING OBJECTIVES:
After reading this chapter and taking the test, you will be able to:

1. Explain five optimal and five undesired outcomes of case management.
2. Describe the roles and responsibilities of case managers.
3. Differentiate between a case manager's leadership roles and personality traits.
4. Describe three approaches to training and education of case managers.
5. List the various necessary topics to be covered in a case management education program.

1. **Which is an outcome from optimal case management regarding quality of care issues?**
   a. minimal recovery
   b. duplication of services
   c. careful monitoring of safety issues
   d. missed risk factors that lead to management issues

2. **Regarding fiscal responsibilities, which is an outcome from inadequate case management?**
   a. reduced acuity on admission
   b. increased length of hospital stays
   c. reduced number of intensive care days
   d. accurate interpretation of benefits for client and facility

3. **For outpatient/community-based management, which is an optimal case management outcome?**
   a. higher readmission rates
   b. increased use of acute facilities
   c. complications during convalescent phase of care
   d. comprehensive and consistent post-hospital follow-up

4. **The role of the case manager in clinical care management includes**
   a. patient selection and identification.
   b. assisting nursing staff with patient care as needed.
   c. ordering equipment and supplies needed by the staff for patient care.
   d. finding out how long the patient would like to stay during his or her hospitalization.

5. **Brokering community resources is an example of which case manager role/responsibility?**
   a. professional activities
   b. information management
   c. management and leadership
   d. financial and resource management

6. **The roles, functions, and responsibilities of case managers are defined by**
   a. professional organizations.
   b. individual advanced case managers.
   c. patient care needs as identified by clinical staff nurses.
   d. a nationally recognized case management job description.

7. **All of the following are included in the "Six Domains of Case Manager's Role and Functions" *except***
   a. case finding and intake.
   b. healthcare facility staffing issues.
   c. psychosocial and economic issues.
   d. vocational concepts and strategies.

8. **The case manager's most important advocacy responsibility and obligation is to the**
   a. payor.
   b. patient.
   c. healthcare institution.
   d. utilization review modality.

9. **A specific action that successful leaders share is**
   a. to admit their mistakes.
   b. to exhibit strong passive behaviors.
   c. the use of "you" messages instead of "I" messages.
   d. to praise others in private and criticize them in public.

10. **A case manager should have all of the following personality traits *except***
    a. risk taking.
    b. emotional intelligence.
    c. openness and flexibility.
    d. aggressive behaviors.

11. **Creativity is a trait that can help strengthen the case manager's role by**
    a. providing a specific fundamental structure to the organization.
    b. helping to solve unusual problems by thinking "outside the box."
    c. adding vibrant colorful surroundings to the environment to uplift emotions.
    d. following strict guidelines imposed by facilities and reimbursement payors.

12. **For the case manager, self-directedness is a/an**
    a. important trait to change into a more passive type of behavior.
    b. difficult personality trait to have because of the need to work under physicians.
    c. good trait to have because of autonomous decision-making done each day.
    d. poor personality trait because of the stringent guidelines that must be followed.

13. **Which of the following is *not* included in the four basic approaches to training and education of case managers?**
    a. graduate level
    b. doctoral level
    c. on-the-job training
    d. school-based non–degree-granting programs

14. Which is an example of a case management continuing education program?
    a. classes on case management included within another larger program of study
    b. training located in a practice setting to learn the specific role for that workplace
    c. annual CMSA conference and contemporary forum lasting one day to one week
    d. advanced education in a full program of theory, leadership, and skills

15. Which should be included in case management education programs as a major topic?
    a. assessment of high-risk populations
    b. interventions for ventilator-dependent patients
    c. setting up community outreach screening programs
    d. primary disease prevention strategies for patient education

16. Which educational program component includes information about tools for process improvement such as pareto charts?
    a. life care planning
    b. case management models
    c. quality management
    d. outcome measurement/variances/guidelines

17. Which is true about academia for case management?
    a. Degree programs for case management began in the late 1980s.
    b. Certification is available since major accrediting bodies added case management.

c. The nursing licensing exam will include case management questions in the near future.
d. Only social work degree programs incorporate case management into their curriculum.

18. "Case Management By Proxy" is
    a. having experienced case managers explain how they managed difficult cases.
    b. going into the field and working with an experienced case manager on a specific case.
    c. having students go out to find people in the community who need case management.
    d. role-playing using sample case studies to assess knowledge, skill, and competencies.

19. Utilization management
    a. should be included in case manager education, but discussed only briefly.
    b. is not a major case manager role and therefore does not need to be taught to students.
    c. needs to be taught in depth to students, including InterQual and Milliman guidelines.
    d. includes issues such as medical directives, surrogates and guardians, and fraud.

20. Which of the following should be a component taught under the topic of "negotiation skills"?
    a. conflict resolution and problem solving
    b. continuous quality improvement (CQI)
    c. self-care concepts and empowerment
    d. change theories such as Rogers, Orem, and King

CHAPTER 3

REIMBURSEMENT CONCEPTS

GENERAL PURPOSE STATEMENT:

To provide case managers and nurses with information about various types of healthcare plan reimbursement programs and the role of the case manager in the United States.

LEARNING OBJECTIVES:

After reading this chapter and taking the test, you will be able to:

1. Describe the various methods of reimbursement for healthcare services.
2. Define prospective payment system.
3. Define managed care organizations.
4. Differentiate between governmental and private (commercial) insurance.
5. Differentiate between Medicare and Medicaid benefit programs.
6. Determine the role of case managers in managed care contracting.
7. List five reimbursement-related responsibilities of case managers.

1. Which of the following provides healthcare services in the United States (U.S.)?
   a. Aid to Families with Dependent Children (AFDC)
   b. preferred provider organization (PPO)
   c. Social Security disability (SSD)
   d. Social Security income (SSI)

2. The two broad types of healthcare reimbursement/insurance programs used in the U.S. healthcare system are
   a. commercial and governmental.
   b. managed care and indemnity plans.
   c. fee-for-service and carve-out plans.
   d. workers' compensation and liability insurance.

3. A generalized structure for the management of use, access, cost, quality, and effectiveness of healthcare services that links patients to providers of healthcare is
   a. indemnity insurance.
   b. liability insurance.
   c. managed care insurance plans.
   d. stop-loss insurance.

4. Government insurance plans that are public programs include Medicaid, Medicare, and
   a. union health.
   b. Veterans' Administration.
   c. liability insurance.
   d. no-fault workers' compensation.

5. Which of the following is true about Medicaid?
   a. Benefits are limited to people over age 65.
   b. Social Security benefits finance Medicaid.
   c. Medicaid is financed by state and federal governments through tax structures.
   d. Eligible individuals include end-stage renal disease patients entitled to Social Security benefits.

6. Mr. J's insurance has paid for 80% of his medical visit, and he is responsible for payment of the remaining 20%. This cost-sharing strategy is called
   a. coinsurance.
   b. co-payment.
   c. deductible.
   d. premium.

7. A carve-out plan is
   a. a deferment of a portion of the medical expenses paid by federally funded coffers.
   b. purchased by an insurance company to protect itself from very expensive cases.
   c. when another type of insurance is responsible for coverage of healthcare costs.
   d. replacement of a portion of the insurance coverage provided to beneficiaries.

8. Which is true about the prospective payment system (PPS)?
   a. It has remained unchanged since it began in 1983.
   b. Hospitals are reimbursed on a fee-for-service schedule.
   c. PPS reimbursement is presently only used in hospital-based care.
   d. Predetermined reimbursement rates are provided based on diagnosis.

9. "Diagnosis-Related Groups" (DRGs)
   a. were originally designed specifically for reimbursement purposes.
   b. do not reimburse for extra days spent in the hospital for any reason.
   c. created a strong need for hospitals to utilize case managers.
   d. reimburse hospitals based on dollar amount and length of stay (LOS).

10. Which type of payment structure bills insurance companies based on actual cost of service provided?
    a. capitation
    b. fee-for-service
    c. per diem reimbursement
    d. pay-for-performance (P4P)

11. When a patient has more than one insurance plan, it is important to
    a. find out first which insurance company is the primary payor.
    b. first bill their public insurance plan, then bill their private insurance plan.
    c. determine which plan reimburses at a higher rate and bill that one first.
    d. bill the insurance plan that has the lower out-of-pocket expense first.

12. Which is true about Medicare Part A?
    a. Part A benefits cannot be taken away, regardless of number of inpatient hospital days.
    b. Lifetime reserve days pay for all hospital expenses without any out-of-pocket expense.
    c. Skilled nursing facility (SNF) care is not covered under any circumstances.
    d. A $1,024 hospital deductible charge is billed to the patient for each new benefit period.

13. Medicare Part B pays for or helps to pay for
    a. hepatitis B vaccine, flu vaccine, and pneumococcal pneumonia vaccines.
    b. erythropoietin only if patient has renal disease but is not on dialysis.
    c. immunosuppressive drugs for the first 5 years after transplant.
    d. oral chemotherapy for cancer, only if drug is not available in injectable form.

14. The Sixth Omnibus Reconciliation Act (SOBRA) became effective in 1987 to provide
    a. Medicaid to pregnant women and children with a family income below the poverty level.
    b. Medicaid to blind and disabled persons who receive SSI.
    c. Medicare supplementation provided by private insurers with a choice of 12 plans.
    d. Medicare to patients with breast or cervical cancer.

15. Tricare is a healthcare program for which of the following groups of people?
    a. workers who get injured while on the job
    b. pregnant women and/or children under 5 years of age
    c. military personnel and their eligible family members or survivors
    d. adults 65 years of age and older who have an income below the poverty level

16. Which HMO (health maintenance organization) model employs the physicians who work exclusively in clinic-type settings for salaries?
    a. group model
    b. staff model
    c. direct contract model
    d. independent practice association (IPA)

17. The prospective payment system (PPS) was established in 1983 to
    a. stop reimbursing hospitals on a fee-for-service basis.
    b. begin an indemnity plan for payment of services by Medicare and Medicaid.
    c. allow for billing of services beyond what a plan pays, and patient must pay difference.
    d. inhibit physicians from billing patients and insurance companies for the same service.

18. The role of case managers in managed care contracting (MCC) includes all of the following *except*
    a. contract negotiation.
    b. denials and appeals processes.
    c. legal interpretation of contract.
    d. utilization review and management procedures.

19. Areas included in the MCC that are related to case management include all of the following *except*
    a. marketing strategies for managed care.
    b. quality/outcomes measurements.
    c. scope of services to be provided.
    d. agreements with other providers.

20. Responsibilities of the case manager with Medicare patients include all of the following *except*
    a. coordinate for necessary services.
    b. discharge planning including post-hospital services.
    c. coordinate care with the Medicare plan's case manager.
    d. tell patient which specific Medicare plans to get.

CHAPTER 4

UTILIZATION MANAGEMENT

GENERAL PURPOSE STATEMENT:
To provide case managers and nurses with information about utilization management.

LEARNING OBJECTIVES:
After reading this chapter and taking the test, you will be able to:

1. Define the terms utilization review and utilization management.
2. Describe the use of criteria and guidelines in the utilization management and review process.
3. Differentiate between the various types of reviews.
4. Determine the role of the case manager in utilization management.
5. Recognize the impact of documentation on utilization management.
6. List five characteristics of case management plans.
7. Identify four goals of case management plans.

1. **What is the process in which medical review determinations are made based on clinical guidelines and structured processes?**
   a. clinical pathways
   b. utilization review (UR)
   c. retrospective authorization
   d. utilization management (UM)

2. **Which is true about UM?**
   a. It is a function independent from case management.
   b. It is an old term that has since been replaced by UR.
   c. It is a process of creating high-quality healthcare by using all resources.
   d. The goal of UM is to use healthcare resources in the most cost-effective and efficient setting.

3. **How does UM differ from UR?**
   a. UM is similar, but has a narrower focus than UR.
   b. UM is practiced in all healthcare settings and UR is not.
   c. UR is a component in case management, but UM is not.
   d. UR is proactive in case management and UM is reactive to medical criteria.

4. **The purpose of UM prospective review is to**
   a. decide if a facility is healing a patient's disorder.
   b. ensure that a decision to admit a patient is appropriate or justified.
   c. determine if the staff at a facility is treating the patients respectfully.
   d. allow patients to have an evaluation tool to rate the care they are receiving.

5. **Which type of review includes the two parameters of "admission review" and "continued stay review"?**
   a. preadmission review
   b. prospective review
   c. concurrent review
   d. retrospective review

6. **Retrospective reviews**
   a. are not useful tools for evaluating quality control.
   b. ensure that criteria are met before discharging a patient from the facility.
   c. allow for intervention to occur to change the course of events for the patient.
   d. are becoming less common due to most services requiring precertifications.

7. **Criteria and guidelines are used in prospective reviews for**
   a. initially determining the patient's hospital length of stay.
   b. finding alternative healing methods for the patient's diagnosis.
   c. selecting the patient's nursing staff during the hospital stay.
   d. determining if patient discharge criteria have been met.

8. **Telephonic reviews**
   a. cost insurance companies more money than other types of reviews.
   b. are the most effective means of UM and rarely have any liability issues.
   c. are usually used for a concurrent review for 24-hour management coverage.
   d. are declining in use, and soon will not be used by any insurance companies.

9. **Practical tips to help with communication with physicians for UM-related interactions include**
   a. focusing on the physician's goals for patient care.
   b. following through on what was discussed with the physicians to gain trust.
   c. discussing a variety of topics with the physicians besides the UM information.
   d. being adversarial and aggressive when approaching the physicians to discuss UM.

10. **The most important skills a case manager in a UM role needs are good communication skills and**
    a. a first-rate clinical databank.
    b. a list of local skilled nursing facilities.
    c. the support of the nursing staff at the facility.
    d. the home phone numbers of all physicians in the facility.

11. **If a physician is a poor documenter, what should the UM nurse do to make sure that inpatient days get paid?**
    a. Teach the physician proper documentation procedures.
    b. Document physician and insurance reviewer conversations.
    c. File a complaint with the hospital to have the physician document properly.
    d. Advise the nursing administrator to contact the insurance company about payment.

12. **Which is an example of thorough and accurate documentation?**
    a. "Mr. J's temperature is elevated today."
    b. "A culture was taken from Mr. J for his fever."
    c. "The result of Mr. J's 3mm, right upper-arm skin biopsy was negative."
    d. "Mr. J was supposed to be transferred today, but now that plan has changed."

13. The Centers for Medicare and Medicaid (CMS) services require all of the following documentation *except*
    a. revisions made to the diagnostic impression.
    b. discharge summary including follow-up arrangements.
    c. history and physical performed within 36 hours of admission.
    d. physician orders of admission status including date and time.

14. Which is true about clinical pathways?
    a. They include timelines for providing interventions.
    b. They encourage practice variations for many diagnoses.
    c. They are orders that prescribe diagnosis-specific activities.
    d. They are algorithms that are an approach to managing a specific diagnosis.

15. Subacute pathways
    a. do not address outcome analysis.
    b. integrate admission criteria but not discharge criteria.
    c. only include nursing-related information.
    d. encourage patient participation through education.

16. Which is an example of a positive variance from the clinical pathway?
    a. The patient responds to the interventions quicker than anticipated.
    b. The patient's original diagnosis has been changed due to test results.
    c. The patient has complications and now needs ventilator assistance.
    d. The patient is not responding and hospital stay is longer than anticipated.

17. All of the following are included as goals of case management plans *except*
    a. improvement in patient/family satisfaction of care.
    b. enhancement of quality of care by addressing any variances early.
    c. incorporation of all disciplines and all-inclusive, supportive care.
    d. allowing patients to develop their own case management plans.

18. Extended care clinical pathways should include
    a. clear benchmarks for measuring quality indicators.
    b. a broad range of patients; clinical and cost issues should not matter.
    c. random participants to form a study group to evaluate improvement.
    d. new ideas implemented on a broad scale to evaluate outcomes.

19. Which example meets InterQual's intensity of service criteria?
    a. The patient needs protective isolation.
    b. The patient has an indwelling urinary catheter.
    c. Oral analgesics are required at least 4 times per day.
    d. The patient needs dressing changes at least 3 times daily.

20. Regarding InterQual's criteria, which is true about what "ISD" stands for?
    a. "I" stands for insurance reimbursement.
    b. "S" stands for service length.
    c. "D" stands for discharge screens.
    d. "ISD" stands for intermediate standards and/or devices.

CHAPTER 5

TRANSITIONAL PLANNING: UNDERSTANDING LEVELS AND TRANSITIONS OF CARE

GENERAL PURPOSE STATEMENT:

To provide case managers and nurses with knowledge about transitional planning, including levels of care and transitions of care within the case management role.

LEARNING OBJECTIVES:

After reading this chapter and taking the test, you will be able to:

1. Define the terms discharge planning, transitions of care, and levels of care.
2. Discuss the relationships between transitions of care and levels of care.
3. Differentiate between the various care settings across the healthcare continuum.
4. Differentiate skilled from nonskilled care.
5. Explain the relationships among transitional planning, utilization management, and reimbursement.
6. Describe the role of the case manager in the various practice settings.
7. Report the impact of case management on care quality and patient safety during transitions of care.

1. Which of the following is focused on "discharging patients from an inpatient hospital setting to another facility or home"?
   a. levels of care
   b. case management
   c. discharge planning
   d. transitional planning

2. To establish an appropriate level of care, all of the below are needed *except*
   a. the right setting.
   b. the right time.
   c. the right provider.
   d. the right social interaction.

3. Regulatory and accreditation standards continue to focus primarily on
   a. levels of care.
   b. discharge planning.
   c. transitional planning.
   d. skilled nursing facility transfers.

4. A role essential to overseeing that provision of care for discharging a patient adheres to standards is the facility's
   a. risk manager.
   b. case manager.
   c. discharging physician.
   d. nursing administrator.

5. When considering discharging a patient from the hospital, in most cases the preferable place to discharge or transfer the patient to is
   a. a skilled nursing facility.
   b. home with family support.
   c. an assisted-living facility.
   d. a rehabilitation center.

6. Since many insurance plans provide home health services based on a patient's condition and needs, it is important to assess
   a. criteria such as being homebound.
   b. the communication needs of the patient.
   c. the availability of various home services.
   d. the doctor's willingness to order home health services.

7. If a patient is discharged from the hospital to an assisted living facility with a need for intravenous (IV) antibiotics, the assisted care facility will
   a. not accept the patient until IV medications are no longer required.
   b. not accept the patient unless the patient can be taken to a physician's office for IV therapy.
   c. accept the patient but home health nurses will need to be retained for IV therapy.
   d. accept the patient because the facility has on-site nursing staff to provide the IV therapy.

8. Which is true about suctioning needs of a patient being discharged?
   a. Skilled nursing facilities (SNFs) will not provide suctioning.
   b. Intermediate care can provide sterile suctioning as needed.
   c. Assisted living facilities will provide simple, nonsterile suctioning.
   d. Rehabilitation facilities will provide frequent tracheal suctioning.

9. When comparing skilled care and nonskilled care, which is true?
   a. Only skilled care providers can apply nonsterile dressings.
   b. Both skilled care and nonskilled care providers take vital signs.
   c. Both skilled care and nonskilled care providers administer medications.
   d. Only nonskilled care providers can perform active range-of-motion exercises.

10. Mandated Medicare criteria must be met before a hospitalized patient can be admitted to a SNF; these criteria include
    a. the care required is based on nursing orders.
    b. the patient is independent for all activities of daily living (ADLs).
    c. the patient's care can also be provided by home healthcare nurses.
    d. the medical condition requires daily skilled services by a licensed professional.

11. After receiving the "Important Message from Medicare" (IM) prior to discharge, a patient or family member can appeal the impending discharge with a/an
    a. attorney's letter to the hospital administrator within the week.
    b. e-mail, letter, or facsimile (fax) to Medicare personnel prior to discharge.
    c. prompt telephone call to the Quality Improvement Organization (QIO).
    d. videotaped message from the patient/family sent to a county court judge.

12. **Definitions of levels of care**
    a. differ from one facility to the next.
    b. are similar in all facilities throughout the United States.
    c. are not an important aspect when transferring a patient.
    d. are standardized regarding what level is offered in each facility.

13. **An example of an acute care facility/agency is a/an**
    a. SNF.
    b. home health agency.
    c. specialty pharmacy provider.
    d. inpatient acute rehabilitation hospital.

14. **The greatest patient benefits are attained when case management focuses on the**
    a. levels of care.
    b. individual patient's needs.
    c. reimbursement methods.
    d. facility's goals of patient care.

15. **The 3-Midnight Rule is**
    a. a Medicare "extended care benefit" that began in the late 1960s.
    b. a requirement that hospitals provide care for a minimum of 3 days
    c. a law that all insurances must pay for 3 days of SNF care after any hospital stay.
    d. a home healthcare reimbursement strategy for Medicare patients.

16. **"The process of moving patients from one level of care to another" is the definition of**
    a. a hand-off.
    b. a hand-over.
    c. transitions of care.
    d. discharge planning.

17. **Care coordination is a/an**
    a. provision of care that is performed by the patient's physician.
    b. duty of the staff nurse caring for the patient in the hospital setting.
    c. effective strategy to make sure that care is uninterrupted during transition encounters.
    d. role of the hospital administration staff to ensure patient discharge is appropriate.

18. **To determine mode of transportation for a patient transferring from the hospital to another facility, the case manager should consider all of the following** *except*
    a. tubes and lines present on patient.
    b. prices and insurance coverage of transportation.
    c. patient and family members opinions.
    d. oral medications that the patient is taking.

19. **The role of the case manager in planning home health care patient services includes**
    a. providing bereavement services and direct patient care as needed.
    b. coordinating services between agencies since no physician is needed to order services.
    c. advising patients they must meet Medicare's eight levels of care for hospice services.
    d. knowing the Medicare standard guidelines for home healthcare and hospice services.

20. **The external case manager needs to**
    a. memorize the reimbursement guidelines of all private insurance companies.
    b. remember that the physician is the key decision-maker for level of patient care.
    c. meet the patient's needs by providing daily hands-on care to the patient in the home.
    d. continue coordinating the level of care the patient currently has despite any complaints.

CHAPTER 6

THE CASE MANAGEMENT PROCESS

GENERAL PURPOSE STATEMENT:
To provide case managers and professional nurses with information about the seven stages of the case management process.

LEARNING OBJECTIVES:
After reading this chapter and taking the test, you will be able to:

1. Describe each stage of the case management process.
2. List five criteria that qualify a patient for case management services.
3. Determine the essential components of a case management assessment.
4. Develop a case management plan of care including establishing goals and prioritization of needs.
5. Describe four strategies which ensure effective implementation of the case management plan of care.
6. Recognize the importance of ongoing monitoring and evaluation of the case management plan of care.
7. Identify three strategies for effective closure of case management services.

1. **Which stage of the case management process eliminates patients who probably will not need case management services?**
   a. case closure
   b. case selection
   c. continuous monitoring
   d. assessment/problem identification

2. **During the case management stage of implementation, the case manager**
   a. refines, revises, and fine-tunes the case plan.
   b. decides which patients meet the intensity of services.
   c. collects data on selected patients, exposing both potential and actual problems.
   d. coordinates and facilitates patient discharge from the hospital to home or to another facility.

3. **Postdischarge telephone calls or personal visits are performed to help make sure all patient and family questions have been answered during the case management stage of**
   a. case selection.
   b. implementation.
   c. evaluation and follow-up.
   d. assessment/problem identification.

4. **Which of the following is a common indicator for case management services in a hospital setting?**
   a. length of stay longer than 5 days
   b. patient is between 40 and 55 years of age
   c. charges for care are approximately $10,000
   d. patient has no spouse, but lives at home with a capable adult child

5. **All of the following are "red flags" that a patient needs case management services** *except*
   a. chronic mental illness.
   b. unintentional overdose.
   c. uncooperative patient behavior.
   d. giving birth to second or third child.

6. **Socioeconomic indicators for case management services include all of the following** *except*
   a. single parent.
   b. out-of-state residence.
   c. admission from an extended care facility.
   d. state- or Medicaid-sponsored health insurance coverage.

7. **Which statement is true regarding nutritional assessments?**
   a. Of the ten leading causes of disease, two are related to nutrition.
   b. Research indicates that malnutrition is a rare problem with hospitalized patients.
   c. A dental/mouth assessment can detect if poor eating is due to ill-fitting dentures.
   d. The case manager should always perform a nutritional assessment independent of a dietician.

8. **What is included in the medication assessment?**
   a. Assess whether the patient is taking the simplest dosing regimen available.
   b. Assess if the patient knows the manufacturer of the medication he/she is taking.
   c. Assess if family members are aware of the medications being taken by patient.
   d. Assess pharmacist profit from the patient's medication purchases.

9. **When the case manager performs a psychosocial assessment, it should include**
   a. the patient's response to the illness or event.
   b. whether the patient can perform hygiene tasks independently.
   c. sanitation of the patient's living space (e.g., rodents, roaches).
   d. whether the patient can meet basic financial obligations (e.g., rent, food).

10. **When developing a case management plan, which information needs to be discussed with the multidisciplinary team?**
    a. location and timeframe of the next level of care
    b. easiest type of care for providers to perform for patient
    c. types of care or equipment needs that will provide the most profit for the facility
    d. tasks to be accomplished by the facility to lower costs of supplies

11. **An appropriate short-term goal for a patient who had hip replacement surgery 2 days ago would include**
    a. returning home safely.
    b. walking 300 feet or more with a walker.
    c. transferring from bed to chair with assistance.
    d. independently performing activities of daily living (ADLs).

12. **When prioritizing goals, the case manager should**
    a. determine the priority of the goals and then advise the patient and family.
    b. determine the most pressing problem for the patient and/or family.
    c. only include patient and family members in prioritization if they are difficult.
    d. explore the patient's prognosis and, if terminal, then prioritize goals for the patient and family.

13. **A strategy that can ensure effective utilization of the case management plan of care includes**
    a. having case managers brainstorm all of the tasks that need to be performed.
    b. maximizing the financial gain of the facility while the patient receives safe care.
    c. having the internal case manager communicate with the external case manager.
    d. documenting every 1 to 2 weeks on patient needs that have been met.

14. **On the day of patient discharge, the internal case manager should**
    a. finalize and confirm transportation pick-up time arrangements.
    b. assess wound care needs of the patient, and order needed supplies.
    c. evaluate pain control and find out if medication can be changed to an oral dosing.
    d. ensure that tests and equipment needed prior to discharge have been ordered.

15. **Implementation of a care plan for an external case manager would include**
    a. written instructions for follow-up appointments with physicians.
    b. educating the patient and family on disease process and hands-on care.
    c. the case manager having written proof of negotiations and pricing agreements.
    d. the review of blood test results that the physician needs prior to patient discharge.

16. **What was the finding of the original landmark 1979 Molter study regarding familial needs?**
    a. The family has a strong need to obtain information about their ill family member.
    b. The need for hope is extremely important when a member of the family is ill.
    c. The equilibrium of the whole familial structure changes when one member is ill.
    d. The family needs to feel a sense of control over the situation.

17. **When appraising the final evaluation of a case, the case manager should assess the impact that case management had on**
    a. staff perceptions of family members.
    b. the financial status of the patient and family members.
    c. updating the family regularly on the patient's progress.
    d. how much durable medical equipment (DME) was ordered for the patient.

18. **A question for the case manager to ask during the evaluation and follow-up process is:**
    a. Were the patient and family members happy with the quality of meals?
    b. Were there any problems with the agencies or companies that were set up?
    c. Did the physician provide adequate communication with patient and family?
    d. Were all ordered test results reviewed by the physician in a timely manner?

19. **One reason for the termination of case management services is**
    a. the case management company closing or relocating.
    b. the case not being resolved within a 2-month period.
    c. an inability to meet the patient's case management goals.
    d. difficult patient or family behaviors that might lead to noncompliance.

20. **When case managers close or terminate a case, they should**
    a. close the case quickly and without a lot of explanations.
    b. refer final patient/family questions to the physician to answer.
    c. explain exactly how much money the insurance company paid for case management.
    d. remind the family of the need to close the case a few days before the last day of involvement.

CHAPTER 7

QUALITY MANAGEMENT AND OUTCOMES

GENERAL PURPOSE STATEMENT:

To provide case managers and professional nurses with information about the relationship between case management, risk management, and quality management services with utilization of core measures, indicators, and outcomes.

LEARNING OBJECTIVES:

After reading this chapter and taking the test, you will be able to:

1. Define the terms performance management, outcomes management, risk management, and core measures.
2. Describe the relationship between case management and quality management.
3. Describe the process of quality reviews.
4. Explain the role of the case manager in quality and outcomes management.
5. List five strategies in case management practice that enhance patient safety.
6. Describe the role of the case manager in the reporting of outcomes (core measures).

1. Which role reacts to actual problems and identifies potential problems with programs such as "pressure ulcer prevention programs?"
   a. performance management (PM)
   b. outcomes management
   c. risk management (RM)
   d. core measures

2. Outcomes management is a
   a. national, standardized performance measurement system.
   b. concept that attempts to meet or exceed the customer's needs.
   c. program that lessens chances of adverse events from happening.
   d. process that allows for the delivery of evidence-based care and treatments.

3. Which is true about core measures?
   a. Core measures were first known as the ORYX measures.
   b. Core measures were first begun by The Joint Commission (TJC) in 1987.
   c. Core measures are quality care-related reports obtained by patient surveys.
   d. The Centers for Medicare and Medicaid Services (CMS) used core measures first.

4. Quality reviews refer to
   a. meeting the needs of the payor for services.
   b. intervening on behalf of patients by case managers.
   c. screening the patient's medical record to see if national standards were met.
   d. identifying circumstances that make patients vulnerable to high-risk situations.

5. Case managers perform all of the following services *except*
   a. acting as a patient and family advocate.
   b. determining if a legal problem exists and applying reactive interventions as needed.
   c. identifying traits in a person that make him or her vulnerable to high-risk situations.
   d. acting as a liaison between the patient, facility, and insurance company.

6. Which of the following oversees all aspects of patient care?
   a. case management
   b. risk management
   c. quality management
   d. performance management

7. During a quality review, which of the following is considered a cardiology clinical indicator?
   a. pericarditis present on admission
   b. planned transfer to special care unit
   c. cardiac arrest not related to any procedure
   d. postoperative bleeding that could not be controlled on a medical floor

8. Which of the following is an example of a quality review?
   a. Hysterectomy patient develops bloody urine; culture reveals bacteria present.
   b. Six-week old infant is admitted for seizures, with a strong family history of epilepsy.
   c. Neonate has an Apgar score of 3, with predelivery diagnosis of placental abruption.
   d. Patient's spleen is removed during a gastrectomy due to surgical splenic artery injury.

9. What is true regarding quality indicators?
   a. They are measurable and specific guides.
   b. They list interventions for case managers to perform.
   c. They can only be written for specific types of medical procedures.
   d. They are utilized after trends in care have already been documented.

10. The National Practitioner's Data Bank has 10 types of claims categories that provide risk managers with
    a. indications of suboptimal care.
    b. measures to avoid mistakes with medications.
    c. advice on how to handle lawsuits within a hospital setting.
    d. guidelines for how to handle difficult patients and/or family members.

11. What is true regarding patient care safety in healthcare organizations?
    a. The first set of National Patient Safety Goals (NPSG) were approved in July 2002.
    b. NSPG goals do not include specific recommendations for quality improvement (QI).
    c. Today, 80% of The Joint Commission (TJC) standards are related to patient safety.
    d. The NPSG were developed by the Institute for Healthcare Improvement.

12. All of the following are strategies that case managers use to enhance patient safety *except*
    a. medication reconciliation.
    b. communication among providers.
    c. timely completion of necessary tests.
    d. providing spiritual patient/family guidance.

13. A national standardized performance measurement system implemented to improve quality health-care is/are
    a. variances.
    b. core measures.
    c. outcomes management.
    d. a potentially compensable event.

14. Which of the following best describes the definition of "outcomes"?
    a. The results and consequences of healthcare services that were or were not received
    b. Adverse events or unusual situations that occur to patients while they are hospitalized.
    c. Four types of outcomes include practitioner, system, community, and patient
    d. Situations occurring frequently to large numbers of patients, which lead to patient risk

15. When the case manager completes an occurrence report, it should be written
    a. with the case manager's judgment about the situation.
    b. with appropriate speculation to give a full subjective point of view.
    c. with objective, factual, clear, and complete statements.
    d. as a personal report to RM, since it will never be used in a court of law.

16. Which is true about QI activities?
    a. QI is a retroactive model.
    b. QI was designed to monitor, prevent, and correct quality deficiencies.
    c. QI is an intermittent process, used only when a problem situation arises.
    d. QI is a process that determines if there is risk for a lawsuit regarding a particular situation.

17. The RM role
    a. reviews current patient charts daily to monitor for problem situations.
    b. determines appropriate outcomes that should be met for each current patient.
    c. controls and minimizes losses through legal methods and public relations efforts.
    d. has an ongoing process of examining and evaluating quality care on a daily basis.

18. A Level II adverse patient outcome (APO) would include which type of situation?
    a. The wrong limb was removed from a patient during surgery.
    b. A patient experienced urinary retention after a total abdominal hysterectomy.
    c. The wrong medication was given, but quickly corrected before any patient harm occurred.
    d. A patient was discharged with pyuria and mild bacteremia, without plans for follow-up care.

19. To anticipate potential problems, case managers
    a. focus on loss prevention activities.
    b. identify potential safety issues in frail and confused patients.
    c. evaluate all hospital risk exposures such as visitor safety and environmental safety.
    d. attempt to minimize cost of liability insurance and liability of claims.

20. Which role ascertains the best plan of care to meet the individual needs of the patient, within the constraints of the payor, using negotiation skills?
    a. case management
    b. RM
    c. quality management
    d. PM

CHAPTER 8

LEGAL ISSUES IN CASE MANAGEMENT

GENERAL PURPOSE STATEMENT:

To provide case managers and professional nurses with information about legal issues in case management.

LEARNING OBJECTIVES:

After reading this chapter and taking the test, you will be able to:

1. Distinguish negligence from malpractice.
2. Recognize the importance of documentation in avoiding risk for litigation.
3. List four strategies to ensure appropriate discharge or case closure.
4. Describe the informed consent process.
5. Explain the role of advanced directives in the planning and case management of patient's care.
6. Identify five strategies case managers may use to reduce legal risk.

1. The failure to act as a reasonable person in a given situation is
   a. negligence.
   b. malpractice.
   c. incompetence.
   d. Affidavit of Merit.

2. All of the following are inclusive of the four elements of negligence *except*
   a. duty
   b. harm
   c. causation
   d. competency

3. Which statement is true regarding malpractice?
   a. Malpractice is a lesser duty than negligence.
   b. Malpractice is considered professional negligence.
   c. Malpractice is a betrayal between two persons who have a written agreement.
   d. Malpractice occurs when a person uses superior skills and knowledge appropriately.

4. Before a professional malpractice case can be filed in court,
   a. there must be proof of the defendant's intention to harm the plaintiff.
   b. an Affidavit of Merit must also be filed, otherwise the lawsuit will be dismissed.
   c. the plaintiff must meet with the defendant to try to determine if settlement is possible.
   d. there needs to be a criminal inquiry to determine if a crime was committed.

5. Which of the following is an example of the appropriate use of the recommended documentation guidelines?
   a. "When I returned from a 'Code Blue' in another room, I found Mr. J on the floor."
   b. "Mr. J is a robust fellow who suddenly fell to the floor with a 'thud' sound."
   c. "Mr. J was lying on the floor when I walked into his messy hospital room."
   d. "I couldn't believe it when I saw Mr. J on the floor after I had just put him in bed!"

6. Which is true about using abbreviations?
   a. Do not use any abbreviations in documentation notes.
   b. Abbreviations that co-workers are familiar with can be used.
   c. Use abbreviations that The Joint Commission (TJC) has approved.
   d. Use abbreviations that have been used in the past by other healthcare professionals.

7. If the case manager forgot to chart a note and remembers a day later, what should he or she do?
   a. Back-date the information when writing it in the chart.
   b. Page back to the appropriate time it should have been charted, and squeeze it in.
   c. Omit the information from the chart since it should have been charted earlier.
   d. Chart at the present date and time, and explain why the entry was delayed.

8. Which statement is an example of appropriate documentation?
   a. "The condition of Mrs. X's home made mobility difficult."
   b. "Mrs. X is a slob and her house is a mess, which can lead to a fall."
   c. "Mr. P was ranting and raving about missing his X-ray appointment."
   d. "Mr. P had a crazy story about why he didn't attend his X-ray appointment."

9. Why is documentation scrutinized by third-party reimbursement payors?
   a. to monitor the quality of care within that facility
   b. to advise patients of their rights while hospitalized
   c. to determine whether a procedure was medically necessary
   d. to evaluate the credibility of the medical staff caring for the patient

10. The best discharge planning starts
    a. at admission to the hospital or medical facility.
    b. after the physician writes the discharge order for the patient.
    c. immediately after an operative procedure or medical treatment.
    d. when the patient begins to show an increase in independence or medical progress.

11. Charges of premature discharge or patient abandonment occur more often due to
    a. hospitals needing more bed space.
    b. adverse payment decisions by third-party payors.
    c. case managers arranging for comprehensive follow-up services.
    d. patients' desires to sign themselves out of the hospital, against medical advice.

12. All of the following are included in the discharge planning of a patient by a case manager *except* the documentation of
    a. patient/family education and teaching.
    b. patient agreement or rejection of recommended services.
    c. any and all changes in the discharge plan and why the change occurred.
    d. core measures that are not needed for medication or discharge planning.

13. **Which is an appropriate statement for discharge planning documentation?**
    a. "Mr. L was given information about his wound before he was sent home."
    b. "Teaching was done by medical staff members prior to Mr. L's discharge."
    c. "A dressing change demonstration was done for Mr. L during his hospitalization."
    d. "Written and verbal wound care instructions were given to Mr. L prior to discharge today."

14. **Informed consent is a legal requirement that is the responsibility of the**
    a. nurse.
    b. physician.
    c. risk manager.
    d. case manager.

15. **Implied consent for medical interventions includes**
    a. difficult patients.
    b. unconscious patients.
    c. patients refusing care.
    d. patients with psychiatric diagnoses.

16. **A patient can be found to be legally incompetent only by**
    a. a court of law and a judge's order.
    b. having two physicians document that the patient is legally incompetent.
    c. having the patient's attending physician and the risk manager sign a legal form.
    d. having the patient's next of kin and physician sign a legal form stating incompetence.

17. **Counseling patients on the right to accept or refuse treatment in hospitals, sub-acute care facilities, hospices, and home health agencies is federally mandated through compliance with the**
    a. Americans with Disabilities Act (ADA).
    b. Patient Self-Determination Act of 1990.
    c. Employee Retirement Income Security Act (ERISA) of 1974.
    d. Health Insurance Portability and Accountability Act (HIPAA) of 1996.

18. **The two most recognized advanced directives are the living will and the**
    a. Affidavit of Merit.
    b. incompetence documentation.
    c. durable power of attorney (POA) for healthcare.
    d. documents from the Offices of Patient Advocacy, ombudsman, or protective services.

19. **Potential case manager negligence cases include**
    a. negligent hiring and retention of employees.
    b. not following recommendations by insurance companies.
    c. sending medical records to other providers as consented to by the patient.
    d. discharging the patient in a timely manner with adequate referrals.

20. **If the case manager is named in a lawsuit and being served with a summons and complaint, he or she should**
    a. avoid receiving the documents.
    b. argue with the process server.
    c. immediately report receipt of the summons and complaint to the employer and attorney.
    d. wait until a trial in a court of law before obtaining or reviewing medical documents.

21. **In most states, how many years is the statute of limitations for adults involved in personal injury cases?**
    a. 1
    b. 2
    c. 5
    d. 10

22. **How can case managers minimize lawsuit risk due to negligent referrals?**
    a. Refer only to organizations that have no evidence of credentialing.
    b. Do not do a cost-analysis or objectively assess providers recommended to patients.
    c. Allow the patient to make the final decision after giving him or her multiple referral options.
    d. Do not consider the cost of a service when providing a referral of service to a patient.

23. **To avoid negligent utilization review activities, the case manager should**
    a. use only criteria of The Joint Commission (TJC) when performing utilization review activities.
    b. apply criteria used by the health insurance plan, such as InterQual.
    c. only apply review criteria intermittently when performing utilization review.
    d. work for a managed care organization (MCO), because they cannot be held liable.

CHAPTER 9

ETHICAL ISSUES IN CASE MANAGEMENT

GENERAL PURPOSE STATEMENT:
To provide case managers and professional nurses with information about identifying and managing ethical dilemmas in case management practice.

LEARNING OBJECTIVES:
After reading this chapter and taking the test, you will be able to:

1. Describe the process of ethical decision making.
2. Recognize ethical dilemmas in case management practice.
3. List four ethical principles important to case management practice.
4. Differentiate between clinical and organizational ethics.
5. Identify five strategies for the effective management of ethical dilemmas.

1. **An example of an ethical dilemma in case management includes**
   a. a patient insists on being discharged home to an unsafe situation.
   b. a physician recommends that a patient have a procedure that is expensive.
   c. an insurance company raises its rates, leading to more people becoming uninsured.
   d. hospital rules state that all admitted patients must understand their rights as a patient.

2. **The impact of the Nancy Cruzan case resulted in the**
   a. Standards of Professional Performance.
   b. Patient Self-Determination Act of 1990.
   c. Code of Professional Conduct for Case Managers.
   d. Guide for the Uncertain Decision-Making Ethics (GUIDE).

3. **Options for evaluating the ethics of a particular patient's situation include all of the following *except* to**
   a. ask for judicial intervention.
   b. call for a family case conference.
   c. ask the institution's ethics committee for assistance.
   d. call the patient's insurance company and follow its recommendation.

4. **Decision-making tools for ethical decisions include**
   a. the use of humor to gain or maintain a sense of perspective.
   b. evaluating the total cost of projected health care for the patient.
   c. having the attending physician decide what is best for the patient.
   d. the use of aggressiveness when dealing with angry patients or family members.

5. **Which of the following is recommended regarding the use of artificial food and hydration for a conscious, irreversibly ill, but not imminently dying patient?**
   a. It is a decision for the family members alone.
   b. The physician and the payor together should make the decision.
   c. Food and hydration are an unreasonable burden, and will not be provided.
   d. The patient can ultimately decide, since he is conscious and capable of decision making.

6. **What is true with regard to decision making?**
   a. Honesty is a very important tool to use with decision making.
   b. Other perspectives are not as important as the attending physician's opinion.
   c. The case manager's opinion of the situation is more important than others.
   d. The perspective that best limits the chance of a lawsuit should be supported.

7. **Clinical ethics committees**
   a. include family members of patient, lawyers, and hospital administrators.
   b. deal with decisions regarding the right to withdraw treatment during end-of-life care.
   c. include experts in utilization management and codes of professional conduct.
   d. review issues regarding resource allocation and appropriateness of the level of care.

8. **Organizational ethics committees review cases or topics that include**
   a. business practices concerning pharmaceutical vendors.
   b. a patient's right to stop medically recommended treatment.
   c. whether a "Do Not Resuscitate" (DNR) order should be in effect for a patient.
   d. dealing with difficult family members who cannot work together to make decisions.

9. **To further investigate a case with an ethical dilemma, during the "Assessment and Problem Identification" phase of the process the case manager should**
   a. list goals and objectives of those involved.
   b. determine the course of action that will produce results most like the ethical ideal.
   c. identify available resources, including ethics committees, clergy, and patient advocates.
   d. determine if the outcome satisfies the parties involved, especially the patient and family.

10. **An ethical dilemma occurs when**
    a. an ethically correct course of action is unclear.
    b. a patient's medical outcome is dependent on their treatment plan.
    c. a physician helps the patient make decisions that are medically in their best interest.
    d. a physician does not agree with a particular diagnosis and performs test to disprove it.

11. **Which of the following is an example of an ethical dilemma?**
    a. Mr. P states that he does not want to be put on a respirator, but when he is unconscious, his wife insists on intubation.
    b. Ms. R wants to have Botox® injections to decrease her wrinkles, but her husband does not think she needs it.
    c. Mr. F wants to have an elective cosmetic procedure but his insurance will not cover it and he cannot afford to pay out-of-pocket.
    d. Mrs. S's family members bring food into the hospital for her to eat that is on her recommended diet.

12. GUIDE
   a. has 25 scenarios defining key issues and conflicts.
   b. takes the place of legal and risk management advisement.
   c. was written in Virginia with its legislation in mind.
   d. was written for ethical decisions pertaining to young pediatric patients.

13. **In 1992, a Delphi study conducted by St. Joseph's Hospital and Medical Center in Phoenix, Arizona, found that**
   a. medical decisions should not be based on chances of survival.
   b. 76% of participants felt that the rationing of health care to the poor was ethical.
   c. 72% of participants agreed that setting a monetary capitation ceiling is ethical.
   d. consumers felt that those who have unhealthy lifestyles should not be charged more.

14. **What was revealed in a 1996 study examining the results of 865 bone marrow transplant patients?**
   a. Of 476 patients who developed two complications, only one survived.
   b. Of 398 patients with a combination of symptoms, there were 156 survivors.
   c. The withdrawing of life support is not recommended for patients with complications.
   d. If patients had a combination of symptoms, the likelihood of survival was still high.

15. **Nurse case managers who are also certified case managers must adhere to all of the following *except***
   a. Standards of Professional Performance.
   b. American Nurses Association's Code of Ethics.
   c. Code of Professional Conduct for Case Managers.
   d. Commission on Rehabilitation Counselor Certification's Code of Professional Ethics.

16. **Case managers are guided by principles of**
   a. veracity.
   b. patient inequality.
   c. unfair distribution of benefits.
   d. dependence on other healthcare professionals.

17. **The case management ethical principle of nonmaleficence includes**
   a. being honest and truthful.
   b. refraining from doing harm to others.
   c. providing personal liberty for patients.
   d. allowing for fair distribution of burdens.

18. **Regardless of the ethical dilemma, the case manager should act based on professional codes of conduct and**
   a. keep the interests of the patient or family above all others.
   b. always stand by the payor's viewpoint of the dilemma.
   c. allow the patient's physician to determine ethical dilemma outcomes.
   d. work closely with the judicial system to solve any hospital-related ethical dilemmas.

19. **Which case manager role did ethicist John Banja compare to an air traffic controller who must coordinate flight patterns so that everyone is not crashing into one another?**
   a. advocacy role
   b. gatekeeping role
   c. cost-containment role
   d. coordinator/facilitator role

20. **False advertisements of outcomes regarding a certain treatment modality require a review by a/an**
   a. patient advocate.
   b. judge in a court of law.
   c. clinical ethics committee.
   d. organizational ethics committee.

CHAPTER 10

CASE MANAGEMENT CREDENTIALS, ORGANIZATIONS, AND STANDARDS

GENERAL PURPOSE STATEMENT:
To provide case managers and professional nurses with information about case management credentials, organizations, and standards.

LEARNING OBJECTIVES:
After reading this chapter and taking the test, you will be able to:

1. Identify professional organizations or societies that are important to case management.
2. Describe accreditation and accreditation agencies affecting case management responsibilities and processes.
3. Identify the various case management credentials and certifications.
4. List the eligibility criteria and examination content for organizations and agencies that provide case management certifications and credentials.
5. Describe case management standards, guidelines, and protocols.

1. **The Case Management Society of America (CMSA)**
   a. is the credentialing body for case managers.
   b. is a nonprofit organization founded in 1990 to support professional case management.
   c. represents more than 200 corporate and individual stakeholders.
   d. provides case management accreditation for healthcare facilities.

2. **Which organization, founded in 1951, is the largest accrediting agency in healthcare?**
   a. The Joint Commission (TJC)
   b. National Committee for Quality Assurance (NCQA)
   c. National Organization for Competency Assurance (NOCA)
   d. American Board of Quality Assurance and Utilization Review Physicians (ABQAURP)

3. **The Disease Management Association of America (DMAA)**
   a. is a certifying body for case managers.
   b. provides accreditation to healthcare facilities related to case management.
   c. promotes a retroactive case manager focus across the care continuum.
   d. strives to improve the population's health through health and wellness promotion.

4. **In 1997, the ORYX initiative was launched by TJC to**
   a. integrate an organization's outcomes with accreditation requirements.
   b. link case management certification requirements with accreditation goals.
   c. ensure credentialing of all staff members in hospital and long-term care facilities.
   d. provide Medicare and Medicaid beneficiaries with quality assurance related to benefits.

5. **Which term is defined as "a process verifying that an organization meets a certain set of nationally recognized standards"?**
   a. credentialing
   b. certification
   c. accreditation
   d. outcomes management

6. **The *Standards of Practice for Case Management* were developed and released by**
   a. TJC in 1997.
   b. CMSA in 1995.
   c. The National Transitions of Care Coalition (NTOCC) in 2006.
   d. The Commission for Case Manager Certification (CCMC) in 1991.

7. **Which section in the *Standards of Practice for Case Management* discusses quality of care, qualifications of a case manager, and research utilization?**
   a. Section I: Introduction
   b. Section II: Standards of Care
   c. Section III: Performance Indicators
   d. Section IV: Definitions

8. **NTOCC assists transitioning patients by**
   a. accrediting facilities that transfer patients on a regular basis.
   b. defining solutions to address the gaps that impact safety and quality care.
   c. establishing a national protocol for case managers regarding patient discharge.
   d. providing a support group for patients who transition their care from one facility to another.

9. **What is true regarding the Certified Case Manager (CCM)?**
   a. The first CCM exam was in the year 2000.
   b. There are approximately 3,000 case managers with the CCM.
   c. CCM is a primary credential that is mandatory to have to work as a case manager.
   d. CCM is a voluntary credential that is increasingly being required for case manager positions.

10. **Which agency provides the Nursing Case Management (RN, CM) credential?**
    a. CCMC
    b. NTOCC
    c. American Nurses Credentialing Center (ANCC)
    d. Certified Professional in Utilization Review (CPUR)

11. **CPUR certification**
    a. is sponsored by CMSA and Sanofi-Aventis.
    b. is the only comprehensive utilization review certification.
    c. has been attained by more than 50,000 healthcare professionals.
    d. offers a 2-week program that includes course work and the certification exam.

12. **The CCMC certification exam includes**
    a. a professional development component.
    b. eight sections that encompass the nursing process.
    c. six core domains of case management knowledge.
    d. a section on the clinical practice of case management nursing concepts.

13. In its four sections, the CPUR certification exam includes
    a. psychosocial and support systems.
    b. vocational concepts and strategies.
    c. current healthcare delivery systems.
    d. management of paper and electronic data.

14. The ANCC certification exam for case management eligibility criteria includes all of the following *except*
    a. at least 30 hours of continuing education in case management.
    b. the equivalent of two years of full-time practice as a registered nurse.
    c. a minimum of 200 hours of clinical practice in case management.
    d. a baccalaureate degree or higher in nursing and an active RN license.

15. Which of the following is one of the main domains of the Certified Professional in Healthcare Quality (CPHQ) exam?
    a. management and leadership
    b. legal and ethical considerations
    c. principles of education/learning
    d. tools of case management practice

16. In 2003, the Healthcare Quality Certification Board (HQCB) changed the CPHQ exam eligibility criteria by
    a. eliminating the minimum education and experience criteria.
    b. increasing experience criteria to 3 years of full-time practice.
    c. increasing the education criteria to the minimum of a master's degree.
    d. decreasing the experience criteria to a minimum of one year of full-time practice.

17. Which of the following is one of the four domains of the Quality Improvement System for Managed Care (QISMC) standards?
    a. Advocacy
    b. Planning
    c. Leadership
    d. Delegation

18. The Utilization Review Accreditation Commission (URAC) has a modular process of accreditation that
    a. only addresses workman's compensation utilization management.
    b. allows organizations to achieve all 22 areas of accreditation and certification.
    c. allows flexibility so an organization can tailor accreditation to the specific services it offers.
    d. strictly adheres to a specific accrediting process that remains unchanged between organizations.

19. Accreditation standards for case management were developed by
    a. QISMC and CCMC in 2003.
    b. URAC and CMSA in 1998.
    c. ABQAURP and the American Nurses Association (ANA) in 2007.
    d. NCQA and the National Association of Social Workers (NASW) in 1990.

20. A set of standardized performance measures designed to assist healthcare purchasers to select managed care plans based on proven performance is the
    a. QISMC.
    b. ORYX.
    c. Health Plan Employer Data and Information Set (HEDIS).
    d. Quality Assessment and Performance Improvement (QAPI).

CHAPTER 11

JOB STRESS AND SUCCESS FACTORS IN CASE MANAGEMENT PRACTICE

GENERAL PURPOSE STATEMENT:

To provide case managers and professional nurses with information about practical applications of case management skills.

LEARNING OBJECTIVES:

After reading this chapter and taking the test, you will be able to:

1. List three strategies for avoiding role conflict.
2. Describe the five steps of problem solving.
3. Recognize subtle approaches to effective time management.
4. Explain the importance of self care.
5. Illustrate five strategies for effective communication.
6. Recommend four techniques for enhancing emotional intelligence skill.
7. Name three effective approaches to multidisciplinary collaboration.

1. To avoid role conflict when implementing a case management program in an organization, the case manager should do all of the following *except*
   a. communicate in newsletters.
   b. provide a training and education session.
   c. communicate in departmental and organizationwide reports.
   d. perform case manager patient tasks prior to organizational role communication.

2. A case manager's communication about the implementation of a case management program should include
   a. a list of global problems within the case manager's facility.
   b. patient feedback about the proposed case management plan.
   c. a list of all facility staff tasks and roles as compared with the case manager role.
   d. a description of how each staff member can assist in the success of the case management program.

3. The first step in problem solving is to
   a. find potentially workable interventions.
   b. brainstorm alternative strategies or approaches.
   c. identify the problem by performing variance analysis.
   d. identify the type of data needed to understand the problem.

4. When problem solving, the case manager should focus on the desired outcome by
   a. evaluating the effect of the plan on the given situation.
   b. first collecting data regarding information that will address the problem or outcome.
   c. identifying other important problems prior to focusing on one single problem and outcome.
   d. beginning with data collection on information indirectly related to the problem or outcome.

5. If no intervention is found during the case management problem-solving process, the case manager should
   a. ask whether the problem needs to be redefined.
   b. interview patients to determine their suggested interventions.
   c. hold case manager conferences until adequate interventions are developed.
   d. allow attending physicians related to the problem to decide on appropriate interventions.

6. Which step of the problem-solving process involves having participants suggest options, resources, and interventions, and then list them in order of feasibility?
   a. step 1: Performing variance analysis
   b. step 2: Focusing on the desired outcomes
   c. step 3: Brainstorming alternative strategies or approaches
   d. step 4: Finding the next intervention

7. Regarding time management skills, what are considered minor distractions?
   a. list inclusions
   b. time robbers
   c. delegation tools
   d. prioritizing skills

8. What is the highest patient priority for a case manager?
   a. a "Code Blue" situation
   b. making insurance calls
   c. confirming tomorrow's discharges
   d. finding resources for patients who will need them in a few days

9. Which of the following is an example of the case manager being succinct?
   a. Be clear and to the point in delivery of information.
   b. Transform a short interaction from a few minutes to a half-hour question-and-answer session.
   c. Respond to each question with very specific detailed statistical information.
   d. Ramble on and talk in circles to allow the other person to have opinions.

10. Delegating includes
    a. assigning tasks that are within the person's scope of training.
    b. allowing the delegated individual to devise his or her own timeframe.
    c. limiting supervision over an assigned task, so that the person feels trusted.
    d. considering the case manager's role instead of the patient when deciding to delegate.

11. Case management self-care refers to
    a. making sure you have time during work to pamper yourself.
    b. making sure you take a lunch break at the same time each day.
    c. asking supervisors for what you need to better perform your job.
    d. asking staff to take over the case management role while you are busy.

12. Regarding case management self-care, which is an example of the author's statement "Get a life!"?
    a. Enjoy your life outside of the case management role.
    b. Spend your time out of the work environment with other case managers discussing work.
    c. Allow the case management process to consume your thoughts all of the time.
    d. Try risky adventures in life that you otherwise would never do, such as skydiving.

13. Which of the following is one of Dr. Stephen Covey's seven habits of highly successful people that can be helpful to the case manager?
    a. "Seek first to be understood, then seek to understand."
    b. "Seek first to understand, then seek to be understood."
    c. "Do not try to listen to understand the perceptions behind someone's words."
    d. "Do not attempt to understand another's perspective until you've identified your perspective."

14. What is essential in establishing a case management plan that reflects the interests, wishes, problems, and goals of the patient and/or family?
    a. understanding the patient and/or family's perceptions
    b. getting the patient and/or family to comprehend the medical diagnoses and needs
    c. providing a support system for the patient and/or family related to the diagnoses
    d. allowing the patient and/or family to participate in as much care as they are able

15. All of the following are recommended as information-gathering techniques for communication *except*
    a. observing the patient's body language.
    b. hearing what the patient is saying to you.
    c. clarifying any discrepancies you notice during your interview with the patient.
    d. using a pad and pencil as a tool to prevent any omissions, but avoiding taking too many notes.

16. Emotional intelligence includes the case manager's ability to
    a. understand the emotional crisis rationale, and then intellectually handle the situation.
    b. help those with impaired cognitive intelligence learn how to compensate emotionally.
    c. use your own emotions and those of others as sources of information for communication.
    d. understand how your emotions are expressed in different ways.

17. Which of the following is *not* included in the essential components necessary to establish effective relationships with other healthcare professionals, patients, and families?
    a. perception and awareness of your feelings and emotions
    b. perception and awareness of other's feelings and emotions
    c. perception and awareness of the effect of these feelings and emotions on the situation at hand
    d. perception and awareness of why feelings and emotions are a critical component to relationships

18. Which of the following is one of the eight truths of change from Collaborative Counseling, Inc.?
    a. To gain you must first give up.
    b. Distress is a sign that something is wrong.
    c. The only way to get rid of the fear of change is to avoid changes.
    d. The more you leave behind, the greater the intensity of sadness.

19. Dr. Robert Eliot developed two rules for keeping things in perspective: "Don't sweat the small stuff" and
    a. "it's all small stuff."
    b. "worry about the big stuff."
    c. "pick your battles with an open mind."
    d. "do not blame the small stuff on others around you."

20. Powell and Tahan explain that the continuous quality improvement technique of consensus is built on the assumption that
    a. it is OK to disagree.
    b. try to be in agreement with your other healthcare coworkers.
    c. you should always follow your planned interventions without anticipating changes.
    d. wasting time planning for changes that may never happen doesn't make sense.

LIPPINCOTT WILLIAMS & WILKINS
CONTINUING EDUCATION ENROLLMENT FORM

Case Management: A Practical Guide for Education and Practice, 3rd Edition

CHAPTER 1
OVERVIEW OF CASE MANAGEMENT

A. REGISTRATION INFORMATION

Last name _____ First name _____ MI _____

Address _____

City _____ State _____ Zip _____

Telephone _____ Fax _____ E-mail_____

- Check here to receive a ❏ Nursing CE certificate ❏ CCM certificate

- ❏ Please fax my certificate(s) to me.

❏ LPN ❏ RN ❏ CNS ❏ NP ❏ CRNA ❏ CNM ❏ Other

Job title _____ Specialty _____

Type of facility _____ Are you certified? ❏ Yes ❏ No

Certified by _____

State of license (1) _____ License # _____

State of license (2) _____ License # _____

❏ Please check here if you do not wish us to send promotions to your e-mail address.

❏ Please check here if you do not wish us to release your name, address, e-mail address to a third party vendor.

Registration deadline: October 31, 2011

RN contact hours: 7 **CCMC hours:** 6 Fee: $50.95
For every 4 tests submitted together, get the lowest priced test free. Submit all 11 tests together for $250, a savings of over 50%.

B. TEST ANSWERS. Darken one circle for your answer to each question.

	a	b	c	d			a	b	c	d
1.	○	○	○	○		11.	○	○	○	○
2.	○	○	○	○		12.	○	○	○	○
3.	○	○	○	○		13.	○	○	○	○
4.	○	○	○	○		14.	○	○	○	○
5.	○	○	○	○		15.	○	○	○	○
6.	○	○	○	○		16.	○	○	○	○
7.	○	○	○	○		17.	○	○	○	○
8.	○	○	○	○		18.	○	○	○	○
9.	○	○	○	○		19.	○	○	○	○
10.	○	○	○	○		20.	○	○	○	○

CM0109

C. COURSE EVALUATION

1. Did this CE activity's learning objectives relate to the general purpose? ❏ Yes ❏ No

2. Was the home study format an effective way to present the material? ❏ Yes ❏ No

3. Was the content relevant to your case management practice? ❏ Yes ❏ No

4. How many minutes did it take you to read the chapter? _____ Study the material? _____ Take the test? _____

D. TWO EASY WAYS TO PAY

❏ Check or money order enclosed (Payable to Lippincott Williams & Wilkins)

❏ Charge my ❏ Mastercard ❏ Visa ❏ American Express

Card # _____ Exp. Date _____

Signature _____

Mail completed test with registration fee to:

Lippincott Williams & Wilkins

CE Group, 333 7th Avenue, 19th floor

New York, NY 10001

Case Management: A Practical Guide for Education and Practice, 3rd Edition

CHAPTER 2

ESSENTIAL CASE MANAGEMENT JOB RESPONSIBILITIES AND SKILLS

A. REGISTRATION INFORMATION

Last name _____ First name _____ MI _____

Address _____

City _____ State _____ Zip _____

Telephone _____ Fax _____ E-mail_____

- Check here to receive a ❏ Nursing CE certificate ❏ CCM certificate

- ❏ Please fax my certificate(s) to me.

❏ LPN ❏ RN ❏ CNS ❏ NP ❏ CRNA ❏ CNM ❏ Other

Job title _____ Specialty _____

Type of facility _____ Are you certified? ❏ Yes ❏ No

Certified by _____

State of license (1) _____ License # _____

State of license (2) _____ License # _____

❏ Please check here if you do not wish us to send promotions to your e-mail address.

❏ Please check here if you do not wish us to release your name, address, e-mail address to a third party vendor.

Registration deadline: October 31, 2011

RN contact hours: 6.5   **CCMC hours:** 6   **Fee:** $47.95

For every 4 tests submitted together, get the lowest priced test free. Submit all 11 tests together for $250, a savings of over 50%.

B. TEST ANSWERS. Darken one circle for your answer to each question.

	a	b	c	d		a	b	c	d
1.	○	○	○	○	11.	○	○	○	○
2.	○	○	○	○	12.	○	○	○	○
3.	○	○	○	○	13.	○	○	○	○
4.	○	○	○	○	14.	○	○	○	○
5.	○	○	○	○	15.	○	○	○	○
6.	○	○	○	○	16.	○	○	○	○
7.	○	○	○	○	17.	○	○	○	○
8.	○	○	○	○	18.	○	○	○	○
9.	○	○	○	○	19.	○	○	○	○
10.	○	○	○	○	20.	○	○	○	○

CM0209

C. COURSE EVALUATION

1. Did this CE activity's learning objectives relate to the general purpose? ❏ Yes ❏ No

2. Was the home study format an effective way to present the material? ❏ Yes ❏ No

3. Was the content relevant to your case management practice? ❏ Yes ❏ No

4. How many minutes did it take you to read the chapter? _____ Study the material? _____ Take the test? _____

D. TWO EASY WAYS TO PAY

❏ Check or money order enclosed (Payable to Lippincott Williams & Wilkins)

❏ Charge my ❏ Mastercard ❏ Visa ❏ American Express

Card # _____ Exp. Date _____

Signature _____

Mail completed test with registration fee to:

Lippincott Williams & Wilkins

CE Group, 333 7th Avenue, 19th floor

New York, NY 10001

Case Management: A Practical Guide for Education and Practice, 3rd Edition

---

CHAPTER 3

REIMBURSEMENT CONCEPTS

A. REGISTRATION INFORMATION

Last name _____ First name _____ MI _____

Address _____

City _____ State _____ Zip _____

Telephone _____ Fax _____ E-mail_____

- Check here to receive a ❏ Nursing CE certificate ❏ CCM certificate

- ❏ Please fax my certificate(s) to me.

❏ LPN ❏ RN ❏ CNS ❏ NP ❏ CRNA ❏ CNM ❏ Other

Job title _____ Specialty _____

Type of facility _____ Are you certified? ❏ Yes ❏ No

Certified by _____

State of license (1) _____ License # _____

State of license (2) _____ License # _____

❏ Please check here if you do not wish us to send promotions to your e-mail address.

❏ Please check here if you do not wish us to release your name, address, e-mail address to a third party vendor.

Registration deadline: October 31, 2011

RN contact hours: 5.5   **CCMC hours:** 4   **Fee:** $41.95
For every 4 tests submitted together, get the lowest priced test free. Submit all 11 tests together for $250, a savings of over 50%.

B. TEST ANSWERS. Darken one circle for your answer to each question.

	a	b	c	d		a	b	c	d
1.	○	○	○	○	11.	○	○	○	○
2.	○	○	○	○	12.	○	○	○	○
3.	○	○	○	○	13.	○	○	○	○
4.	○	○	○	○	14.	○	○	○	○
5.	○	○	○	○	15.	○	○	○	○
6.	○	○	○	○	16.	○	○	○	○
7.	○	○	○	○	17.	○	○	○	○
8.	○	○	○	○	18.	○	○	○	○
9.	○	○	○	○	19.	○	○	○	○
10.	○	○	○	○	20.	○	○	○	○

CM0309

C. COURSE EVALUATION

1. Did this CE activity's learning objectives relate to the general purpose? ❏ Yes ❏ No

2. Was the home study format an effective way to present the material? ❏ Yes ❏ No

3. Was the content relevant to your case management practice? ❏ Yes ❏ No

4. How many minutes did it take you to read the chapter? _____ Study the material? _____ Take the test? _____

D. TWO EASY WAYS TO PAY

❏ Check or money order enclosed (Payable to Lippincott Williams & Wilkins)

❏ Charge my ❏ Mastercard ❏ Visa ❏ American Express

Card # _____ Exp. Date _____

Signature _____

Mail completed test with registration fee to:

Lippincott Williams & Wilkins

CE Group, 333 7th Avenue, 19th floor

New York, NY 10001

Case Management: A Practical Guide for Education and Practice, 3rd Edition

CHAPTER 4

UTILIZATION MANAGEMENT

A. REGISTRATION INFORMATION

Last name _____ First name _____ MI _____

Address _____

City _____ State _____ Zip _____

Telephone _____ Fax _____ E-mail_____

- Check here to receive a ❏ Nursing CE certificate ❏ CCM certificate

- ❏ Please fax my certificate(s) to me.

❏ LPN ❏ RN ❏ CNS ❏ NP ❏ CRNA ❏ CNM ❏ Other

Job title _____ Specialty _____

Type of facility _____ Are you certified? ❏ Yes ❏ No

Certified by _____

State of license (1) _____ License # _____

State of license (2) _____ License # _____

❏ Please check here if you do not wish us to send promotions to your e-mail address.

❏ Please check here if you do not wish us to release your name, address, e-mail address to a third party vendor.

Registration deadline: October 31, 2011

RN contact hours: 8.5   **CCMC hours:** 6   **Fee:** $59.95

For every 4 tests submitted together, get the lowest priced test free. Submit all 11 tests together for $250, a savings of over 50%.

B. TEST ANSWERS. Darken one circle for your answer to each question.

	a	b	c	d			a	b	c	d
1.	O	O	O	O		11.	O	O	O	O
2.	O	O	O	O		12.	O	O	O	O
3.	O	O	O	O		13.	O	O	O	O
4.	O	O	O	O		14.	O	O	O	O
5.	O	O	O	O		15.	O	O	O	O
6.	O	O	O	O		16.	O	O	O	O
7.	O	O	O	O		17.	O	O	O	O
8.	O	O	O	O		18.	O	O	O	O
9.	O	O	O	O		19.	O	O	O	O
10.	O	O	O	O		20.	O	O	O	O

CM0409

C. COURSE EVALUATION

1. Did this CE activity's learning objectives relate to the general purpose? ❏ Yes ❏ No

2. Was the home study format an effective way to present the material? ❏ Yes ❏ No

3. Was the content relevant to your case management practice? ❏ Yes ❏ No

4. How many minutes did it take you to read the chapter? _____ Study the material? _____ Take the test? _____

D. TWO EASY WAYS TO PAY

❏ Check or money order enclosed (Payable to Lippincott Williams & Wilkins)

❏ Charge my ❏ Mastercard ❏ Visa ❏ American Express

Card # _____ Exp. Date _____

Signature _____

Mail completed test with registration fee to:

Lippincott Williams & Wilkins

CE Group, 333 7th Avenue, 19th floor

New York, NY 10001

Case Management: A Practical Guide for Education and Practice, 3rd Edition

CHAPTER 5

TRANSITIONAL PLANNING: UNDERSTANDING LEVELS AND TRANSITIONS OF CARE

A. REGISTRATION INFORMATION

Last name _____ First name _____ MI _____

Address _____

City _____ State _____ Zip _____

Telephone _____ Fax _____ E-mail_____

- Check here to receive a ❑ Nursing CE certificate ❑ CCM certificate

- ❑ Please fax my certificate(s) to me.

❑ LPN ❑ RN ❑ CNS ❑ NP ❑ CRNA ❑ CNM ❑ Other

Job title _____ Specialty _____

Type of facility _____ Are you certified? ❑ Yes ❑ No

Certified by _____

State of license (1) _____ License # _____

State of license (2) _____ License # _____

❑ Please check here if you do not wish us to send promotions to your e-mail address.

❑ Please check here if you do not wish us to release your name, address, e-mail address to a third party vendor.

Registration deadline: October 31, 2011

RN contact hours: 8.5   **CCMC hours:** 6   **Fee:** $59.95

For every 4 tests submitted together, get the lowest priced test free. Submit all 11 tests together for $250, a savings of over 50%.

B. TEST ANSWERS. Darken one circle for your answer to each question.

	a	b	c	d			a	b	c	d
1.	O	O	O	O		11.	O	O	O	O
2.	O	O	O	O		12.	O	O	O	O
3.	O	O	O	O		13.	O	O	O	O
4.	O	O	O	O		14.	O	O	O	O
5.	O	O	O	O		15.	O	O	O	O
6.	O	O	O	O		16.	O	O	O	O
7.	O	O	O	O		17.	O	O	O	O
8.	O	O	O	O		18.	O	O	O	O
9.	O	O	O	O		19.	O	O	O	O
10.	O	O	O	O		20.	O	O	O	O

CM0509

C. COURSE EVALUATION

1. Did this CE activity's learning objectives relate to the general purpose? ❏ Yes ❏ No

2. Was the home study format an effective way to present the material? ❏ Yes ❏ No

3. Was the content relevant to your case management practice? ❏ Yes ❏ No

4. How many minutes did it take you to read the chapter? _____ Study the material? _____ Take the test? _____

D. TWO EASY WAYS TO PAY

❏ Check or money order enclosed (Payable to Lippincott Williams & Wilkins)

❏ Charge my ❏ Mastercard ❏ Visa ❏ American Express

Card # _____ Exp. Date _____

Signature _____

Mail completed test with registration fee to:

Lippincott Williams & Wilkins

CE Group, 333 7th Avenue, 19th floor

New York, NY 10001

Case Management: A Practical Guide for Education and Practice, 3rd Edition

CHAPTER 6
THE CASE MANAGEMENT PROCESS

A. REGISTRATION INFORMATION

Last name _____ First name _____ MI _____

Address _____

City _____ State _____ Zip _____

Telephone _____ Fax _____ E-mail_____

- Check here to receive a   ❑ Nursing CE certificate   ❑ CCM certificate

- ❑ Please fax my certificate(s) to me.

❑ LPN   ❑ RN   ❑ CNS   ❑ NP   ❑ CRNA   ❑ CNM   ❑ Other

Job title _____ Specialty _____

Type of facility _____ Are you certified? ❑ Yes ❑ No

Certified by _____

State of license (1) _____ License # _____

State of license (2) _____ License # _____

❑ Please check here if you do not wish us to send promotions to your e-mail address.

❑ Please check here if you do not wish us to release your name, address, e-mail address to a third party vendor.

Registration deadline: October 31, 2011

RN contact hours: 7   **CCMC hours:** 6   **Fee:** $50.95
For every 4 tests submitted together, get the lowest priced test free. Submit all 11 tests together for $250, a savings of over 50%.

B. TEST ANSWERS. Darken one circle for your answer to each question.

	a	b	c	d			a	b	c	d
1.	○	○	○	○		11.	○	○	○	○
2.	○	○	○	○		12.	○	○	○	○
3.	○	○	○	○		13.	○	○	○	○
4.	○	○	○	○		14.	○	○	○	○
5.	○	○	○	○		15.	○	○	○	○
6.	○	○	○	○		16.	○	○	○	○
7.	○	○	○	○		17.	○	○	○	○
8.	○	○	○	○		18.	○	○	○	○
9.	○	○	○	○		19.	○	○	○	○
10.	○	○	○	○		20.	○	○	○	○

CM0609

C. COURSE EVALUATION

1. Did this CE activity's learning objectives relate to the general purpose?　❏ Yes　❏ No

2. Was the home study format an effective way to present the material?　❏ Yes　❏ No

3. Was the content relevant to your case management practice?　❏ Yes　❏ No

4. How many minutes did it take you to read the chapter? _____ Study the material? _____ Take the test? _____

D. TWO EASY WAYS TO PAY

❏ Check or money order enclosed (Payable to Lippincott Williams & Wilkins)

❏ Charge my　❏ Mastercard　❏ Visa　❏ American Express

Card # _____ Exp. Date _____

Signature _____

Mail completed test with registration fee to:

Lippincott Williams & Wilkins

CE Group, 333 7th Avenue, 19th floor

New York, NY 10001

Case Management: A Practical Guide for Education and Practice, 3rd Edition

CHAPTER 7

QUALITY MANAGEMENT AND OUTCOMES

A. REGISTRATION INFORMATION

Last name _____ First name _____ MI _____

Address _____

City _____ State _____ Zip _____

Telephone _____ Fax _____ E-mail_____

- Check here to receive a ❏ Nursing CE certificate ❏ CCM certificate

- ❏ Please fax my certificate(s) to me.

❏ LPN ❏ RN ❏ CNS ❏ NP ❏ CRNA ❏ CNM ❏ Other

Job title _____ Specialty _____

Type of facility _____ Are you certified? ❏ Yes ❏ No

Certified by _____

State of license (1) _____ License # _____

State of license (2) _____ License # _____

❏ Please check here if you do not wish us to send promotions to your e-mail address.

❏ Please check here if you do not wish us to release your name, address, e-mail address to a third party vendor.

Registration deadline: October 31, 2011

RN contact hours: 4   CCMC hours: 4   Fee: $32.95
For every 4 tests submitted together, get the lowest priced test free. Submit all 11 tests together for $250, a savings of over 50%.

B. TEST ANSWERS. Darken one circle for your answer to each question.

	a	b	c	d			a	b	c	d
1.	○	○	○	○		11.	○	○	○	○
2.	○	○	○	○		12.	○	○	○	○
3.	○	○	○	○		13.	○	○	○	○
4.	○	○	○	○		14.	○	○	○	○
5.	○	○	○	○		15.	○	○	○	○
6.	○	○	○	○		16.	○	○	○	○
7.	○	○	○	○		17.	○	○	○	○
8.	○	○	○	○		18.	○	○	○	○
9.	○	○	○	○		19.	○	○	○	○
10.	○	○	○	○		20.	○	○	○	○

CM0709

C. COURSE EVALUATION

1. Did this CE activity's learning objectives relate to the general purpose?   ❏ Yes   ❏ No

2. Was the home study format an effective way to present the material?   ❏ Yes   ❏ No

3. Was the content relevant to your case management practice?   ❏ Yes   ❏ No

4. How many minutes did it take you to read the chapter? _____ Study the material? _____ Take the test? _____

D. TWO EASY WAYS TO PAY

❏ Check or money order enclosed (Payable to Lippincott Williams & Wilkins)

❏ Charge my   ❏ Mastercard   ❏ Visa   ❏ American Express

Card # _____ Exp. Date _____

Signature _____

Mail completed test with registration fee to:

Lippincott Williams & Wilkins

CE Group, 333 7th Avenue, 19th floor

New York, NY 10001

Case Management: A Practical Guide for Education and Practice, 3rd Edition

CHAPTER 8

LEGAL ISSUES IN CASE MANAGEMENT

A. REGISTRATION INFORMATION

Last name _____ First name _____ MI _____

Address _____

City _____ State _____ Zip _____

Telephone _____ Fax _____ E-mail_____

- Check here to receive a ❑ Nursing CE certificate ❑ CCM certificate

- ❑ Please fax my certificate(s) to me.

❑ LPN ❑ RN ❑ CNS ❑ NP ❑ CRNA ❑ CNM ❑ Other

Job title _____ Specialty _____

Type of facility _____ Are you certified? ❑ Yes ❑ No

Certified by _____

State of license (1) _____ License # _____

State of license (2) _____ License # _____

❑ Please check here if you do not wish us to send promotions to your e-mail address.

❑ Please check here if you do not wish us to release your name, address, e-mail address to a third party vendor.

Registration deadline: October 31, 2011

RN contact hours: 8   **CMC hours:** 6   **Fee:** $56.95
For every 4 tests submitted together, get the lowest priced test free. Submit all 11 tests together for $250, a savings of over 50%.

B. TEST ANSWERS. Darken one circle for your answer to each question.

	a	b	c	d			a	b	c	d
1.	O	O	O	O		13.	O	O	O	O
2.	O	O	O	O		14.	O	O	O	O
3.	O	O	O	O		15.	O	O	O	O
4.	O	O	O	O		16.	O	O	O	O
5.	O	O	O	O		17.	O	O	O	O
6.	O	O	O	O		18.	O	O	O	O
7.	O	O	O	O		19.	O	O	O	O
8.	O	O	O	O		20.	O	O	O	O
9.	O	O	O	O		21.	O	O	O	O
10.	O	O	O	O		22.	O	O	O	O
11.	O	O	O	O		23.	O	O	O	O
12.	O	O	O	O						

CM0809

C. COURSE EVALUATION

1. Did this CE activity's learning objectives relate to the general purpose?   ❏ Yes   ❏ No

2. Was the home study format an effective way to present the material?   ❏ Yes   ❏ No

3. Was the content relevant to your case management practice?   ❏ Yes   ❏ No

4. How many minutes did it take you to read the chapter? _____ Study the material? _____ Take the test? _____

D. TWO EASY WAYS TO PAY

❏ Check or money order enclosed (Payable to Lippincott Williams & Wilkins)

❏ Charge my   ❏ Mastercard   ❏ Visa   ❏ American Express

Card # _____ Exp. Date _____

Signature _____

Mail completed test with registration fee to:

Lippincott Williams & Wilkins

CE Group, 333 7th Avenue, 19th floor

New York, NY 10001

Case Management: A Practical Guide for Education and Practice, 3rd Edition

CHAPTER 9

ETHICAL ISSUES IN CASE MANAGEMENT

A. REGISTRATION INFORMATION

Last name _____ First name _____ MI _____

Address _____

City _____ State _____ Zip _____

Telephone _____ Fax _____ E-mail_____

- Check here to receive a ❏ Nursing CE certificate ❏ CCM certificate

- ❏ Please fax my certificate(s) to me.

❏ LPN ❏ RN ❏ CNS ❏ NP ❏ CRNA ❏ CNM ❏ Other

Job title _____ Specialty _____

Type of facility _____ Are you certified? ❏ Yes ❏ No

Certified by _____

State of license (1) _____ License # _____

State of license (2) _____ License # _____

❏ Please check here if you do not wish us to send promotions to your e-mail address.

❏ Please check here if you do not wish us to release your name, address, e-mail address to a third party vendor.

Registration deadline: October 31, 2011

RN contact hours: 4.5   **CCMC hours:** 4   **Fee:** $35.95
For every 4 tests submitted together, get the lowest priced test free. Submit all 11 tests together for $250, a savings of over 50%.

B. TEST ANSWERS. Darken one circle for your answer to each question.

	a	b	c	d			a	b	c	d
1.	○	○	○	○		11.	○	○	○	○
2.	○	○	○	○		12.	○	○	○	○
3.	○	○	○	○		13.	○	○	○	○
4.	○	○	○	○		14.	○	○	○	○
5.	○	○	○	○		15.	○	○	○	○
6.	○	○	○	○		16.	○	○	○	○
7.	○	○	○	○		17.	○	○	○	○
8.	○	○	○	○		18.	○	○	○	○
9.	○	○	○	○		19.	○	○	○	○
10.	○	○	○	○		20.	○	○	○	○

CM0909

C. COURSE EVALUATION

1. Did this CE activity's learning objectives relate to the general purpose?   ❏ Yes   ❏ No

2. Was the home study format an effective way to present the material?   ❏ Yes   ❏ No

3. Was the content relevant to your case management practice?   ❏ Yes   ❏ No

4. How many minutes did it take you to read the chapter? _____ Study the material? _____ Take the test? _____

D. TWO EASY WAYS TO PAY

❏ Check or money order enclosed (Payable to Lippincott Williams & Wilkins)

❏ Charge my   ❏ Mastercard   ❏ Visa   ❏ American Express

Card # _____ Exp. Date _____

Signature _____

Mail completed test with registration fee to:

Lippincott Williams & Wilkins

CE Group, 333 7th Avenue, 19th floor

New York, NY 10001

Case Management: A Practical Guide for Education and Practice, 3rd Edition

CHAPTER 10
CASE MANAGEMENT CREDENTIALS, ORGANIZATIONS, AND STANDARDS

A. REGISTRATION INFORMATION

Last name _____ First name _____ MI _____

Address _____

City _____ State _____ Zip _____

Telephone _____ Fax _____ E-mail_____

- Check here to receive a ❑ Nursing CE certificate ❑ CCM certificate

- ❑ Please fax my certificate(s) to me.

❑ LPN ❑ RN ❑ CNS ❑ NP ❑ CRNA ❑ CNM ❑ Other

Job title _____ Specialty _____

Type of facility _____ Are you certified? ❑ Yes ❑ No

Certified by _____

State of license (1) _____ License # _____

State of license (2) _____ License # _____

❑ Please check here if you do not wish us to send promotions to your e-mail address.

❑ Please check here if you do not wish us to release your name, address, e-mail address to a third party vendor.

Registration deadline: October 31, 2011

RN contact hours: 4.5   **CCMC hours:** 4   **Fee:** $35.95

For every 4 tests submitted together, get the lowest priced test free. Submit all 11 tests together for $250, a savings of over 50%.

B. TEST ANSWERS. Darken one circle for your answer to each question.

	a	b	c	d		a	b	c	d
1.	○	○	○	○	11.	○	○	○	○
2.	○	○	○	○	12.	○	○	○	○
3.	○	○	○	○	13.	○	○	○	○
4.	○	○	○	○	14.	○	○	○	○
5.	○	○	○	○	15.	○	○	○	○
6.	○	○	○	○	16.	○	○	○	○
7.	○	○	○	○	17.	○	○	○	○
8.	○	○	○	○	18.	○	○	○	○
9.	○	○	○	○	19.	○	○	○	○
10.	○	○	○	○	20.	○	○	○	○

CM1009

C. COURSE EVALUATION

1. Did this CE activity's learning objectives relate to the general purpose? ❑ Yes ❑ No

2. Was the home study format an effective way to present the material? ❑ Yes ❑ No

3. Was the content relevant to your case management practice? ❑ Yes ❑ No

4. How many minutes did it take you to read the chapter? _____ Study the material? _____ Take the test? _____

D. TWO EASY WAYS TO PAY

❑ Check or money order enclosed (Payable to Lippincott Williams & Wilkins)

❑ Charge my ❑ Mastercard ❑ Visa ❑ American Express

Card # _____ Exp. Date _____

Signature _____

Mail completed test with registration fee to:

Lippincott Williams & Wilkins

CE Group, 333 7th Avenue, 19th floor

New York, NY 10001

Case Management: A Practical Guide for Education and Practice, 3rd Edition

CHAPTER 11

JOB STRESS AND SUCCESS FACTORS IN CASE MANAGEMENT PRACTICE

A. REGISTRATION INFORMATION

Last name _____ First name _____ MI _____

Address _____

City _____ State _____ Zip _____

Telephone _____ Fax _____ E-mail_____

- Check here to receive a ❏ Nursing CE certificate ❏ CCM certificate

- ❏ Please fax my certificate(s) to me.

❏ LPN ❏ RN ❏ CNS ❏ NP ❏ CRNA ❏ CNM ❏ Other

Job title _____ Specialty _____

Type of facility _____ Are you certified? ❏ Yes ❏ No

Certified by _____

State of license (1) _____ License # _____

State of license (2) _____ License # _____

❏ Please check here if you do not wish us to send promotions to your e-mail address.

❏ Please check here if you do not wish us to release your name, address, e-mail address to a third party vendor.

Registration deadline: October 31, 2011

RN contact hours: 5 **CCMC hours:** 4 **Fee:** $38.95

For every 4 tests submitted together, get the lowest priced test free. Submit all 11 tests together for $250, a savings of over 50%.

B. TEST ANSWERS. Darken one circle for your answer to each question.

	a	b	c	d			a	b	c	d
1.	○	○	○	○		11.	○	○	○	○
2.	○	○	○	○		12.	○	○	○	○
3.	○	○	○	○		13.	○	○	○	○
4.	○	○	○	○		14.	○	○	○	○
5.	○	○	○	○		15.	○	○	○	○
6.	○	○	○	○		16.	○	○	○	○
7.	○	○	○	○		17.	○	○	○	○
8.	○	○	○	○		18.	○	○	○	○
9.	○	○	○	○		19.	○	○	○	○
10.	○	○	○	○		20.	○	○	○	○

CM1109

C. COURSE EVALUATION

1. Did this CE activity's learning objectives relate to the general purpose? ❑ Yes ❑ No

2. Was the home study format an effective way to present the material? ❑ Yes ❑ No

3. Was the content relevant to your case management practice? ❑ Yes ❑ No

4. How many minutes did it take you to read the chapter? _____ Study the material? _____ Take the test? _____

D. TWO EASY WAYS TO PAY

❑ Check or money order enclosed (Payable to Lippincott Williams & Wilkins)

❑ Charge my   ❑ Mastercard   ❑ Visa   ❑ American Express

Card # _____ Exp. Date _____

Signature _____

Mail completed test with registration fee to:

Lippincott Williams & Wilkins

CE Group, 333 7th Avenue, 19th floor

New York, NY 10001